NURSING ISSUES
in the 21st CENTURY

Perspectives From the Literature

Edited by **Eleanor C. Hein, R.N., Ed.D.**

Professor Emerita
University of San Francisco School of Nursing
San Francisco, California

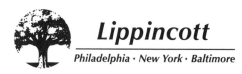
Lippincott
Philadelphia · New York · Baltimore

Acquisitions Editor: Margaret Zuccarini
Editorial Assistant: Helen Kogut
Project Editor: Debra Schiff
Senior Production Manager: Helen Ewan
Production Coordinator: Patricia McCloskey
Art Director: Carolyn O'Brien
Manufacturing Manager: William Alberti
Compositor: Pine Tree Composition, Inc.
Printer: R. R. Donnelley

9 8 7 6 5 4 3 2 1

Library of Congress Cataloging-in-Publication Data
   Nursing issues in the 21st century : perspectives from the literature / edited by Eleanor C. Hein.
      p. cm.
   Includes bibliographical references and index.
   ISBN 0-7817-3017-1 (alk. paper)
      1. Nursing—Social aspects—United States.   2. Nursing—Practice—United States.   3.
   Nursing—United States—Forecasting.   I. Hein, Eleanor C.
RT86.5.N875 2001
610.73'0973—dc21
                                                                                    00-063971

FOREWORD

*F*ive major elements are extraordinarily impacting the nursing profession today. Although the elements have always existed, they have never before been so dramatic or *influential*. It can be observed today that:

Nursing is a dynamic profession, with the word *dynamic* referring to the constant change occurring both internally and externally to the profession. It is essential the professional nurse be fluid within these dynamics.

As with many professions, nursing exists because of the needs and demands of society. Society and its problems have evolved and will continue to evolve, placing increased demands on an already pressured health care system. From this evolution, consumers, out of necessity, have become actively involved in their health care, and, ultimately, consumers may be in control. Due in large part to information technology, consumers of health care have access to and utilize the bounty of facts and advice available to them on most aspects of health promotion and disease prevention, as well as palliative and curative care.

Nursing knowledge and essential skills have increased at a dramatic rate. Recent exploration on the subject speculates that the knowledge increase in the last 10 years is equal to that gained in the previous 100 years. Never before has it become so essential for the nurse to become both an active and life-long learner. Not only has the knowledge base increased, but also the teaching-learning process has changed. Today a nurse may enroll in continuing education at almost any level of advanced education online. Technology in all aspects of the profession continues to advance, and for the professional nurse to deliver up-to-date care safely and competently, its utilization is crucial. For example, the Internet has become a valuable source of information for patients and consumers. Nurses are challenged to know as much as, if not more than, the client does.

Nursing as a profession is global. In all societies someone exists to perform the duties of a "nurse." These individuals, whether they are in developed or developing countries, contribute to established and accepted standards of practice. It is essential that we nurses know what these standards are and utilize them in our day-to-day practice.

Nursing is a collaborative profession existing in a complex health care system. It is a system that at one time had as its concern only *three* influencing factors: cost, access, and quality. Today there are five influencing factors: cost, access, cost, quality, and cost. This change has yielded new care and ethical issues.

In her book, Dr. Eleanor C. Hein has included classic literature that addresses these five elements. Dr. Hein's contribution will be useful not only for baccalaureate nursing students, but for the practicing nurse as well. The book does not answer *specific questions* regarding any of the current issues confronting the profession, but stimulates the reader to think critically, thereby basing decisions, values, and beliefs on a sound knowledge base. It also generates in the reader the realization that all questions do not have concrete or "black and white" answers and that more than one correct response may exist.

Dr. Hein is not only pragmatic in her approach, but visionary as well. She begins each chapter with an historical overview giving the reader a context of the issues within the chapter itself. She includes current professional and practice-based literature, readings for further investigation of a topic, questions for discussions, and Internet resources. In addition to articles from prestigious journals, Dr. Hein includes approximately 45 non-nursing sources (eg, *Hastings Center Report, Newsweek, The Village Voice* and *Harper's*). Non-nursing literature was carefully selected based on the prevailing non-nursing perspective of current health care issues together with real and potential nursing ramifications. For these reasons, Dr. Hein's book will be a valuable contribution to the education of nursing students and to all those nurses who actively seek to grow in their knowledge and practice.

John M. Lantz, R.N., PhD.
Dean and Professor
School of Nursing
University of San Francisco

PREFACE

The purpose of this book is to expose baccalaureate nursing students to provocative points of view on issues relevant to professional nursing and health care. The issues facing us today are formidable, multifaceted, and sometimes difficult to comprehend, much less solve. We are experiencing a world increasingly conflicted in its values, beliefs, and ideas, that are all too often spurred on by impassioned and inflammatory rhetoric. For nursing students about to enter this world, mastery of basic nursing content is not enough. More will be required of them, not less. What is evident is that nurses about to enter this conflicted arena must be as knowledgeable about the world of ideas and the issues at hand as they are about the fundamentals of their nursing practice. They must be able to use fairly sophisticated critical thinking abilities to explore divergent ideas, generate dialogue, and help formulate solutions to the health care issues facing us. Nursing students who can actively engage in this process will be nurses with a professional future.

To prepare themselves for this eventuality, nursing students must make use of the liberalizing and humanistic elements of their baccalaureate education. In baccalaureate nursing programs throughout the country, nursing students are not only dealing with a rapidly changing and often chaotic health care delivery system, they are also required to master content that 5 to 10 years ago was considered appropriate only for senior students. The time students have to master nursing content is compressed and limited. Because of this, it is not always possible to consistently expose students to health care issues throughout their nursing program. There is even less time to expose them to other points of view outside of nursing and do so in a way that is readily accessible, timely, and relevant. Exposure to differing or provocative points of view should begin early in the educational process. It is from this exposure that students can stretch their critical thinking skills as they examine the more diverse and complex health care issues facing us today. This book provides that opportunity.

Several criteria guided the development of this book. First, I did not want the readings in this book to duplicate basic nursing content. While the overall issues themselves are not new, and are a part of most baccalaureate nursing curricula, the specific topics within each issue are relatively recent and do not repeat the core content of baccalaureate nursing curricula. What the readings do offer students is additional knowledge and perspectives that gives them the opportunity to apply their basic nursing content more broadly. Second, the issues chosen for this book were selective. The issues were chosen because they represent immediate and growing concerns about problems and perceptions related to health and well being. Third, for this book to be relevant, its readings must be current and incorporate different, sometimes opposing points of view from a variety of disciplines. This criterion was achieved. Three fourths of the readings in this book were published in 1999 and 2000, with approximately half of the readings divided between the nursing literature and other disciplines. Helping students to challenge, invigorate, and sharpen their thinking about divergent points of view was of primary importance in the selection of readings. Readings drawn from nursing, philosophy, journalism, ethics, history, sociology, politics, business, and economics offer students the opportunity to question, disagree, challenge, and debate the issues and problems that emerge from what they have read and that will ultimately affect their professional practice. The final criterion for this book was that it should coincide with the overall goal of baccalaureate education by providing a liberalizing, humanistic dimension to the educational process of nursing students. I believe the balance of readings, divided as they are between nursing and other disciplines, meets this criterion.

The organization of this book is divided into five major sections. To facilitate an understanding of the interrelationships of one or more issues with others, the issues presented in this book have been arranged in relevant clusters. In this way, students can see how loosely related issues such as politics, economics, and managed care fit together as a conceptual unit. Each cluster presents a theme reflective of the issues in that section. Part One, Nurses and Their Professional Heritage, begins with selective milestones highlighting significant achievements from nursing's history that provide an historical context from which to gauge today's achievements in nursing. How nurses see themselves, how others perceive them, their working conditions, and the problems and issues with which they are confronted in the service of others comprise the remainder of this section. Access and boundaries are the themes in Part Two. Issues related to privacy have captured the attention and concern of the public and have become a major issue for health care professionals. The ease with which privacy and confidentiality can be violated through increased access to computer technology is the focus of discussion in the first part of this section. The financial and moral limits of health care are explored in discussions of health care rationing and the uncharted moral boundaries of genetic engineering. Woven into these issues are the values, limits, and uses of computer technology and the Internet in health care now and in the future. The themes of vulnerability and safety are the focus of Part Three. The impact of homelessness and the uninsured upon our health care resources have become more worrisome as their numbers mount. Additionally, the increased numbers of HIV-infected elderly and the resurgence of tuberculosis in this country have brought the plight of vulnerable populations into sharper focus for health care professionals. With all these issues before us, the imminent health care needs of our rapidly growing aging population loom on the horizon. Their needs will also add to the financial strain that providing health care resources will create and will become worse as planning for that eventuality is delayed. Encompassing all the issues related to vulnerability is the pervasive spread of violence in this country. Violence is a threat to our most basic safety needs, not only for those already disenfranchised, but for everyone for whom safety and protection from added vulnerability is an issue. The themes in Part Four focus on health care reform. In this section, the myths surrounding managed care and the problems within it serve as the basis for the examination of managed care as a mode of health care delivery. The public's growing frustration and dismay with managed care is compounded by the spiraling cost of prescription drugs, which have risen beyond reason. The need for reform in both these areas is clearly evident, but the political will of Congress is not. This section explores the interrelationship of health care reform, its economics, and the political process that will determine whether reforms of any kind will take place. Envisioning the future is the concluding theme of Part Five. The future of nursing is explored from the vantage point of the past. Beginning in 1950 and spanning the course of the decades that follow, nurses explore the issues facing their profession and share their hopes for the future of nursing. The extent to which professional nursing has succeeded is for today's nurses to determine.

The five major parts of this book can be read in any order and at any level in students' baccalaureate nursing programs. Introductory remarks set the stage for each chapter. An overview prefaces each chapter providing students with an historical perspective for the readings in that chapter. Each chapter concludes with a series of discussion questions to stimulate thought, exchange viewpoints, and encourage dialogue. Further suggested readings and Web site resources are also included at the end of each chapter. These Web site resources are specific to the topics in each chapter, and also include general search engine Web sites, health Web sites and professional journal Web sites.

◾ ACKNOWLEDGMENTS

My thanks and appreciation to Lippincott Williams & Wilkins for its continued and wholehearted support in the development of this book. To Margaret Zuccarini and Helen Kogut of the Nursing Education Division, my thanks and appreciation for their counsel and assistance. This book would not be possible without the cooperation of various journals and authors who granted me permission to use their material. My thanks to all of them. I particularly wish to acknowledge the help of Joseph Garity and Marion Gin, reference librarians at the University of San Francisco. Without their assistance, my ability to navigate the Internet and find the resources I needed would have taken twice as long. I wish to again single out two individuals whose support and feedback I have come to rely upon over the years. They are Dr. Ellene Egan, R.N., Ed.D., Assistant Professor of Nursing, University of

San Francisco; and Christine Wachsmuth, R.N., M.S., Assistant Administrator, Paramedic and Emergency Services, San Francisco General Hospital, San Francisco, California. Their candor and insights continue to be invaluable. My thanks also to Dr. John M. Lantz, Dean, University of San Francisco School of Nursing, for graciously consenting to write the foreword for this book. Finally, to the many nursing students who are at the threshold of their professional careers in the 21st century. May the path you choose in the service of others be one that nurtures and celebrates life.

Eleanor C. Hein, R.N., Ed.D.
Professor Emerita

CONTENTS

PART **ONE**

NURSES AND THEIR PROFESSIONAL HERITAGE

CHAPTER **1**

Links to the Past   1

CHAPTER **2**

Nurses: A Professional Reality Check   53

CHAPTER **3**

Cultural Diversity: A Celebration of Differences   120

PART TWO

ISSUES OF ACCESS AND BOUNDARIES

CHAPTER **8**

Living Longer: Are We Ready? 357

CHAPTER **9**

Violence: Is Anyone Safe? 384

PART FOUR

ISSUES OF HEALTH CARE REFORM

CHAPTER **10**
Delivering Health Care: At What Cost? 421

CHAPTER **11**

Economics: Dollars and "No Sense"? 457

CHAPTER **12**

Politics: Do We Make a Difference? 484

PART **FIVE**

ENVISIONING THE FUTURE

PART ONE

NURSES AND THEIR PROFESSIONAL HERITAGE

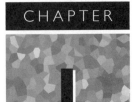

CHAPTER

1

Links to the Past

History is not everyone's cup of tea. For some people, it's a waste of time and irrelevant. But history matters. It gives us a chronology of past events, a testament of where we came from, who we were, and what we achieved. Without that chronology, we have no historical home and nothing upon which to anchor our present or future.

History is tradition and continuity handed down from one generation to another. Some may think of history as a gloomy chronicle of humanity's follies and misadventures. To others, however, it is a spacious dwelling filled with the greatness and achievements of its statesmen, artists, musicians, scientists, and philosophers. Their ideas and voices come alive, helping us to learn from the past so that we may live more wisely in our present world. Given the centuries during which humanity is chronicled, the lessons history offers us are inexhaustible.

While the same can be said of nursing's history, much of it still remains a mystery to many nurses. As more and more knowledge is packed into nursing programs, there are fewer and fewer attempts, if any, to include even some of the basic elements of nursing's history into nursing curricula. It is not uncommon for nurses to know nothing about their professional heritage much less nursing's past accomplishments. Significant events from the past become trivialized and eventually ignored. Even Florence Nightingale, with all her achievements, has become a caricature—a vague-looking, expressionless woman holding a lamp in some dark, faraway place. This is hardly a worthy or accurate picture of a woman who produced an enormous body of work as a reformer, statistician, and researcher. The continuity of nursing and its traditions cannot be passed on to future generations of nurses if the present generation of nurses know nothing about their professional heritage.

Ours is a rich cultural heritage, one filled with numerous accomplishments and noteworthy events. Chronicled in its history are the experiences, hopes, and dreams of past nurses, all of whom tried to make the world a better place than they found it. They were remarkable women with an abundance of courage and perserverance who did extraordinary things to advance nursing in a world not yet ready to accept them as equals among equals. Their experiences should not be trivialized.

The readings in this chapter are historical snapshots capturing moments from the past that illuminate our heritage. They set the stage of examining the dilemmas women faced as they tried to forge new roles for themselves in both society and nursing. Florence Nightingale's life and achievements illustrate the difficulties many women faced as they tried to carve out a role for themselves in a rigid and constricted society. Overcoming the impact of social forces upon nursing illustrates nurses' resiliency and the progress they made in advancing nursing's goals. Because of them, nursing has moved ahead, expanded its knowledge, refined its practice, and created new roles for itself. How can that be irrelevant?

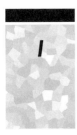

The Risk of Not Understanding Nursing History

Karen E. Ogren

A people without history
Is not redeemed from time, for history is a pattern[1]
                                        —T.S. Eliot

Disillusioned with a health care system that provides care unequally and expensively, Americans are clamoring for reform. As the largest group of health care providers in the United States, nurses can play a key role in transforming the health care system. Maraldo optimistically asserted, "The next century will see the nursing model of care integrated more fruitfully into priorities and policies of the health care delivery system."[2(p228)] Also, Lynaugh and Fagin[3] pointed out that nurses provide the family-centered, holistic care that many reformers, dissatisfied with the disease-centered medical model of care, are envisioning. Nurses, as a group, must be politically active now if they are to become leaders in health care reform.

Historically, nurse leaders such as Florence Nightingale, Sojourner Truth, and Lillian Wald have provided role models for political action. For example, Nightingale, politically adept, was able to integrate many of her beliefs about health care into the accepted practices of her time. Mason pointed out Truth was also politically active, saying, "Sojourner Truth was a nurse who used her political skills to move a society to embrace the connections between freedom and health."[4(p12)] Wald, also politically skillful, "used power and politics to further her vision of the connection between health and social conditions."[4(p12)] These and other nursing leaders made significant contributions to health care reform.

Unfortunately, nurses historically have lost many opportunities for leadership in health care policy formation. A review of nursing history reveals some political successes and many more failures. Exploring their history will help nurses learn from the past and avoid previously encountered pitfalls

Karen E. Ogren was a nursing student, Department of Nursing, Saint John Fisher College, Rochester, New York.

Reprinted from *Holistic Nursing Practice*, 8(2), 8–14, 1980, with permission of Aspen Publishers, Inc., © 1994.

while building on successes. Studying nursing history can be risky because history's lessons can be discouraging; however, ignoring that history presents a much greater risk. By not studying and understanding nursing history, nurses again risk being left out of health care reform in the United States. Nurses must now risk using their own history.

■ DEFINITION AND PURPOSE OF HISTORY

Simply stated, history is the study of the past; however, because inherently fallible human beings with their individual opinions provide this study, history is not the absolute truth. Therefore, history is an interpretation of the past. Hamilton explained the value of history: "History allows humans to slip the bonds of their own time and memories and to perceive a broader canvas of human actions, thoughts and feelings."[5(p45)] By studying history, people understand their own lives more fully. Also, Lynaugh and Reverby pointed out, "The intellectual pleasure of history comes from the discovery of the 'connectedness' and pattern of events in time and within interpretive frameworks."[6(p4)] History allows people and groups to appreciate how their lives fit into a pattern and, thus, history helps people to more fully understand the present. Individually and collectively, nurses have much to gain from studying their history.

Church stated emphatically that nurses must study their history, saying, "Historical awareness should be viewed as a prerequisite to a professional mentality and identity."[7(p94)] In other words, nurses must understand their history before they can effectively tackle the many issues currently facing nursing. Furthermore, Mauksch implored nurses to examine their history, maintaining, "Our past offers an abundance of learning if only we study it, and building our future will be infinitely more effective if we know how we arrived at today."[8(p483)] Therefore an examination of history will allow nurses to more fully understand critical issues facing nursing today. This understanding can empower nurses to demand leadership roles in health care policy formation. Succinctly stated by Donahue, "In a very real sense, nursing can find its past in the present and its present in the past."[9(p9)]

More specifically, nurses can use historical study to understand and, thereby, improve particular conditions affecting nursing. Baer described the usefulness of history for understanding current issues: "Using the method of history, the researcher can seek a problem's root, trace its changes through various eras, and identify its main components."[10(16)] Brown and D'Antonio concurred, remarking that history provides "not only a broader understanding of the origins of our current successes and dilemmas, but also provides an analytical approach to complex clinical and professional issues that defy simplistic explanations."[11(p319)] Nurses have much to learn from experiences of their ancestors because present conditions are deeply rooted in the past; therefore, restricted explanations of current conditions that ignore the past offer little hope for solutions. Donahue identified several key nursing concerns requiring historical examination: "Many of the topics of concern today—financial security for nurses, regulation of nursing practice, and the nursing shortage—were being discussed more than 100 years ago."[9(p9)]

■ HISTORICAL EXAMINATION OF CURRENT ISSUES

Nursing's economic dilemma grows out of nursing's "order to care in a society that refuses to value caring"[12(p1)] as identified by Reverby. Caring was considered to be a woman's duty and, accordingly, economic reward was not considered to be necessary. Minkowski supported the view that nursing is a woman's duty: "Healing has always been regarded as the natural responsibility of mothers and wives."[13(p288)] Further complicating the pay issue is nursing's roots in religious orders. Hughes asserted,

> The correlation between nursing and a religious calling and the resultant belief that willing self-sacrifice was essential to nursing practice provided the justification needed to support the low pay and long hours of labor that historically characterized the nurse's employment.[14(p65)]

Further, relatively low pay for nurses is related to the traditionally female gender of nurses. Women's work is generally lower paid than men's work. The conflict between service to others and economic needs has persisted throughout the history of nursing in the United States, although the role of nurses in health care has not remained constant. Referring to nurses, Brider pointed out, "At each step in the evolution of health care in this country, they have taken the stage in a new role that transformed the way they performed without resolving their economic dilemma."[15(p77)] Historical study offers further insight into the economic issue facing nursing.

Historical study also provides insight into an extremely divisive issue in nursing—education. Ever since formal training of nurses in the United States began in hospitals during the 1870s, education of nurses has caused controversy among nurses. How much education does a nurse require? The original debate began between newly formally trained nurses and older nurses who learned their skills on the job before formal training was available. Each group attempted to maintain their position in the profession. When several leaders during the 1920s recommended university education for nurses, this controversy over the amount and type of training required to be a nurse intensified. According to Baer, "Once again groups of nurses acted against each other out of fear rather than working together to find solutions acceptable to all."[10(p20)] Further, this debate again intensified in 1965 when the American Nurses Association (ANA) recommended that a baccalaureate degree should be the minimum qualification for registered nurses. This recommendation was opposed by associate degree registered nurses, hospital-based schools of nursing and licensed practical nurses.[16] Baer urged nurses to recognize the different training options as one aspect of diversity in nursing, declaring, "It can be a great strength if we negotiate our diversity and sustain our unified institutional strength, as did the nursing leaders of 1900."[17(p319)]

An issue related to education is regulation of nursing practice. One of Nightingale's goals for nursing was establishing ethical and conduct codes.[2] This desire to maintain or improve the quality of nursing care by establishing rules for practice continued throughout nursing history. Regulation of nursing also caused controversy. For example, according to Friedman, when nursing leaders called for licensure during the 1890s, "Many old-style nurses saw it as a way of putting them out of business."[16(p2854)] Regulation comes from within and outside of nursing. Accordingly, from within, the ANA Code for Nurses[18] prescribes ethical principles for nursing practice and, from without, nurses must be licensed by respective state boards of nursing. Current regulation of nursing has historic antecedents.

One further problem facing present-day nurses is shortage. Nursing shortages are associated with other issues confronting nurses, especially financial issues. Throughout the 20th century, nursing in the United States has experienced repeated periods of shortage because of the many problems facing nurses. Friedman explained, "It is the most populous profession in health care, with 2.1 million registered nurses alone; yet it has undergone repeated cycles of shortage and oversupply, with shortage being the current order of the day."[16(2851)] The causes of nursing shortages are complex; however, an examination of history offers insight and possible solutions.

Besides providing insight into current, divisive issues affecting the profession, history helps develop a clearer definition of nursing. Church asserted that nurses do not generally understand their history, claiming, "This absence of a historical perspective could account for the current dilemma that relates to redefining nursing and determining its parameters of professional responsibility within the health care arena."[19(p275)] Studying history can enable nurses to more clearly understand their role in providing health care and, thereby, assist them to clearly define their role. Friedman further illustrated the need for a clear definition of nursing: "A persistently vague and constantly shifting definition of nursing practice has long complicated nursing's effort to define itself and thus create a professional identity."[16(p2851)] Without a clear definition of what nursing is, nurses risk being left out of health care reform in the United States.

Nurses must also assert their autonomy as a means of being included in health care reform. Historically, nurses have been powerless in the health care system, and much of this powerlessness relates to the predominance of women, a traditionally powerless group, in the profession. Also, Reverby maintained, "Nurses were expected to act out an obligation to care, taking on caring more as an identity than as work, and expressing altruism without thought of autonomy either at the bedside or in their profession."[20(p5)] Nurses are still struggling for autonomy. This lack of autonomy results, in part, from the public perception of nurses being subordinate to physicians. Nurses have an obligation to educate the public about their role, and, thereby, assert their autonomy. Church claimed studying history is an important step in establishing autonomy because "ignorance of the past contributes to the inability to identify one's boundaries properly and retards the development of the essential autonomy that accompanies professional self-determination."[19(p275)] By exercising their autonomy as professionals, nurses can be leaders in health care reform.

Moreover, nurses must unite in order to assert their control in health care reform. Unfortunately, the nursing profession has not yet achieved unity. Because nurses come from a wide variety of backgrounds and have diverse interests, nurses as a group have difficulty expressing themselves as a unified voice. Friedman claimed, "nursing has been divided internally from the beginning" and continues, "Often its members have spent more time fighting each other than any outside enemies."[16(p2851)] Nurses must stop fighting each other and unite to battle for their common interests. A unified nursing profession can lead the United States in health care reform. Church pointed the way to unity for nursing: "The study of history represents the potential for the discovery of a unity and continuity of one's identity."[19(p275)] Church said that history unifies because "having determined a collective past, one can look to developing a sense of unity."[19(p277)] History has much to offer nursing with regard to having a unified voice in health care reform.

■ LESSONS FROM NURSING HISTORY

Unfortunately, many nurses have little knowledge about their history. Education for nurses rarely includes history, except for occasional graduate-level courses. Additionally, finding historical information about nurses can be difficult because nurses have traditionally been female. Unfortunately, information about the daily lives of females was rarely recorded and passed on, and achievements in domestic arts, including nursing, was not considered to be important.[21] Nonetheless, interest in nursing history is growing, and increasing numbers of resources concerning nursing history are becoming available.

Studying nursing history provides nurses with role models for political action. Donahue pointed out, "The fact is that many of the early leaders in nursing were involved in the social issues of the times including women's suffrage, child labor laws, public health, and national defense."[22(p77)] Mason used Nightingale, Truth, and Wald as examples of politically active and influential nurses, saying, "They were all expert nurses and recognized the power of their expertise."[4(p14)] Mason urged present-day nurses to be politically active and to be leaders in health care reform: "Nurse leaders throughout history have been astute political players. Many have used their power and political skills to change the face of health care and other social issues of the times."[4(p16)] Nurses can use the lessons taught by history to develop ways of influencing health care reform.

For example, history teaches nurses the importance of working together. Previous divisions within the profession have undermined its political power. Lynaugh and Fagin urged nurses to cooperate with each other: "Together we can ensure that there is enfranchisement and expanded authority for all nurses while we struggle to agree to a different and more unified future."[3(p189)]

In addition to presenting a unified front, nurses must educate the public about their role in the health care system. Hughes asserted, "Nursing potential has not been fully recognized or utilized by the public, and this has led to wasted nursing talent and inadequate care for society."[14(p55)] Baer blamed this lack of public understanding on nurses themselves. "Because nurses expect approval and appreciation for their work to occur automatically because their work is 'good,' they spend less time explaining their work and fighting for its piece of the health care pie."[10(p18)] Nurses must assert themselves and explain their role to the public. Moreover, nurses can have an important role in the changes in the health care system, especially if the public understands the role of nurses.

Furthermore, nurses will be able to accomplish more if they work with other groups. Reverby stated, "The dilemma of nursing is too tied to society's broader problems of gender and class to be solved solely by political or professional efforts of one occupational group."[20(p10)] A historical examination of problems facing nursing today illustrates their complexities. This understanding points to the need for nursing to cooperate with other groups to more effectively establish their place in health care reform.

Nurses must study their history. An examination of history provides insight into and direction for addressing problems currently affecting the profession, such as pay, regulation, shortage, education, defining nursing practice, autonomy, and unity. Historical study also reveals role models for political action in such nurse leaders as Nightingale, Truth, and Wald. History can also dictate a blueprint for action. Without understanding nursing history, current nurses cannot effectively address present-day conditions. Specifically, nurses must risk a sometimes painful examination of history in order to achieve political power.

Examining history allows nurses to more fully appreciate their important role in the health care system of the United States. Therefore by not understanding nursing history, nurses risk being left out of health care reform—again. Friedman asserted, "Nursing, more than at any point in its history, has the chance to exercise enormous power in society."[16(p2858)] Nurses must become more politically active. Nurses can assert themselves individually or in organized groups. For example, in 1992, Eddie Bernice Johnson became the first registered nurse elected to the United States Congress. Previously, as a Texas State Senator, Johnson used her political power to enact health care reform. Collectively, during the 1992 elections, nurses influenced local and national elections by endorsing candidates through the ANA and state and local nurses' associations. Nurses also must educate lawmakers about nursing and continue to openly communicate with elected officials. Nurses must make themselves heard. Nurses have much to offer to health care, and this country will not realize its health care potential without leadership from the nursing profession.

References

1. Eliot TS. *Four Quartets.* London, England: Faber & Faber; 1944.
2. Maraldo PJ. NLN's first century. *Nursing and Health Care.* 1992; 13:227–228.
3. Lynaugh JE, Fagin CM. Nursing comes of age. *Image: Journal of Nursing Scholarship.* 1988;20:184–190.
4. Mason DJ. Nursing and politics: a profession comes of age. *Orthopaedic Nursing.* 1990;9:11–17.
5. Hamilton DB. The idea of history and the history of ideas. *Image: Journal of Nursing Scholarship.* 1993;25:45–48.
6. Lynaugh JE, Reverby S. Thoughts on the nature of history. *Nursing Research.* 1987;36:4,69.
7. Church OM. New knowledge from old truths: problems and promises of historical inquiry in nursing. In: McCloskey JC, Grace HK, eds. *Current Issues in Nursing.* St. Louis, MO: Mosby; 1990.
8. Mauksch IG. Understanding our past to build our future. *Oncology Nursing Forum.* 1989;16:483–487.
9. Donahue MP. The past in the present. *Journal of Professional Nursing.* 1990;6:9.
10. Baer ED. American nursing: 100 years of conflicting ideas and ideals. *Journal of the New York State Nurses Association.* 1992;23(3):16–21.
11. Brown JM, D'Antonio P. Nursing history and scholarship—critical issues for the discipline. *Journal of Professional Nursing.* 1990;6:319.
12. Reverby SM. *Ordered To Care: The Dilemma of American Nursing, 1850–1945.* New York, NY: Cambridge; 1987.
13. Minkowski WL. Women healers of the Middle Ages: selected aspects of their history. *American Journal of Public Health.* 1992;82:288–295.
14. Hughes L. The public image of the nurse. *Advances in Nursing Science.* 1980;2(3):55–72.
15. Brider P. The struggle for just compensation. *American Journal of Nursing.* 1990;90(10)77–88.
16. Friedman E. Troubled past of "invisible" profession. *JAMA: Journal of the American Medical Association.* 1990;264:2851–2858.
17. Baer ED. Of exclusion and divided houses. *Nursing Research.* 1990;39:318–319.
18. American Nurses' Association. *American Nurses' Association: Code for Nurses with Interpretive Statements.* Washington, DC: ANA; 1985.
19. Church OM. Historiography in nursing research. *Western Journal of Nursing Research.* 1987;9:275–279.
20. Reverby SM. A caring dilemma: womanhood in nursing in historical perspective. *Nursing Research.* 1987;36:5–11.
21. Bullough VL, Bullough B, Wu YB. Achievement of eminent American nurses of the past: a prosopographical study. *Nursing Research* 1992;41:120–124.
22. Donahue MP. Why nursing history? *Journal of Professional Nursing.* 1991;7:77.

2

A Caring Dilemma: Womanhood and Nursing in Historical Perspective

Susan Reverby

"**D**o not undervalue [your] particular ability to care," students were reminded at a recent nursing school graduation.[1] Rather than merely bemoaning yet another form of late twentieth-century heartlessness, this admonition underscores the central dilemma of American nursing: The order to care in a society that refuses to value caring. This article is an analysis of the historical creation of that dilemma and its consequences for nursing. To explore the meaning of caring for nursing, it is necessary to unravel the terms of the relationship between nursing and womanhood as these bonds have been formed over the last century.

■ THE MEANING OF CARING

Many different disciplines have explored the various meanings of caring.[2] Much of this literature, however, runs the danger of universalizing caring as an element in female identity, or as a human quality, separate from the cultural and structural circumstances that create it. But as policy analyst Hilary Graham has argued, caring is not merely an identity; it is also work. As she notes, "Caring touches simultaneously on who you are and what you do."[3] Because of this duality, caring can be difficult to define and even harder to control. Graham's analysis moves beyond seeing caring as a psychological trait; but her focus is primarily on women's unpaid labor in the home. She does not fully discuss how the forms of caring are shaped by the contexts under which they are practiced. Caring is not just a subjective and material experience, it is a historically created one. Particular circumstances, ideologies, and power relations thus create the conditions under which caring can occur, the forms it will take, the consequences it will have for those who do it.

Susan Reverby, assistant professor and director, Women's Studies Program, Wellesley College, Wellesley, Massachusetts.

The basis for caring also shapes its effect. Nursing was organized under the expectation that its practitioners would accept a duty to care rather than demand a right to determine how they would satisfy this duty. Nurses were expected to act out of an obligation to care, taking on caring more as an identity than as work, and expressing altruism without thought of autonomy either at the bedside or in their profession. Thus, nurses, like others who perform what is defined as "women's work" in our society, have had to contend with what appears as a dichotomy between the duty to care for others and the right to control their own activities in the name of caring. Nursing is still searching for what philosopher Joel Feinberg argued comes prior to rights; that is, being "recognized as having a claim on rights."[4] The duty to care, organized within the political and economic context of nursing's development, has made it difficult for nurses to obtain this moral and, ultimately, political standing.

Because nurses have been given the duty to care, they are caught in a secondary dilemma: forced to act as if altruism (assumed to be the basis for caring) and autonomy (assumed to be the basis of rights) are separate ways of being. Nurses are still searching for a way to forge a link between altruism and autonomy that will allow them to have what philosopher Larry Blum and others have called "caring-with-autonomy," or what psychiatrist Jean Baker Miller labeled "a way of life that includes serving others without being subservient."[5] Nursing's historical circumstances and ideological underpinnings have made creating this way of life difficult, but not impossible, to achieve.

■ CARING AS DUTY

A historical analysis of nursing's development makes this theoretical formulation clearer. Most of the writing about American nursing's history begins in the 1870s when formal training for nursing was introduced in the United States. But nursing did not appear de novo at the end of the nineteenth century. As with most medical and health care, nursing throughout the colonial era and most of the nineteenth century took place within the family and the home. In the domestic pantheon that surrounded "middling" and upper-class American womanhood in the nineteenth century, a woman's caring for friends and relatives was an important pillar. Nursing was often taught by mother to daughter as part of female apprenticeship, or learned by a domestic servant as an additional task on her job. Embedded in the seemingly natural or ordained character of women, it became an important manifestation of women's expression of love of others, and was thus integral to the female sense of self.[6] In a society where deeply felt religious tenets were translated into gendered virtues, domesticity advocate Catherine Beecher declared that the sick were to be "commended" to a "woman's benevolent ministries."[7]

The responsibility for nursing went beyond a mother's duty for her children, a wife's for her husband, or a daughter's for her aging parents. It attached to all the available female family members. The family's "long arm" might reach out at any time to a woman working in a distant city, in a mill, or as a maid, pulling her home to care for the sick, infirm, or newborn. No form of women's labor, paid or unpaid, protected her from this demand. "You may be called upon at any moment," Eliza W. Farrar warned in the *The Young Lady's Friend* in 1837, "to attend upon your parents, your brothers, your sisters, or your companions."[8] Nursing was to be, therefore, a woman's duty, not her job. Obligation and love, not the need of work, were to bind the nurse to her patient. Caring was to be an unpaid labor of love.

■ THE PROFESSED NURSE

Even as Eliza Farrar was proffering her advice, pressures both inward and outward were beginning to reshape the domestic sphere for women of the then-called "middling classes." Women's obligations and work were transformed by the expanding industrial economy and changing cultural assumptions. Parenting took on increasing importance as notions of "moral mothering" filled the domestic arena and other production labor entered the cash nexus. Female benevolence similarly moved outward as women's charitable efforts took increasingly institutional forms. Duty began to take on new meaning as such women were advised they could fulfill their nursing responsibilities by managing competently those they hired to assist them. Bourgeois female virtue could still be demonstrated as the balance of labor, love, and supervision shifted.[9]

An expanding economy thus had differing effects on women of various classes. For those in the growing urban middle classes, excess cash made it possible to consider hiring a nurse when circumstances, desire, or exhaustion meant a female relative was no longer available for the task. Caring as labor, for these women, could be separated from love.

For older widows or spinsters from the working classes, nursing became a trade they could "profess" relatively easily in the marketplace. A widow who had nursed her husband till his demise, or a domestic servant who had cared for an employer in time of illness, entered casually into the nursing trade, hired by families or individuals unwilling or unable to care for their sick alone. The permeable boundaries for women between unpaid and paid labor allowed nursing to pass back and forth when necessary. For many women, nursing thus beckoned as respectable community work.

These "professed" or "natural-born" nurses, as they were known, usually came to their work, as one Boston nurse put it, "lately" when other forms of employment were closed to them or the lack of any kind of work experience left nursing as an obvious choice. Mehitable Pond Garside, for example, was in her fifties and had outlived two husbands—and her children could not, or would not, support her—when she came to Boston in the 1840s to nurse. Similarly Alma Frost Merrill, the daughter of a Maine wheelwright, came to

Boston in 1818 at nineteen to become a domestic servant. After years as a domestic and seamstress, she declared herself a nurse.[10]

Women like Mehitable Pond Garside and Alma Frost Merrill differed markedly from the Sairy Gamp character of Dickens' novel, *Martin Chuzzlewit*. Gamp was portrayed as a merely besotted representative of lumpenproletarian womanhood, who asserted her autonomy by daring to question medical diagnosis, to venture her own opinions (usually outrageous and wrong) at every turn, and to spread disease and superstition in the name of self-knowledge. If they were not Gamps, nurses like Garside and Merrill also were not the healers of some more recent feminist mythology that confounds nursing with midwifery, praising the caring and autonomy these women exerted, but refusing to consider their ignorance.[11] Some professed nurses learned their skills from years of experience, demonstrating the truth of the dictum that "to make a kind and sympathizing nurse, one must have waited, in sickness, upon those she loved dearly".[12] Others, however, blundered badly beyond their capabilities or knowledge. They brought to the bedside only the authority their personalities and community stature could command. Neither credentials nor a professional identity gave weight to their efforts. Their womenhood, and the experience it gave them, defined their authority and taught them to nurse.

■ THE HOSPITAL NURSE

Nursing was not limited, however, to the bedside in a home. Although the United States had only 178 hospitals at the first national census in 1873, it was workers labeled "nurses" who provided the caring. As in home-based nursing, the route to hospital nursing was paved more with necessity than with intentionality. In 1875, Eliza Higgins, the matron of Boston's Lying-In Hospital, could not find an extra nurse to cover all the deliveries. In desperation, she moved the hospital laundress up to the nursing position, while a recovering patient took over the wash. Higgins' diaries of her trying years at the Lying-In suggest that such an entry into nursing was not uncommon.[13]

As Higgins' reports and memoirs of other nurses attest, hospital nursing could be the work of devoted women who learned what historian Charles Rosenberg has labeled "ad hoc professionalism," or the temporary and dangerous labor of an ambulatory patient or hospital domestic.[14] As in home-based nursing, both caring and concern were frequently demonstrated. But the nursing work and nurses were mainly characterized by the diversity of their efforts and the unevenness of their skills.

Higgins' memoirs attest to the hospital as a battleground where nurses, physicians, and hospital managers contested the realm of their authority. Nurses continually affirmed their right to control the pace and content of their work, to set their own hours, and to structure their relationships to physicians. Aware that the hospital's paternalistic attitudes and practices toward its "inmates" were attached to the nursing personnel as well, they fought to be treated as workers, "not children," as the Lying-In nurses told Eliza Higgins, and to maintain their autonomous adult status.[15]

Like home-based nursing, hospital nurses had neither formal training nor class status upon which to base their arguments. But their sense of the rights of working-class womanhood gave them authority to press their demands. The necessity to care, and their perception of its importance to patient outcome, also structured their belief that demanding the right to be relatively autonomous was possible. However, their efforts were undermined by the nature of their onerous work, the paternalism of the institutions, class differences between trustees and workers, and ultimately the lack of a defined ideology of caring. Mere resistance to those above them, or contending assertions of rights, could not become the basis for nursing authority.

■ THE INFLUENCE OF NIGHTINGALE

Much of this changed with the introduction of training for nursing in the hospital world. In the aftermath of Nightingale's triumph over the British army's medical care system in the Crimea, similar attempts by American women during the Civil War, and the need to find respectable work for daughters of the middling classes, a model and support for nursing reform began to grow. By 1873, three nursing schools in hospitals in New York, Boston, and New Haven were opened, patterned after the Nightingale School at St. Thomas' Hospital in London.

Nightingale had envisioned nursing as an art, rather than a science, for which women needed to be trained. Her ideas linked her medical and public health notions to her class and religious beliefs. Accepting the Victorian idea of divided spheres of activity for men and women, she thought women had to be trained to nurse through a disciplined process of honing their womanly virtue. Nightingale stressed character development, the laws of health, and strict adherence to orders passed through a female hierarchy. Nursing was built on a model that relied on the concept of duty to provide its basis for authority. Unlike other feminists at the time, she spoke in the language of duty, not rights.

Furthermore, as a nineteenth-century sanitarian, Nightingale never believed in germ theory, in part because she refused to accept a theory of disease etiology that appeared to be morally neutral. Given her sanitarian beliefs, Nightingale thought medical therapeutics and "curing" were of lesser importance to patient outcome, and she willingly left this realm to the physician. Caring, the arena she did think of great importance, she assigned to the nurse. In order to care, a nurse's character, tempered by the fires of training, was to be her greatest skill. Thus, to "feminize" nursing, Nightingale sought a change in the class-defined behavior, not the gender, of the work force.[16]

To forge a good nurse out of the virtues of a good woman and to provide a political base for nursing, Nightingale sought to organize a female hierarchy in which orders passed down from the nursing superintendent to the lowly probationer. This separate female sphere was to share power in the provision of health care with the male-dominated arenas of medicine. For many women in the Victorian era, sisterhood and what Carroll Smith-Rosenberg has called "homosocial networks" served to overcome many of the limits of this separate but supposedly equal system of cultural division.[17] Sisterhood, after all, at least in its fictive forms, underlay much of the female power that grew out of women's culture in the nineteenth century. But in nursing, commonalities of the gendered experience could not become the basis of unity since hierarchial filial relations, not equal sisterhood, lay at the basis of nursing's theoretical formulation.

Service, Not Education

Thus, unwittingly, Nightingale's sanitarian ideas and her beliefs about womanhood provided some of the ideological justification for many of the dilemmas that faced American nursing by 1900. Having fought physician and trustee prejudice against the training of nurses in hospitals in the last quarter of the nineteenth century, American nursing reformers succeeded only too well as the new century began. Between 1890 and 1920, the number of nursing schools jumped from 35 to 1,775, and the number of trained nurses from 16 per 100,000 in the population to 141.[18] Administrators quickly realized that opening a "nursing school" provided their hospitals, in exchange for training, with a young, disciplined, and cheap labor force. There was often no difference between the hospital's nursing school and its nursing service. The service needs of the hospital continually overrode the education requirements of the schools. A student might, therefore, spend weeks on a medical ward if her labor was so needed, but never see the inside of an operating room before her graduation.

Once the nurse finished her training, however, she was unlikely to be hired by a hospital because it relied on either untrained aides or nursing student labor. The majority of graduate nurses, until the end of the 1930s, had to find work in private duty in a patient's home, as the patient's employee in the hospital, in the branches of public health, or in some hospital staff positions. In the world of nursing beyond the training school, "trained" nurses still had to compete with the thousands of "professed" or "practical" nurses who continued to ply their trade in an overcrowded and unregulated marketplace. The title of nurse took on very ambiguous meanings.[19]

The term, "trained nurse," was far from a uniform designation. As nursing leader Isabel Hampton Robb lamented in 1893, "the title 'trained nurse' may mean then anything, everything, or next to nothing."[20]

The exigencies of nursing acutely ill or surgical patients required the sacrifice of coherent educational programs. Didactic, repetitive, watered-down medical lectures by physicians or older nurses were often provided for the students, usually after they finished ten to twelve hours of ward work. Training emphasized the "one right way" of doing ritualized procedures in hopes the students' adherence to specified rules would be least dangerous to patients.[21] Under these circumstances, the duty to care could be followed with a vengeance and become the martinet adherence to orders.

Furthermore, because nursing emphasized training in discipline, order, and practical skills, the abuse of student labor could be rationalized. And because the work force was almost entirely women, altruism, sacrifice, and submission were expected, encouraged, indeed, demanded. Exploitation was inevitable in a field where, until the early 1900s, there were no accepted standards for how much work an average student should do or how many patients she could successfully care for, no mechanisms through which to enforce such standards. After completing her exhaustive and depressing survey of nursing training in 1912, nursing educator M. Adelaide Nutting bluntly pointed out: "Under the present system the school has no life of its own."[22] In this kind of environment, nurses were trained. But they were not educated.

Virtue and Autonomy

It would be a mistake, however, to see the nursing experience only as one of exploitation and the nursing school as a faintly concealed reformatory for the wayward girl in need of discipline. Many nursing superintendents lived Nightingale ideals as best they could and infused them into their schools. The authoritarian model could and did retemper many women. It instilled in nurses idealism and pride in their skills, somewhat differentiated the trained nurse from the untrained, and protected and aided the sick and dying. It provided a mechanism for virtuous women to contribute to the improvement of humanity by empowering them to care.

For many of the young women entering training in the nineteenth and early twentieth centuries, nursing thus offered something quite special: both a livelihood and a virtuous state. As one nursing educator noted in 1890: "Young strong country girls are drawn into the work by the glamorer [sic] thrown about hospital work and the halo that sanctifies a Nightingale."[23] Thus, in their letters of application, aspiring nursing students expressed their desire for work, independence, and womanly virtue. As with earlier, nontrained nurses, they did not seem to separate autonomy and altruism, but rather sought its linkage through training. Flora Jones spoke for many such women when she wrote the superintendent of Boston City Hospital in 1880, declaring, "I consider myself fitted for the work by inclination and consider it a womanly occupation. It is also necessary for me to become self-supporting and provide for my future."[24] Thus, one nursing superintendent reminded a graduating class in 1904: "You have become self-controlled, unselfish, gentle, compassionate, brave, capable—in fact, you have risen from the period of irresponsible girlhood to that of womanhood."[25] For women like Flora Jones, and many of nursing's early leaders, nursing was the singular way to grow to maturity in a womanly profession that offered meaningful work, independence, and altruism.[26]

Altruism, Not Independence

For many, however, as nursing historian Dorothy Sheahan has noted, the training school, "was a place where . . . women learned to be girls."[27] The range of permissible behaviors for respectable women was often narrowed further through training. Independence was to be sacrificed on the altar of altruism. Thus, despite hopes of aspiring students and promises of training school superintendents, nursing rarely united altruism and autonomy. Duty remained the basis for caring.

Some nurses were able to create what they called "a little world of our own." But nursing had neither the financial nor the cultural power to create the separate women's institutions that provided so much of the basis for women's reform and rights efforts.[28] Under these conditions, nurses found it difficult to make the collective transition out of a women's culture of obligation into an activist assault on the structure and beliefs that oppressed them. Nursing remained bounded by its ideology and its material circumstances.

■ THE CONTRADICTIONS OF REFORM

In this context, one begins to understand the difficulties faced by the leaders of nursing reform. Believing that educational reform was central to nursing's professionalizing efforts and clinical improvements, a small group of elite reformers attempted to broaden nursing's scientific content and social outlook. In arguing for an increase in the scientific knowledge necessary in nursing, such leaders were fighting against deep-seated cultural assumptions about male and female "natural" characteristics as embodied in the doctor and the nurse. Such sentiments were articulated in the routine platitudes that graced what one nursing leader described as the "doctor homilies" that were a regular feature at nursing graduation exercises.[29]

Not surprisingly, such beliefs were professed by physicians and hospital officials whenever nursing shortages appeared, or nursing groups pushed for higher educational standards or defined nursing as more than assisting the physician. As one nursing educator wrote, with some degree of resignation after the influenza pandemic in 1920: "It is perhaps inevitable that the difficulty of securing nurses during the last year or two should have revived again the old agitation about the 'over-training' of nurses and the clamor for a cheap worker of the old servant-nurse type."[30]

First Steps Toward Professionalism

The nursing leadership, made up primarily of educators and supervisors with their base within what is now the American Nurses' Association and the National League for Nursing, thus faced a series of dilemmas as they struggled to raise educational standards in the schools and criteria for entry into training, to register nurses once they finished their training, and to gain acceptance for the knowledge base and skills of the nurse. They had to exalt the womanly character, self-abnegation, and service ethic of nursing while insisting on the right of nurses to act in their own self-interest. They had to demand higher wages commensurate with their skills, yet not appear commercial. They had to simultaneously find a way to denounce the exploitation of nursing students, as they made political alliances with hospital physicians and administrators whose support they needed. While they lauded character and sacrifice, they had to find a way to measure it with educational criteria in order to formulate registration laws and set admission standards. They had to make demands and organize, without appearing "unladylike." In sum, they were forced by the social conditions and ideology surrounding nursing to attempt to professionalize altruism without demanding autonomy.

Undermined by Duty

The image of a higher claim of duty also continually undermined a direct assertion of the right to determine that duty. Whether at a bedside, or at a legislative hearing on practice laws, the duty to care became translated into the demand that nurses merely follow doctors' orders. The tradition of obligation almost made it impossible for nurses to speak about rights at all. By the turn of the century necessity and desire were pulling more young women into the labor force, and the women's movement activists were placing rights at the center of cultural discussion. In this atmosphere, nursing's call to duty was perceived by many as an increasingly antiquated language to shore up a changing economic and cultural landscape. Nursing became a type of collective female grasping for an older form of security and power in the face of rapid change. Women who might have been attracted to nursing in the 1880s as a womanly occupation that provided some form of autonomy, were, by the turn of the century, increasingly looking elsewhere for work and careers.

■ A DIFFERENT VISION

In the face of these difficulties, the nursing leadership became increasingly defensive and turned on its own rank and file. The educators and supervisors who comprised leadership lost touch with the pressing concern of their constituencies in the daily work world of nursing and the belief systems such nurses continued to hold. Yet many nurses, well into the twentieth century, shared the nineteenth-century vision of nursing as the embodiment of womanly virtue. A nurse named Annette Fiske, for example, although she authored two science books for nurses and had an M.A. degree in classics from Radcliffe College before she entered training, spent her professional career in the 1920s arguing against increasing educational standards. Rather, she called for a reinfusion into nursing of spirituality and service, assuming that this would result in nursing's receiving greater "love and respect and admiration."[31]

Other nurses, especially those trained in the smaller schools or reared to hold working-class ideals about respectable behavior in women, shared Fiske's views. They saw the leadership's efforts at professionalization as an attempt to push them out of nursing. Their adherence to nursing skill measured in womanly virtue was less a conservative and reactionary stance than a belief that seemed to transcend class and educational backgrounds to place itself in the individual character and workplace skills of the nurse. It grounded altruism in supposedly natural and spiritual, rather then educational and middle-class, soil. For Fiske and many other nurses, nursing was still a womanly art that required inherent character in its practitioners and training in practical skills and spiritual values in its schools. Their beliefs about nursing did not require the professionalization of altruism, nor the demand for autonomy either at the bedside or in control over the professionalization process.

Still other nurses took a more pragmatic viewpoint that built on their pride in their workplace skills and character. These nurses also saw the necessity for concerted action, not unlike that taken by other American workers. Such nurses fought against what one 1888 nurse, who called herself Candor, characterized as the "missionary spirit . . . [of] self-immolation" that denied that nurses worked because they had to make a living.[32] These worker-nurses saw no contradiction between demanding decent wages and conditions for their labors and being of service for those in need. But the efforts of various groups of these kinds of nurses to turn to hours' legislation, trade union activity, or mutual aid associations were criticized and condemned by the nursing leadership. Their letters were often edited out of the nursing journals, and their voices silenced in public meetings as they were denounced as being commercial, or lacking in proper womanly devotion.[33]

In the face of continual criticism from nursing's professional leadership, the worker-nurses took on an increasingly angry and defensive tone. Aware that their sense of the nurse's skills came from the experiences of the workplace, not book learning or degrees, they had to assert this position despite continued hostility toward such a basis of nursing authority.[34] Although the position of women like Candor helped articulate a way for nurses to begin to assert the right to care, it did not constitute a full-blown ideological counterpart to the overwhelming power of the belief in duty.

The Persistence of Dilemmas

By midcentury, the disputes between worker-nurses and the professional leadership began to take on new forms, although the persistent divisions continued. Aware that some kind of collective bargaining was necessary to keep nurses out of the unions and in the professional associations, the ANA reluctantly agreed in 1946 to let its state units act as bargaining agents. The nursing leadership has continued to look at educational reform strategies, now primarily taking the form of legislating for the B.S. degree as the credential necessary for entry into nursing practice, and to changes in the practice laws that will allow increasingly skilled nurses the autonomy and status they deserve. Many nurses have continued to be critical of this educational strategy, to ignore the professional associations, or to leave nursing altogether.

In their various practice fields nurses still need a viable ideology and strategy that will help them adjust to the continual demands of patients and an ever more bureaucratized, cost-conscious, and rationalized work setting. For many nurses it is still, in an ideological sense, the nineteenth century. Even for those nurses who work as practitioners in the more autonomous settings of health maintenance organizations or public health offices, the legacy of nursing's heritage is still felt. Within the last two years, for example, the Massachusetts Board of Medicine tried to push through a regulation that health practitioners acknowledge their dependence on physicians by wearing a badge that identified their supervising physician and stated that they were not doctors.

Nurses have tried various ways to articulate a series of rights that allow them to care. The acknowledgment of responsibilities, however, so deeply ingrained in nursing and American womanhood, as nursing school dean Claire Fagin has noted, continually drown out the nurse's assertion of rights.[35]

Nurses are continuing to struggle to obtain the right to claim rights. Nursing's educational philosophy, ideological underpinnings, and structural position have made it difficult to create the circumstances within which to gain such recognition. It is not a lack of vision that thwarts nursing, but the lack of power to give that vision substantive form.[36]

■ BEYOND THE OBLIGATION TO CARE

Much has changed in nursing in the last forty years. The severing of nursing education from the hospital's nursing service has finally taken place, as the majority of nurses are now educated in colleges, not hospital-based diploma schools. Hospitals are experimenting with numerous ways to organize the nursing service to provide the nurse with more responsibility and sense of control over the nursing care process. The increasingly technical and machine-aided nature of hospital-based health care has made nurses feel more skilled.

In many ways, however, little has changed. Nursing is still divided over what counts as a nursing skill, how it is to be learned, and whether a nurse's character can be measured in educational criteria. Technical knowledge and capabilities do not easily translate into power and control. Hospitals, seeking to cut costs, have forced nurses to play "beat the clock" as they run from task to task in an increasingly fragmented setting.[37]

Nursing continues to struggle with the basis for, and the value of, caring. The fact that the first legal case on comparable worth was brought by a group of Denver nurses suggests nursing has an important and ongoing role in the political effort to have caring revalued. As in the Denver case, contemporary feminism has provided some nurses with the grounds on which to claim rights from their caring.[38]

Feminism, in its liberal form, appears to give nursing a political language that argues for equality and rights within the given order of things. It suggests a basis for caring that stresses individual discretion and values, acknowledging that the nurse's right to care should be given equal consideration with the physician's right to cure. Just as liberal political theory undermined more paternalistic formulations of government, classical liberalism's tenets applied to women have much to offer nursing. The demand for the right to care questions deeply held beliefs about gendered relations in the health care hierarchy and the structure of the hierarchy itself.

Many nurses continue to hope that with more education, explicit theories to explain the scientific basis for nursing, new skills, and a lot of assertiveness training, nursing will change. As these nurses try to shed the image of the nurse's being ordered to care, however, the admonition to care at a graduation speech has to be made. Unable to find a way to "care with autonomy" and unable to separate caring from its valuing and basis, many nurses find themselves forced to abandon the effort to care, or nursing altogether.

■ *ALTRUISM WITH AUTONOMY*

These dilemmas for nurses suggest the constraints that surround the effectiveness of a liberal feminist political strategy to address the problems of caring and, therefore, of nursing. The individualism and autonomy of a rights framework often fail to acknowledge collective social need, to provide a way for adjudicating conflicts over rights, or to address the reasons for the devaluing of female activity.[39] Thus, nurses have often rejected liberal feminism, not just out of their oppression and "false consciousness," but because of some deep understandings of the limited promise of equality and autonomy in a health care system they see as flawed and harmful. In an often inchoate way, such nurses recognize that those who claim the autonomy of rights often run the risk of rejecting altruism and caring itself.

Several feminist psychologists have suggested that what women really want in their lives is autonomy with connectedness. Similarly, many modern moral philosophers are trying to articulate a formal moral theory that values the emotions and the importance of relationships.[40] For nursing, this will require the creation of the conditions under which it is possible to value caring and to understand that the empowerment of others does not have to require self-immolation. To achieve this, nurses will have both to create a new political understanding for the basis of caring and to find ways to gain the power to implement it. Nursing can do much to have this happen through research on the importance of caring on patient outcome, studies of patient improvements in nursing settings where the right to care is created, or implementing nursing control of caring through a bargaining agreement. But nurses cannot do this alone. The dilemma of nursing is too tied to society's broader problems of gender and class to be solved solely by the political or professional efforts of one occupational group.

Nor are nurses alone in benefiting from such an effort. If nursing can achieve the power to practice altruism with autonomy, all of us have much to gain. Nursing has always been a much conflicted metaphor in our culture, reflecting all the ambivalences we give to the meaning of womanhood.[41] Perhaps in the future it can give this metaphor and, ultimately, caring, new value in all our lives.

References

1. Wticher, Gregory. "Last Class of Nurses Told: Don't Stop Caring," *Boston Globe,* May 13, 1985, pp. 17–18.
2. See, for examples, Larry Blum et al., "Altruism and Women's Oppression," in *Women and Philosophy,* eds. Carol Gould and Marx Wartofsy (New York: G. P. Putnam's, 1976), pp. 222–247; Nel Noddings, *Caring.* Berkeley: University of California Press, 1984; Nancy Chodorow, *The Reproduction of Mothering.* Berkeley: University of California Press, 1978; Carol Gilligan, *In a Different Voice.* Cambridge: Harvard University Press, 1982; and Janet Finch and Dulcie Groves, eds., *A Labour of Love, Women, Work and Caring.* London and Boston: Routledge, Kegan Paul, 1983.
3. Graham, Hilary, "Caring: A Labour of Love," in *A Labour of Love,* eds. Finch and Groves, pp. 13–30.
4. Feinberg, Joel. *Rights, Justice and the Bounds of Liberty* (Princeton: Princeton University Press, 1980), p. 141.
5. Blum et al., "Altruism and Women's Oppression," p. 223; Jean Baker Miller, *Toward a New Psychology of Women* (Boston: Beacon Press, 1976), p. 71.
6. Ibid; see also Iris Marion Young, "Is Male Gender Identity the Cause of Male Domination," in *Mothering: Essays in Feminist Theory,* ed. Joyce Trebicott (Totowa, NJ: Rowman and Allanheld, 1983), pp. 129–146.
7. Beecher, Catherine. *Domestic Receipt-Book* (New York: Harper and Brothers, 1846), p. 214.
8. Farrar, Eliza. *The Young Lady's Friend—By a Lady* (Boston: American Stationer's Co., 1837), p. 57.

9. Beecher, Catherine, *Miss Beecher's Housekeeper and Healthkeeper.* New York: Harper and Brothers, 1876; and Sarah Josepha Hale, *The Good Housekeeper.* Boston: Otis Brothers and Co., 7th edition, 1844. See also Susan Strasser, *Never Done: A History of Housework.* New York: Pantheon, 1982.

10. Cases 2 and 18, "Admissions Committee Records," Volume I, Box 11, Hone for Aged Women Collection, Schlesinger Library, Radcliffe College, Cambridge, Mass. Data on the nurses admitted to the home were also found in "Records of Inmates, 1858–1901," "Records of Admission, 1873–1924," and "Records of Inmates, 1901–1916," all in Box 11.

11. Dickens, Charles. *Martin Chuzzlewit.* New York: New American Library, 1965, original edition, London: 1865; Barbara Ehrenreich and Deirdre English, *Witches, Nurses, Midwives: A History of Women Healers.* Old Westbury: Glass Mountain Pamphlets, 1972.

12. Penny, Virginia. *The Employments of Women: A Cyclopedia of Women's Work* (Boston: Walker, Wise and Co., 1863), p. 420.

13. Higgins, Eliza. Boston Lying-In Hospital, *Matron's Journals, 1873–1889,* Volume I, January 9, 1875, February 22, 1875, Rare Books Room, Countway Medical Library, Harvard Medical School, Boston, Mass.

14. Rosenberg, Charles, "'And Heal the Sick': The Hospital and the Patient in 19th Century America," *Journal of Social History* 10 (June 1977):445.

15. Higgins, *Matron's Journals,* Volume II, January 11, 1876, and July 1, 1876. See also a parallel discussion of male artisan behavior in front of the boss in David Montgomery, "Workers' Control of Machine Production in the 19th Century," *Labor History* 17 (Winter 1976):485–509.

16. The discussion of Florence Nightingale is based on my analysis in *Ordered to Care,* chapter 3. See also Charles E. Rosenberg, "Florence Nightingale on Contagion: The Hospital as Moral Universe," in *Healing and History,* ed. Charles E. Rosenberg. New York: Science History Publications, 1979.

17. Smith-Rosenberg, Carroll. "The Female World of Love and Ritual," *Signs: Journal of Women in Culture and Society* 1 (Autumn 1975):1.

18. Burgess, May Ayers. *Nurses, Patients and Pocketbooks.* New York: Committee on the Grading of Nursing, 1926, reprint edition (New York: Garland Publishing Co., 1985), pp. 36–37.

19. For further discussion of the dilemmas of private duty nursing, see Susan Reverby, "'Neither for the Drawing Room nor for the Kitchen': Private Duty Nursing, 1880–1920," in *Women and Health in America,* ed. Judith Walzer Leavitt. Madison: University of Wisconsin Press, 1984, and Susan Reverby, "'Something Besides Waiting': The Politics of Private Duty Nursing Reform in the Depression," in *Nursing History; New Perspectives, New Possibilities,* ed. Ellen Condliffe Lagemann. New York: Teachers College Press, 1982.

20. Robb, Isabel Hampton. "Educational Standards for Nurses," in *Nursing of the Sick 1893* (New York: McGraw-Hill, 1949), p. 11. See also Janet Wilson James, "Isabel Hampton and the Professionalization of Nursing in the 1890s," in *The Therapeutic Revolution,* eds. Morris Vogel and Charles E. Rosenberg. Philadelphia: University of Pennsylvania Press, 1979.

21. For further discussion of the difficulties in training, see JoAnn Ashley, *Hospitals, Paternalism and the Role of the Nurse.* New York: Teachers College Press, 1976, and Reverby, *Ordered to Care,* chapter 4.

22. *Educational Status of Nursing,* Bureau of Education Bulletin Number 7, Whole Number 475 (Washington, D.C.: Government Printing Office, 1912), p. 49.

23. Wells, Julia. "Do Hospitals Fit Nurses for Private Nursing?" *Trained Nurse and Hospital Review 3* (March 1890):98.

24. Boston City Hospital (BCH) Training School Records, Box 4, Folder 4, Student 4, February 14, 1880, BCH Training School Papers, Nursing Archives, Special Collections, Boston University, Mugar Library, Boston, Mass. The student's name has been changed to maintain confidentiality.

25. Snively, Mary Agnes. "What Manner of Women Ought Nurses to Be?" *American Journal of Nursing 4* (August 1904):838.

26. For a discussion of many of the early nursing leaders as "new women," see Susan Armeny, "'We Were the New Women': A Comparison of Nurses and Women Physicians, 1890–1915." Paper presented at the American Association for the History of Nursing Conference, University of Virginia, Charlottesville, VA, October 1984.

27. Sheahan, Dorothy. "Influence of Occupational Sponsorship on the Professional Development of Nursing." Paper presented at the Rockefeller Archives Conference on the History of Nursing, Rockefeller Archives, Tarrytown, NY, May 1981, p. 12.

28. Freedman, Estelle. "Separatism as Strategy: Female Institution Building and American Feminism, 1870–1930," *Feminist Studies 5* (Fall 1979):512–529.

29. Dock, Lavinia L. *A History of Nursing,* volume 3 (New York: G. P. Putnam's, 1912), p. 136.

30. Stewart, Isabel M. "Progress in Nursing Education during 1919," *Modern Hospital 14* (March 1920):183.

31. Fiske, Annette. "How Can We Counteract the Prevailing Tendency to Commercialism in Nursing?" *Proceedings of the 17th Annual Meeting of the Massachusetts State Nurses' Association,* p. 8. Massachusetts Nurses Association Papers, Box 7, Nursing Archives.

32. Candor, "Work and Wages," Letter to the Editor, *Trained Nurse and Hospital Review 2* (April 1888):167–168.

33. See the discussion in Ashley, *Hospitals, Paternalism and the Role of the Nurse,* pp. 40–43, 46–48, 51, and in Barbara Melosh, *"The Physician's Hand": Work Culture and Conflict in American Nursing* (Philadelphia: Temple University Press, 1982), passim.

34. For further discussion see Susan Armeny, "Resolute Enthusiasts: The Effort to Professionalize American Nursing, 1880–1915." Ph.D. dissertation, University of Missouri, Columbia, Mo., 1984, and Reverby, *Ordered to Care,* chapter 6.

35. Feinberg, *Rights,* pp. 130–142; Claire Fagin, "Nurses' Rights," *American Journal of Nursing 75* (January 1975):82.

36. For a similar argument for bourgeois women, see Carroll Smith-Rosenberg, "The New Woman as Androgyne: Social Disorder and Gender Crisis," in *Disorderly Conduct* (New York: Alfred Knopf, 1985), p. 296.

37. Boston Nurses' Group, "The False Promise: Professionalism in Nursing," *Science for the People 10* (May/June 1978):20–34; Jennifer Bingham Hill, "Hospital Nightmare: Cuts in Staff Demoralize Nurses as Care Suffers," *Wall Street Journal,* March 27, 1985.

38. Bonnie Bullough, "The Struggle for Women's Rights in Denver: A Personal Account," *Nursing Outlook 26* (September 1978):566–567.

39. For critiques of liberal feminism see Allison M. Jagger, *Feminist Politics and Human Nature* (Totowa, NJ: Rowman and Allanheld, 1983), pp. 27–50, 173, 206;

Zillah Eisenstein, *The Radical Future of Liberal Feminism*. New York and London: Longman, 1981; and Rosalind Pollack Petchesky, *Abortion and Women's Choice* (Boston: Northeastern University Press, 1984), pp. 1–24.

40. Miller, *Toward a New Psychology;* Jane Flax, "The Conflict Between Nurturance and Autonomy in Mother-Daughter Relationships and within Feminism," *Feminist Studies* 4 (June 1978):171–191; Blum et al., "Altruism and Women's Oppression."

41. Fagin, Claire, and Donna Diers, "Nursing as Metaphor," *New England Journal of Medicine* 309 (July 14, 1983):116–117.

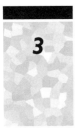

3

Florence Nightingale: Reformer, Reactionary, Researcher

Irene Sabelberg Palmer

Florence Nightingale, extolled as the greatest woman England produced in the nineteenth century, has been proclaimed with Lister and Simpson as one of three notables of that century identified for the magnitude of their everlasting contributions to the welfare of mankind (Cook, 1913, p. 439).

Two geniuses emerged from the Crimean War: Todleben, the Russian defender of Sebastopol, and Florence Nightingale, who was the only person to emerge from England's disaster with a reputation enhanced (Trevelyan, 1947, p. 653). Trevelyan (1947) and Churchill (1958 vol. 4, p. 61) said that through Florence Nightingale major efforts were made in the education and improvement in the position of women.

This paper discusses the development of Nightingale's character and philosophy and the roles through which she has been historically recognized.

■ INFLUENCES ON THE NIGHTINGALE CHARACTER

The Victorian World. Nightingale was born into a society characterized by widely disparate social structures. At one end of society the carefree, complacent upper class lived in a state of isolated affluence; at the other end was the victimized, oppressed lower stratum. The lot of British working and lower classes was characterized by pauperism, the workhouse, famine, drunkenness, and despicable working conditions which fostered disease, disability, and early death. The lord and lady bountiful concept was prevalent. Customary efforts at reform made by the aristocracy assumed the form of charity bazaars, balls, and other social benefits to raise money. Except for fund rais-

---

Irene Sabelberg Palmer (Jersey City Medical Center School of Nursing, Jersey City, New Jersey; Ph.D., New York University, New York) is dean, Philip Y. Hahn School of Nursing, University of San Diego, San Diego, California.

ing, few attempts at substantive reform or concern were made by the well-to-do. Nightingale's mother was known to make the rounds of the village poor, taking them the leftovers from the family table, handing the donations to them from her carriage, disdaining to step into the hovels they called homes. Florence was born into this socioeconomic milieu.

The Formation of the Nightingale Character and Philosophy. Florence Nightingale's heritage amply fitted her for the roles she was to play in history. Her parental lineage evidenced the strong characteristics of a love of the arts; dissent from religious orthodoxy; practical tenderness and sympathy for the underprivileged; and a reflective, developed intellect.

Nightingale received a meticulous education, especially through the direction and personal efforts of her father. This education afforded her with knowledge and perspective far surpassing that of other men and women of the era. Coupled with a background derived from extensive travel, Nightingale was an accomplished linguist; informed in the arts, mathematics, and statistics; well-read in philosophy and history; and perceptive about politics, economics, and government. She exercised her eager and keen intelligence constantly as she furthered her inquiry into her own varied interests which included religion, philosophy, land-use systems, liberty, freedom, social conditions, and institutions (Cook, 1913). The value of informed action, based on extensive knowledge, is well illustrated by the Nightingale personality.

Nightingale's beliefs and philosophy emerged in the first third of her life largely as a function of her extensive education and travel; from her belief that she had received a call from God to do His work; from the strict Victorian upbringing and narrow scope of activities socially acceptable to well-born women at that time; and from her compassionate sensitivity to the predicaments, sorrows, and miseries of people less well situated than her family.

As a youthful scholar, Nightingale became aware of those intellectual thoughts and philosophic ideologies developing in the world about her. She pursued these ideas to understand more fully the meaning of life, truth, and the Will of God. While she realized that service meant helping mankind, the exact nature of her life's work became formulated and clarified over years devoted to developing her philosophy and interpretation of the work God called her to do (Nightingale, 1869b, passim).

As Nightingale developed her beliefs, she became convinced that man's knowledge of truth released him from blind acceptance of authority and enabled him to act freely, consciously, and intelligently. She rejected the prevalent standards of divine revelation, authority, and majority opinion, and substituted as her criteria conscience, feeling, sense of justice, and experience.

Nightingale (1873a) was in the vanguard of the human rights movement and a proponent of that concept identified today as holistic man. She believed that man is creative, with inherent rights to the pursuit of his own development, interest, and goals; she strongly objected to man's being used as a passive pawn driven at the will of another (Nightingale, 1860b, vol. I, p. 76). In her opinion, creative man has the ability to alter his lot in life and modify his destiny. She espoused the brotherhood of man and believed that God's plan for man is not that God "should give man what he asked for, but that mankind should obtain it for mankind"; she urged that "a better world . . . will not be given to us; let us then begin without delay to make one" (Nightingale, 1860b, vol. II, p. 77). Believing that it is fatal to all human progress to remain in the position God placed the individual, Nightingale (1860b, vol. II, p. 88; 1873b) gave expression to the philosophic credo underlying her reforming nature when she said, "We MUST ALTER the 'state of life,' [not conform to it]" (p. 33).

Nightingale was tolerant of religious beliefs in a society torn by bigotry; she placed a higher value on deed than creed and considered the person of primary importance, transcending status, creed, and disease. Her recognition of the hardships suffered by the poor and her deep compassion for human beings was a constant in her life and shaped her work. The debutante Nightingale identified nursing as the means through which she could bring relief and succor to the oppressed and thereby live a meaningful life of service to God.

Of incisive intellect, charming, witty, and besought by suitors, Florence Nightingale was an alien spirit in the rich and aristocratic social sphere of Victorian England. She was a "herald of revolt . . . against the barriers of convention, both in thought and conduct" (Mantrip, 1932, passim). Bound by inflexible convention more crippling than physical disability and by the unremitting handicap of being a woman, she was hindered from realizing her personal objectives. She determined to overcome these obstacles. She rejected the brilliant social circle of patrician England.

Nightingale's characteristics of tenderness, compassion, and sensitivity melded with her constructive zeal, unwavering beliefs, great reliance on the value of personal experiences, extreme discontent with the status quo, the philosopher's desire for a higher order; and, her brilliant, quenchless intellect provided the backdrop for her extraordinary social contributions.

Nightingale's reactionary character actually had two facets: constructive reform and obstructive action. Her insatiable curiosity and probing, analytical mind formed the basis for her research role.

■ THE NIGHTINGALE PERSONALITY

Nightingale, the Reformer. Nightingale's zeal as a reformer originated in her great dissatisfaction with the present and her intense desire for social improvement. Throughout her life her uniform response to the status quo was that of constructionist or revisionist. Her constructive role in reformation can be seen by her constant objection to the stultifying mode of the Victorian woman's life with its limited social choices, namely indolence, marriage, or servitude, and to existing social conditions, abject poverty or affluence

(Nightingale, 1860b, vol. II). Nightingale was extremely frustrated with these conditions and constantly demanded corrective actions.

She believed that negative or solitary dissent was a mistake. Nightingale's (1873b) motto was, "Create and do not criticize" (p. 36); she wrote, "Every great reformer began by being a solitary dissenter. . . . But in every case it was a *positive* dissent; ending not in a protest, but in a great reform" (p. 26). She believed that the past cried out for man to make the future different, and she resolved that she would seek a better life for women in, as well as out of, marriage. Her philosophic belief of service to God through service to man, her constructive criticism, and her reaction to her social sphere compelled Nightingale to make her own way in the world, to be independent, to acquire a profession or occupation to utilize all her faculties.

Nightingale found ultimate release in her creation and development of a new estate that incorporated an unheard of system of education, a respectable livelihood, and the constructive social utilization of women.

Upon this philosophic basis and through this constructive zeal, the profession of nursing was conceived and born. Nightingale, the reformer, got her greatest opportunity when the British government asked her to go to Scutari to be responsible for nursing the British soldiers. Nightingale's significant reforms began in Scutari when she came face to face with the greatest organizational mismanagement recorded in history (for further information on Nightingale in the Crimea, see Palmer, 1976).

The military hospitals run by the British government lacked elementary supplies, a system of identifying the British soldier who could not identify himself, a system of maintaining hospital records and vital statistics, and a system of providing the soldier with any care approaching humane standards. Her strong administrative ability became apparent as she initiated corrective action quickly and directly while never losing sight of the wider horizon.

Achieving these reforms, she went further and established a laundry; reading rooms and classes for the soldiers; wholesome forms of recreation; a banking system so the soldier could save his pay instead of squandering it on women and drink; a hospital for the wives, women, and children of soldiers who accompanied them to war and were often neglected by military authorities; and a system of corresponding with the soldier's family back home. In brief, Nightingale was the original Red Cross Grey Lady, dietitian, banker, laundress, supply clerk, teacher, social service worker, occupational therapist, recreational therapist, hospital executive officer, chief nurse, Army quartermaster, Army sanitarian, military registrar, and the soldier's nurse.

With her eye on her major purpose of national health and Army reform, she communicated all her findings with her recommendations for improvement to her staunch ally, Sir Sidney Herbert, Secretary at War, and to everyone else of influence whom she knew. By the time the war was over, she was a formidable opponent to those who advocated the continuance of the status quo, an unquestionable proponent of hospital and military reform, and an irrefutable authority on everything concerning the soldier, the entire Army medical system, and military administration. She did not rest on her achievements, realizing only too well that unless the entire civilian and military hospital system was changed, all would come to naught since military hospitals were but a cross-section of their civilian counterparts. She had the great wisdom to recognize that the most effective way to promote the health and welfare of the British soldier was to improve the health of the British population which was the source of the British Army. Nightingale set out to achieve major reforms which were initiated in the five-year period immediately following the Crimean War and were based largely on her vivid and devastating experiences there.

Nightingale knew she possessed exemplary characteristics of the reformer: great popular appeal as a national heroine and expert knowledge in matters of health, sanitation, military medicine, hospitals, nursing, and the care of the soldier.

The astute Nightingale knew that crusted conservatism would never countenance a woman directly carrying out the reforms so sorely needed in Britain. She was forced by social custom to use others to accomplish the wide scope of her primary goal of improving the health of the British population and at the same time improving the lot of the British soldier, establishing a respectable system of nursing, and improving the social position of women. She used people as a means to an end by involving them in goal identification and goal achievement. Because she was a woman, an open partnership in the affairs of state was denied her, yet those reforms so vital to the nation were actually state affairs (August, 1975, pp. 207–208). She used the power of her prestige to push for the reforms she realized were essential to her major purpose, and she had her reforms carried out by persons whom she or her colleagues knew in all positions of social and political leadership, including the Queen.

In essence, her method for reform was to: select influential leaders who would initiate the appropriate questions; persuade cabinet ministers to appoint commissions to address the issues; have people she knew were interested and politically strong appointed as commissioners; present them with material compiled in lucid, graphic detail so the conclusions were unmistakable and would be recommended; persuade officials other than commissioners to carry out the recommendations; not leave to chance the dissemination of official reports but publish privately these reports and information for consumption by the British people; and use the press to publish her letters to the editor and articles on timely topics associated with necessary reforms.

Nightingale's reforms are evidenced in attitudinal, organizational, educational, and sociopolitical changes stemming from her efforts.

Attitudinal Changes. Prime among the shifts in opinion that can be attributed to Nightingale were those affecting the British soldier, women, nurses, and care of the sick poor (Trevelyan, 1943, pp. 548–549). In the post-Nightingale era the British soldier was no longer treated as an insensate brute but was considered one of Her Majesty's subjects and, as such, entitled to common decency, adequate rations, suitable provisions, quarters sufficient to support life and health, and appropriate medical treatment when he was ill or wounded.

Through Nightingale's successful demonstration of the efficacy of carefully supervised nursing and her system of training women to be nurses, the public's attitude of nursing was raised from that of a disreputable pastime to a worthy and dignified occupation in which women of good repute and family might safely seek work.

The "humane barbarity," as described by Russell (1966, p. 90), characteristic of the treatment of the sick in hospitals and the poor in workhouses and infirmaries, was eliminated.

Organizational Changes. The major organizational reform initiated by Nightingale was that of pinpointing responsibility. An improved, streamlined Army administration, and hospital management, hospital construction following sanitary principles, pinpointing Army medical responsibility, the initiation of a system of vital statistics for civil and military hospitals, as well as evaluating Army medical officers according to competency and not seniority were some of the organizational changes introduced by Nightingale. Through her work, hospitals were converted from pesthouses and hellholes to places where those in need could once again receive hospitable and humane help.

Educational Changes. Two main educational changes emerged from Nightingale's reform: the education of women for respectable occupations and the creation of an Army Medical School for the training of Army medical officers. Also, her great concern for the peasants in India led her to develop a plan whereby they could be educated so they could improve their lot in life.

Sociopolitical Changes. Nightingale was a great political scientist. She tested the waters of public opinion and governmental requirements and identified those needs of the Empire which should be resolved to assure the welfare of the British subject. Alterations in cabinet and ministerial responsibilities attest to her success. She was also deeply concerned about India and proposed measures to: correct the abuses of money lending, alleviate the need for irrigation, establish a system of representative government, and help prevent starvation (Nightingale, 1874, 1878, 1883a, b).

Nightingale's great energies for these kinds of constructive reforms also made it possible for her to be an obstructionist.

Nightingale, the Reactionary. Nightingale, an effective change agent, rejected and opposed with all the vigor she could muster those propositions and ideas incongruent with her own knowledge, beliefs, and experiences upon which she placed great reliance.

She was in intimate of some of the greatest social activists, academicians, and scholastics of the Victorian age. To a great extent, she lived in the intellectual world and thrived on her associations with the mental giants of her age. She conversed with these contemporaries on her favorite learned topics, such as the nature of man, philosophy, religious thought, and social reform. Living in an era which saw the traditional bastions of knowledge and experience challenged, Nightingale remained disdainful of those new scientific tenets in conflict with her own ideas and convictions. She was unshakeable and unyielding in her beliefs and rejected what she could not see, even in the face of new evidence.

While she was alert to the stimulating, burgeoning world of scientific thought and social progress swirling around her, she flatly spurned those propositions and movements not consistent with her experiences and beliefs (Nightingale, 1873a, b). Particularly in the later half of her life, she attempted to retard progress in a world of rapidly accelerating change and was no longer able to keep pace or look ahead of the times of which she was a part.

Several explanations are possible: She was a product of an aristocratic, sheltered, Victorian upbringing, and reverted in her later life to these inculcated precepts; the vivid experiences which she had to deal with and resolve in the early years of life indelibly imbedded in her mind the value of cleanliness and sanitary practices; and the successful results achieved through her own observations and analyses of her rich and varied experiences convinced her of the rectitude of her values, opinions, and beliefs.

There are several notable progressive movements to which Nightingale was unalterably opposed, despite data supporting an opposite point of view. She unequivocally spurned the concepts that illness and disease could be the result of specific microorganisms rather than of dampness and dirt (Nightingale, 1858a, p. 7; 1873a, p. 575).

Nightingale was adamant on the germ theory of disease, and dispensed with the idea simply by comparing that notion with a medieval concept of witchcraft as a cause of sickness. She disclaimed Huxley, a contemporary man of science, for his "belief in things not verified by the senses," and criticized his advocacy of scientific progress as similar to superstition (Nightingale, 1873a, p. 568). She cemented her position with the statement, "The germ hypothesis, moreover, is directly at variance in its results with ascertained sanitary experience" (Nightingale, 1882, pp. 62–63). She rejected bacteriology, antisepsis, and the germ theory of disease while living in the contemporary society of Darwin, Mendel, Huxley, Pasteur, John Stuart Mill, Snow, Lister, and others.

Another contemporary progressive movement was education for women. Nightingale, who in her youth had acutely desired a university education, supported the movement of opening universities to women. She was a strong proponent of founding women's colleges and the revolutionary force behind the improved social position of women (Churchill, 1958; Trevelyan, 1947). She was only 28 year old when Queen's College opened in London and offered women a liberal school training as well as a six-year course of college education (Chambers's, 1890, vol. 8, p. 526). Queen's College is identified as Britain's first women's college. Her recognition of the significance and national importance of the movement in the education of women is seen in her correspondence. However, she did not visualize that an educational system for nursing, an occupation she designed for women, might be taught in a university rather than learned in a hospital (Nightingale, 1881, p. 10; 1883c, pp. 1038–1043).

Nightingale's vision and goal for social reform for women and nursing stopped short of educating nurses at a college or university (Nightingale, 1858b). Her experiences fully convinced her of the value of the hospital as the school of experience and training for the preparation of the nurse, and she never wavered from this belief (Nightingale, 1881, 1883c). Nightingale lacked the foresight or wisdom to predict the ultimate outcomes of university education for nurses while advocating university education for women. She (1867, p. 6) never conceived of an education for nurses paralleling the extensive education to which she was heir. Nor did she recognize that the reforms she was instrumental in effecting were in no insignificant measure a real function of her own excellent education.

Another major aspect of Florence Nightingale's reactionary trait arose from the popularity of the nursing movement she had pioneered. Nightingale raised nursing from, as she put it, "the sink it was" and got it well established as a respectable venture, as a calling similar to a religious vocation. She left it there and concentrated her efforts in spheres of higher intellectual order. As the efficacy of the trained nurse and hospital management became recognized, Nightingale developed negative ideas about the role of nursing. To the end of her days she thought of nursing more a spiritual calling than a profession in its own right, parallel to other professions and based on a comprehensive education.

Her admonishments to her followers carry frequent warnings about making nursing a book-and-examination business. She relentlessly opposed associations, certificates, examinations, and the term "graduates," as having any value in establishing the fitness of the woman to nurse (Newton, 1949, p. 213).

Nightingale's opposition to state registration for nurses in Great Britain held the profession back for many years. Yet, the basic reason advocated for nurse registration was to assure some quality control over those so engaged, which was the harsh struggle Nightingale originally waged to establish nursing as a work based on some training.

Nursing to Nightingale was largely action-oriented, concerned primarily with creating order and procedure, with elementary problem solving, not to be overly burdened by book learning and theoretical inquiry, despite her frequent admonishments and prescriptions of the need for the nurse to know reasons underlying her action. Hear her say,

> Training is to teach not only what is to be done but how to do it. The physician or surgeon orders what is to be done. Training has to teach the nurse how to do it to his order; and to teach not how to do it but *why* such and such

> a thing is done and not such and such another. . . . The trained power of attending on one's own impressions made by one's own senses so that these should *tell* the nurse how the patient is, is the *sina qua non* of being a nurse at all . . . (Nightingale, 1883c, p. 1038).

Nightingale's reliance on observation, fact, and experience as validation of what is necessary is most apparent. However, in her prescription for nursing she forgot that her personal basis for validation of observation was her own extensive education, not a year of practical training in a hospital ward.

The speculation can be raised why Nightingale stopped where she did with nursing considering her power, prestige, intellect, and drive. It is difficult to suggest that she envisioned nursing as the cutting edge of social reform or scientific progress. It may be she did not foresee nursing as an intellectual endeavor sufficient to occupy her mind or of sufficient stature to develop the keen intellect of others in nursing.

The answer may also be found in her heroic efforts and extraordinary experiences at Scutari and the Crimea. Through almost all her life, the welfare of the British soldier was her all-engrossing passion. Nightingale saw all efforts in district and rural nursing, midwifery, hospital, sick and health nursing directed toward raising the level of wellness of the British subject and in so doing preserving her commitment to the British soldier to fight his cause, rather than devoting her energies to the professionalization of nursing.

The strict Victorian attitudes and culture rejected by the young Nightingale were accepted by her in later life and her semicloistered living may have contributed to her role as obstructive reactionary.

Nightingale, the Researcher. Participation in research activities was a natural outcome of Nightingale's keen, perceptive intellect and her multiple interests. She possessed in abundance the qualities of the good researcher: insatiable curiosity, command of her subject, familiarity with methods of inquiry, a good background in statistics, and ability to discriminate and abstract.

Nightingale's greatest skills as a researcher were her extraordinary capability to maintain detailed and copious anecdotal notes and records on a wide variety of occurrences and events, her gift for expressive communication, her aptitude for ordering and codifying her observations, her talent in using statistics, her skill in graphic protrayal of data, and her ability to extrapolate. Her outstanding capacity to conceptualize, infer, analyze, and synthesize was revealed time and again as she reviewed multiple sources of complex data and abstracted meaningful information, related data to a larger universe, and explained it clearly.

Nightingale had a fantastic ability to codify her observations in a systematic way that made them useful to others. Story has it that she and John Snow were colleagues in the London cholera epidemic of August 1854, and that the records Nightingale maintained on the origins of the victims helped Snow pinpoint the role of the Broad Street pump.

Nightingale's reliance on statistics was based on the orderliness of her nature and her great attention to detail (Nightingale, 1871). Her statistical evidence which could not be refuted was one reason why corrective reforms and actions were taken. Her statistical studies opened her eyes to the mortality of the British Army at home, in the Crimea, and in India. Convinced of the practical value of statistics, she used them to drive her messages home.

It was Nightingale who laid to rest forever the myth that the British soldier died of wounds. Her "cox combs" are a hallmark in which she separately diagrammed deaths in the Army from wounds and from other diseases and compared them to the deaths which occurred in England (Nightingale, 1859b).

It was Nightingale who drew to the attention of the world the lack of hospital and military statistics which prevented the Army from ascertaining its true fighting strength at any time. Comparing similar situations that occurred in civilian hospitals, she had the extraordinary vision to propose a system of hospital record keeping and disease nomenclature. Although not adopted because of the expense involved, the Nightingale influence of a century ago can be seen in the standard nomenclature and system used internationally today.

Nightingale possessed vast information about the British Army in India and the nature and causes of premature and preventable mortality with which it was afflicted. She obtained these data by conducting studies with the India Office. She participated in designing the questionnaire and reviewed all the returns from the British Army in India (Nightingale, 1863, pp. 347–370). Her brilliant analysis of the health of the British Army in India led to many corrective actions. Her inescapable conclusion, however, that "existing sanitary negligence" was such "that unless the health of the British troops in India be improved and the death rate decreased . . . the Empire will never be able to hold India with a British Army . . ." (Nightingale, 1864, pp. 501–502).

Hear the researcher criticize official mortality statistics as she defines the entire population in contradiction to the partial finding of 69 deaths per 1,000 per annum of the Army in India: "This death rate is in fact understated, for it says nothing of the invalids sent home from India who die at sea, or within a short time of their arrival at home; nor of the loss to the service by destroyed health; nor of the mutiny years" (Nightingale, 1864, p. 503).

Driving her point home with a clarity of understanding meaningful to the British public, Nightingale asserted, "Few people have an idea of what a death rate of 69 per 1,000 represents—the amount of inefficiency from sickness—of invaliding . . ." (1864, p. 503). She then stated that the quoted death rate meant the Army would lose, on an average, 5,037 men a year or the equivalent of an entire brigade. In her inexorable fashion she said, "It may lose, some years, half that number. But in other years, it will lose two such brigades" (p. 503). Lest the point escape the common man, Florence Nightingale (1864) drew the stark conclusion in the question, "And where are we to find 10,000 recruits to fill up the gap of deaths of a single unhealthy year?" (p. 503).

Nightingale, a past master in the art of research, incorporated historical, explanatory, descriptive, comparative, and field methods in her investigative work. Nor were her inquiries limited to hospitals and health, for by the time she left for Scutari she had analyzed the theological precepts underlying both Anglican and Roman religions as well as prevalent concepts of Egyptian mythology (Cook, 1913).

Nightingale (1858a) used the force of history when she compared morbidity and mortality statistics of the British Army under the Duke of Wellington to that occurring in the Crimean War and in analyzing the hazards which lying-in hospitals on the continent and in Great Britain presented to the puerperal woman (Nightingale, 1871).

Her explanatory methods were most in evidence as she recounted experiences at Scutari and Balaclava for the Secretary at War, or retold the story of the lime juice, or cited the lack of medical rations and clothing (Nightingale, 1858a). When the question arose of how effective the Army purveyor was in distributing drawers or diets, she brought forth the unfilled requisitions and supplied the information on the items she provided from her stores; detailed the futile steps, confusing procedures, and inherent hazards in requisitioning official material; and concluded by recommending simple solutions. She refuted official testimony, and one of her best illustrations is seen when the Select Committee was reviewing the adequacy of medical comforts for the sick or wounded British soldier in Crimea. She made the total supplies available in a six-month period meaningful in terms of medical comforts available to one soldier during that time and revealed by that method that the sick British soldier's ration for six months was provisioned at seven bottles of wine, six pounds of sugar, 1¼ pounds of tea, 2½ pounds arrowroot, ¾ pounds mutton, and so on (Nightingale, 1858a).

The question of the availability of lime juice for the British soldier in Scutari is chronicled with meticulous detail from the first request on November 17 through the honeycomb and maze of officialdom, to the eventual procurement and disbursement on January 29 of the elusive lime juice (Nightingale, 1858a).

Realizing that corrective reform in the absence of irrefutable data was most improbable, Nightingale (1858a, c; 1859a; 1863) used research to gather accurate information, presented facts with her own caustic inferences, and drew unassailable conclusions. Leaving little to the imagination or chance interpretation, she diagrammed data graphically and explained the subject cogently, with a terseness, stark lucidity, and vividness seldom surpassed. Through her attention to detail, her ability to mass data, synthesize, and order it in relation to a universe with which she was intimately familiar, she was able to apply enormous amounts of incontestable information for the initiation of tremendous corrective action.

One of the world's most inspired and inspirational people, Florence Nightingale knew what she wanted to accomplish in her life and set out to do so, leaving a heritage rarely surpassed and seldom approximated in the history of women and of nations.

References

August, Eugene, ed. *John Stuart Mill, a Mind at Large*. New York, Charles Scribner's Sons, 1975.

Chamber's Encyclopedia: A Dictionary of Useful Knowledge. New edition London, William and Robert Chambers, 1890, vol. 8.

Churchill, W.S. *A History of the English-Speaking Peoples*. New York, Dodd, Mead Co., 1958, vol. 4.

Cook, Sir Edward. *The Life of Florence Nightingale, Volume One*. London, Macmillan, 1913.

Mantrip, J.C. Florence Nightingale and religion. *London Q Rev* 157:318–325, July 1932.

Newton, M.E. *Florence Nightingale's Philosophy of Life and Education*. Stanford, Calif., Stanford University, 1949. (Unpublished doctoral dissertation)

Nightingale, Florence. *Notes on Matters Affecting the Health, Efficiency and Hospital Administration of the British Army, Founded Chiefly on the Experience of the Late War*, presented by request to the Secretary of State for War. London, Harrison and Sons, 1858.(a)

———. *Subsidiary Notes as to the Introduction of Female Nursing into Military Hospitals in Peace and in War*, presented by request to the Secretary of State of War. London, Harrison and Sons, 1858.(b)

———. (Evidence and appendix LXXII) In *Report of the Commissioners Appointed to Inquire into the Regulations Affecting the Sanitary Condition of the Army, the Organization of Military Hospitals, and the Treatment of the Sick and Wounded*. Presented to both Houses of Parliament by command of Her Majesty. London, H. M. Stationery Office, 1858.(c)

———. *Notes on Hospitals;* being two papers read before the National Association for the Promotion of Social Science, at Liverpool in October 1858. *With Evidence Given to the Royal Commissioners on the State of the Army in 1857*. 2d ed. London, John W. Parker and Sons, 1859.(a)

———. *A Contribution to the Sanitary History of the British Army During the Late War with Russia*. London, John W. Parker and Sons, 1859.(b)

———. Hospital statistics appendix proposal for a uniform plan of hospital statistics. In *Programme of the Fourth Session of the International Statistical Congress* to be held in London on July 16th, 1860, and five following days. London, H. M. Stationery Office, 1860.(a)

———. *Suggestions for Thought to the Searchers after Truth among the Artizans of England, 3 volumes*. London, George E. Eyre and William Spottiswoode, 1860.(b)

———. Observations on the evidence contained in the stational returns. Dated Nov. 21, 1862. In *The Royal Commission on the Sanitary State of the Army in India, 2 volumes*. London, H. M. Stationery Office, 1863.

———. *How People May Live and not Die in India*. London, Longman, Green, Longman, Roberts, and Green. 1864.

————. *Suggestions for the Improvement of the Nursing Service of Hospitals and on the Method of Training Nurses for the Sick Poor.* London, Spottiswoode and Co., 1867.

————. *Introductory Notes on Lying-in Institutions.* London, Longmans, Green and Co, 1871.

————. A note of interrogation. *Fraser's Mag* (New Series) 7:567–577, May 1873.(a)

————. A sub-note of interrogation; what will our religion be in 1999? *Fraser's Mag* (New Series) 8:25–36, July 1873.(b)

————. Irrigation and means of transit in India. (Letter to the editor) *Illus Lond News,* 65:99, Aug. 1, 1874.

————. The people of India. *Nineteenth Cent* 4:193–221, Aug. 1878.

————. *Trained Nursing for the Sick Poor.* London, Spottiswoode and Co., 1881.

————. Remarks. In *Infection,* by Sir J. C. Jervoise, Bt. 2d ed. London, Vacher and Sons, 1882.

————. Our Indian stewardship. *Nineteenth Cent* 14:329–338, Aug. 1883.(a)

————. The dumb shall speak and the dear shall hear, or the Ryot, the Zemindar, and the government. A paper presented at the General Sessions of the East India Association, June 1, 1883. *J East India Assoc* 15:163–238, July 1883.(b)

————. Nurses, training of: (and) nursing the sick. In *A Dictionary of Medicine,* ed. by Richard Quain. London, Longmans, Green and Co., 1883, (c) vol. 2

Palmer, I. S. Florence Nightingale and the Salisbury incident. *Nurs Res* 25:370–377, Sept.-Oct. 1976.

Russell, W. H. *Russell's Despatches from the Crimea.* 1854–1856, ed. by Nicholas Bentley. New York, Hill and Wang, 1966.

Trevelyan, G. M. *English Social History.* London, Longmans, Green and Co., 1943.

————. *History of England.* New York, Longmans, Green and Co., 1947, p. 653.

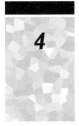

4

The Fateful Decade, 1890–1900

Teresa E. Christy

*T*here is probably no 10-year span in nursing's history during which so many important events occurred or so many fateful decisions were made than in the period between 1890 and 1900. It was a time of unprecedented growth in American nursing, a period of emergence of several of our most important nursing leaders, an era of tremendous proliferation of schools of nursing, and the decade of the greatest organizational strides for the fledgling profession.

Only 17 years earlier, in 1873, the first three schools of nursing were opened in this country. At the start of the decade, in 1890, there were 35 schools, with 1,552 pupil nurses, and by 1900 there were 432 schools with 11,164 students[1]. Hospitals were recognizing the value of trained nurses in the care of the sick and were quick to see the advantages of staffing the institutions with nurses-in-training.

It was obvious to such leading nursing educators of the time as Isabel Adams Hampton and Lavinia L. Dock that most of these training schools were being opened with little thought for educational principles and even less thought to any standards for curriculum development. Both of these women were at what was in 1890 probably the best American school, Johns Hopkins Hospital Training School for Nurses in Baltimore, Md. There was no official organization of nurses or nurse educators, and although Isabel Hampton was moderately well known, she alone did not as yet have sufficient power or prestige to exert much control over the situation.

An opportunity presented itself in 1893, when Ms. Hampton was appointed chairman of a committee to arrange a congress of nurses under the auspices of the International Congress of Charities, Correction, and Philanthropy at the Chicago World's Fair. At the congress, Ms. Hampton delivered a paper in which she protested the lack of uniformity of instruction in training schools and the completely inadequate education being provided[2]. In attendance were a number of superintendents of training schools from the United

Teresa Christy, R.N., Ed.D., associate professor at the University of Iowa College of Nursing, earned her doctorate in historiography. She was a member of the ANA Bicentennial Committee.

States and Canada. And while the congress was still in session Ms. Hampton organized a committee to form an association of superintendents, one objective of which would be the establishment and maintenance of a universal standard of training. This association became the first official, organized group of nurses, adopting in 1894 the name of "American Society of Superintendents of Training Schools for Nurses." In 1912 the society changed its name to the National League of Nursing Education, and in 1952 it was again reorganized under the present National League for Nursing.

In this same year, 1893, two other nurses were embarking on a mission that was to have equally far reaching effects. Lillian D. Wald and Mary Brewster moved into a tenement on New York's lower east side. Supported by private philanthropists, they began serving their neighbors through diagnosing and treating human responses, teaching, counseling, and providing nursing care. This was the origin of the famous Henry Street Settlement and the beginning of public health nursing in the United States.

Within the next few years, Isabel Hampton (now married to Dr. Hunter Robb), a firm believer in the power of organized effort, saw the need to unite practitioners of nursing. The Society of Superintendents included only educators, and Ms. Robb now set out to bring all nurses together in an association attuned to general needs and common welfare. In 1896, she was successful in founding the Associated Alumnae of the United States and Canada, the organization that in 1911 became known officially as the American Nurses' Association.

Isabel Hampton Robb has been described as a visionary and, with the assistance of other great leaders like Louise Darche, Irene Sutliffe, Edith Draper, Mary E.P. Davis, Isabel McIsaac, Anna Maxwell, Annie Goodrich, and M. Adelaide Nutting, she set out in the next four years to accomplish two other dreams.

From its inception in 1893, the Society of Superintendents had discussed the need for some way to establish standards for curricula in nursing schools. Ms. Robb, a trained teacher prior to her entrance into nursing, discussed with her colleagues the desirability of a program of some sort to prepare nurses to teach. A committee was formed to investigate the possibilities of setting up some sort of course in an institute for pedagogy. At the sixth annual convention of the Society of Superintendents, in May 1899, the committee—Ms. Robbs, Ms. Nutting, Linda Richards, Mary Agnes Snively, and Lucy L. Drown—reported the successful completion of their mission. In October 1899, two nurses entered the hospital economics course at Teachers College, Columbia University. Thus, the first program for nurses under the auspices of a university was begun.

But the decade was not over, and these women, who had already accomplished so much, had one more goal in mind. They wanted to create an official means of communication for nurses, a periodical of some sort which would be conducted by and for nurses. With Ms. Davis as the business arm, Sophia Palmer as the editorial arm, Ms. Robb, Ms. Nutting, Ms. Dock, and several others as financial supporters, these determined women launched the first issue of the *American Journal of Nursing* in October 1900.

The courage and fortitude of these early nurses was truly amazing, and the impact of these accomplishments is almost immeasurable. It is doubtful that as much was accomplished in any other 10-year period of the one hundred years of American nursing. And in the two hundred years of United States history, both for the American public that is served and for the nurses of today, it was indeed the "Fateful Decade."

References

1. U.S. Bureau of Education. *Annual Report of the Commissioner of Education, 1909.* Washington, D.C., U.S. Government Printing Office, 1909, p. 1077.
2. Hampton, I. A. Educational standards for nurses. In *Hospitals, Dispensaries and Nursing.* Papers and discussions in the International Congress of Charities, Correction and Philanthropy, Section III, Chicago, June 12–17, 1893. Baltimore, Johns Hopkins Press, 1894.

5

Nursing and the Great Depression

M. Louise Fitzpatrick

"Not all the results of the depression and unemployment have been bad," May Ayres Burgess wrote in 1932(1).

The stock market crash in the autumn of 1929 did, to be sure, usher in a decade characterized by severe economic depression, unemployment, and multiple hardships that pervaded every facet of American life. However, the years of recovery that followed—and culminated in the passage of the Social Security Act—marked the beginning of increased government involvement in many matters affecting citizens' personal lives, and health became a major focus.

During the twenties, the need for expanded health services to rural areas was recognized, and measures were attempted to meet the demands. Demonstration projects like one in Cattaraugus County, N.Y., provided models for expanding public health nursing services through county health departments, but financing problems jeopardized their viability.

There were many attempts to recruit nurses and nursing students into rural work, but most nurses were not educationally prepared to take part in rural public health programs. The challenge of rural services was primarily met by the Red Cross Public Health Nursing Service (formerly the Red Cross Town and Country Nursing Service). That service was begun in 1912 to provide care to people in areas of the country which had no established health or nursing resources of their own(2). It was estimated that, of the 3,000 counties in the United States, 2,500 were rural and few had health programs comparable to those in urban areas(3). The need was particularly apparent in the South. There the incidence of infant mortality, communicable diseases such as typhoid, and such deficiency diseases as scurvy and pellagra was extremely high.

At the time of this article, M. Louise Fitzpatrick, R.N., Ed.D., was an assistant professor at Columbia University Teachers College, where she earned her doctorate. Her dissertation was a history of the National Organization for Public Health Nursing.

At no time in history had nursing encountered a worse employment situation. The demand for community nursing services was increasing, but agencies were not in a position to hire. Voluntary agencies, which provided most public health nursing service, were also in perilous financial straits. These agencies depended on philanthropic contributions, and when donors had to retrench, so did many programs.

Further, the vast majority of nurses worked in private duty. When the financial crisis hit their clientele, there was a sharply decreased demand for their services.

A positive note in the midst of all this adversity was the manner in which the nursing community responded. Nursing organizations, recognizing that a problem of such magnitude required concerted effort, set aside their vested interests. The Joint Committee on the Distribution of Nursing Services developed out of this concern, and studies were begun in conjunction with the ANA Registry Committee to find solutions to nurse unemployment(4).

Some nursing leaders like Adelaide Nutting and Emilie Sargent believed that the unemployment was not wholly due to the depression and were quick to remind nurses that the problem had been predicted(5,6). They referred to the 1923 Report of the Rockefeller Foundation study, *Nursing and Nursing Education in the United States*, which warned that the number of nurses was being increased too rapidly. Later in 1928, the first report of the Committee on the Grading of Nursing Schools, *Nurses, Patients and Pocketbooks* also pointed to the problem of over-production, the saturation of the private duty field, the shortage of nurses in some of the newer specialties, and the serious maldistribution of nurses, with far too few in rural areas(7). Unfortunately, it took a major crisis to bring the point home. Hundreds of nurses in industry and offices were being let go and inactive married nurses attempted to return to work—both saturating the private duty field even more(8).

Out of necessity, the depression stimulated a serious re-evaluation of nursing and nurse education. It forced nursing to look anew at the apprenticeship system which had evolved over the years. It also provided the catalyst needed to bring about the closing of hundreds of small schools of nursing which flooded the field with thousands of nurses each year. And it stimulated increased concern for the quality of nursing care and standards of practice.

Nursing organization determined several possible ways to ease the employment situation. One was the reduction of the numbers of students, which would make it possible to use funds allocated for student allowances to employ graduate nurses in hospitals. Another measure was the institution of the eight-hour work day for special duty nurses. The fees, of course, were reduced, but work opportunities were available for more nurses. It was also recognized that fields such as public health work in rural areas might be able to absorb some of the unemployed. However, frequently nurses were unwilling to leave the overcrowded field of private duty, and those who were willing needed help in retooling for a very different kind of practice(9).

■ *FEDERAL PROGRAMS*

In 1933, soon after President Roosevelt took office, programs to rescue the country from its difficulties were authorized. The passage of the Federal Emergency Relief Act in May 1933 and the creation of the Civil Works Administration the following November held special significance for nurses in general and for public health nursing in particular.

Under FERA Rules and Regulation #7, bedside care for the indigent was made a legitimate claim on public relief funds and permitted contracting for this service with existing voluntary nursing services(10). The stipulations were not mandatory, so that state and local relief boards might or might not adopt them. But when they were adopted, the provision made it possible for voluntary nursing agencies to be reimbursed for service to patients who were unable to pay. Funds for nursing care came out of the total FERA budget and were expected to augment rather than replace state and local funding for health programs.

Through the influence of Harry Hopkins, director of the FERA program and a friend of the NOPHN's general director, Katharine Tucker, the provision of nursing services to the indigent and unemployed was strongly encouraged. The use of official registry nurses to supplement the number of agency nurses was permitted, and in some instances bedside nursing services developed where none had previously existed(11). The result was jobs for nurses and care for those in need of it.

When the CWA was organized, Mr. Hopkins suggested that states, in consultation with the U.S. Public Health Service, set up relief projects for unemployed nurses. Pearl McIver, USPHS chief nurse analyst, was the special consultant responsible for the program. Under CWA, nurses were involved in developing and providing a wide variety of community-based services, many of which were established in those rural areas which had earlier been identified as needing expanded public health resources. In addition to bedside care and preventive family health services, nurses were employed in Children's Bureau projects covering the full range of child and school health services. Antepartal and child health conferences were established, a variety of clinics were staffed, and classes in home hygiene were conducted. Nurses were also employed to conduct state and county surveys to determine service needs in relation to communicable diseases, malnutrition, and chronic illness(12). The ANA became the primary nursing organization responsible for interpreting the relief employment program to nurses(13).

To qualify for work in a CWA project, nurses had to be unemployed and in financial need of work. Because the projects were designed to help all nurses regardless of their specialization areas, large numbers were inadequately prepared for the jobs, since most projects involved some form of public health nursing. The NOPHN was concerned that standards of public health nursing practice be maintained. It worked closely with the federal government in delineating guidelines for the projects and urged that qualified nursing supervisors be provided for the nurses. In addition, it provided consultation and materials for these official programs(14).

The projects were highly successful. By 1934, there was a definite improvement in the employment situation of nurses, and official public health nursing services had been successfully expanded.

More than 10,000 nurses were given work under CWA and many were able to retain their positions permanently(15). In 1935 the CWA projects were assumed by the Works Progress Administration, and the number of unemployed nurses continued to be reduced. In 1936, WPA Projects were providing work in 16 states for 6,000 nurses(16,17).

Another important result of this particular recovery project was the stimulation it gave to tax-supported public health nursing services throughout the country. Because nurses working under CWA projects had to be associated with official agencies, many projects were developed within them, and emphasis was thereby placed on the responsibility of government to provide health care for the public. Other beneficial outcomes included a better distribution of nurses and increased collaboration among the various nursing organizations.

The passage of the Social Security Act in 1935, with its provisions of great significance for public health nursing, was undoubtedly an event of major importance during the second half of the decade. It promoted the concept of health and social services under government auspices and reinforced the thrust of the programs begun during the period of national recovery.

Provisions for crippled children and maternal and child health services in Title V of the act underlined the need for more and better prepared workers to carry out the programs that federal grants to the states would help establish.

With the guidance and consultation of Surgeon General Parran and Pearl McIver of the USPHS and Naomi Deutsch, nurse director of the Childrens' Bureau, generalized community health nursing programs under official auspices were encouraged, and cooperative effort between official and voluntary nursing agencies were begun.

Under the Social Security Act, a large sum of federal money was assigned to the USPHS and a substantial proportion of this was given to states as grants-in-aid for establishing and maintaining adequate public health services and for training personnel. Through scholarship funds allocated to states, 1,000 nurses were able to take advantage of educational programs during 1936(18,19). By the end of the next year others were availing themselves of the training funds, and by 1938 nearly 3,000 public health workers had received preparation for their work through the provisions of the Social Security Act(20).

Federal help to the states had a tremendous vitalizing effect on both official and voluntary nursing agencies. In some states new services were established; in others services were expanded. Cooperative endeavors between local voluntary and official agencies were embarked on, and nurses and other health workers had benefited from the educational assistance given to them to prepare for the challenges which were anticipated in the future.

By the end of the decade official nursing services were so well established that it was possible for the Red Cross to leave the responsibility for local service in the hands of local governments. With continued assistance of nursing consultants from the Children's Bureau, USPHS, NOPHN, and the Metropolitan and John Hancock Life Insurance Companies, local communities were able to inaugurate and strengthen community nursing services. The precedents set by government during the Great Depression and through the programs of the New Deal changed the complexion of all that was to follow in health care and nursing services.

References

1. Burgess, M. A. Quality Nursing. *Am. J.Nurs.* 32:1050, Oct. 1932.
2. Havey, I. M. The American Red Cross meets the challenge of rural nursing. *Am.J. Nurs.* 32:1129–1131, Nov. 1932.
3. Tromenhauser, Eleanor. While waiting. *Am.J.Nurs.* 32:837, Aug. 1932.
4. Committee (editorial) *Am.J.Nurs.* 30:1546, Dec. 1930.
5. (Goodrich, A. W., Nutting, M. A., and Wald, L. D.) Past, present, and future of nursing, by M. S. Gardner. *Am.J.Nurs.* 31:1385–1394, Dec. 1931.
6. Sargent, E. G. The nursing profession works for recovery. *Am.J.Nurs.* 33:1165–1172, Dec. 1933.
7. Committee on the Grading of Nursing Schools. *Nurses, Patients and Pocketbooks: Report—of a Study of the Economics of Nursing.* May A. Burgess, director. New York, The Committee, 1928.
8. Ashmun, Margaret. Cause and cure of unemployment in the nursing profession. *Am.J.Nurs.* 33:653, July 1933.
9. *Ibid.*
10. Federal Emergency Relief Act. *Rules and Regulations No. 7.* Washington, D. C., 1933. (also can be found in N.O.P.H.N. Archive, microfilm no. 11 located at National League for Nursing, New York)
11. Tax money for privately administered public health nursing services. *Public Health Nurs.* 25:373–377, July 1933.
12. The significance of the FERA Program to public health nursing. *Public Health Nurs.* 26:517, Oct. 1934.
13. Haupt, A. C. Some new emphasis in public health nursing. *Public Health Nurs.* 27:624–629, Dec. 1935.
14. Fitzpatrick, M. L. *The National Organization for Public Health Nursing 1912–1952: Development of a Practice Field.* (Publication No. 11–1510) New York, National League for Nursing, 1975. p. 112–113.
15. Woodward, E. S. Federal aspects of unemployment among professional women. *Am.J.Nurs.* 34:534, June 1934.
16. WPA nursing projects. *Public Health Nurs.* 29:50–51, Jan. 1937.
17. WPA projects for registered nurses. *Am.J.Nurs.* 37:35, Jan. 1935.
18. Social security act. (Forward in 1937) *Am.J.Nurs.* 37:4, Jan. 1935.
19. McIver, Pearl. Public nursing under the Social Security Act: developments under the U.S. Public Health Service. *Public Health Nurs.* 28:585–590, Sept. 1936.
20. Tobey, J. A. *Public Health Law.* New York, The Commonwealth Fund. 1939, p. 33.

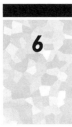

The Lasting Impact of World War II on Nursing

Bonnie Bullough

Placing nurses at or near the battle zone was a controversial issue in earlier wars; by the time of World War II there was no longer any question about it. Nurses of various nationalities played a significant role in the war effort and had a share in creating a different balance of fighting power.

The more sophisticated fire power of the day increased casualties to both soldiers and civilians, but greatly improved health care helped cut the mortality from communicable diseases and wound infections that had characterized earlier wars. Thus health manpower began to assume an importance in successful warfare approaching that of arms and bearers of arms. Although this fact is seldom discussed, it has undoubtedly had an impact on subsequent governmental decisions about nursing and medicine.

The war in Europe was preceded by a protracted preparatory phase in which German and Italian expansionism was seen as a danger to other European nations. The British and French finally declared war in 1939 when Germany invaded Poland.

In this country the possibility of involvement was hotly debated, but the decision was made for us in December 1941 when the Japanese attacked our naval base at Pearl Harbor in Honolulu. Eventually, all of the industrialized nations in the world were drawn into the conflict, which did not end until August 1945, after the Americans dropped atomic bombs on Hiroshima and Nagasaki in Japan(1).

From the beginning, organized nursing supported the war effort. Not that nurses favored the war before it started, but documents suggest that they believed it was inevitable so they might as well prepare.

At the 1938 American Nurses' Association convention, the Army Nurse Corps announced it had increased its strength from 600 to 675(2). In 1940, Julia C. Stimson, ANA president and former head of the Army Nurse Corps,

At the time of this article, Bonnie Bullough, R.N., Ph.D., was an associate professor in the School of Nursing at California State University at Long Beach.

convened a meeting of representatives of all of the national nursing organizations, various federal agencies, and the American Red Cross, a coordinating body known at first as the Nursing Council on National Defense, later as the National Nursing Council for War Service(3,4). It performed many services in coordination and communication, but perhaps its most lasting contribution was to sponsor the first reasonably accurate national census of registered nurses.

Realizing that state board lists were often out of date and included nurses who were registered in more than one state, the NNCWS conducted a mail survey and, in 1941, reported that there were an estimated 289,286 registered nurses in the country and that 173,055 of this number were employed(5).

By the time the war ended, 100,000 nurses had volunteered and 76,000 had actually served in the Army or Navy Nurse Corps(6). Their war experiences were as varied as the areas in which they served. While some of the nurses who were stationed in the Philippines were evacuated when the islands fell, 66 remained behind. Members of this group were in a hospital attacked by the Japanese; 37 months later they again came under fire when the Americans recaptured the area(7). Nurses went ashore with the invading troops in North Africa; they landed under fire at Anzio, and they moved into the beachhead at Normandy four days after the invasion. Dressed in fatigues rather then dress uniforms, they became a familiar sight wherever American troops were stationed(8,9).

As they served, their role and status in the armed forces changed. In the legislation under which the Army Nurse Corps was created in 1902 and the Navy Nurse Corps in 1908, the nursing units were envisioned as somewhat separate from the regular forces, and the law specified female nurses. They were recruited by the Red Cross rather than the services themselves, and nurses had no clear position in the military hierarchy.

In 1920, Army nurses and, in 1942, Navy nurses were given a status called relative rank, which meant that they carried officers' titles but were accorded less power and pay than their male counterparts. In the midst of the war, relative rank was temporarily abandoned, the recruitment responsibilities were removed from the Red Cross, and nurses were brought more closely into the military services system.

In 1947, full commissioned status was sanctioned, and the segregation of Negro nurses was ended. The last vestige of discrimination in the Army Nurse Corps was finally removed in 1954, when men were admitted with full rank as officers(10,11,12).

On the surface, this struggle for rank may seem to have only symbolic significance; it was actually a real struggle to gain the power that was needed to plan and deliver good nursing care. Most of the discrimination against nurses was subtle and paternalistic; it was nevertheless real. Nurses' ambiguous status in the highly structured military system led to inefficiency and indirection. What they won when regular rank was finally achieved was the right to manage nursing care, including both the care they themselves delivered and nursing functions carried out by the enlisted corpsmen. In gaining this managerial power, military nurses set the direction for all members of the nursing profession to move toward more autonomy and more responsible managerial positions.

The vigorous recruitment by the armed forces created serious shortages in the civilian sector, and the manner in which this problem was solved had several long-range consequences. The movement to stratify nursing started before the war, but the wartime experience in both military and civilian hospitals was the deciding factor in changing nursing from a single entity to a multi-level system.

During the war the Red Cross and the Office of Civilian Defense trained more than 200,000 volunteer nurse's aides. At first these aides were used only for non-nursing tasks, such as serving food and water or running errands, but the shortage of help forced them to take on some nursing functions. Eventually many of these aides switched from volunteer to paid status, and their cost effectiveness in the basic bedside role did much to stimulate the permanent development of nurses' aides and licensed practical nurses(13,14).

The second approach to the shortage was governmentally sponsored refresher courses to bring inactive nurses back into the work force. Since many of these women were married and had significant family responsibilities, they were available only part time. They were accepted on these terms, and employers found they could make significant contributions. As a consequence some of the old prejudices against married and part-time nurses crumpled.

The third strategy was to bring massive numbers of students into nursing schools, not only to prepare them for nursing after graduation, but also to use their services while they were in training. Because students had been the major source of nursing manpower since the beginning of the hospital training school movement in the last quarter of the nineteenth century, this was in no way precedent setting. The new element in the program was the large-scale federal assistance to schools and students which was furnished by the Cadet Nurse Corps.

Established in 1943, the Cadet Nurse Corps had by 1945 allocated funds to 1,125 schools and 170,000 students. Since the corps forbade discrimination on the basis of race or marital status and set minimum educational standards, it was a significant factor in improving the educational system(15,16). The federal assistance set a precedent for governmental cooperation in nursing education and, although in the post-war years that assistance varied with administrations and national conditions, the funds that were granted helped the schools as they moved into the mainstream of American education. Federal funds gave educators stronger bargaining power with colleges as they sought affiliations for nursing schools.

In summary, the events of World War II had a lasting impact on nursing. The contributions made by nurses to the war effort were significant; in fact, they helped to make the health care team a crucial factor in any modern combat force. Many old prejudices were abandoned, and nurses gained power and prestige. The one-to-one "primary nursing" role gave way to a stratified nursing team which in the post-war years pushed many registered nurses away from direct patient contact into managerial roles.

Paradoxically, the Cadet Nurse Corps, which used students as workers, set precedents for federal aid to nursing education which later helped the schools escape from the apprenticeship system.

References

1. Bullough, V. L. *Man in Western Civilization.* New York, Holt, Rinehart, and Winston, 1970, p. 436–448.
2. Federal government section. (Report of the Biennial) *Am.J.Nurs.* 38:686–687, June, 1938.
3. Nursing Council on National Defense. *Am.J.Nurs.* 40:1013, Sept. 1940.
4. Newell, Hope. *The History of the National Nursing Council.* New York, National Organization for Public Health Nursing, 1951.
5. The national survey. *Am.J.Nurs.* 41:929–930. Aug. 1941.
6. The nurses' contribution to American victory, facts and figures from Pearl Harbor to VJ Day. *Am.J.Nurs.* 45:683–686, Sept. 1945.
7. Clarke, A. R. Thirty-seven months as prisoners of war. *Am.J.Nurs.* 45:342–345, May 1945.
8. Army nurses in ETO. *Am.J.Nurs.* 45:386–387. May 1945.
9. Roberts, M. M. *American Nursing: History and Interpretation.* New York, Macmillan Co., 1954, pp. 342–351.
10. Aynes, E. A. *From Nightingale to Eagle: An Army Nurse's History.* Englewood Cliffs, N. J., Prentice-Hall, 1973.
11. Flikke, J. O. *Nurses in Action.* Philadelphia, J. B. Lippincott, 1943.
12. Bullough, Vern, and Bullough, Bonnie. *The Emergence of Modern Nursing.* 2d. ed. New York, Macmillan Co., 1969, pp. 199–206.
13. ———.The causes and consequences of the differentiation of the nursing role. In *Varieties of Work Experience,* ed. by Phyllis L. Stewart and Muriel Cantor, New York, John Wiley & Sons, 1974, pp. 292–300.
14. Lippman, H. B. The future of the Red Cross volunteer nurse's aide corps. *Am.J.Nurs.* 45:811–812, Oct. 1945.
15. Petry, Lucile. The U.S. Cadet Nurse Corps. A summing up. *Am.J.Nurs.* 45:1027–1028. Dec. 1945.
16. U.S. Public Health Service. *The U.S. Cadet Nurse Corps and Other Federal Nurse Training Programs, 1943–1948.* Washington D. C., U.S. Government Printing Office, 1950.
17. Roberts, *op. cit.,* pp. 383–393.

Discussion Questions

1. Evaluate one historical theme from nursing's past and the degree to which that theme continues today.

2. What aspect of nursing's history appeals to you the most? Explain.

3. Reverby (Article 2) makes a case for altruism with autonomy. Is this possible in today's practice setting?

4. Are the dilemmas cited by Reverby still experienced by nurses today? Explain. If so, what are they?

5. What social forces in the Victorian era contributed to Florence Nightingale's reactionary stance? What social forces today play a part in nursing's stance on various health care issues?

6. What elements of Miss Nightingale's philosophy of nursing continue to prevail in nursing today?

7. In your opinion, what were the most compelling human factors that made 1890–1900 a fateful decade?

8. What impact did the Great Depression have on nursing?

9. Of the legacies nursing generated as a result of the Great Depression, which one do you feel contributed the most to the development of nursing as a profession?

10. What changes during World War II are still operative in nursing today? In what way have those changes improved professional nursing?

11. Discuss the role of the federal government in upgrading nurses and professional nursing during World War II. What role does the federal government play today in advancing professional nursing?

Further Readings

Attewell, A. (1998). Florence Nightingale's relevance to nurses. *Journal of Holistic Nursing, 16*(2), 281–291.

Friedman, E. (1990). Troubled past of "invisible" profession. *JAMA, 264*(22), 2851–2858.

Kalisch, P. A. & Kalisch, B. J. (1995). *The advance of American nursing* (3rd ed), Philadelphia: J. B. Lippincott.

Shannon, M. L. (1975). Our first four licensure laws. *American Journal of Nursing, 75*(8), 1327–1329.

Smith, F. T. (1981). Florence Nightingale: Early feminist. *American Journal of Nursing, 81*(5), 9–12.

Welch, M. (1990). Florence Nightingale—the social construction of a Victorian feminist. *Western Journal of Nursing Research, 12*(3), 404–407.

Web Site Resources for Links to the Past

American Association for the History of Nursing   www.aahn.org
Brownson's Nursing Notes   http://members.tripod.com/~diannebrownson/history.html
Florence Nightingale Museum   www.florence-nightingale.co.uk/
The History of Nursing   http://gnv.fdt.net/~dforest/hxindex.htm
The History of Nursing Archives   www.bu.edu/speccol/nursing.htm

General Search Engine Web Sites

About.com   www.about.com
All the Web   www.alltheweb.com
Direct Hit   www.directhit.com

Health Web Sites

On Health   www.onhealth.com
Med Explorer   www.medexplorer.com
Self Care   www.selfcare.com

Professional Journal Web Sites

MedWebPlus   www.medwebplus.com
The Nurses Portal   www.nursinglife.com

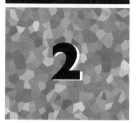

Nurses: A Professional Reality Check

It was evening as the nurse sat at the patient's bedside and held his hand while waiting for his fever to abate. Every few minutes she applied cold compresses to his forehead to ease his discomfort. She had worked all day and was tired, but despite being off duty, she felt it was her duty to stay with him. She would not fail him.

Ms. Smith was a model nurse. Her uniform was always clean and neat and her disposition was pleasing and cheerful. Even in the most difficult situations, she was poised, tactful, and unruffled. When doctors made their rounds, she was always available, holding the patient charts as she accompanied the physicians on their rounds.

Are these nurses real? Not to us, perhaps, but to the public they are. The public's image of nurses has not essentially changed since nursing's inception. Many articles in nursing, some written as early as 1928, speak to the concerns nurses have had about what they know to be their image and what the public believes their image to be. The concerns continue and so do the myths about nursing. "Nice girls don't do nursing!," "If you have a strong back and a weak mind, be a nurse," "Nursing is the road to matrimony," and "Personality is all you need to be a nurse," are just a few examples. Myths are powerful. The reason they influence the public to such a great extent is that myths make life easier. Use exaggeration, distort to simplicity all the widely held beliefs about nursing, spread them through the media, and you have a myth that won't go away. But it needs to go away, and quickly.

And what is the real image of nurses today? Patients know. They can see that nursing is grueling work. They know what harried nursing care feels like. They see it in the tired, worn, stressed faces of their nurses—when they see one. Nurses know, too. They know they are not the insipid image the media continues to send out. They know they are educated, committed, and compassionate professionals. They know they are not and never will be all things to all people, but they are deeply troubled that they cannot be just some things to their patients.

These contradictory images of nurses have far-reaching consequences for all of us. They affect the health care labor market, enrollments in nursing programs, the quality and stability of health care, and the morale of nurses who provide that care. If the public does not know what nurses do, what is the incentive to become a nurse? If one becomes a nurse, what is the incentive to stay in nursing given the present state of health care delivery? Clearly something has to change. These are the issues that are explored in this chapter. All of the readings selected for this chapter illustrate one clear and troubling message: that nurses are, if not already becoming, an endangered species. Should that happen, what images will we have then?

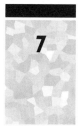

7

The Public Image of the Nurse

Linda Hughes

*T*he scope and function of nursing practice have expanded over the past century, yet nurses continue to be bound by myths, traditions and archaic ideas about their role in health care delivery. Although many nurses are now assuming independent and innovative roles in health care, the public continues to view the physician as the sole authority and as the primary provider of health care. Nursing potential has not been fully recognized or utilized by the public, and this has led to wasted nursing talent and inadequate care for society.

A historical study was recently conducted to determine the public opinion of the nurse and the nursing profession during the period 1896 to 1976.[1] Data from popular magazines, novels and newspapers were obtained to formulate generalizations and identify themes that emerged during that period. The mass media have not only reflected but have also directed public opinion about the nurse and the nursing profession. From a historical perspective, the image of the nurse that has been projected through the mass media has been a distortion of reality, grounded in mythical beliefs and traditional ideas that for too long have gone unchallenged and unquestioned by the general public and by many nurses. The public image of the nurse may account, at least partially, for the failure of the public to fully utilize the services of the nurse in health care delivery.

■ HISTORICAL STUDY OF PUBLIC OPINION

Social and cultural changes evolve slowly and the effects of these changes are felt over a long period of time. Examination of historical records can give the researcher the advantage of discovering significant truths about human na-

At the time of this article, Linda Hughes, R.N., M.S., was an instructor in nursing, Oklahoma Baptist University, Shawnee, Oklahoma.

Reprinted from *Advances in Nursing Science*, 2(3) 55–72, 1980, with permission of Aspen Publishers, Inc., © 1980.

ture and social action. "The historian's advantage is that he is apt to see the whole Gestalt of circumstances which serves as a matrix for the ensuing behavior."[2(p34,35)] For this reason, the historical study of public opinion is valid. Indeed, the concept of public opinion was identified by a historian over 2,000 years ago: "Thucydides, in his *History of the Peloponnesian War*, organized his book around three closely related but different themes, the distribution of public opinion, the processes of opinion formation, and the impact of opinion upon government decisions."[3(p117,118)]

In his essay on the study of public opinion, Benson defined the historical approach to be "the use of procedures to secure data from documents that the researcher locates and selects but does not create, directly or indirectly. By selecting documents and . . . interrogating their author, historical researchers generate data designed to answer questions about past public opinion."[3(p109)]

Garraghan also discussed the value of documents in generating ideas about public opinion: The historian, he wrote, is able to "construct clear and distinct ideas or images of persons, events, institutions, and other things about which the document informs us."[4(p330)]

Sources

Standard sources utilized by historians often do not reflect the opinion and popular ideas held by the mass population. Opinions expressed in newspaper and magazine editorials cannot always be assumed to reflect the opinion of the general public. The historian is well advised to look for data about public opinion in other sources such as school books, pulp fiction, comic books, fan magazines, novels and popular magazines.[5]

Vincent characterized the concept of public opinion as elusive and one that requires the researcher to utilize many and varied sources in order to make accurate and valid generalizations. He also pointed to the difficulty of determining exactly what public opinion was at a given time. He cautioned that "a large portion of the mass accepts its opinions from others"—and that those "others" may be a small but vociferous minority.[6(p281,282)]

The ability of the historian to know and understand the men and women of the past is dependent upon the traces left behind. The historian must utilize every possible method of historical inquiry to come to the highest attainable degree of truth about the past. The following statement, by a historian, points out the importance of making inferences and generalizations in the study of public opinion.

> [T]he men and women who have left records were not the common people; they were the literate, the people in positions of power and influence of one kind or another. The were, in brief, not representative of the entire population, though certainly they may have been representative of their own class or group. The problem of knowing the ordinary man . . . is compounded by the

scant records in which those people set forth their feelings and concerns. The historian is often left to infer from the records of literate people what the ordinary man thought about himself and about those who directed the course of his actions by domestic and diplomatic decisions.[5(p58)]

Nursing "Poorly Understood"

Nurses have recognized the necessity of public understanding and cooperation in elevating the status of the nursing profession and initiating changes within the health care system. In 1928 the *American Journal of Nursing* requested its readers to define the major professional aim for the coming year. Public cooperation and understanding of the nursing profession was identified by many of the respondents as the major aim toward which the nursing profession should address itself. As one nurse commented, "the task of obtaining community understanding and, through it, community cooperation is indeed a challenge for, as nurses and as a profession, we are still poorly understood. For the most part, the community does not consider nursing an essential service for which it has a responsibility."[7(p52)]

Despite an additional 52 years of evolution, the nursing profession is still poorly understood. Kinlein, describing the inception of her independent nursing practice, observed in 1977: "In the minds of the public, nursing was an adjunct to medicine, and any time they approached a nurse for care, or a nurse approached them to give care, the need had flowed from the medical condition of the person...."[8(p43)] Kinlein's observation about the publicly perceived close tie between nursing practice and medical practice bears a remarkable similarity to a comment made 100 years ago. The readers of *Nineteenth Century* were told in 1880 that "Nursing is doctoring.... Any one who will set himself to define the function of the nurse as distinct from that of the doctor will very soon find himself involved in absurdity."[9(p1092)]

Public opinion, though elusive, is a powerful factor influencing the consumer's utilization of nursing care. In light of the current public dissatisfaction with the health care system, nursing has the opportunity to assume a more beneficial role in health care delivery. To ensure more efficient and effective utilization of nursing care, the public must be cognizant of and receptive to the actual and potential role of the nurse in health care. Historical study can provide insight into factors that have influenced past public opinion toward the nursing profession. This knowledge can facilitate the nursing profession's development in the future.

■ DEFINITION OF TERMS

The following terms were defined for the purpose of studying public opinion regarding the nurse and the nursing profession.

Historical development—the chronological series of events, nursing and nonnursing, that have had a direct bearing upon the nursing profession.

Historical method—the effective gathering of source materials about past ideas of groups, appraising them critically, and presenting an interpretation of the results obtained.

Public opinion—a persistent, general orientation of society toward some individuals, groups or institutions which may or may not be based upon legitimate, correct or informed knowledge.

Nurse—one who provides preventive, curative or rehabilitative care to an individual or a group of individuals for the purpose of obtaining economic, educational or emotional remuneration. (This definition is based on the public's perception of the nurse and is not necessarily consistent with the nursing profession's definition.)

■ METHODOLOGY

The author used the historical method of research to analyze the problem. The collection of data was limited to literature obtainable in libraries of the southwestern United States. *Readers' Guide to Periodical Literature*, 1896 through 1976, was used to obtain data from secular magazines pertaining to the nurse and the nursing profession. *The New York Times*, 1895 through 1976, was systematically examined to obtain data about the nursing profession. The author also examined selected lay novels pertaining to the nurse and the nursing profession. These data were analyzed to provide an understanding of the public view of the nurse and her role. The author then drew inferences, generalizations and conclusions regarding public opinion of the nurse and the nursing profession.

To determine a relationship between nursing practice and the public opinion of the nurse, the author examined the professional organ of the American Nurses Association, the *American Journal of Nursing*, 1900 through 1976, as well as the professional organ of the National League of Nursing, *Nursing Outlook*, 1953 through 1976. Major trends within nursing practice were identified along with specific major social, legislative and economic factors that have influenced nursing practice. On the basis of these findings, the author determined the effect of nursing practice upon the public opinion of the nurse.

■ OVERVIEW OF FINDINGS

Woman's Work

The public consistently identified nursing as "work peculiarly suited to the dainty, delicate-minded woman."[10(p974)] Indeed, the nursing role and the mothering role were seen as historically interrelated. Innate maternalism and womanly qualities were publicly viewed as essential characteristics of the ideal nurse. Since women were mothers, it naturally followed that women were better suited for the nursing role than men both psychologically and emotionally. The public assumed that all women had a natural affinity for nursing work and that providing care for the sick came as second nature to any woman. As one nurse observed in 1883, the public "consider[s] hardly any training at all necessary for our nurses . . . the generality of people think that any woman can nurse."[11(p310)]

Victorian Roots

Training schools for nurses were established and a professional association for nurses in the United States was developed during the closing years of the Victorian Era. Victorian ideology "defined women's proper social roles in narrow and restricted ways . . . women's actions had to be consistent with moral sensibility, purity, and maternal affection, and no other code of behavior was acceptable."[12(p14)] Victorian ideology dictated that women exhibit specific womanly qualities and subordinate all personal interests and activities to the maintenance of the home and the family.[12,13] Educational and career opportunities for women were restricted because endeavors in these areas were believed to detract the woman from the execution of her responsibilities as a wife and mother. Women were expected to be passive, conservative, submissive and obedient to masculine authority. Society viewed competitiveness, aggressiveness, independence and initiative as masculine attributes. Such attributes were considered unattractive when exhibited in a woman. Women hesitated to engage in activities that could make them appear "unladylike" and thereby detract from their womanliness. Social respectability was stressed in Victorian ideology, and the vast majority of women made every effort to earn and maintain respectability by their actions and their manner.

> Nineteenth-century women were not always the passive, submissive and pure creatures of popular idealizations, but neither were they ever completely free from this stereotype. Its most pervasive and effective form of control was through the social and individual demand for respectability. . . .[13(pxix)]

Virtue Personified

As a predominantly woman's profession, nursing was deeply influenced by Victorian ideas about women and their proper place in society. The public image of the ideal nurse mirrored the public image of the virtuous woman.[12,13,15] Nurses were depicted in the secular literature as the epitome of true womanhood and the embodiment of all good womanly qualities. As the readers of *Good Housekeeping* were told in 1915, nursing is "that very high development of the qualities known as 'womanly' . . . [the nurse] seems to be a sort of embodied womanhood raised to the nth power."[16(p736)]

In light of the restrictions historically placed upon women in terms of their roles outside the home, equating nurses with true womanhood in the public literature served to tell women, in effect, that nursing was one occupation in which they could utilize their potential without compromising their social respectability. In fact, many articles written about nursing in the popular literature encouraged women to enter the nursing profession precisely because it *was* a woman's profession and nursing was one field in which women could rise to top positions and be well compensated for their achievements. Outlining the advantages of nursing as a suitable occupation for women, one nurse commented in 1904 that nursing "is also unique in being perhaps the only profession unreservedly assigned to women . . . in which they occupy all the higher positions. In every other line of life women either struggle in ineffectual competition with men or occupy the subordinate and less well-paid posts."[17(p310)]

In 1915 a lay writer informed the public that a nursing career was available to women simply because men allowed it. This writer again commented on the absence of competition from men: "it is still a tussle to get a footing at all, [in other leading professions] because of 'Keep Off the Ladder' signs posted in masculine handwriting. But here is a profession to which nobody nowadays denies women full access."[16(p729)]

Thirty years later this theme was repeated in an effort to recruit women for nursing during World War II. Women were told: "The opportunity . . . to advance to posts of responsibility in nursing is relatively great because of the size of the field and lack of competition from men."[18(p18)]

These statements in relation to a predominantly woman's profession cast insight into the secondary role which women historically were forced to assume. They reveal that competition with men was seen as useless and hardly worth the woman's efforts. Competitiveness was not a womanly quality and nursing was obviously seen as an avenue for women to realize their potential without appearing unwomanly.

Unwholesome Reputation

Advertising nursing as a virtuous and womanly occupation had a beneficial effect, at least initially, upon the nursing profession. Before the establishment of training schools for nurses in this country, nurses had a particularly unwholesome reputation. Criminals, prostitutes, and intemperate and immoral women were commonplace among the ranks of those calling themselves nurses. By the very nature of the work, nursing was seen as menial labor barely befitting consideration by domestic servants. Women who were forced to earn a living and who were unable to secure any other form of work engaged in nursing.

In *Martin Chuzzlewit*, published in 1844, Dickens provided a representative example of the "professional nurse" of the time in the fictitious character of Sairey Gamp: "it was difficult to enjoy her society without becoming conscious of a smell of spirits . . . she took to [her profession] very kindly; insomuch, that setting aside her natural predilections as a woman, she went to a lying-in or a laying-out with equal zest and relish."[19(p302)]

The sick who fell subject to the ministrations of these "Sairey Gamps" were victims more often than they were recipients of nursing care. Dominated by women of such questionable reputation, nursing did not attract any respectable or well-qualified women. An English nurse provided the following summation of pre-Nightingale nursing:

> . . . nursing . . . was at a low ebb; arduous and ill-paid, neither religious nor professional, it only attracted people who were quite unfit for any other occupation, often drunken and brutal, almost invariably inefficient. Particularly feeble paupers were . . . made night nurses, because the pittance so earned would enable them to buy better food than the ordinary workhouse fare.[20(p587,588)]

Nurses in the United States were of no higher caliber than those of England. Prior to 1873 the trained nurse did not exist in this country. Any woman who desired to nurse the sick could do so; indeed, many women were coerced into nursing work. One physician wrote that, prior to the trained nurse, "some of the nursing in Bellevue Hospital . . . was done by drunken prostitutes who in the Police Court were given the option of going to prison or to hospital service. No wonder they were often found in drunken sleep under the beds of their dead patients whose liquor they had stolen."[21(p71)]

Nursing work was not only confined to women of questionable reputation, but convalescent patients also provided much of the nursing care in the early hospitals. One New York physician reminisced: "when I was an interne in a large hospital in 1875 . . . nurses were far inferior to the average domestic servant. Not a few of them had been patients who when convalescent had been elevated to the position of nurses. Some of them were faithful souls and did their best, but most of them had a fondness for Sairey Gamp's teapot and smelt of Sairey Gamp's tea."[22(p164,165)]

Changing the Public Image

With the establishment of training schools in the United States, the public image of the nurse underwent a slow process of change. Early nursing educators were intent upon upgrading the social status and the public image of the nurse. These early nurses attempted to keep the temperamentally unfit out of the profession by carefully screening applicants to training schools and rigidly enforcing a standard of exemplary behavior in pupil nurses. As one hospital manager reported in 1908, "no matron would choose her probationers from applicants with marked physical blemishes . . . she would wisely give preference to those who were personally pleasing."[23(p824)]

The power of the public press also served to facilitate the improvement in the image of the nurse by publicly placing the nurse on a compatible social level with the good Victorian woman. Elevating the social status of the nurse enhanced the ability of the nursing profession to attract women of a higher quality for nursing work. Had nursing not come to be positively viewed by the public as a womanly occupation, many respectable and intelligent women never could have been induced to enter the nursing profession.

Thus defining the ideal nurse as an example of true womanhood in the public literature did exert a positive influence upon the nursing profession. However, the close public correlation between the ideal nurse and the true woman had some damaging effects upon the profession as well. Longstanding social beliefs about women and their role in society became the foundation for several mythical beliefs that were associated with the nursing profession. The confining image of the nurse which developed on the basis of social beliefs about women hampered the growth of nursing as a profession and promoted restrictions in the scope of nursing practice.[24,25]

▪ THE IDEAL NURSE

The mass media created a mythical image of the ideal nurse, and the public historically expected all practicing nurses to adhere to that image. Many popular magazines depicted the nurse as little more than a "starched white figure moving romantically in hospital wards and operating rooms."[26(p74)] The ideal nurse was portrayed in lay publications as pretty, preferably young, cool and calmly efficient, clean and crisp in her uniform and possessing a pleasing personality.

Emphasis on Personality

The personality of the nurse was given a great deal of emphasis in the public literature. The personality characteristics of the ideal nurse paralleled the personality characteristics of the good Victorian woman. Womanly qualities were stressed as essential to the successful performance of the nursing role. In 1942, for example, *Occupations* ran an article, directed to high school students, which summarized the qualities of the ideal nurse as "neatness, tact, reliability, good judgment, poise, accuracy, dependability, honesty, common sense, and emotional stability. A nurse should also be loyal, conscientious, and cooperative. She should have initiative, dignity, imagination, and a timely sense of humor. She should be alert . . . [and] interested in her patients. . . ."[27(p280)]

While these qualities provided an excellent description of a fictitious nurse like Cherry Ames, they neither accurately nor realistically described actual nurses engaged in day-to-day nursing practice. Given the best of circumstances, it would be difficult for any person to display all of these qualities consistently, since situations and interactions are never static.

Much of the popular literature implied that if the nurse had a pleasing personality, then her mental capabilities were of secondary importance. As the public was told in 1941, "the personality and appearance of the nurse reacts subtly but genuinely upon the sick person."[28(p9)] While that is true, the intellectual and technical abilities of the nurse react subtly with the sick person as well. However, the public literature tended to stress the nurse's personality almost to the point of negating the intellectual and educational requirements of nursing practice.

In light of the importance placed upon the personality of the nurse, the implication was often made that education could not compensate for the absence of pleasing personality characteristics in the nurse. The public was told that "No amount of training will make a coarse-minded woman a dainty nurse."[10(p974)] Arguing that state registration of the nurse would not improve the quality of the practicing nurse, a hospital administrator made the following assertion in 1902: "far more attention is paid to and value put upon the character of the nurses than on their success in the technical part of their training."[29(p772,773)] In 1956 *Reader's Digest* repeated that statement when it reported that "The responsiveness of a nurse comes more from her personality than from her formal education . . ." though the nurse was required to "perform delicate tasks and exercise the kind of judgment that until recent years were the exclusive prerogatives of doctors."[30(p82)]

While a pleasing personality is essential for any professional person seeking to serve the public, this qualification alone could hardly be considered adequate to aid the nurse in exercising judgment, day in and day out, upon which the patient's life could depend. The inconsistency of statements such as these was not, however, seriously questioned by the public, primarily because the public had a limited understanding of the role of the nurse in patient care.

Overlooking Abilities and Knowledge

Nurses have had their role defined to the public in terms of the performance of rote and repetitive tasks. In 1955 *Look* defined the functions of the nurse as "giving injections, back rubs and bed baths, [and] making a neat hospital bed."[31(p62)] As recently as 1971 *Life* reported that, as a student nurse, one "learns the right way to take a blood pressure, read thermometers—and even empty a bedpan."[32(p47)] Given this limited view of the role of the nurse in health care, it is little wonder that the public failed to recognize intellectual abilities and a sound knowledge base as necessary requirements for excellence in nursing practice.

Intellectual abilities again assumed a secondary place in light of the qualification of physical fitness for nursing work. Besides being dainty, delicate minded and womanly, the nurse was expected to be a hard worker. Physical strength and stamina were consistently seen as basic requirements for the ideal nurse. Women were told in 1915 that to be considered eligible for nurses' training they must be "guaranteed sound of body by a physician, sound of morals by a clergyman, and sound of teeth by a dentist."[16(p732)] In 1943 potential applicants for nursing schools were told that they would have to "pass a rigid physical test, probably intelligence and aptitude tests."[33(p67)]

A Bedside Voice

Even the timbre of the nurse's voice was given consideration by the public. In a letter to the *American Journal of Nursing* in 1906 a former patient encouraged nurses to cultivate a soft speaking voice because "a well-modulated voice is a blessing" in the sick room.[34(p104)] In 1917 *Literary Digest* quoted a physician as saying that upon the nurse's voice depended much of her usefulness, and that "if she has not a good 'bedside' voice by inheritance and home-training, she should proceed to acquire it at all costs."[35(p27)]

Unrealistic Expectations

The image of the ideal nurse projected through the mass media was a figment of public imagination. This image created an unrealistic expectation of the practicing nurse. The nursing profession historically faced public criticism because actual nurses often failed to measure up to the idealistic standard that was projected through the mass media. In addition, the public image of the ideal nurse did not advance the ability of the profession to gain public support for needed improvements in legislation and education for the practicing nurse.

■ NURSING AS A CALLING

For centuries the responsibility for providing nursing care to the sick poor was assumed by religious orders. The early association between nursing and religion resulted in the public identification of nursing as a charitable and merciful gesture to humankind. This belief about nursing continued after it became a secular occupation for women. Many nurses and the general public alike historically equated nursing with a religious calling that required its followers to display the qualities of devotion, dedication, obedience to authority, willing self-sacrifice and self-effacement. Ethel Fenwick, first president of the International Council of Nurses, elaborated upon the woman's motivation in choosing the nursing profession as a career: "I believe that a large proportion [of nurses] adopt this calling from the highest motives and the heart-felt desire to fulfil the Divine command to tend the sick."[36(p326)]

Nonnursing groups often expressed the opinion that, in the absence of the religious motivations Fenwick described, no nurses could hope to attain any measure of success in their work. As one hospital manager concluded in 1902, "it will never be possible to have perfect nursing without willing self-sacrifice."[29(p772)]

In working for reforms to elevate the economic and professional status of the profession, nurses were often judged as being selfish, self-centered and failing to live up to the religious instincts that were felt to be natural to their calling. Nurses were often viewed as subject to "small feminine vanities," believed to be "strangely out of place when allied with a calling concerned with issues so grave."[23(p824)] Typifying the attitude of many of his colleagues, one hospital administrator blatantly declared that nurses must subordinate themselves to the duties of their calling. In his words,

> . . . nursing is a calling demanding of its followers, if they are to excel, a measure of self-obliteration which to minds dominated by ideas of personal advantage and advancement may appear foolishness, but is essential to the true nurse. This does not mean that the woman who takes up nursing must be necessarily indifferent to matters affecting her own health and well-being. . . . But she must be capable of giving them their rightful, which is a secondary, place.[28(p825)]

The natural and inevitable result of viewing nursing as a calling led to the belief that, for their labors, nurses received heavenly rather than earthly rewards. Isabel Stewart, a prominent nursing educator, concluded in 1927 that nurses had been persuaded to believe that the "only satisfactions . . . ever expect[ed] in nursing are the satisfactions that come through self-sacrifice."[37(p538)] An article run in *Good Housekeeping* in 1961 summarized this belief in this way: "despite long hours, low pay, and more grind than glamour, the moments when [the nurse's] compassion and skill help relieve a patient's suffering more than compensate for the drawbacks of her profession."[38(p35)]

The correlation between nursing and a religious calling and the resultant belief that willing self-sacrifice was essential to nursing practice provided the justification needed to support the low pay and long hours of labor that historically characterized the nurse's employment. Of greater importance, this belief was supported by male-dominated groups within the health care system, groups that exerted external control over the practice and the education of the nurse. By advocating this belief, these groups attempted to provide legitimate rationalization for the exploitation of women's labors in the health care system.

■ MYTHICAL THEMES ASSOCIATED WITH THE NURSING PROFESSION

The public image of the nurse has been intricately related to several mythical beliefs that have been projected to the public as repeated themes throughout the history of the nursing profession. Mythical beliefs have a powerful influence on society in part because of their adherence to cultural beliefs and also because they are generalized to an entire society or group within society. Despite the connotation of the term falsity, myths exist because the majority of society believe in their authenticity and validity. By responding to consciously and unconsciously held beliefs and values, myths transmit their validity and justify their existence and their perpetuation.

The Born Nurse

The public has historically viewed nursing work as a special area in which women could excel because of their innate "womanliness." As a result of this belief, the need to educate women for nursing work was publicly minimized. Maternal instincts and womanly qualities were God-given, and a woman was born with them or without them. Even after training schools were established in this country, the belief existed that the nurse was born, not made; thus leading to the assumption that no amount or kind of training could instill in a woman the essential qualities of the ideal nurse. As a hospital manager asserted in 1902, "No training, whether the hours be long or short, will endow a young woman with gifts which Nature has failed to bestow upon her. . . . Maternal instincts and nursing instincts are much the same, and women are born with them or without them."[29(p771,772)]

The argument that the nurse was born and not made was used throughout nursing's history as justification for limiting the educational preparation of student nurses. Nursing education in the United States developed as a manifestation of apprenticeship training. Training schools for nurses were affiliated with a specific hospital. Student nurses functioned as the nursing service department of the hospital. Following a specified time of service, the student nurse received a diploma from the training school and was discharged from the hospital as a graduate trained nurse. Student nurses, in effect, traded their labor on the hospital wards for their training as a nurse.

Hospital administrators were quick to recognize the economic value of the hospital-based training school for nurses. Staffing the hospital wards with student nurses provided a plentiful and inexpensive source of labor. Moreover, admitting women to the training school every six months or every year provided the hospital with a fresh group of workers to staff the hospital wards. In fact, in many training schools, student admission occurred year-round depending on the labor needs of the hospital. If one student nurse dropped out, another was readily admitted.

Functioning as the nursing service department of the hospital, the vast majority of student nurses did not receive the educational opportunities needed to adequately prepare them for nursing work. The educational needs of the student nurse assumed a secondary place in light of the nursing service needs of the hospital. Many training schools for nurses offered no semblance of an education for their students. Student nurses worked as many as 105 hours a week; lectures, of which there were few, were offered in the evening after a full day of work; classroom and laboratory facilities were virtually nonexistent, and few schools provided even one paid instructor.[25]

Nonnursing groups, especially hospital administrators, who had an economic investment in the type and amount of training student nurses received, were the primary advocates of the born-nurse myth. Defending the limited educational preparation of the student nurse, one hospital authority stated in 1908 that "no amount of training will transform a probationer wanting in personal suitability into a good nurse. . . . Inefficiency in a nurse is much more often due to want of character than to a lack of intelligence or a capacity to learn the mere technicalities of her art. . . ."[23(p830)]

The born-nurse myth appeared in the popular literature in relation to the educational preparation of the nurse as recently as 1968. *Look,* reporting on an apparent nursing shortage, reported that the "aggravating factor" was the recommendation made in 1965 by the American Nurses' Association that the baccalaureate degree should be the basic requirement for beginning entry into professional nursing practice. "Your ability to like people depends on your basic personality," opined an anonymous hospital authority. "Love and concern are God-given; they're not handed out with a college degree."[39(p29)]

The born-nurse myth contributed to the difficulties faced by the nursing profession as attempts were made to improve the educational opportunities available to prepare women for nursing work. Although nursing educators repeatedly argued that nurses were only as good as their education, they had little impact upon a belief that had been ingrained in the minds of the public for the better part of the century. The propagation of the born-nurse myth has been a persuasive argument used to thwart the attempts of the profession to elevate nurses' educational and professional standards. Following a study of medical education in 1910, standards for medical education were developed and medical schools were quickly established in the university setting. As a general rule, however, collegiate affiliations for nursing education were not established until some 40 years later.

The New Road to Marriage

Marriage and motherhood have been the traditional societal expectation of women. Since nursing has traditionally been predominantly a woman's profession, it was inevitable that the marriageability of nurses would receive the attention of the public, especially young women seeking to enter the profession. The promise of marriage as an attractive fringe benefit of nursing work pervaded popular literature. Articles published about nursing, geared to the young woman, often implied that becoming a nurse would improve one's chances for marriage, especially marriage to physicians. Nursing was defined as the "new road to matrimony" in 1897,[40(p31)] and 70 years later, *Mademoiselle* advised young women "in search of a physician-husband" that they "would do well to conduct the search in hospital corridors, for a homely nurse is more likely to marry a young physician or medical student than is a homely secretary or teacher."[41(p134)]

While an attractive salary, fringe benefits and opportunities for career advancement have been the usual selling features for most vocations, marriage was the primary selling feature for the nursing profession in the popular literature. Particularly during the war years when the need for nurses was especially great, advertising the improved marriageability of nurses went into high gear. Recruitment campaigns conducted especially during World War II promised women that if they became nurses and volunteered for overseas duty they could expect romantic encounters that could well culminate in marriage. Based on an interview with a nurse recruiter during World War II, *The New York Times* informed women that on overseas military bases marriages were occurring at the rate of four per day.[42] Women were told that "nurses were never inclined to be old maids very much. Why, most nurses can hardly avoid marrying doctors. . . ."[43(p4)]

Many women, having been conditioned to view nursing work as a temporary and, at best, stop-gap occupation, entered nursing with little desire to maintain a long-term commitment to the profession. Nursing schools historically trained thousands of women, many of whom remained in nursing work for only a short period of time. Moreover, many nurses were satisfied to tolerate the low pay and poor working conditions that throughout history have plagued the working nurse because they viewed their employment as temporary and anticipated eventual withdrawal from nursing practice.

Nurse as Physician's Helpmate

The public has viewed nurses as being wedded to physicians. Nursing practice, in the minds of the public, has been and continues to be subordinately linked to medical practice. The public has for many years watched nurses faithfully carry out physicians' orders, respond to physicians' demands and idiosyncrasies, prepare patients and the sickroom for physicians' visits and clean up after physicians following their departure from the sickroom. As a result, the public has believed that the physician is the "master and controller of both nurse and patient."[44(p1105)] In a more recent era, *Today's Health* reported on flight nurses in Vietnam with the observation that "romance is flourishing. . . . To date, five nurses have married men they met at war, and almost all others are being energetically courted."[45(p60)]

Women were also told that undergoing nurse's training would be excellent preparation for marriage and motherhood. Women had nothing to lose by completing nurses' training because, whether they chose to practice as nurses or not, they could use the knowledge gained to aid them in their role as wives and mothers. For a nominal tuition and "three years of interesting work, [the woman] could buy herself . . . perfect preparation for marriage and motherhood."[46(p116)]

As mentioned before, Victorian ideology dictated that woman not assume careers that could interfere with the execution of their responsibilities as wives and mothers. Consistent with this ideology, the subtle implication was made throughout the popular media that, after marriage, women were no longer expected to remain in active nursing practice. Marriage provided a legitimate exit from the profession. Several "true" stories about nurses were published in the popular literature which depicted the ideal nurse who, though deeply gratified by her service to humanity, planned to marry and retire from the profession.[47,48] As recently as 1960 *Today's Health* reported that "if later [nurses] should trade their caps for a wedding ring, what better preparation would there be for marriage and motherhood?"[49(p66)]

This image of the nurse led to the assumption that nurses functioned only under physician supervision. The public has viewed nurses as being totally dependent upon physicians to guide everyday nursing practice. Indeed, the public has been led to believe that any action by a nurse that had not been approved by a physician could result in harm to the patient. The public was told that "A fundamental principle of the nurse's existence is that she gives nursing care only under the direction of a licensed physician. . . . Infringement, with the best intentions in the world, may lead to misunderstanding, harm, even danger to the patient. . . ."[50(p206)]

To the detriment of the public and the nursing profession alike, the public has never identified nursing care as separate and distinct from physician care. In fact, the public has historically assumed that the major role of the nurse is to aid physicians in their efforts to provide medical services. The public has never equated nursing care with health care, rather it has viewed nursing care as a watered-down version of physician care. The nurse has been seen as an extension of the physician, performing simple medical procedures in the sickroom. As an editorial in *The New York Times* stated in 1921, the nurse "is trained to exercise judgment and assume responsibility in many minor matters, and so enables her chief to devote himself more fully to the major functions of his profession."[51(p14)] This notion was repeated 55 years later when nurse practitioners were defined as "trained assistants and [physician] surrogates" whose function was to "free the highly trained modern physician from . . . routine and often repetitious tasks."[52(p532)]

The mythical belief in the nurse's subordination to the physician, projected through the popular media, has led to public depreciation of the role of the nurse in health care. Nursing care has always existed with or without physician supervision. The failure of the public to recognize this has had a damaging effect upon the growth of nurses as professional practitioners and upon the utilization of nurses to their fullest potential in health care.

■ *EDUCATING THE PUBLIC*

The need for public education has been dramatically demonstrated by the media's interpretation of the recent expansion of many nurses into more independent and health-oriented roles. For example, in the words of two popular magazines, nurses in expanded roles are performing "routine tasks that we've come to associate with physicians,"[53(p21)] tasks that "bore more M.D.'s, yet take up so much of their expensive time."[54(p35)] The public continues to view the nurse as dependent upon physician supervision and unable to function without medical direction. As recently as 1975 *McCalls* reported that independent nurse practitioners "generally have to be associated with doctors in some way since, despite their independence, they are really an extension of good medical service."[54(p35)]

Nursing care continues to be equated with the performance of tasks and, for the most part, is not associated with the use of decision-making skills and independent thinking. Reporting on the development of an independent nurse practitioner program in 1966 *Time* quoted a physician to say that the nurse "doesn't have to know the specific difficulty . . . she simply has to know enough to say to herself. . . . this one is for the doctor."[55(p71)]

Any profession that seeks to serve the public must concern itself with public opinion. Public opinion has been and continues to be a powerful tool to promote change in society. The nursing profession has been aware of the need to maintain a well-educated and informed public. The American Nurses' Association, for example, declared 1978 as the Year of the Nurse and conducted a nationwide campaign to educate the public to the role of the nurse in health care.

To be beneficial, however, public education must be a constant process that gives the public consistent and repetitive exposure to the nursing profession. Although some nurses have utilized the public press, they have been well in the minority. Lack of journalistic knowledge and insecurity in their literary ability have kept many nurses from attempting to communicate with the public through the press. As a result, nursing's efforts to educate the public have proved to be haphazard, thus ineffectual.

The importance of establishing a positive public image is especially great at this time in history. Debates about the crisis in health care are common and many of the inadequacies of the present health care system are being publicly exposed. As consumers of health care, the public is expressing dissatisfaction with the high cost and the poor quality of services available to them. This social climate will inevitably lead to changes in the health care delivery system.

Because of the nursing profession's intimate association with the existing health care system, changes in this system will have a direct bearing on nursing practice. Public opinion of the nurse has had and will continue to have an effect on the ability of the nursing profession to provide a unique and beneficial service to the public. The general public is the consumer of health care, and its demand for and utilization of nursing services will determine the extent to which nurses will function in nontraditional roles in the future. For example, the ability to function as professional practitioners mandates that third party payment and direct reimbursement for nursing services be established. This form of reimbursement must compensate nurses for more than just the performance of tasks and the execution of the physician's orders.

If the nursing profession believes that it has a valuable service to offer in the area of health care, this must be communicated to the public through the mass media. There is no one more capable or better qualified to inform the public of contributions the nursing profession can make in the area of health care than nurses themselves. By openly communicating with the public, nurses can dispel the myths that have long surrounded the nursing profession and begin to project an image that accurately and positively reflects what nursing is. As one nurse commented half a century ago, "we have unequalled opportunities for service and instruction. . . . Whether we justify our existence, whether we convince the public that we are really essential, rests with us."[56(p819)]

References

1. Hughes, L. "Nursing and the Public: Images and Opinions of the Profession 1896–1976." Master's thesis, Texas Woman's University 1978.
2. Ware, C. *The Cultural Approach to History* (New York: Columbia University Press 1940).
3. Benson, L. *Toward the Scientific Study of History* (Philadelphia: J. B. Lippincott Co. 1972).
4. Garraghan, G. *A Guide to Historical Method* (Westport, Conn.: Greenwood Press 1940).
5. Stephens, L. *Probing the Past* (Boston: Allyn and Bacon 1974).
6. Vincent, J. *Historical Research* (New York: Franklin Reprints 1974).
7. Roberts, A. "Aims for 1928." *Am J Nurs* 28:1 (January 1928) p. 52.
8. Kinlein, M. L. *Independent Nursing Practice with Clients* (Philadelphia: J. B. Lippincott Co. 1977).
9. Sturges, O. "Doctors and Nurses." *Nineteenth Century* 7:40 (June 1880) p. 1089–1096.
10. Rae, L. "The Question of the Modern Trained Nurse." *Nineteenth Century* 51:304 (June 1902) p. 972–974.
11. Craven, F. "Servants of the Sick Poor." *Nineteenth Century* 13:74 (April 1883) p. 667, 668.
12. Rothman, S. *Woman's Proper Place* (New York: Basic Books 1978).

13. Hymowitz, C. and Weissman, M. *A History of Women in America* (New York: Bantam Books 1978).

14. Vicinus, M. *A Widening Sphere* (Bloomington: Ind.: University Press 1977).

15. Kalisch, P. and Kalisch, B. *The Advance of American Nursing* (Boston: Little, Brown and Co. 1978).

16. Comstock, S. "Your Daughter's Career: If She Wants to Be a Nurse." *Good Housekeeping* 61:6 (December 1915) p. 728–736.

17. Ferguson, H. "State Registration of Nurses." *Nineteenth Century* 55:324 (February 1904) p. 310–317.

18. "Says U.S. Will Have 48,000 Nurses in '48 with Post-War Jobs for All." *New York Times* (June 11, 1945) p. 18.

19. Dickens, C. *Martin Chuzzlewit* (New York: Dutton Press 1968).

20. Moss, M. "The Evolution of the Trained Nurse." *Atlantic Monthly* 91:1047 (May 1903) p. 587–599.

21. Worchester, A. *Nurses and Nursing* (Cambridge: Harvard University Press 1927).

22. Bristow, A. T. "What Registration Has Done for the Medical Profession." *Am J Nurs* 3:3 (December 1903) p. 161–167.

23. Rawlings, B. "Nurses in Hospitals." *Nineteenth Century* 64:381 (November 1908) p. 824–836.

24. Bullough, B. "Barriers to the Nurse Practitioner Movement: Problems of Women in a Woman's Field" in Bullough, B. and Bullough, V., eds. *Expanding Horizons for Nurses* (New York: Springer Publishing Co. 1977) p. 307–318.

25. Ashley, J. *Hospitals, Paternalism, and the Role of the Nurse* (New York: Teachers College Press 1976).

26. Stafford, J. "Operation Nurse." *Science Newsletter* 51:5 (February 1, 1947) p. 74–75.

27. Madison, L. "What I Want to Be." *Occupations* 30:4 (January 1952) p. 280–281.

28. McLaughlin, K. "Needed: More Nurses." *New York Times Magazine* (March 9, 1941) p. 9+.

29. Holland, S. "The Case for Hospital Nurses." *Nineteenth Century* 51:303 (May 1902) p. 770–779.

30. Reynolds, Q. "Young Women in White." *Reader's Digest* 69:415 (November 1956) p. 79–83.

31. "Twin Nurses." *Look* 19:9 (May 3, 1955) p. 62.

32. "A Man in Blue Dons Nurse's White." *Life* 70:18 (May 14, 1971) p. 47, 48.

33. Hawes, E. "There's a Career in Nursing." *Woman's Home Companion* 70:1 (January 1943) p. 66, 67.

34. "The Nurse from a Patient's Point of View." *Am J Nurs* 7:2 (November 1906) p. 104.

35. "The Nurse's Voice." *Literary Digest* 55:19 (November 10, 1917) p. 27.

36. Fenwick, E. "Nurses a la Mode." *Nineteenth Century* 41:240 (February 1897) p. 325–332.

37. Stewart, I. "Educating Nurses." *Survey* 58:10–12 (August 15–September 15, 1927) p. 537, 538.

38. Markel, H. "Student Nurse." *Good Housekeeping* 153:1 (July 1961) p. 32+.

39. Berg, R. "Where Did All the Nurses Go?" *Look* 32:2 (January 23, 1968) p. 26+.

40. Priestley, E. "Nurses a la Mode." *Nineteenth Century* 41:239 (January 1897) p. 28–37.

41. Hoffman, R. "The Angel of Mercy Is Dead." *Mademoiselle* 66:2 (December 1976) p. 134+.

42. "Col. Clement Hails Army Nurses in Pacific: Homemaking Skills in Jungle Is Stressed." *New York Times* (May 17, 1944) p. 22.
43. "Higher Learning Urged for Nurses." *New York Times* (December 8, 1940) sec. 2, p. 4.
44. Lonsdale, M. "Doctors and Nurses." *Nineteenth Century* 7:40 (June 1880) p. 1105–1108.
45. Martin, L. "Angels of Vietnam." *Today's Health* 45:8 (August 1967) p. 16+.
46. Mayor, M. "How to Get Nurses Galore." *Reader's Digest* 56:334 (February 1950) p. 116–118.
47. Acuille, J. "I Had to Grow Up—in a Hurry." *Woman's Home Companion* 82:10 (October 1955) p. 36–38.
48. Villet, B. "More than Compassion." *Life* 72:14 (April 1972) p. 68.
49. Conley, V. "R.N.—Those Magic Initials," *Today's Health* 38:12 (December 1960) p. 38+.
50. Deming, D. "Nursing by Leg Power." *Survey* 63:4 (November 15, 1929) p. 205, 206.
51. Editorial Comment. "Nursing as a Profession." *New York Times* (May 19, 1921) p. 14.
52. Birenbaum, A. "New Health Practitioner in Primary Care." *Intellect* 105:2374 (April 1976) p. 532–534.
53. Safran, C. "Their Patients Call Them Supernurses." *Today's Health* 53:7 (July–August 1975) p. 20+.
54. "The New Family Doctor Is a Nurse." *McCalls* 103:1 (October 1975) p. 35.
55. "Where Doctors Don't Reach." *Time* 88:4 (July 22, 1966) p. 71.
56. "Minutes of the Proceedings of the Thirteenth Annual Convention of the Nurses' Associated Alumnae of the United States." *Am J Nurs* 19:10 (July 1910) p. 817–819.

8

The Missing Voices
in Coverage of Health

Bernice Buresh

*E*arlier this year a University of Pennsylvania research group reported that a noninvasive intervention could prevent the repeated hospitalizations of high-risk elderly patients, improve their overall care, and save taxpayers millions of dollars.

Sound like a candidate for a good health story? The editors of The Journal of the American Medical Association thought so. They chose it as the top item for the packet of news releases sent out to reporters about articles in the February 17 issue of JAMA.

But this story didn't get the kind of play JAMA studies often do. It did not go entirely unnoticed—it went on the Associated Press wire, National Public Radio did a report on it, and a handful of newspapers gave it a paragraph or two. The Philadelphia Inquirer's Michael Vietz developed the JAMA study into a piece on the care needs of the rapidly expanding number of elders who live with multiple chronic illnesses, and the Inquirer ran the piece on the front page. By and large, though, the media were uninterested.

There may have been several reasons why other journalists ignored the study. Perhaps old people aren't an appealing subject even though their care has a tremendous impact on health care costs, the allocation of social services and the demands on family caregivers. Maybe there was a lot of competing news that day. But as someone who has watched this happen time and time again, I can't help but think that the determining factor was that the university researchers were nurses and the intervention they tested was nursing care.

This conclusion stems from many years of writing about nursing and monitoring the coverage of this profession. Nurses are so consistently overlooked in news coverage about health and health care that it is hard not to

Bernice Buresh is a freelance writer who has been a reporter for The Milwaukee Sentinel *and a correspondent and Bureau Chief for* Newsweek. *She taught journalism for many years at Boston University and has been a Knight Journalism Fellow at Stanford and a fellow in the Joan Shorenstein Center on the Press, Politics and Public Policy at Harvard's John F. Kennedy School of Government.*

Reprinted from *Nieman Reports*, 53(3) 52–55, with permission of the Nieman Foundation, © 1999.

think that prejudice is at least partly responsible. In a study I led nine years ago, my colleagues and I found nurses and nursing to be all but absent in the health coverage of three of the nation's top newspapers. Not surprisingly, physicians accounted for almost one-third of 908 sources who were directly quoted in the stories we analyzed. However, sources from government, business, education, nonprofits, even patients and family members as well as non-professional hospital workers also were quoted more often than nurses. The voices and views of nurses came through in only 10 of the 908 quotes.

A broader study commissioned in 1997 by the nursing honor society Sigma Theta Tau International found little improvement. Named for the late Nancy Woodhull, a news executive and expert on women and the media, the recent study, like ours, found numerous examples of nurses being passed over in favor of other sources—even when it is clear that nurses would be the most logical sources. For example, a Chicago Tribune article (September 14, 1997) focuses on lay midwives and the legal prohibitions which prevent them from practicing in Illinois if they don't have a nursing degree. The article's sources included lay midwives and a physician but no practicing certified nurse midwives.

Nurses' invisibility in the news is noticeable in all aspects of health coverage. My analyses indicate that one-fourth to one-third of health news reports are devoted to coverage of research findings. That's a conservative estimate if you also count the spinoffs—backgrounders, columns and features—prompted by research studies. It is very difficult, if not impossible, to identify a column, television health program, or health section that regularly includes findings from nursing studies in its reportage.

Lack of attention to nursing research is a serious oversight because much of this burgeoning field is devoted to the most significant health care issue of our time—the care and treatment of those with chronic illness. Thanks to the many biomedical, surgical and acute care advances of the last half century, instead of being quickly killed by serious illness, large portions of our population live for lengthy periods and into advanced age with chronic diseases or conditions. These include cancer, heart disease, arthritis, high blood pressure, birth abnormalities, osteoporosis, diabetes and so on. Increasingly the "diagnosis and cure" medical model is inadequate in this environment. Ongoing care and management of these conditions is needed, and that care is the crux of nursing research.

A case in point is the JAMA study. Penn nursing researchers randomly divided 363 sick and frail elderly hospital patients into two groups. The control group received routine discharge planning and, if referred, standard home care. Those who were in the second group were visited within 48 hours of being admitted to the hospital and then every 48 hours during the hospitalization by an advance-practice nurse who specialized in geriatrics. Once the patient was discharged, the same nurse visited him or her at home at least twice and was available in person or by phone for the next month. These nurses focused on the patients' medications, symptoms, diet, activities, sleep, medical follow-up and emotional status. They collaborated with physicians to adjust therapies, obtained referrals for needed services, set up support systems, and helped the patients and their families adjust to life at home.

The outcomes tell us a lot about the efficacy of this approach. Six months after discharge, 20 percent of the group with master's-degree nurses was hospitalized again compared with 37 percent of the control group. Only 6.2 percent of the group monitored by nurses had multiple hospital readmissions, compared with 14.5 percent of the control group. When they occurred, hospital stays were much shorter for the first group—1.5 hospital days per patient compared with 4.1 days for the control group. Health care costs for the group with transitional care were $600,000 less than costs for the control group. Medicare was saved an average of $3,000 per patient. At a time when the mounting costs of health care are routinely covered on the business pages and on television news, the fact that evidence such as this was ignored is peculiar.

Patients and their families know how devastating cycling in and out of a hospital can be. As Mary D. Naylor, associate professor of nursing and the lead author of the study said, "We're still relying on hospitals to respond to what we know are, in many cases, preventable readmissions. Our system of care is not responsive to the needs of the older community." Nursing research identifies responsive care. Yet health writers seem to have little acquaintance with nursing research. One 25-year veteran of the medical and health beat who reads several medical journals told me he couldn't think of the name of a single nursing journal. Another health editor responded to a colleague of mine who raised the subject with, "Nursing what?" Even when nursing research receives the imprimatur of medicine by appearing in a top medical journal, it is still likely to be ignored.

As journalist Suzanne Gordon pointed out in her recent book, "Life Support: Three Nurses on the Front Lines," when coverage focuses exclusively on medicine, it reinforces the notion that illness is an event rather than a process. When journalists cover health innovations only as medical interventions they create a simplistic and inaccurate picture of health care. If journalists were to ask nurses how new treatments really affect patients they would have a truer picture of not only the efficacy of these treatments, but of the needs that patients have for care before, during and after medical encounters. While medical researchers and physicians develop these new treatments, nurses administer many of them and monitor their immediate and ongoing effect on patients. Nurses are the ones who know what impact these medical advances have not only on patients' cells, tissues and organ systems, but on their lives.

For patients and policymakers, a gaping informational hole remains even from the vigorous coverage of managed care. As a recent Kaiser Family Foundation study confirmed, reporters have brought the denials of treatments, medications and experimental procedures under managed care to the public's attention. They have exposed the HMO's that have tried to prevent physicians from candidly discussing a patient's condition and appropriate treatment options. They have attended to the patient backlash as well. Even nursing won a moment in the news as part of managed care coverage. A rash of stories reported that hospitals were "downsizing" and "deskilling." But few journalists examined what these cutbacks meant in terms of patient care.

Pittsburgh Post-Gazette medical writer Steve Twedt is one who did. He spent a year researching this question and talking to nurses, nursing researchers, patients, families, aides, physicians, attorneys and policymakers. "In hospital after hospital across the country," Twedt wrote in his resulting 1996 four-part series, "nurses with years of experience are being replaced by unlicensed aides who get only minimal training before caring for patients." His investigation, he wrote, produced "example after example of hospital patients throughout the nation who were injured or killed by the mistakes or negligence of aides performing duties they weren't equipped to handle." His most troubling conclusion was, "Despite the profound impact on patients, no one is systematically monitoring this sweeping change in health care."

It has similarly escaped the notice of journalists that proposed remedies to the problems of managed care do not address nursing care. The so-called patient bills of rights in state legislatures and Congress focus on medical care. With limited exceptions (childbirth and mastectomies), these bills do not constrain insurers and hospitals from restricting patients' access to nursing care. The bills that do address nursing care—those that mandate minimum levels of nurse staffing in hospitals and nursing homes—have gotten very little attention.

Reports on the effects of Medicare cuts in the balanced Budget Act of 1997 are also too narrowly focused. For example, Bob Herbert in his New York Times column (April 15, 1999) discussed the disastrous impact reduced Medicare payments are having on teaching hospitals and their ability to educate future physicians. Nursing was not mentioned once in his description of the dire effects the cuts are having on staff levels, hospital treatment and care, and professional education.

Yet teaching hospitals are nursing institutions as much as they are medical institutions. Hospitals are the primary site of nursing education. Nursing education suffers when hospital revenues drop. In fact, one of the major missed stories of this decade has been the effect of the dismissal of clinical nurse specialists and other hospital nurse educators on nursing education and practice. Nursing education has taken a direct hit in other ways, not the least of which is the reluctance of good candidates to enter a field that is being decimated and abused by market-driven health care.

Not surprisingly, the country now faces a serious nursing shortage. Although this has been reported largely as a demographic aging-of-the-nursing-workforce phenomenon, it is much more complex and interesting as evidenced by the frenzied recruiting hospitals are engaging in even while, in some cases, continuing to lay off nurses. To be sure, it is not easy to cover nursing. Although some nursing organizations and nursing schools have knowledgeable media specialists who understand the needs of journalists, in general nursing research studies and innovations in nursing practice don't arrive in the newsroom in prepackaged print or electronic form. It takes work to ferret out significant stories.

Then there is the problem of getting nurses to talk. Reporters need to understand that most nurses are employees of large institutions, and many are afraid of retribution if they say anything. Even a very small percentage of those theoretically protected by unions will go on the record. Then, too, some nurses feel so rejected by the press they have given up trying to interest journalists in developments in their discipline.

With 2.6 million members, nursing is our largest health care profession. There are many reasons to cover nursing, including the fact that press scrutiny tends to keep any important field on its toes and accountable to the public. Like medicine, nursing should be covered warts and all. One more thing to think about. Editors should lose the nurse nostalgia bit. Not long ago the Atlantic Monthly inserted sentimentalized images of nurses complete with angels' wings into a book excerpt on contemporary nursing, and Working Woman illustrated a nurse employment trend piece with a decades-old picture of a lineup of nurses in starched uniforms and cap. What editor today would illustrate a medical story with a doctor wearing an otolaryngeal mirror strapped around his head? Registered nurses haven't worn white caps since the 1970's, yet such pictures abound. These images lose their romantic appeal when you realize that you wouldn't want a nurse with a 19th Century or even 1950's education and training to take care of you any more than you would want a surgeon with training limited to those periods to operate on you.

It's time for the journalistic community to recognize nurses for what they are—flesh and blood professionals who, unlike angels, need to be paid for the extremely hard and critical work that they do and who, like their patients, are endangered in our health care system. By reporting on the vital roles nurses play in patient treatment and care and by seeking out their perspectives in any coverage of health care, journalists would add critical dimensions to the ongoing debates about what health care is going to be like for Americans in the 21st Century.

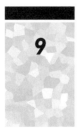

9

Nurse, Interrupted

Suzanne Gordon

It's May 13, the day after Florence Nightingale's birthday, and as part of the annual celebration of Nurses' Week—established in part to commemorate Nightingale's role in the development of professional nursing—members of the Massachusetts Nurses Association have asked me to speak to a group of registered nurses (RNs) at the University of Massachusetts Memorial Health Care Campus in Worcester. Usually, such events are upbeat—occasions for flowery praise of America's largest predominantly female profession, which is also the largest profession in the health care system. Not today. The 30 or so middle-aged nurses who straggle into a bare auditorium look like they're attending a wake.

In a sense, they are. These RNs entered the profession with high expectations and a strong sense of purpose several decades ago, but the field they work in is no longer either patient- or nurse-friendly terrain. The health care system has changed, and nurses like the weary ones at this event feel they are unable to fulfill their historic mission of caring for the sick. "Nurses are simply exhausted," explains Kate Maker, an RN for 16 years, who works on an intensive care unit (ICU). "Patients can't survive without our services. But today we can't give them those services" because they are sicker, and there are more patients for each nurse to take care of.

In the ongoing public debate about the quality of market-driven medicine, most criticism has focused on the deterioration of physician autonomy and of the doctor-patient relationship under "managed care." But health care cost cutting and competition are having an ever-more damaging impact not just on doctors but on the nation's 2.6 million RNs.

Hospital restructurings and down-sizings have slashed bedside nursing staff—the backbone of the hospital—and have replaced RNs with poorly trained and poorly paid nursing assistants. Those RNs who remain at the bedside must now care for greater numbers of sicker patients who are assembly-

Suzanne Gordon, B.A., is an author and journalist in Boston, Massachusetts.

lined through the hospital in shorter and shorter periods of time. Ironically, in an era when much attention is focused on the problem of medical errors, nurses no longer have time to be patients' 24-hours-a-day early-warning and early-intervention system. They no longer have time to get to know patients and respond to their needs. Even as the medical system as a whole becomes increasingly impersonal, nurses can no longer provide the level of comfort and compassion they once did.

The consequences of cuts in nursing care are extremely serious. Patients who could recover, don't. Preventable complications escalate. Some patients die. Moreover, as nurses are stretched too thin in the hospital and as patients are denied expert nursing care at home, the burden of care is shifted to unpaid, ill-prepared family caregivers.

Largely because of current conditions, veteran nurses are leaving the field and potential new entrants are being discouraged from joining the profession. Just as the population is aging and in need of more nursing care, the nation now faces a new nursing shortage.

■ MORE PATIENTS, FEWER NURSES

As hospitals compete for managed care contracts and try to gain clout with insurers, cost cutting is moving more and more money away from the bedside. Faced with lower fees from both HMOs and Medicare, hospitals are desperate to save money. Since RNs represent 23 percent of the hospital work force and are the biggest share of labor costs (and are only 10 percent unionized), downsizing RN staff has become an irresistible cost-reduction strategy.

Over the past decade, hospitals have turned to expensive consultants who assure anxious hospital CEOs that their product is just like any other easily definable, measurable commodity. Change the production process, make operations more efficient, replace expensive employees with cheaper ones, and help those who remain to be more productive—you'll save money without sacrificing quality, consultants say.

Hospitals have thus downsized their RN staffs through layoffs or by attrition. They have also replaced RNs, who in 1996 earned on average $37,738 plus benefits, with unlicensed assistive personnel (UAPs), who earn 20 to 40 percent less.

No states regulate the education of nurse assistants. So someone with no high school diploma and a few hours of on-the-job training may change sterile dressings, insert urinary catheters, or clean tracheostomy tubes. Meanwhile these nursing assistants are actually practicing under the supervising RN's license; under state licensure rules, the RN can be held responsible for any mistakes made by aides working under his or her direction—and can lose his or her license as a result of those mistakes.

To make sure workers are productive, hospitals may also cross-train janitors, housekeepers, transport workers, and security guards to do nursing work. (That person changing your tracheostomy tube may be a janitor!) Studies report that hospital nursing staffs, which once consisted of 85–95 percent registered nurses and only 5–15 percent aides, are now only 80, 70—sometimes 50—percent registered nurses and up to 50 percent aides.

Hospitals often dispute nurses' claims that restructuring has resulted in fewer nurses at the bedside. The American Hospital Association (AHA), for example, contends that the number of RNs employed in hospitals actually rose from 858,909 in 1992, to 901,198 in 1997. But the association does not take account of where in the hospitals RNs are working. Hospitals provide the AHA only with aggregate FTEs (full-time equivalent positions), a number that includes all RNs regardless of whether they're involved in providing direct care or have purely administrative functions, such as dealing with insurance companies.

"Hospitals now have a cadre of RNs who are taking care of the charts, not the patients," says Jean Chaisson, a clinical nurse specialist at the Beth Israel Deaconess Medical Center in Boston. "On a floor with fewer RNs spread thinner, when I'm busy rushing one patient to the operating room, these case managers or utilization reviewers are not there to help make sure another patient isn't falling on the floor."

Besides, even according to the AHA's own statistics, when RN FTEs are calculated on a per-admission basis—reflecting the volume of patients and intensity of the patients' needs—their number declines slightly. This report explains that there are "fewer RNs particularly in markets with high managed care penetration."

Nurses like Chaisson tell us that their workload has increased and that they may be taking care of two or three times the number of patients they took care of in the past—perhaps 10 to 16 patients on medical surgical floors or three to four patients in ICUs.

The Institute for Health and Socio-Economic Policy (IHSP) recently analyzed 18.2 million California hospital discharge records and other data collected from state agencies and the hospital industry for the California Nurses Association. Between 1994 and 1997, there was an 8.8-percent increase in the average number of patients for which an RN cared, a 7.2-percent decrease in the number of RNs employed, and a 7.7-percent jump in the number of patients per staffed bed between 1995 and 1998.

The New York State Nurses Association reported similar findings when it surveyed its state's RNs. Twenty-two percent of the nurses who responded said they were responsible for 10 or more patients. Hospital surgical nurses reported an average patient load of 9.4 patients, and critical care nurses, 3.14 patients. Forty-six percent of the nurses said they couldn't provide the level of nursing care patients needed.

What Jane Smith faces when she gets to work at night on an orthopedic floor in a southern community hospital is typical for today's restructured nurse. (Note: Some of the names in this article have been changed.) With only one aide, she routinely cares for up to 20 frail, elderly patients who have just emerged from the operating room after having total hip or knee replacements. Her patients are completely immobilized and may be in excruciating pain. Smith has to take their vital signs frequently, draw their blood, and every few hours inject drugs (such as pain relievers, or heart or ulcer medications) into their veins.

It is now well-known that insufficient pain medication jeopardizes a patient's ability to heal. It is also well-known that pain medication should be administered well before patients are turned or do their physical therapy. But Smith says, "If you have a really heavy patient load, you don't have time to do it. They ask for pain medication, and I tell them I'll be there as soon as I can. I recently had five patients in a row who needed meds, and I had to put them on a list. You run in there and give them meds, and get a pain scale, and ask if there's anything you can do and they'll say, 'You're too busy. I don't want to ask you.'"

Orthopedic surgeon William Marshall works with Jane Smith and shares her frustrations. Because nurses are so overloaded, he says, "you order a unit of blood at 6:30 in the morning, and you find out that at 5:30 in the evening it still has not been given. You find patients [who were] calling for medicine for pain, and it wasn't given to them until an hour-and-a-half later."

Marshall says that "cuts to the bone" are driving individual nurses to despair. "There are people with whom I've worked for 10 or 15 years," he explains with mounting distress, "and I find them in tears, saying, 'I can't stand it anymore. I'm going to leave.'"

■ SICKER PATIENTS, BUSIER NURSES

Another cost-cutting measure—shortened length of hospital stay—is changing the nature of patient needs and making it more difficult for nurses to minister to them.

For almost every operation, treatment, or diagnostic procedure requiring hospitalization, length of stay has been shortened. Although getting patients out of the hospital and back home is touted as a wonderful thing for patients, it actually makes it harder to care for those who are hospitalized.

In the past, people came into the hospital for surgery the day before their operations and stayed in the hospital until they were well on the road to recovery. Today, the 91-year-old woman who is on Jane Smith's unit (after a hip replacement operation) does not come in the day before surgery for tests, but arrives at the hospital on the day of the operation. Nor will the woman remain in the hospital until she recovers. She's out in three days. Which means she is much sicker while she's in the hospital, as are all the other patients nurses care for.

When length of stay is so truncated, the hospital becomes like a Midas muffler shop. Forty to 50 percent of the total patients admitted to a hospital may be discharged in 24 hours. Barbara Norrish of Samuel Merritt College,

Department of Nursing, and Thomas Rundall of the University of California, Berkeley's School of Public Health, have demonstrated that patients' shortened length of stay increases nurses' *cumulative* patient load. "A typical nurse may come onto her unit at 7:00 in the morning and take care of seven patients with an aide," says Norrish. "But four of those patients are discharged at noon, and four new patients are admitted at 1:00 P.M. The nurse manager who sees the patients at 1:00 P.M. will argue that the nurse only has seven patients. But she doesn't; she has 11."

Plus, with all these admissions and discharges, activity on the unit—not just at the bedside—also escalates with nurses spending as much time talking to home care agencies, rehabilitation facilities, nursing homes, or family members, negotiating the hand-off of the patient, as they do for direct patient care.

Erica Wilson, who works in an oncology clinic in a prestigious teaching hospital in a major metropolitan area in the Northeast, is a case in point. In her clinic, the same number of RNs now see more patients than ever before. Half of Wilson's patients are on experimental treatments. She must spend more time reviewing treatment plans and double-checking calculations of drug dosages. Because the side effects of experimental drugs aren't well-known, those drugs must be infused more slowly. Wilson also has to closely monitor patients, respond to any hint of an adverse reaction, and review with patients complex schedules for chemotherapy.

Many of her patients now take highly toxic drugs—drugs that used to be administered in a hospital or clinic—at home. If they experience side effects, they call the clinic. Wilson must leave patients to respond to these calls. At the same time, patients who have been discharged from the hospital while they are still ill are bringing more serious problems to the clinic. And the increased volume of sicker patients leads to more clinic emergencies like cardiac and respiratory arrests. As a result of the volume and acuity of patients, "things are being missed," she says. "If we aren't making major mistakes, it's by the skin of our teeth."

Such heavy caseloads don't only detract from patient care; they erode the quality of the nurses' working life. Harried RNs say they have no time to go to the bathroom, eat lunch, or have a cup of coffee much less get off the unit to attend essential educational seminars.

One stressed-out emergency room nurse explains that she has more than once almost fainted because she can't find a moment in her eight-hour shift to get a bite to eat. Another RN tells me she won't drink tea or coffee on the job because caffeine just makes her go to the bathroom, and she has no time to take a toilet break. More say they suffer from stress-related illnesses, like ulcers, colitis, and hypertension. Because they are unable to get help turning and moving patients, many report back injuries.

According to the Bureau of Labor Statistics, 700,000 health care workers suffered an injury or illness in 1996—twice as many as were reported in 1990. The rate of injuries surpassed that of manufacturing, construction, and mining, which are well-known high-hazard industries. Of the 91 categories of workers the Bureau of Labor Statistics measures, RNs ranked fourth in days lost at work due to nonfatal illnesses and injuries. Only "stock handlers and baggers," "freight and stock material handlers," and "laborers/construction workers"—all primarily male—had more illnesses and injuries. In Minnesota, between 1990 and 1994, when restructuring efforts reduced nursing by 9.2 percent, there was a 65-percent increase in RN work-related injuries and illnesses.

Nurses' morale is also plummeting because of an increased use of "floating" and mandatory overtime, scheduling practices that nurses have long deplored as unsafe to patients and demeaning to nurses. When nurses float, they are moved from the unit where they usually work to one with which they may not be familiar. For example, if a cardiac nurse calls in sick or goes on vacation, managers may send an oncology nurse to replace him or her. "Would you ask an ear, nose, and throat doctor or dermatologist to cover cardiology for the day and expect high quality care?" Jean Chaisson asks. "I don't think so."

Today, after an exhausting 8- or 12-hour shift, a nurse may also suddenly learn that he or she has to work an extra 8 or 12 hours. For a largely female work force with child care and family responsibilities, this is particularly onerous.

"You work from 3:00 in the afternoon to 11:00 at night. You have arranged for someone to take care of your kids," says Kate Maker, a nurse at the University of Massachusetts Medical Center in Worcester. "So at 10:00 you're told you have to work mandatory overtime. Well, just like the hospital can't pull nurses out of the sky to suddenly work 11 to 7, we can't pull babysitters out of the sky at 11:00 at night to take care of our kids. We're put in the terrible position of having to choose between abandoning our patients and abandoning our children." If RNs protest that these assignments are unsafe for their patients, they are often warned that refusing the assignments will constitute "patient abandonment"—a charge that can lead to a disciplinary action by the state Board of Registration in Nursing.

Perhaps more than anything else, nursing morale has bottomed out because RNs say they no longer have time to really "care" for their patients. "Before, I was able to sit in a room and teach patients about their care and listen to them," an ICU nurse in the Midwest told me. "But today, you can't have any kind of interaction with patients. You don't have time to talk with them, or hold their hand, or be with them. Today, we only have time to take care of their tubes." This nurse eventually left the hospital.

■ LOSING NURSES, LOSING LIVES

Not surprisingly, patients and their family members are feeling the side effects of the disorganization of nursing care. Madge Kaplan is the Boston-based Health Desk editor for National Public Radio's *Marketplace* show. Last winter, her 81-year-old father had a stroke and was hospitalized at a major northeastern teaching hospital. He then spent a total of three months in its inpatient and rehabilitation units. The medical aspects of his care, Kaplan explains, were excellent.

But Kaplan adds, "If my father or the three other patients in his room needed to go to the bathroom, if they needed to reposition themselves to eat a meal, if they needed help in adjusting their position in a wheelchair, if they needed help unwrapping utensils to eat a meal, that help was not forthcoming."

It was "tragic," Kaplan says, to watch "these frightened, frail elderly patients push themselves to the limit of their energy to get someone to pay attention to them. Pleading with someone to get a glass of water or to wipe someone up when they had spilled something on their bed."

Kaplan, like Jane Smith's patients, understood that the nursing staff were overwhelmed. "Nurses seemed to have their hands full—so much so that I always came away feeling that staff seemed tense, stretched, and in no mood to engage with patients and the people visiting them."

Although boosters of market-driven health care insist that "consumers" like Kaplan and her father will vigorously advocate for themselves when they don't get the service they expect, neither complained to hospital administration. Why? Because when people are sick, vulnerable, and totally dependent, they are loath to alienate those who hold their lives in their hands.

Patients do, however, register their concerns when they are not immediately dependent on their hospital for care. In 1996, the AHA sent its members a confidential report entitled "Reality Check: Public Perceptions of Health Care and Hospitals." The report summarized data gathered in focus groups with 300 patients in 12 states plus an opinion survey of another 1,000 patients. "The key indicator that people referred to as a measure of quality of their hospital care," the report stated, "was the nurse."

The report went on to say that those surveyed

> hold a strong belief that skilled nurses are being systematically replaced by poorly trained and poorly paid aides. Their perspective on the "thinness" of hospital nurse staffing was reflected in a universally mentioned experience: "If I hadn't stayed in the hospital room with my mother, child, or spouse, they would never have gotten the correct medication or care on time." People believe the profit motive is behind the reduction in nursing care. They are angry at the reversal in health care priorities this represents.

In the face of patient and nurse complaints, the hospital and insurance industries often argue that nurses have not proven their worth and that their critical role in patient care has not been scientifically documented.

Nothing could be further from the truth. While nursing's contributions—like those of other predominantly female occupations—have hardly received the kind of research attention devoted to the highly male medical profession, there is, in fact, a considerable body of scientific literature that explains what nurses do and why it is critical to patient health.

Jeffrey H. Silber and his colleagues at the University of Pennsylvania School of Medicine are studying an important variable in determining patient mortality—what they call "failure to rescue." These researchers report that among hospitals with comparably adjusted case mixes, some are better at "rescuing" patients than others. Working with researchers Linda Aiken and Julie Sochalski of the University of Pennsylvania School of Nursing, they have identified the critical factors in patient rescue. Hospitals need to have enough educated staff who recognize a problem when they see it. Those staff must be with patients enough of the time and must have enough status and authority in the institution to mobilize resources and deal with crises. Nurses, the researchers explain, are the educated eyes-on/hands-on, 24-hour-surveillance-and-intervention system in hospitals.

When, as other recent studies confirm, hospitals employ enough educated nurses and give them ample time with patients, patients have fewer urinary tract infections, falls, pneumonias, and bedsores. And they are less likely to die. When Aiken and her colleagues analyzed the care of AIDS patients, they documented that "an additional 0.5 nurse per patient per day—or an additional nurse for every six patients on each eight-hour shift—would be expected to reduce the likelihood of [patients] dying by roughly one-third."

In October, Michael Rie, an anesthesiologist and intensive care physician at the University of Kentucky, presented a quality-assurance analysis of ICU readmissions in one university hospital. (The data were collected in response to findings that the average length of ICU stay for patients with respiratory problems was longer than that suggested by a nationally accepted benchmark.) The study found that patients at low risk of death and/or readmission to ICU—who had been discharged to regular hospital floors—were being readmitted at a seemingly elevated rate. Patients with a predicted low risk of death, 10 percent, had an actual mortality rate of 24 percent.

When investigators explored why patients were readmitted to the ICU, they discovered that 80 percent of these patients had potentially preventable ICU readmissions. The problem was they weren't receiving enough basic respiratory care on non-ICU floors. A plausible inference is that there weren't enough staff in this hospital to suction patients' lungs and help them cough.

Not only is this endangering patients' health and sometimes their lives; it's not even cost-effective. In this particular hospital, for example, the nonlabor costs for the ICU readmission of only 79 patients was $1.6 million—or 35 percent of the cost of their entire hospitalization. If labor costs were added to this figure, it would be two to three times as high. (This points to the need not just for better staffing but also for intermediate care units that provide a level of services less intensive than in ICUs but more intensive than on general care floors.) The fact that cutting nursing services doesn't save money is confirmed in other studies about hospital restructuring.

Laying off RNs and replacing them with aides works only for so long. Eventually hospitals have to hire additional RNs. But today, when they try to fill vacancies, many hospitals are finding it more and more difficult to attract new recruits. In a report on the new nursing shortage, even the AHA concludes that "RN Dissatisfaction May Be Driving the Current Shortage in Hospitals."

This increasingly well-publicized dissatisfaction with working conditions and concern about the quality of patient care is driving young women and men away from studying nursing in the first place. In an era of low unemployment, especially when women have more career options than ever before, why would anyone want to spend the time and money involved in getting a nursing education for the privilege of being part of a cheap, disposable labor force? And why would more men decide to enter a "women's profession" that even women are finding unattractive? It is hardly surprising that the number of young people interested in entering four-year nursing programs has been steadily declining over the past four years and fell by 5.5 percent in 1998.

■ WHAT CAN BE DONE

For the past several years, nurses have tried to focus public attention on the erosion of their working conditions. This summer, both Massachusetts and California passed whistle-blower bills. And after intense pressure from the California Nurses Association, California Governor Gray Davis recently signed the first safe-staffing law anywhere in the country (and he did it despite the opposition of the state's hospital industry). This measure requires that, by the year 2002, the state Department of Health implement safe nurse-to-patient ratios and limit the floating of nurses between units.

But while legislation like California's can help alleviate the nation's persistent nursing crisis, it is only a short-term solution. Many other, more fundamental changes need to be made in both the financing and delivery of health care. As long as we have a job-based, employer-dominated private health insurance system in which billions of dollars are siphoned off every year for unnecessary advertising, marketing, and administrative costs (not to mention insurance and drug company profiteering), those who provide hands-on care will always be starved for resources.

But though national health insurance is a necessary first step toward improvement, it is not in itself a sufficient condition for quality nursing care. Even if America eventually provides tax-supported coverage as Canadians have had since the 1970s, nursing care may still be a cost-cutting target (as it has been in Canada lately) if the value that nurses add to the health care system is not recognized.

In other words, despite recent curbs on physician autonomy and specialist referrals, most people—even under the degraded conditions of managed care—regard *medically necessary care* as an entitlement. There is, however, no parallel conception of *necessary nursing care.* If such a concept did exist, the training and deployment of nurses and the organization of nursing care within hospitals would be seen as no less important to patient outcomes than medicine's role in diagnosis and treatment. The dangers of both radically reduced hospital stays and insufficient nursing care in other settings would be more widely understood. And there would be better pay for and treatment of nurses as well as greater social recognition and respect.

Our contract with RNs would be, in effect, that we must care about *them* if we want them to care for us.

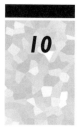

10

Nursing Schools Perplexed by Falling Enrollments

Katherine S. Mangan

Celia Collins has wanted to become a nurse since she was six, when she lived in a small town in Jamaica. Her family's next-door neighbor, a nurse and midwife, would lift her over the hibiscus-covered fence between their homes and let her tag along on house calls.

A dozen years later, as a high-school senior in Boston, Ms. Collins eagerly accepted Boston College's offer of admission to its School of Nursing, where she is now a junior. Her mother, a single parent who had barely eked out a living teaching in Jamaica, had moved to Boston to be near relatives.

Ms. Collins also does some recruiting for Boston College, and when she enters high schools, she finds that few students share her passion for nursing. More and more students are turning their backs on the field, which could spell trouble for the nation's health-care system.

HELPING AN AGING POPULATION

The number of students enrolled in bachelor's-degree programs at U.S. nursing schools has slid 17 per cent in the past four years, according to a survey by the American Association of Colleges of Nursing. Enrollment in master's-level nursing programs, which had been climbing steadily, dropped 2 per cent in 1998. The findings are based on the responses of 531, or 80 per cent, of the U.S. nursing schools with bachelor's- and graduate-degree programs.

The declining interest in nursing careers comes at a time when they should be an easy sell. The nation's elderly population is expanding rapidly, and the average age of nurses is also rising, meaning that there may soon be too few nurses to go around. The U.S. Bureau of Labor statistics has predicted that job opportunities for registered nurses will grow by 21 per cent by 2006, compared with a 14-per-cent increase for all other occupations. If current enrollment trends continue, the nation will face a nursing shortage beginning in 2010, according to the Division of Nursing of the U.S. Department of Health and Human Services.

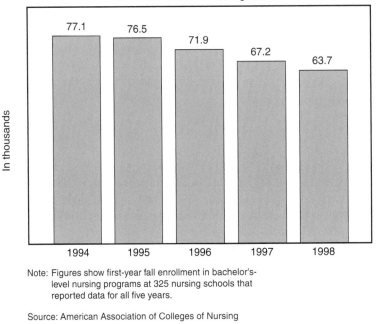

Enrollment Trends at Nursing Schools

Note: Figures show first-year fall enrollment in bachelor's-
level nursing programs at 325 nursing schools that
reported data for all five years.

Source: American Association of Colleges of Nursing

Chronicle chart by Jasmine Stewart

Experts cite a number of reasons why enrollment is sliding, even as job prospects improve. Among the explanations are:

- The perception among students that the number of nursing positions will decline as hospitals consolidate their services and merge.
- The fear that managed care, with its emphasis on cost cutting and efficiency, is pushing patients out of hospitals more quickly, reducing the demand for nurses.
- The enrollment caps that some nursing schools have established. Due to budget cuts, many schools say they do not have enough faculty members to teach classes, or to oversee students' clinical training.
- The several years of stagnating or falling wages for nurses. The average annual salary for registered nurses employed by hospitals—about $40,000—dropped 1.5 per cent per year from 1994 to 1997.

Much of the bad press is yesterday's news. Amid a wave of hospital mergers in the early 1990s, thousands of nurses lost their jobs. In Boston, for example, 10 major hospital systems have been reduced to four, creating a widespread perception in the city that nursing is a dead-end profession. But many hospitals in Boston and elsewhere have found that they cut too close to the bone, and they have recently stepped up their hiring, several national studies show.

"Part of the problem is just bad publicity," says Barbara Munro, dean of nursing at Boston College. "People hear that hospitals are closing and that there are fewer jobs, and that's just not true.

"Many hospitals cut their nursing staffs more than they should have, and under-anticipated the number of patients they'd have today. Now, they are having to go back and reopen units that were closed, and rehire nurses," she says.

But with the number of nursing graduates declining, some hospitals are having a tough time filling those positions, she says. Among the hardest hit sections of hospitals are critical care, labor and delivery, and emergency-room care.

At Beth Israel Deaconess Medical Center, where Ms. Collins assists the nursing staff as part of her clinical training, the nurses are often stretched to the limit. When she's not answering patients' call lights, she's hustling from room to room to help nurses.

"Every nurse is pulling you, asking 'Can you help me in this room?'" she says. "You rarely get to take a break."

Still, she remains enthusiastic about a profession that many of her peers seem to be rejecting.

"Seeing the condition people are in when they walk into the hospital, and seeing them leave with their families. I know I'm part of something very important," says Ms. Collins. "It's very uplifting."

Nursing schools hope that kind of enthusiasm will spread. Boston College, which enrolled only 40 new nursing students in 1997—less than half the number that matriculated during an average year in the early 1990s—is sending students such as Ms. Collins back to their high schools to try to convince skeptical students that nursing really is a good career path. The aggressive recruiting increased the size of last fall's entering class to 70 students.

Boston College went even further this winter, writing to students who had expressed interest in nursing on their PSAT to invite them to spend a weekend meeting faculty members. The students were put up in dormitories and given tours of the campus and city. The college's efforts seem to be paying off—18 of the 19 students who attended the weekend event have applied for early admission.

■ REDUCING CLASS SIZE

The College of Nursing at the University of Cincinnati responded to declining interest in the field by intentionally reducing the size of its entering class—from 120 in 1997 to 96 in 1998. Applications for the 1998 class were down 20 percent, and college officials worried that the quality would suffer if they had to dip too deeply into the candidate pool to fill a class.

"There is a demand and a need for nurses, but a lot of people have this misconception that there's an oversupply," says Andrea R. Lindell, dean of nursing at Cincinnati and president of the American Association of Colleges of Nursing.

Beth Mancini, senior vice-president for nursing administration at Parkland Hospital in Dallas, says some hospitals in her area are reporting that as many as 12 per cent of their available nursing positions remain unfilled.

Many other hospitals that have laid off registered nurses, who must pass a state licensing examination, and replaced them with cheaper workers are finding that the new workers are not as efficient. "When they tried to use less-expensive personnel, they found that it was more expensive, not less," says Ms. Munro, of Boston College.

In fact, several national advisory groups have urged nursing schools to expand advanced-level programs, to produce more nurses who are comfortable with medicine's ever-increasing complexity. The National Advisory Council on Nurse Education and Practice, which advises the federal Division of Nursing, has recommended that at least two-thirds of nurses have bachelor's degrees by 2010. Currently, fewer than a third do.

Enrollment in programs that train nurse practitioners—higher-level nurses who assume many of the primary-care functions of physicians—increased 1 per cent from 1997 to 1998, to 19,190, according to the study by the nursing-college association.

Mary Daugherty, a second-year student enrolled in a master's program in nursing offered jointly by Samuel Merritt College and Saint Mary's College of California, says she chose the field largely because of the employment outlook. "The job prospects are excellent, because there's such an overwhelming demand for nurse practitioners," says Ms. Daugherty, who is studying in Oakland, California.

An aging work force should make that demand even greater in the next decade, according to experts. The average age of nurses rose from 40 in 1980 to 44 in 1998.

"Due to the aging of the work force alone, I believe we will have a large reduction in the number of nurses in the market, a problem we haven't had to deal with in the past 20 to 30 years," says Peter I. Buerhaus, director of the Harvard Nursing Research Institute and an assistant professor at the Harvard School of Public Health.

■ PROVIDING CLINICAL TRAINING

Among the biggest challenges in educating nurses is finding clinical-training sites, and preceptors who want to work with students.

As medical schools shift more of their training toward primary care, they're competing directly with nursing schools for clinical sites. At the same time, some health-maintenance organizations that train nursing students have cut back on their training hours.

As a consequence, some nursing schools have cut their enrollments simply because they have no place to train new students.

And preceptors who used to work free are increasingly demanding wages, arguing that in an era of managed care, they cannot afford to have their productivity and efficiency hampered.

The problem is, many nursing schools can't afford to pay them.

"We could not absorb that kind of a hit," says Rita Carty, dean of the College of Nursing and Health Science at George Mason University. "We would have to pass that cost directly on to the students."

Ms. Munro says if current trends continue, the quality of health care will be seriously compromised.

"I've spent my life in nursing education," she says. "When the time comes that I need a nurse, I'll be very upset if no one is available."

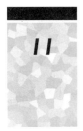

The Struggle for Just Compensation

Patricia Brider

"Are [our] ideals incompatible with sound business principles?"

A Johns Hopkins nurse put the question to *AJN* in 1914, adding that in her opinion, "It is not in any way unworthy or contemptible for nurses to look on their life-work as professional people look on theirs." How can nursing attract talented women who must support themselves, she asked, when those who choose other fields "reach a greater earning capacity at a much younger age than a nurse can, and keep it to a greater age?"

From its beginnings, the nursing profession has grappled with its own ambivalence: how to reconcile the ideal of selfless service with the necessity of making a living.

It's no accident that for nearly a century, nurses have been at the center of almost continual crisis, with "shortages" alternating regularly with unemployment. In journals, memoirs and letters to *AJN*, nurses down the years have recorded both their joy in productive careers and their disappointment with the way their work was valued.

Nursing scholars have passed some harsh judgments. The common charge is that nursing's early conditioning was acquired in schools that "exploited" students as a labor pool. Others trace nurses' economic status to a classic male-female competition in which physicians and hospitals have usually held the winning hands. Nurses have been subjected to group psychoanalysis in dozens of studies that came to the same unsurprising conclusion: They would like to apply their skills more freely and pay their bills more promptly.

It's no wonder that nurses early on developed an unparalleled skill at "role-playing." At each step in the evolution of health care in this country, they have taken the stage in a new role that transformed the way they performed, without resolving their economic dilemma.

Patricia Brider, news editor, American Journal of Nursing, *New York.*

■ STUDENTS AS CAREGIVERS

"The discipline was military. . . ."

More than one nurse of the early 1900s recalled her education in those terms.

It all began with Florence Nightingale's determination to replace hospitals' untrained and often disreputable "attendants" with a corps of efficient and respectable young women. They were to learn on the hospital wards how to apply "trained powers of observation and reflection."

America's early schools, at first independently run, were soon absorbed into the hospital's administrative structure. By 1900, the pattern was entrenched; undergraduates supplied the care under the supervision of senior students. The school's superintendent was often the only graduate nurse on the premises.

Students were typically housed three to a room in dormitories, subject to early curfews and battalions of regulations. In return for an $8- to $12-a-month "allowance," they rose at dawn and worked 10–15 hours, often seven days a week. Formal instruction accounted for about 2% of the curriculum; most spare time was spent sewing bandages, washing windows and cleaning floors.

"There are so many rules, such miles and miles of red tape," seethed a student in a 1908 diary entry. "To say that any tendency to experiment and find a better way of doing things is discouraged is putting it very mildly indeed."

"It oughtn't to be necessary to break down one's health to become a graduate nurse, but that is what it amounts to," she added. Some did succumb to typhoid, scarlet fever, pneumonia or diphtheria. As late as 1932, a University of Minnesota study found that 84% of its students reacted positively to the tuberculin test.

Almost from the start, nurses raised their voices against grinding routines that left little energy for learning. A New York graduate recalled one practice as especially frustrating: "We were sent out on private duty for which the hospital received $16 a week, and we received nothing. Some spent almost all their second and third years on cases, losing the greater part of their operating room training."

"Industrial slavery" was the term applied to early nursing schools by the vice president of the New York Academy of Medicine, Arthur Bristow, in 1906.

At that time, "a man or woman could be expected to spend seven or eight years (including high school) in preparation for a life-work if the income afterward was to be $1,500 or $2,000," said Bristow. But after talking to many nurses, he had discovered to his "utter astonishment" that their earnings would average $650. Because the work was so "severe," he was told, the average nurse could expect a career of 10 years at the most. "Do the returns warrant the outlay?" he asked.

■ THE FREE-LANCE NURSE

"Private duty is too much a game of chance . . ."

An Ohio RN delivered the verdict as she quit the profession in 1928.

Veterans of the era agree on the "ghastly hours" and the "soul-crushing exhaustion." They also have warm remembrances of the "wonderful friends" . . . "entering a home where all is confusion and getting things straightened out" . . . "seeing a patient after a hard night drop into an hour of restful sleep."

For decades, nursing essentially meant taking care of patients in the home. Through the 1920s, private-duty nurses still accounted for over 50% of the RN workforce.

Most worked on a 24-hour basis, snatching two hours' sleep when they could. They were responsible for the family's morale as well as the patient's, and often for cooking and cleaning too. When operations were performed at home, they were the ones who set up the dining table or operating-board and sterilized equipment in the family wash boiler.

The conventional wisdom was that those who had the knack of falling in with a family's ways prospered in private-duty practice; others did not. By the standards of the day, those who worked steadily were well-paid, and even envied by women in other lines of work. They were apt to earn $20 to $25 a week, for example, in the years from 1900 to 1910, when sirloin steak cost 22¢ a pound and a good striped work dress could be had for $3.

But the 1920s saw the average private-duty nurse out of work five months out of 12 and clearing about $1,300 in the other seven months. By comparison, New York City schoolteachers started at $1,500 a year in 1926 and in-

TABLE 11-1. RNs Bring Up the Rear in Career Gains

Occupation	Average Starting Salary ($)	Average Maximum Salary ($)	Salary Progression (%)
Accountants	22,073	68,252	209.2
Attorneys	36,365	118,601	226.1
Engineers	29,340	83,248	183.7
Personnel Specialists	22,229	53,816	142.1
Registered Nurses	24,605	41,662	69.3

RNs' pay "makes limited progress over a typical career," says ANA, citing BLS figures that show maximum salaries averaging only 68% over starting pay.
Copyright © 1990, J. B. Lippincott. Reprinted with permission from the *American Journal of Nursing*, 90(10), 77–80, 83–88, Oct. 1990.

creased their earnings to $2,800 after 13 years. The nurse's earnings seldom increased and were likely to fall off toward the end of her career.

Moreover, most private-duty nurses supported at least one family member. For those not living with a family on long-term cases, room rent consumed 25–30% of their income. "Boots and walking skirts wear out as if they were alive and had a grudge to pay off; hats look a fright in two months if they must be worn out, rain or shine," wrote Wisconsin nurse Grace Holmes in 1907. Holmes advised spending at least 25¢ for lunch: "It is poor economy to eat too cheap lunches."

Many "live from hand to mouth . . . never knowing from day to day what their income will be," concluded a 1928 study.

Nurses' recollections stress the wrenching uncertainty of the work: "Scrubwomen have steady employment, always get $4 per day and work only eight hours" . . . "I have never made more than $1,000 in any one year" . . . "I will land in the poorhouse; I hope to go back to secretarial work" . . . "There is no protection, no bonus, no vacation with pay; the compensation leaves very little for retirement and living expenses."

Before pensions and Social Security were dreamt of, independent careers were especially precarious for those who stayed single. Calculations vary, but agree that 60 to 80 percent of nurses through 1930 were unmarried. In middle age, these women were often invalided by the cumulative impact of 24-hour shifts. All eventually discovered that "doctors and hospitals demand young, energetic nurses," as one maturing California nurse noted wryly.

The American Nurses' Association pleaded with its members to save money, invest and buy annuities. Many failed to do so, and letters to *AJN*, described their "appalling condition." One told of "Miss S, a very superior and successful nurse": "Though she has been nursing almost steadily since graduation, she has only $200 laid by. She is alone in the world. She longs for rest, but there is no rest in sight. . . . Loved ones needed her help and she gave it. But what is to become of *her*?"

■ THE PUBLIC HEALTH CRUSADER

"Public health is the supreme adventure . . ."

A Pennsylvania nurse saw it that way in the 1920s, when a fourth of the nation's nurses were working to improve maternity and infant care, eradicate TB and take health care into rural areas.

The field evolved apart from the medical-oriented mainstream, emphasizing preventive care and offering the chance to practice with a unique degree of autonomy. Public health nurses also upgraded their economic status; as one said, "I have never borrowed money since I gave up private duty." In 1926, PHNs reported a starting average of $1,450 a year and an overall average of $1,700, compared to the private-duty nurse's $1,300 and the $2,079 computed for the graduate nurses then beginning to be hired in larger numbers by hospitals.

Paychecks improved as the focus of public health shifted from voluntary agencies to hospitals and municipal health departments. Then, under increasing budget pressures, the public health workforce gradually declined to about 7% of the RN population. By 1988, a public health staff nurse's income was running 10% behind hospital norms, and the recent escalation in hospital pay substantially widened the gap.

■ THE FRACTIONAL NURSE

"Work grows scarce, with short cases. What is to become of older nurses?"

The question was posed by a New York nurse, describing a job market that was anything but roaring. To stay employed in the 1920s, many nurses had to cast themselves in unaccustomed roles as hourly or group practitioners.

What happened to private-duty nursing was an open secret. With hospitals increasingly the focus of health care, their schools churned out nursing graduates without regard to the nation's need for all of them. While the medical profession was cutting back its numbers of students, the number of hospital nursing schools grew from 432 in 1900 to 2,155 in 1926. The nurse-physician ratio reversed itself: in 1900, there were 90 nurses for every 1,000 physicians; by 1920, there were 1,029 nurses per 1,000 physicians.

"Hourly nursing" was not a new idea; nursing leaders at the turn of the century had called for "sliding scales," pointing out that the then-prevailing weekly charge of $20 to $25 was more than the average breadwinner earned in a week. Thirty years later, surveys showed that only 9% of U.S. families had hired private-duty nurses over the previous three years.

Seeking economic leverage for private-duty nurses, ANA promoted a network of nurse-run registries and backed experiments in "group" nursing that had special-duty RNs dividing their time among two or three hospital patients. As well as a way of broadening the market, the group plan was a means of spreading work among more nurses.

Special-duty shifts had by then shortened to 12 hours in most hospitals. Because typical group plans called for cutting the standard $6 to $7 fee for 12 hours to $4 or $5 for 8 hours, the scheme met with mixed reactions among the nursing ranks.

More effective than most of these moves was a steady barrage of criticism of schools for flooding the market with graduates that most hospitals refused to employ. In a landmark 1928 study, the Committee on the Grading of Nursing Schools corrected some misconceptions; only 2,151 out of 7,416 hospitals were running schools. But those 2,151 hospitals housed 60 percent of acute-care beds; most others were staffed mainly by "attendants."

By the committee's standards, hundreds of schools were woefully under-staffed and short of clinical facilities. They existed, it was charged, only be-cause "it is cheaper to run a poor school than it is to pay graduate nurses."

The committee called for action to "grade" schools and weed out inferior ones. The study's director, May Burgess, said the system made no sense: "Who can imagine a bank openly preferring to staff its offices with utterly un-trained students, teach them all it can in three years, and as soon as they have learned the rudiments of banking, discharge them all and seek a new supply of untrained students to take their places?"

■ STAFF NURSES: THE HOSPITAL'S NEW BACKBONE

"I appreciate my clean bed, my somewhat regulated life . . ."

The California nurse who made the comment had switched from private duty to hospital work ten years before. "Self-preservation is the law of nature," she noted. "Have gained 25 pounds. Don't look as old as I did nine years ago. Have been able to accumulate some property. Have been ill only three days in ten years."

The great Depression of the 1930s effectively ended the argument about how health care should be staffed. In 1927, most hospitals that sponsored schools depended entirely on student labor. A decade later, almost all of them employed some graduate nurses.

Meantime, private-duty nurses' earnings had plunged to an average $737 a year, according to an ANA survey. Some registries calculated that the RNs on their rolls averaged less than two months' employment in 1932. Nursing groups all over the country asked *AJN* to caution RNs against moving in their direction. "Cases are short and far between," wrote Albuquerque's registry. "Nurses are advised not to come to Seattle expecting work," warned the King County association.

Stiffening the competition for jobs, industrial and office nurses were laid off. Married nurses, who once could be depended on to retire permanently, streamed back to work in earnest when their husbands were laid off.

Weaker schools began to close as ANA launched a drive to increase em-ployment of graduate nurses. Hospital heads began to debate the costs of a stable staff vs. the expense of upgrading schools enough to satisfy their critics.

Tipping the balance was the desperation of many RNs who accepted pay cuts and, in some cases, worked without pay in return for room and board, then valued at $10 a week "at least."

In the spirit of economy, the 8-hour day and the 48-hour week began to dawn. Cincinnati hospitals conformed to the pattern in 1934, dividing the two

12-hour special-duty shifts then prevalent into three 8-hour shifts. The $15 charge for the shift was split among three nurses instead of two.

On the same principle, hospitals like Ellis in Schenectady decided to employ five 8-hour nurses for every three who were then on staff on 10-hour schedules, spreading the salaries for the three current employees among the five. With the reduced pay, "we now have all our general staff nurses on 8-hour shifts at an average salary of about $50 [a month]," the hospital reported.

Shortened schedules were the tradeoffs for cuts in pay. On the whole, however, hospital salaries stayed in line with those for other professional women of the 1930s. The grading committee, updating its work in 1932, urged nurses to consider "the physical comforts hospitals give": "The salary of $60 a month with maintenance in a high-grade hospital is equivalent to at least $140 a month without maintenance."

Though a free-lance nurse could get by on less than $20 a week in the mid-1930s, the trick was to find the $20. The transition to the relative security of institutional work, once undertaken, was usually a permanent one. Many who made it recorded, in letters and surveys, their relief and satisfaction with the "regular pay and hours" . . . "work that's full of interest" . . . "the companionship of other nurses" . . . "the homelike conditions when off duty."

Not all who took refuge in hospitals were thrilled with the structured environment and "heavy responsibility." A California nurse voiced a key complaint to be echoed down the years: "I was nearly always expected to do more than it was possible to do, and my off-duty time found me in a state of exhaustion so that I was unable to act or feel like a normal individual."

▨ THE COLLECTIVE NURSE

"Florence Nightingale was a scrapper, too!"

That assertion signaled a new point of view on the RN's role. The president of the California Nurses Association, Mary Stanley, said it in 1966 as San Francisco RNs decided to try something new—peaceful informational picketing for a raise in pay, then barely over $400 a month at the starting level.

The step was not taken lightly. For over 50 years, nurses had disparaged labor unions as "unprofessional."

Some minds began to change with the transition to jobs in hospitals. Those who moved out of the isolation of private duty soon realized that professionals in other fields were making economic and social gains denied to nurses.

Social Security was an especially sore point; nurses at that time were excluded from the legislation that gave most U.S. workers the protection of some retirement income and unemployment compensation. In 1946, the Bureau of Labor Statistics reported "a widespread feeling of insecurity" among institutional nurses. The majority by then were living outside of hospital quarters. Most had no pension plan, and only industrial nurses could count on unemployment and old-age benefits. Two in five were covered by a hospitalization plan, but most had to pay for it. Over half those who worked overtime got no extra pay. Off-shift differentials were still the exception. One of the nurses quoted calculated that after allowing for childcare, income tax and carfare, she netted 30¢ for a day's work.

Judging that the time had come, the American Nurses' Association offered itself as a vehicle for salary reform that could also speak with authority to professional issues. ANA adopted a national Economic Security program in 1946 and campaigned for more equitable salaries and a 40-hour week. But Congress narrowed the program's reach by passing the 1947 Taft-Hartley Act, which exempted nonprofit hospitals from bargaining.

While ANA fought to roll back the law, nursing's economic status slipped steadily. A 1955 study showed general-duty RNs starting at about $250 a month and making $70 less, on the average, than factory workers. Eight years later, general-duty salaries were averaging $86.50 a week—$1,465 a year less than teachers' and next to lowest of the professional and technical occupations.

Long-simmering frustrations exploded in the spring of 1966. California Nurses Association members at three private San Francisco hospitals confronted managers with 40 pages of grievances. The move roused nurses at other area hospitals. Over 30 hospitals were drawn into the confrontation, which climaxed with nearly 2,000 RNs submitting resignations. A fact-finding panel granted 30–40% raises that made San Francisco nurses the highest-paid in the U.S., at rates ranging from $600 a month for beginners to $700 after five years.

The San Francisco success ignited uprisings across the country. Salaries began to climb as ANA announced a national starting goal of $6,500 in 1966 and rescinded the no-strike policy it had adopted in 1950. Within four years, 45 state nurses' associations had established employment standards and 32 had negotiated 333 contracts for 40,200 nurses. Working with labor groups, ANA won repeal of the hospital exemption in 1974, allowing SNAs to organize nonprofit institutions.

The state associations have guarded their members' economic welfare in good times and bad, through contracts that usually set the standard in their communities. SNAs have also successfully tackled practice issues through mechanisms like the "professional performance" committees that became the centerpiece of CNA's contracts.

Better benefits were a focus from the first. Under continued pressure, most hospitals have gradually upgraded their policies; according to a new Hewitt Associates survey, over three-fourths now offer a "defined-benefit" pension plan as well as health insurance; over half cover 80–100% of hospital bills minus a $100 or $200 deductible.

Much of the impetus for change has come from the 139,000 ANA members now enrolled in 841 bargaining units in 27 states. Smaller numbers, totaling about 190,000, belong to a variety of labor unions. More than 1,000,000 RNs remain uncovered by any kind of contract. Organizers charge that efforts to recruit these nurses have been undermined by policies of the National Labor Relations Board that allow hospitals to stall unionizing moves. Whether they can continue to evade organizing will likely be decided by the Supreme Court, which has been asked to rule on a new NLRB policy that would ease the process of setting up all-RN units.

With the great majority of nurses still unrepresented, the pace of overall salary growth has been controlled by shifting trends in hospital spending.

As a University of Texas survey gauges it, staff nurse salaries since 1972 have nearly tripled at the starting level, climbing from an average $8,172 to $23,488. At the top, the increase was more than triple: from $10,152 to $35,300. But those increases are put in perspective by an ANA analysis (see Table 11-2) that matches salaries with inflation and calculates that beginning pay has actually declined by 9%, in real terms, while top-level salaries grew by 105.

Even the current upsurge has failed to override the inflation factor; the spectacular increases are coming in the big cities, at major medical centers and their competitors, and at hospitals where nurses have representation. "The most recent finding is that collective bargaining increases salary 7–10%," says a University of Delaware economist, Charles Link, who is studying nursing salaries.

In the most significant advances, starting pay passed the $30,000 mark last year in Los Angeles, Boston, New York, and San Francisco. The New York State Nurses Association crashed through traditional salary ceilings, negotiating pay scales with increases of $500–$750 a year over 20–40 years—a rate that's elevated salaries for some veteran nurses to $50,000 or more.

▥ NURSES UNLIMITED

"We started as entrepreneurs and we may be coming full circle . . ."

So it seems to nurse-entrepreneur Ellen Sanders, who chairs ANA's Commission on Economic & General Welfare. "Young nurses can't conceive of working 12 hours a day for $4,000 a year—as many of us did—and it's just as hard to them to realize that nurses weren't always employees of hospitals."

In one of the striking developments of the decade, nurses are finding new careers in HMOs and PPOs, insurance companies, peer review groups, and pharmaceutical and supply firms. Some leaders are convinced the future lies this way, with more and more RNs recapturing the independence of free-lance work in more sophisticated, and more profitable, forms of practice: as entrepreneurs, as nurse practitioners, in nursing centers, and as members of groups that contract with hospitals for their services.

The dramatic growth of such opportunities has already heightened the pressures on supply and salaries, as have the growing numbers who prefer to work through agencies.

Sanders points out that the spread of ambulatory care centers alone has enormously expanded the choice of practice sites. If nursing groups are united in their dealings with the political system, she thinks, they can negotiate reimbursement policies supporting the nurse in search of "full autonomy."

Whether or not total autonomy is a target for most nurses, sufficient numbers have recently voted with their feet to make it clear that they want a fuller professional role with the economic security that other professional roles command. The likelihood, however, is that many will continue to let others carry the battle—not because they shrink from it but because they find consistent satisfaction in caring for people, despite the obstacles often put in their way. The system has always been able to count on nurses like the one who summed up her career half-a-century ago:

"I have had plenty of knocks; I have worked like a horse; been fatigued almost to the point of unconsciousness; but I will be blessed if I ever stopped liking it. I have been kicked out one door for distemper only to politely walk in another and start in again."

AJN asked some top economists what they viewed as the hard facts and the broad trends, given nurses' sometimes self-defeating attitudes toward their personal welfare.

The numbers still show that hospitals employ two-thirds of the nation's working RNs—the same proportion computed in the 1970s. By now, that percentage signifies over a million hospital nurses.

Institutions are apt to remain the dominant sources of services and jobs, predicts Linda Aiken, a University of Pennsylvania nurse-scholar who tracks salary ups and downs. Given population shifts that point to a soon-declining workforce, Aiken argues that hospitals must restructure so that they can operate with "fewer, better-paid" nurses.

The hope is that hospitals have learned a lesson from their miscalculations during the recession and early DRG years, when they shaved nursing services to the bone. In response, school enrollments started dropping, just as it was realized that the acuity of illness was shooting so high that staffs had to be replenished and trained for expanded ICUs and floors full of critically ill patients. By last year, a Commonwealth Fund study of 15,000 RNs in six cities discovered that nearly 40% of them were working in critical care.

"That figure blew our minds," says Columbia University economist Eli Ginzberg, one of the study group. "It must have dawned on administrators that such operations couldn't be run without nurses and that it made no sense to pour money into agencies instead of paying decent salaries."

Ginzberg sees salaries now as "more realistic, for the first time since ever"—at least in key cities like New York and Los Angeles, "and to a lesser extent in other places." But the industry remains overbedded, he emphasizes;

TABLE 11-2. Inflation Undermines Nurses' Salary Growth/1973–1989

	Average Starting Salary	Salary Increase (%)	Change Adjusted for Inflation (%)	Average Maximum Salary (%)	Salary Increase (%)	Change Adjusted for Inflation (%)
1989	23,488	4.8	0.0	35,330	9.9	5.1
1987	20,964	3.1	−0.5	29,088	4.8	1.2
1985	19,440	3.6	0.0	26,604	5.3	1.7
1983	18,084	2.9	−0.3	24,348	4.6	1.4
1981	16,068	12.3	2.0	21,408	15.8	5.5
1979	12,492	5.9	−5.4	16,356	7.6	−3.7
1977	10,944	5.2	−1.3	14,040	6.8	0.3
1975	9,672	6.3	−2.8	12,288	8.1	−1.0
1973	8,508	4.1	−2.1	10,512	3.6	−2.6

Data from the University of Texas Medical Branch at Galveston, National Survey of Hospital and Medical School Studies. Increases in starting pay for RNs have lagged behind inflation changes, reports ANA in this analysis of salary growth over the past 16 years.
Copyright © 1990, J. B. Lippincott. Reprinted with permission from the *American Journal of Nursing, 90*(10), 77–80, 83–88, Oct. 1990.

a wave of closures could depress salaries again. And the impact of suddenly rising enrollments is problematic: "The worst way to improve economic returns to a group is to increase the supply."

University of Delaware economist Charles Link raises doubts about recent gains in experience differentials. Link's latest information shows no progress: "Perhaps our next survey will pick up a change, but data through 1988 present an age-earnings profile that's still very flat compared to professions like engineering and accounting." Link is also finding "practically no economic advantage" in earning a BSN in addition to an ADN.

How to differentiate salaries will probably continue to spark debate, though the surge in shift premiums has been generally welcomed. The economic incentives for managers are still viewed as too meager to tempt many to assume those responsibilities.

Bonuses for specialists are a sensitive point; the Hospital Compensation Service calculates that 53% of ICU nurses were paid at the same grade level as general-duty RNs last year. Some of the opposition comes from staff nurses themselves and from unions that want to spread pay raises equally over the staff.

Still an open question is whether the pay-equity and comparable-worth movements were, and will be, crucial factors in pushing up nursing salaries.

Throughout the 1970s and 1980s, both ANA and many SNAs attacked inequities in state employees' pay and won important victories in Pennsylvania, Illinois and Washington State. The National Committee on Pay Equity reports some progress; women now earn 66¢ for every $1 men are paid, compared to the 59¢ share found for women less than 10 years ago.

Finally, wider acceptance of collective bargaining could make the critical difference. Managements will be working harder than ever to control outlays for benefits and salaries. The California Nurses Association, for example, is fighting an attempt to change state laws so that hospitals could institute 12-hour shifts without their staffs' consent. "We worked too hard for the 8-hour day to see it eroded now," says Mary Foley, the San Francisco staff nurse who headed ANA's Commission on Economic & General Welfare for three years.

Nurses need a choice of schedules, Foley emphasizes: "This is still a woman's profession. When 12 hours becomes the norm for a hospital, we lose a whole population of older nurses and many of those with school and family obligations."

CNA bargainers are promoting clinical ladders as the solution for nurses who want to stay at the bedside. "It's exciting," says Foley, "to see nurses realizing that this is a tangible benefit that offers alternative places to go in the system. That's what we can offer through concerted action—a practical way to take control of the workplace and the clinical issues."

12

Trouble in the Nurse Labor Market?
Recent Trends and Future Outlook

Peter I. Buerhaus and Douglas O. Staiger

Nursing personnel play a central role in producing and coordinating patient care in both acute and nonacute care settings, and recent vigorous efforts to lower and control costs have greatly affected nurses' employment, earnings, and clinical practice. Registered nurses (RNs), in particular, have been involved if reluctant participants in hospitals' efforts to restructure patient care delivery in the 1990s. Many RNs assert that they are working harder than ever, that work satisfaction and morale are suffering, and that the quality of patient care has deteriorated over the past few years.[1] They also complain that employment opportunities are disappearing rapidly in acute care hospitals, where historically two-thirds of all RNs have been employed.[2]

The perceived decline in hospital employment has been balanced to some extent by the shift of patient care delivery into nonacute care settings. Many in the nursing profession believe that health care delivery has been overly concentrated in acute care settings and thus have welcomed this shift.[3] Moreover, the greater use of nonhospital settings has generated an expectation of new employment opportunities for nurses. Nursing education programs throughout the country are scrambling to revise their curricula to prepare nurses for new jobs and expanding opportunities in nonhospital settings.[4] However, some question the capacity of nonacute providers to employ all of the RNs leaving hospitals as a result of downsizing, consolidation, and efforts to gain greater efficiency.[5]

These and many other problems besetting the nurse workforce were brought before the Institute of Medicine's (IOM's) Committee on the Adequacy of Nurse Staffing in Hospitals and Nursing Homes in 1996 and the President's Advisory Commission on Consumer Protection and Quality in the Health Care Industry in 1998.[6] Throughout their deliberations, the commit-

Peter Buerhaus is the director of the Harvard Nursing Research Institute and an assistant professor at the Harvard School of Public Health in Boston, Massachusetts. Douglas Staiger is an associate professor of economics at Dartmouth College in Hanover, New Hampshire, and faculty research fellow at the National Bureau of Economic Research in Cambridge, Massachusetts.

tees faced a crucial lack of empirical data regarding the effects of hospital restructuring and other health system changes on nurse staffing. Thus, both committees called for public and private efforts to collect and analyze data on the nurse workforce.

In our earlier work, which analyzed data available through 1994, we found that the spread of managed care had slowed employment growth for RNs in some states and shifted employment toward nonhospital settings, particularly home health.[7] Despite these emerging trends, the national impact on nurse employment and earnings was slight. Since 1994 there has been a surge in the growth of managed care, and it is likely that the national impact on the nurse workforce has grown.[8]

In this paper we examine employment and earnings trends for nursing personnel using data through 1997. Our analysis focuses on two questions. First, to what extent has the recent growth in managed care affected the employment of nurses nationwide? Have the emerging trends seen in our earlier work appeared more broadly, and have new trends emerged? Second, what do these trends imply for the future nurse workforce? In particular, are employment and earnings likely to be adversely affected over the next few years as health maintenance organizations (HMOs) and other forms of managed care spread?

■ DATA AND METHODS

Data Sources

Data were obtained from the U.S. Bureau of the Census Current Population Survey (CPS) Outgoing Rotation Group Annual Merged Files. The CPS, a household-based survey administered monthly by the Census Bureau, is widely used by researchers and by the U.S. Department of Labor to estimate current trends in unemployment, employment, and earnings. The CPS covers a nationally representative sample of more than 100,000 persons, and every month one-quarter of the sample (the outgoing rotation group) is asked detailed questions about current employment status, hours worked, earnings, occupation, and industry of employment. These data offer several advantages over other data commonly used to analyze the nurse workforce (for example, the American Hospital Association Personnel Surveys and the federal government's National Sample Surveys of the Population of Registered Nurses). Specifically, the CPS is the only source of annual data for all nursing personnel (RNs, licensed practical nurses, or LPNs, and aides) employed in both hospital and other settings. In addition, using CPS data enables comparisons of employment and earnings trends between nursing and other occupations.

We used CPS data on nursing employment and earnings for the period 1983–1997. The data set included all persons ages twenty-one to sixty-four who reported their occupation as RN (N = 47,996), LPN (N = 12,115), or aide, orderly, or attendant (N = 45,126). Hourly wages were calculated as usual weekly earnings divided by usual weekly hours. Wages were adjusted for inflation using the Consumer Price Index for all goods in urban areas (CPI-U) and are reported in constant 1997 dollars. Employment was measured as full-time equivalents (FTEs) (that is, the number of full-time employees plus one-half the number of part-time employees), where full-time employment is defined as working thirty or more hours per week. For each category of nursing personnel, data on earnings, employment, and employment setting were aggregated at the annual level. As a validity check, estimates of RN employment based on CPS data were compared with corresponding estimates from the 1984, 1988, 1992, and 1996 National Sample Surveys of the Population of Registered Nurses and found to be quite similar.[9]

In some analyses we categorized states into high versus low enrollment in HMOs according to the proportion of citizens enrolled in HMOs in 1994. We did this to be consistent with our earlier analysis of nurse employment and earnings trends and to enable us to determine whether trends that were emerging in 1994 continued in later years. The high-HMO-enrollment states (sixteen states and the District of Columbia) contain approximately one-half of the U.S. population and had an average HMO enrollment three times higher than the thirty-four low-enrollment states in 1994 (24 percent versus 8 percent).[10] HMO enrollment has grown in all states since 1994, but it has been more rapid in the low-enrollment states.

Data Limitations

Although the CPS data have many advantages, they have a few limitations that bear upon our analysis. First, the survey instrument used to gather data for the CPS was revised in January 1994. As a result, interviewers probe more thoroughly for jobs in which the person worked only a few hours in the week of the survey. This change probably resulted in an increase in the number of nursing personnel, particularly part-time workers, who reported being employed, and it may have slightly affected estimates of earnings and occupation.[11] Thus, some caution must be used when comparing our 1994–1997 estimates with those of earlier years.

A second limitation of the CPS data is that home health care, freestanding clinics, and HMO settings are combined in the industry definition "Health Services, Not Elsewhere Classified" (NEC). Comparing employment data from the 1992 and 1996 National Sample Surveys of the Population of Registered Nurses with the CPS indicates that employment in the NEC category consists largely of home health care providers. Similarly, other U.S. Bureau of Labor Statistics (BLS) data obtained from employer surveys indicate that home health accounts for nearly two-thirds of all employment in the NEC sector.[12] We are confident, therefore, that analyses of CPS data for the NEC category largely reflect employment and earnings trends for nurses employed by home health care providers.

Our analysis of CPS data relies on annual estimates. To make estimates representative of the U.S. noninstitutionalized population, we used sampling weights provided by the CPS. Because of the large samples being used, all trends reported in this paper are precisely estimated. For RNs and aides, the standard errors are about 2 percent for employment estimates and 1 percent for wage estimates. For LPNs, standard errors are about twice as large. As a result, for all outcome variables reported, one can reject the null hypotheses that there were no changes over time and no differences between high- and low-HMO-enrollment states at the .01 level.[13]

■ RESULTS

Employment and Earnings

Employment of RNs and aides grew impressively between 1983 and 1994 (Table 12-1). Growth averaged 3–4 percent per year, nearly double the rate of employment growth among all occupations over the same period. In contrast, LPN employment declined slightly over this period. Since 1994, employment growth for RNs has slowed to just under 2 percent, while employment growth for LPNs and aides has increased slightly.

What is behind the recent slowdown in RN employment growth? The overall slowdown since 1994 is largely the result of a lack of employment growth in hospitals, a sector that until recently employed more than two-thirds of RNs and experienced annual growth rates of 2–3 percent in RN employment. In contrast, hospital employment of LPNs and aides, which declined sharply throughout the 1980s and early 1990s, declined less (and even increased for aides) after 1994. This suggests that hospitals may have increasingly substituted less-skilled nursing personnel for RNs. Despite these changes, RN staffing levels per hospital bed have continued to increase since 1994 (as the number of beds has declined).[14]

Given the declines in hospital employment of LPNs and aides, and the recent stagnation of hospital employment of RNs, where have jobs been created? Although home health (the NEC sector) is a much smaller industry that the hospital industry, it has been the fastest-growing employment setting for all nursing personnel throughout the 1980s and 1990s. In fact, the NEC sector has been the primary source of new employment for LPNs and aides since 1983 and for RNs since 1994.

The deceleration in the rate of employment growth for RNs (both total and hospital employment) during the past several years coincides with a noticeable decrease in earnings (Table 12-1). RNs experienced strong yearly growth in inflation-adjusted hourly wages through 1990 (averaging 2.7 percent per year), but wage growth leveled off between 1990 and 1994 and

TABLE 12-1. Growth of Employment and Earnings for Nursing Personnel, 1983–1997

	Selected Years				Average Annual % Change			Percent Change, 1983–1997
	1983	1990	1994	1997	1983–1990	1990–1994	1994–1997	
Employment (thousands of FTEs)								
All sectors								
RNs	1,201	1,483	1,735	1,836	3.1	4.0	1.9	52.9
LPNs	399	398	361	363	−0.1	−2.4	0.2	−9.0
Aides	1,015	1,228	1,372	1,521	2.8	2.8	3.5	49.9
Hospital sector								
RNs	879	1,040	1,182	1,184	2.4	3.2	0.1	34.8
LPNs	250	195	141	126	−3.5	−7.8	−3.7	−49.7
Aides	419	386	294	336	−1.1	−6.6	4.5	−19.7
NEC sector								
RNs	69	112	179	232	7.1	12.3	9.1	234
LPNs	9	22	32	55	13.0	10.6	19.7	501
Aides	47	137	262	364	16.4	17.6	11.6	671
Wages (in 1997 dollars)								
All sectors								
RNs	16.00	19.25	19.45	18.61	2.7	0.3	−1.5	16.3
LPNs	11.33	12.19	12.97	12.29	1.0	1.6	−1.8	8.4
Aides	8.30	8.74	8.38	8.36	0.7	−1.0	−0.1	0.7

SOURCE: U.S. Bureau of the Census, Current Population Survey (CPS), Outgoing Rotation Group Annual Merged Files, 1983–1997.
NOTES: FTE is full-time equivalent, RN is registered nurse, LPN is licensed practical nurse. NEC is "not elsewhere classified" and includes home health care, freestanding clinics, and health maintenance organizations. "Aides" include nurse aides, orderlies, and assistants.

then fell 1.5 percent annually over the next three years. Wage growth for LPNs was less impressive through the 1980s, and since 1994 LPNs have experienced a similar decline in earnings. Real wages for aides have grown very little during the past fifteen years, despite impressive growth in total employment. In fact, wage growth for aides has been quite similar to that of all nonnursing occupations, in which real wages changed little between 1983 and 1997.

Role of Managed Care

To investigate the effect of managed care on employment and earnings trends, we compared growth rates for employment and earnings of RNs in states with high HMO enrollment with those of states with low HMO enrollment. RNs are of particular interest because they constitute the largest professional component of the nurse workforce. Data for LPNs and aides show fewer systematic differences between high- and low-enrollment states and are not reported here.

Our 1996 analysis of trends through 1994 found a marked slowdown in RN employment growth and a shift out of hospitals occurring primarily in states with high HMO enrollment.[15] If managed care in fact caused these changes, then we would expect that these trends would have continued in states with high HMO enrollment and also would begin to appear in states that had low enrollment as of 1994. In other words, trends that were observed first in high-enrollment states should be indicative of what happens later in other states as managed care spreads.

This is precisely the pattern we found. The slowdown in employment growth, which occurred around 1990 in states with high HMO enrollment, occurred in the low-HMO-enrollment states beginning around 1994 (Figure 12-1). This pattern is even more striking in the hospital sector, where employment first flattened out in the high-enrollment states and then flattened out a few years later in the low-enrollment states (Figure 12-2). Similarly, wages began falling in states with high HMO enrollment after 1991, while wages continued to rise in states with low HMO enrollment through 1993 (Figure 12-3). However, wages have declined in all states since 1993.

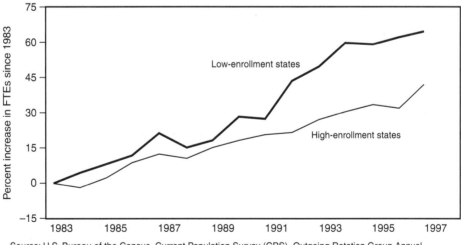

Source: U.S. Bureau of the Census, Current Population Survey (CPS), Outgoing Rotation Group Annual Merged Files, 1983–1997.
Note: RN is registered nurse. HMO is health maintenance organization. FTE is full-time equivalent.

FIGURE 12-1. Employment growth of RNs since 1983 in states with high and low HMO enrollment, 1983–1997.

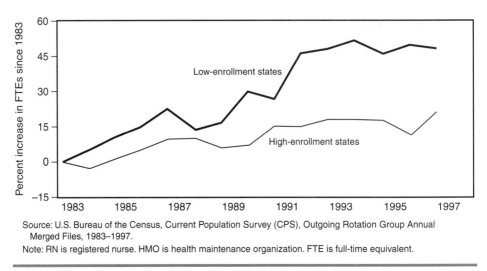

Source: U.S. Bureau of the Census, Current Population Survey (CPS), Outgoing Rotation Group Annual Merged Files, 1983–1997.
Note: RN is registered nurse. HMO is health maintenance organization. FTE is full-time equivalent.

FIGURE 12-2. Employment growth of RNs since 1983 in the hospital sector in states with high and low HMO enrollment, 1983–1997.

Because trends in the high-enrollment states indicate what the rest of the nation can expect as managed care spreads, recent developments in these states are worth noting. There is some indication of a resurgence in employment growth in 1997, but it is impossible to know whether this is an aberration or an emerging trend (Figure 12-1). More importantly, since 1992 there has been a clear slowdown in employment growth in the home health (NEC)

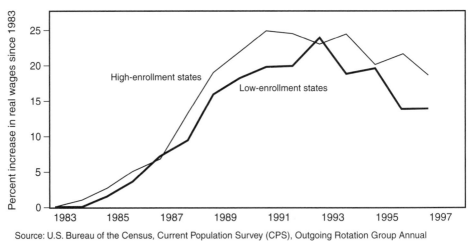

Source: U.S. Bureau of the Census, Current Population Survey (CPS), Outgoing Rotation Group Annual Merged Files, 1983–1997.
Note: RN is registered nurse. HMO is health maintenance organization.

FIGURE 12-3. Wage growth of RNs since 1983 in states with high and low HMO enrollment, 1983–1997.

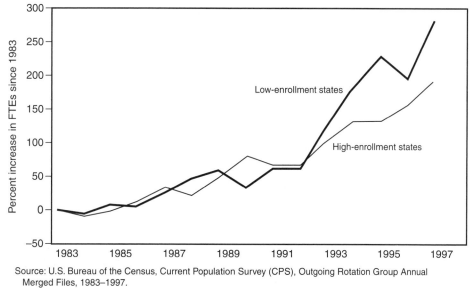

Source: U.S. Bureau of the Census, Current Population Survey (CPS), Outgoing Rotation Group Annual Merged Files, 1983–1997.
Note: RN is registered nurse. NEC is "not elsewhere classified" and primarily includes home health care. HMO is health maintenance organization. FTE is full-time equivalent.

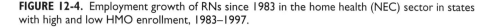

FIGURE 12-4. Employment growth of RNs since 1983 in the home health (NEC) sector in states with high and low HMO enrollment, 1983–1997.

sector in the high-HMO states relative to the low-HMO states (Figure 12-4). It appears that managed care is beginning to adversely affect employment opportunities in this key sector.

▪ DISCUSSION AND IMPLICATIONS

We undertook this analysis to address two overriding questions. First, to what extent has the recent growth in managed care affected the employment and earnings of nurses nationwide? Second, what does this imply for the future? In particular, can we expect employment and earnings of nurses to be adversely affected over the next few years as HMOs and other forms of managed care spread?

Has Managed Care Affected Nurse Employment and Earnings?

Labor-market conditions for nursing personnel, and RNs in particular, have worsened over the past few years. Our findings suggest that this trend is attributable to growth in managed care, which has adversely affected the employment and earnings of nurses nationwide. In particular, it appears that managed care has reduced demand for RNs, first in hospitals and more recently in home health, and as a result has led to a decline in RN earnings. The slowdown in hospital employment and wage growth, first observed in states with high HMO enrollment in the early 1990s, has now emerged in all states. The slowdown in the rate of home health employment growth has emerged only in the past few years in states with high HMO enrollment.

Trouble Ahead? Implications for the Future

Recent trends in states with high HMO penetration provide a good guide to likely employment and earnings trends for RNs in the near future. Based on the recent experience of these states, RNs can expect little employment growth in hospitals, a deceleration of employment growth in home health, and a continued gradual decline in wages over the next few years. These effects should be particularly pronounced in areas of the country that have only recently experienced the spread of managed care.

In the longer term, trends in employment and earnings of nurses will depend largely on how the maturing managed care market affects employment opportunities in the hospital and home health sectors. In both sectors the longer-term employment prospects for nurses are less clear.

Outlook for Hospital Employment

Because hospitals are the largest sector of the nurse labor market, particularly for RNs, a change in employment growth in this sector will have a disproportionate effect on overall employment and earnings trends. The trends since 1994 in high-HMO states show little growth in hospital employment of RNs, but there is also no evidence of the drastic employment reductions that some have forecasted for the hospital sector.[16] On the other hand, very recent evidence suggests that hospital employment of RNs may be growing once more in the high-HMO states. Between 1996 and 1997 RN employment grew 8.2 percent in the states with high HMO enrollment, with much of this growth coming from hospital employment. At the same time, in 1998 there have been a number of reports of RN shortages throughout the country, suggesting that hospitals may be beginning to increase the size and elevate the skill of their nursing staffs.[17]

What might account for this recent upturn in RN employment? One possibility is that the slowdown in RN employment growth was temporary as hospitals passed through a transitional period in which they implemented downsizing initiatives aimed at improving efficiency. Thus, we may now be observing a resumption of employment growth as the high-HMO states move out of this transitional period. Some support for this view is provided by interviews of health executives in Minnesota and Oregon—which experienced early growth in managed care—who reported a rebound in RN employment in the early 1990s following a tumultuous period of rapid hospital downsizing and restructuring.[18]

Alternatively, the recent upturn in RN employment might represent a short-term correction for past cuts. Hospitals may have scaled back the number of RNs and reduced the skill mix of nursing personnel to a point at which it was no longer possible to appropriately treat a growing number of older and acutely ill patients. This view was strongly expressed by many nurses' organizations that offered testimony in 1995 to the IOM Committee on the Adequacy of Nurse Staffing in Hospital and Nursing Homes. Hospitals in high-enrollment states also may have become increasingly concerned about their nurse staffing as a result of rising public mistrust and growing media attention to perceptions of declining quality of care, as well as by the groundswell of consumer protection legislation introduced throughout the states.[19]

Does the increase in hospital employment of RNs in 1997 represent an emerging trend, a short-term correction for past cuts, or perhaps even a statistical aberration? Until data on RN employment for 1998 and later years become available, it is impossible to know which is the case or to what extent these new developments may offset the substantial slowing in the rate of employment growth for RNs that we otherwise expect.

Outlook for Home Health Employment

Perhaps the most important new trend to emerge since 1994 has been the slowdown in RN employment growth in the home health (NEC) sector in states with high HMO enrollment. This change suggests that employment growth in this key sector might soon begin to decelerate nationwide. In addition, Medicare's implementation of a prospective payment system for the home health care industry during the next four years will place new economic pressure on providers and reinforce the slowing effect of managed care. Given that home health has been the fastest-growing sector for nurse employment in the 1990s, a slowing of employment growth in this sector could substantially blunt future employment opportunities for RNs (and other nursing personnel).

The forces transforming the health care delivery system during the 1990s have significantly affected the nurse labor market. The slowdown in employment growth and falling earnings observed over the past several years are likely to continue in the near term, but nursing still looks like a good career option, with employment growth and earnings continuing to be high relative to other occupations. The longer-term outlook for the nurse labor market is less clear. The next few years will be critical as we begin to observe the effects of a maturing managed care industry on the nursing profession.

Nurses occupy the front ranks in the delivery of personal health care services, playing vital roles as coordinators of care and as patient advocates. According to a recent national survey, more than 80 percent of Americans believe that nurses are doing a "good job" of serving health care consumers. Roughly 65 percent hold the same view about physicians, pharmaceutical companies, and hospitals, and only 34 percent, about HMOs and managed care companies.[20] How successfully nurses, employers, educators, and policymakers handle the coming challenges in the nurse labor market will be critical not only to maintaining the public's trust in the nursing profession but to preserving the public's confidence in the health care system as a whole.

This study was supported by a grant from the Robert Wood Johnson Foundation. The authors appreciate the able assistance of David Auerbach.

Notes

1. P. Brider, "Morale Skidding with Restructuring," *American Journal of Nursing* 96, no. 2 (1996): 62, 64; P. Brider, "$3 Million Suit Exposes 'De-Skilling'," *American Journal of Nursing* 96, no. 11 (1996): 70; C. Helmlinger, "A Growing Physical Workload Threatens Nurses' Health," *American Journal of Nursing* 97, no. 4 (1997): 64–66. M. Gillilan, "Workforce Reductions: Low Morale, Reduced Quality Care," *Nursing Economics* 15 no. 6 (1997): 320–322; A. Greiner, *Cost and Quality Matters: Workplace Innovations in the Health Care Industry* (Washington: Economic Policy Institute, 1995); Peter D. Hart Research Associates, Inc., "Health Profession's View of Quality: A National Survey presented to the President's Advisory Commission on Consumer Protection and Quality" (17 December 1997); and J. Greene and A.M. Nordhaus-Bike, "Nurse Shortage, Where Have All the RNs Gone?" *Hospital and Health Networks* (August 1997): 78–80.

2. P. Brider, "Enrollment Boom Ends as Job Hunts Lengthen," *American Journal of Nursing* 96, no. 2 (1996): 61, 65.

3. D.G. Knauth, "Community Nursing Centers: Removing Impediments to Success." *Nursing Economics* 12, no. 3 (1994): 140–145; and M.E. Zotti, P. Brown, and R.C. Stotts, "Community-Based Nursing versus Community Health Nursing: What Does It All Mean?" *Nursing Outlook* 44, no. 5 (1996): 211–217.

4. See, for example, *The Essentials of Baccalaureate Education for Professional Nursing Practice* (Washington: American Association of Colleges of Nursing, 1998).

5. L. H. Aiken, J. Sochalski, and G.F. Anderson, "Downsizing the Hospital Nursing Workforce," *Health Affairs* (Fall 1996): 88–92; P.I. Buerhaus and D.O. Staiger, "Future of the Nurse Labor Market According to Health Executives in High Managed-Care Areas of the United States," IMAGE: *Journal of Nursing Scholarship* 29, no. 4 (1997): 313–318; and E. H. Hadley, "Nursing in the Political and Economic Marketplace: Challenge for the 21st Century," *Nursing Outlook* 44, no. 1 (1996): 6–10.

6. Institute of Medicine, *Nursing Staff in Hospitals and Nursing Homes: Is It Adequate?* (Washington: National Academy Press, 1996); and *Engaging the Health Care Workforce* (Washington: Advisory Commission on Consumer Protection and Quality in the Health Care Industry, 17 January 1998).

7. P.I. Buerhaus and D.O. Staiger, "Managed Care and the Nurse Workforce," *Journal of the American Medical Association* 276, no. 18 (1996): 1487–1493.

8. G. Jensen et al., "The New Dominance of Managed Care: Insurance Trends in the 1990s," *Health Affairs* (January/February 1997): 125–136.

9. E. Moses, *The Registered Nurse Population: Findings from the National Sample Survey of Registered Nurses.* (Rockville, Md.: Division of Nursing, Bureau of Health Professions, Health Resources and Services Administration, 1984, 1988, 1992, 1996).

10. The states with high enrollment in HMOs in 1994 are Arizona, California, Colorado, Connecticut, District of Columbia, Florida, Hawaii, Maryland, Massachusetts, Michigan, Minnesota, New Mexico, New York, Oregon, Pennsylvania, Washington, and Wisconsin. Enrollment data provided by InterStudy Publications, Bloomington, Minnesota, unpublished documents, 1995.

11. A.E. Polivka, "The Redesigned Current Population Survey," *Journal of Economic Perspectives* (Summer 1996): 169–180.

12. Bureau of Labor Statistics, *Employment and Wages, Annual Averages,* 1994 (Washington: U.S. Department of Labor, November 1995), Table 2.

13. Conventional standard errors and statistical tests assume independence across observations. The independence assumption may be violated, however, because multiple individuals within a household are sampled and because it is possible that the same individual could appear in the sample twice. For our data, treating each household as a cluster and correcting for arbitrary intracluster correlation (along the lines of Huber) had a negligible impact on the estimated standard errors and p-values. Therefore, for simplicity we report only conventional standard errors and statistical tests. See P.J. Huber, "The Behavior of Maximum Likelihood Estimates under Non-Standard Conditions," *Proceedings of the Fifth Berkeley Symposium on Mathematical Statistics and Probability,* no. 1 (1967), 221–233. Also, see *Stata Reference Manual,* Release 3.1, 6th ed., vol. 2, no. 2 (College Station, Tex.: Stata Corporation, 1993), 405–414.

14. Based on bed data from *1998 Hospital Statistics* (Chicago: American Hospital Association, 1998) and our estimates of RN employment from Exhibit 1, the ratio of RNs per hospital bed was 0.651 in 1983, 0.857 in 1990, 1.048 in 1994, and 1.115 in 1996 (the most recent bed data available).

15. Buerhaus and Staiger, "Managed Care and the Nurse Workforce."

16. Pew Health Professions Commission, *Critical Challenges: Revitalizing the Health Profession for the Twenty-first Century* (San Francisco: University of California, San Francisco, Center for the Health Professions, 1995).

17. M. Chandler, "Preventative Treatment in RN Shortage," *Miami Herald,* 2 February 1998, 7; M. Hawke, "Needed by 2005: More (Good) Nurses," *Nursing Spectrum* (New England Edition), 26 January 1998, 2, 4–5; Greene and Nordhaus Bike, "Nurse Shortage;" and American Organization of Nurse Executives, "AONE Develops Issue Brief on Nursing Shortage," *AONE News Update* 4, no. 12 (1998): 1.

18. Buerhaus and Staiger, "Future of the Nurse Labor Market According to Health Executives."

19. M. Brodie, L.A. Brady, and D.E. Altman, "Media Coverage of Managed Care: Is There a Negative Bias?" *Health Affairs* (January/February 1998): 9–25; and R.J. Blendon et al., "Understanding the Managed Care Backlash," *Health Affairs* (July/August 1998): 80–94.

20. Blendon et al., "Understanding the Managed Care Backlash."

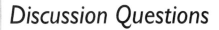

Discussion Questions

1. What is your assessment of the public's image of nurses today?

2. Which media images of nurses are accurate? Which are inaccurate? What are the gaps in reality in the images that are inaccurate?

3. What needs to be done to inform the public about what nurses really do? Where would you begin?

4. If you were writing the script for a television program that included nurses, how would you portray them?

5. In the last year, how many newspaper articles and/or TV programs have you read or seen about nursing?

6. What news items would you like to see in the media about the nursing profession?

7. What kind of media coverage is there about nursing on your campus? If there is little or no coverage, how would you go about getting coverage?

8. Based on your observations in a practice setting, to what extent do you agree or disagree with Gordon's view of nurses (Article 9)? Support your observations.

9. How do the nurses with whom you work cope with their workloads?

10. What needs to be done to improve the working conditions of nurses?

11. What were your reasons for entering nursing? To what degree do your reasons correspond to the themes in Mangan (Article 10)?

12. What suggestions do you have for encouraging others to enter nursing?

13. What do you consider just compensation for a professional nurse?

14. Given the uncertain outlook for hospital employment cited in Buerhaus and Staiger (Article 12), what other job options in nursing would you consider? Explain your reasons.

15. What concerns do you have about future employment in nursing?

Further Readings

Baugh, S. (1999). Why do women choose nursing? *Journal of Nursing Education, 38*(4), 156–161.

Friedman, E. (1990). Nursing: Breaking the bonds? *JAMA, 264*(24), 3117–3125.

Gordon, S. (1997). What nurses stand for. *Atlantic Monthly, 279*(2), 81–88.

Kalisch, P.A. & Kalisch, B.J. (1982). The image of the nurse in motion pictures. *American Journal of Nursing, 82*(4), 609–611.

Kalisch, P.A. & Kalisch, B.J. (1981). When nurses were national heroines: Images of nursing in American films, 1942–1945. *Nursing Forum, 10*(1), 14–61.

Meier, E. (1999). The image of the nurse: Myth vs reality. *Nursing Economics, 17*(5), 273–275.

Meissner, J. E. (1999). Are we still eating our young? *Nursing 99, 29*(2), 42–43.

Peterson, C. A. (1999). Nursing supply and demand. *American Journal of Nursing, 99*(7), 57–58.

Sullivan, E. J. (1999). The invisible majority: Nurses in the media. *Journal of Professional Nursing, 15*(4), 203–204.

Web Site Resources for Nurses: A Professional Reality Check

All Nurses   www.allnurses.com
American Nurses Association   www.ana.org
National League for Nursing   www.nln.org
Nursing Center   www.nursingcenter.com
The Nursing Network   www.nursingnetwork.com
Nursestat   http://www.nursestat.com
Nurse Week   www.nurseweek.com/
The Nursing Student WWW Page   www2.csn.net/~tbracket/htm.htm
Nursing World   www.nursingworld.org
SN: Student Nurse   http://studentnurse.hypermart.net/

General Search Engine Web Sites

AltaVista   www.altavista.com
Hot Bot   www.hotbot.com

Health Web Sites

Health Answers   www.healthanswers.com
Health Gate   www.healthgate.com

Professional Journal Web Sites

Achoo   www.achoo.com
American Journal of Nursing   www.nursingcenter.com
Nursing Outlook   www.mosby.com
Nursing Research   www.nursingcenter.com
Pediatric Nursing   www.ajj.com
Nursing Forum   www.nursecominc.com
Nursing Management   www.springnet.com
Online Journal of Issues in Nursing   www.nursingworld.org

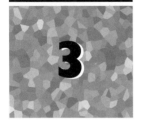

Cultural Diversity:
A Celebration of Differences

We live in a world of differences. Different cultures, different lifestyles, different ethnic groups, and different religions. While we share many common human traits that connect us with one another, our differences can and do separate us. And those differences matter. Instead of celebrating the unique character inherent in cultural and ethnic diversity, those differences have led to intolerance, misperceptions, and conflict. They spill over spreading everywhere. Black churches are burned; swastikas are painted on synagogue walls; Catholics and Protestants fight each other in Northern Ireland; Serbs and Albanians slaughter each other in Kosovo. All because of differences.

When did our country's "melting pot" become a container of oil and water? When did our sense of values become locked in the gated community of our minds, where ethnic and cultural differences are not welcome and need not apply? Why have ethnic and cultural differences become a battleground of passion and violence instead of a celebration of diversity and the gifts of human understanding they offer us?

In every corner of our country, and with every segment of its ethnically and culturally diverse population, nursing celebrates differences through nursing practice. In doing so, however, another issue emerges. What is the message we are sending if we, as a profession, are predominantly white, serving a multicultural population? How will our multicultural population make their health beliefs understood to someone not of their culture? For the answers to these questions, we must first look at our own history and examine the extent to which diversity exists within our profession. The first part of this chapter begins with an historical overview tracing black nurses' efforts to achieve recognition, acceptance, and inclusion as colleagues and members of the American Nurses Association. That history sets the stage for the readings that follow in which questions are raised and criticisms voiced about whether nursing itself is as ethnically and culturally diverse as it could be.

The remaining readings in this chapter focus on the growing interest of health care consumers in alternative and complementary medicine. Many health care practices associated with alternative and complementary medicine have been used for centuries in other cultures. Today, they have found a home in this country. These health care practices offer us the chance to learn more about how other cultures view and treat health problems. Its holistic philosophy is particularly appealing as health care consumers become increasingly disenchanted with traditional medicine. As the use of alternative and complementary medicine grows, so do the issues surrounding its use. Our responsibility is to understand the issues that surround them, and then translate them to our patients so that these practices can be used safely. The emergence of alternative and complementary medicine brings us a new world of beliefs and practices. Both the health care practices we know and the health care practices that are still a mystery can give us the best of two worlds and another opportunity to celebrate differences.

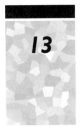

13

Black Nurses in the United States: 1879–1992

M. Elizabeth Carnegie

■ EDUCATION

Schools exclusively for Blacks did not exist until 1886 with the establishment of the diploma program at Spelman College in Atlanta, Georgia. In the 97 years between 1886 and 1982, when the last diploma program for Blacks closed (Grady Hospital School of Nursing in Atlanta), 90 such schools had existed (Carnegie, 1991). With the exception of eleven schools in five northern states, the majority of schools of nursing were in the South. Therefore most of the Black diploma graduates in the United States are products of these segregated Black schools.

Howard University in Washington, D.C. established the first baccalaureate program for Blacks in 1922, but closed it in 1925. The oldest ongoing baccalaureate program at a historically Black institution is at Florida A & M University in Tallahassee, having graduated its first class of three with bachelor's degrees in 1941. The number of baccalaureate programs at historically Black colleges and universities had grown to 23 in 1992. There are other baccalaureate programs in nursing in newer institutions that are also predominantly Black, such as Chicago State University, University of the District of Columbia, and Medgar Evers College of the City University of New York.

Associate degree programs in nursing did not come on the scene until 1952, with an experimental project by Mildred Montag of Teachers College, Columbia University, New York. One of her experimental programs was at a Black institution—the Norfolk Division of Virginia State College.

Several other associate degree programs were developed at historically Black colleges and universities: Alcorn State University, Natchez, Mississippi; Mississippi Valley College; Itta Bena, which existed from 1964 to 1979; Kentucky State University, Frankfort; Bluefield State University, West Virginia;

M. Elizabeth Carnegie, D.P.A., R.N., F.A.A.N., is Editor Emerita, Nursing Research, and author, The Path We Tread, Blacks in Nursing, 1854–1990.

Reprinted with permission from the Journal of the Black Nurses Association, 6(1) 13–18, Fall/Winter, 1992.

Lincoln University, Missouri; and Tennessee State University, Nashville. Because most associate degree programs are in community colleges there are many that are located in predominantly Black areas that have a high enrollment of Black students. As neighborhoods change, the complexion of the student body usually changes.

There are four historically Black colleges and universities with master's degree programs, all accredited by the National League for Nursing: Hampton University, Hampton, Virginia; Howard University, Washington, D.C.; Bowie State University, Bowie, Maryland; and Albany State College, Albany, Georgia.

The first known Black nurse to earn a master's degree was Estelle Massey Riddle Osborne in 1931 from Teachers College, Columbia University, New York. For years she remained the only Black nurse with this distinction. The first Black nurse to hold a doctorate was Elizabeth Lipford Kent; she earned it in 1955 at the University of Michigan, Ann Arbor. Dr. Kent is also the product of two Black schools. She held a bachelor's degree from Spelman College in Atlanta, Georgia before entering St. Philip Hospital School of Nursing in Richmond, Virginia.

The latest directory of nurses with doctorates was published in 1984 by the American Nurses Association. Although the nurses' race was not included, 77 were identifiable as Black. Listings were based on voluntary responses to a questionnaire, so the numbers are not necessarily accurate.

Since 1974, the American Nurses Association has been funded by the federal government (National Institute of Mental Health) to help minority nurses earn doctoral degrees. Since that time, nearly 130 minority nurses (mostly Black) have graduated from the most prestigious universities in the country. A good estimate of the 5,415 nurses in the United States with earned doctorates, 300, or 5 percent, are Black (National Sample Survey, 1988). This is significant because the national survey for that same year indicated that of the 2,033,032 registered nurses in the United States, only 73,647, or 3.6 percent, were Black.

A few of these Black nurses with doctoral degrees have pursued postdoctoral education to enhance their skills in research, educational and service administration, and various clinical areas.

■ *EMPLOYMENT*

When the first white nurses completed their training at the hospital schools in the late 19th century, their only avenue of employment was private duty nursing in homes. The situation was no different for Black nurses. Mary Mahoney, for example, spent her entire career as a private duty nurse.

After Lillan Wald established public health as a distinct discipline in nursing in 1893, nurses found employment in this area. The first Black public health nurse in the United States was Jessie Sleet Scales who, after months of seeking employment, was hired in 1900 by the Charity Organization Society, New York. Mrs. Scales was an 1895 graduate of Provident Hospital School of Nursing, a Black school in Chicago. Another early Black public health nurse was Elizabeth Tyler Barringer, a Freedmen's graduate who, in 1906, was appointed to the staff of the Henry Street Visiting Nurse Service in New York City.

By 1911, public health agencies were beginning to be established in counties throughout the country. In fact, in 1915 North Carolina passed a law requiring public and private hospitals, sanitariums, and institutions where colored patients were admitted for treatment to hire colored nurses to care for these colored patients (Consolidated Statutes of North Carolina, 1915). Such laws were typical all over the country, but especially in the South. Because of discrimination in the North and South hospitals servicing Black patients hired Black nurses. Some of the white hospitals had separate wards, floors, or wings designated for Black patients. Black nurses were hired to care for them.

As indicated earlier, schools for Black nurses were established toward the end of the 19th Century. Those operated by Blacks had Black faculty. In some, like Lincoln School for Nurses in New York, although established for Blacks, had white administration and faculty. In some southern states with Black and white schools under the same aegis, the white faculty taught both races separately. All of these schools have been closed.

At the end of 1990, forty-five Black deans of baccalaureate and higher degree programs were identified; 20 headed those in the 23 historically Black colleges and universities (Carnegie, 1991). This means that the majority (25), were deans of schools that were not historically Black. Four Black nurses hold vice-presidencies for academic affairs—they are at Hampton University, Virginia; Kentucky State University, Frankfort; University of Kentucky, Lexington; and Indiana University of Pennsylvania.

In the early years, employment of Black nurses in the federal government—the military, the U.S. Public Health Service, and the Veterans Administration—followed the established pattern of racial segregation. During World War I, although Black nurses had volunteered their services, they were not accepted until after the Armistice had been signed in 1918. Only 18 nurses were accepted. At the beginning of the United States' involvement in World War II, the Army set a quota for the acceptance of Black nurses. The number was 56. It took years of efforts by Black nurses and civil rights organizations to combat this discrimination. The Army did not lift this quota until near the end of the war. The Navy at first refused to enlist Black nurses, but relaxed its policy in early 1945 by accepting four Black nurses.

Today, Black nurses are serving without discrimination in all areas of the military. Both Hazel Johnson Brown and Clara Adams-Ender have been promoted to the top nursing position possible in the Army, Chief of the Army Nurse Corps with the rank of Brigadier General. After retiring from the Army

Nurse Corps in 1991, Brigadier General Clara Adams-Ender became the first nurse and woman to command an Army Post—Fort Belvoir in Virginia.

Black nurses in the Navy, both men and women, have attained senior rank and hold high level positions within nursing administration. Additionally the Air Force has six Black nurses with the rank of full colonel.

In 1919 the country had a major influenza epidemic. During that year trained nurses were employed in the hospital nursing service of the Public Health Service. Charity Collins Miles was employed as its first Black nurse. She was a 1906 graduate of Spelman College School of Nursing in Atlanta. Since that time, Black nurses have held key positions in the Public Health Service in this and other countries.

In 1923, a Veterans Administration facility was opened in Tuskagee, Alabama to serve Black veterans. Until 1941, this was the only Veterans Administration facility that would appoint Black nurses. Around this time, a few Black nurses were transferred from Tuskagee to other facilities but were assigned to segregated units. In 1954, because of the successes in the civil rights forces movement, the Veterans Administration ordered the end of segregation in all its hospitals. Today, there are no barriers. Indeed a Black nurse, Vernice Ferguson, holds the title of Assistant Chief Medical Director for Nursing Programs of the VA Nursing Services. Additionally Black nurses are holding top-level positions in many community health facilities, hospitals, and educational institutions, and others are doing well in private practice.

■ *ORGANIZED NURSING*

Nurses were not organized on a national level until 1893 when the American Society of Superintendents of Training Schools for Nurses in the United States and Canada (forerunner of the National League for Nursing) was founded. The literature does not indicate the involvement of Black nurses at that time. Neither is there indication of Black nurses' involvement when the American Nurses Association was founded in 1896.

A Black nurse, Martha Franklin, who had been graduated from the Women's Hospital in Philadelphia in 1897, became concerned about the welfare of Black nurses throughout the country. She wrote to all those she knew suggesting to organize so that they could: (1) achieve higher professional standards; (2) breakdown discriminatory practices in schools of nursing, in jobs, and in nursing organizations; and (3) develop leadership among Negro nurses. Miss Franklin called a meeting in New York in 1908 and 52 Black nurses were in attendance. This became the first organizational meeting of the National Association of Colored Graduate Nurses (NACGN).

From 1908 until 1951, when NACGN dissolved, this organization fought discrimination on all fronts but especially for integration of the Black nurse into the American Nurses Association (ANA). Beginning in 1916, when ANA became a federation of states, with the state becoming the membership unit, the southern states barred Blacks. It was not until 1961 that all states accepted Blacks, thereby giving all nurses membership in ANA.

In 1948, Estelle Massey Riddle Osborne, who was the president of NACGN, was elected to the Board of Directors of ANA. Mrs. Osborne was the first Black elected official of ANA. Since then, there has been a Black president, Barbara Nichols, who served two terms, 1978–1982. Other Blacks have served since then in elected and appointed positions.

Between the year of 1951 (when NACGN dissolved) and 1970 there was a void in Black nurses leadership in ANA. Additionally ANA did not seem to be concerned about any issues of importance to Black nursing or Black health care. Therefore at the 1970 ANA Convention in Miami, Florida, most of the 200 Blacks present caucused and formed an organized body of what became the National Black Nurses Association. NBNA was officially established in 1971, and incorporated in 1972. Dr. Lauranne Sams became the first national president of NBNA. With headquarters in Washington, D.C., NBNA has thousands of members in over 50 chapters throughout the country working to provide quality health care for the Black community. It also has an official refereed journal entitled, *Journal of the National Black Nurses Association.*

In 1986, a group of Black faculty in institutions of higher education met to determine how to best meet their professional needs. This resulted in the creation of the Association of Black Faculty in Higher Education. Dr. Sallie Tucker-Allen became its first president. Like other professional organizations, ABNF has an official journal, which is also refereed.

Although established as a sorority in 1932, Chi Eta Phi functions as a professional organization of registered nurses in the United States, Africa, and the Caribbean. It is also a member of the ANA Nursing Organizational Liaison Forum. The latest group of Black nurses to organize is the Association of Seventh Day Adventist Black Nurses.

When the early nursing organizations were founded, there were only a few that accepted Blacks as members. Those few that did accept Blacks restricted their participation to followers, not leaders, hence the need for Blacks to form their own organizations. Today, though Black nurses are accepted without racial restrictions in organizations, there is still a place for Black-run organizations to meet special needs. The average Black nurse recognizes the American Nurses Association as the organization of professional nurses and belongs to it, as well as, to other specialty groups—clinical, non-clinical, religious, gender, and ethnic/racial. NBNA, for example, is not a substitute for ANA nor a re-creation of NACGN but an organization established to meet certain needs of Black nurses and the Black community.

Black nurses forged ahead since 1879 when Mary Mahoney graduated. They have exemplified courage, commitment, dedication, assertiveness, accountability, and an unwavering belief in the integrity of humankind. Because of these pioneers, Black nurses are practicing today with dignity in all areas of nursing.

References

Carnegie ME (1991). *The Path We Tread, Blacks in Nursing, 1854–1990,* 2nd Edition, New York, National League for Nursing.

Consolidated Statutes of North Carolina (1915), Raleigh.

National Sample Survey of Registered Nurses (1988), Bureau of Health Professions, Division of Nursing, Department of Health and Human Services.

14

Diversity in Nursing:
A Challenge for the Profession

Susan Cole and Lori Stutte

Statistics show that nearly 90 percent of the total Registered Nurse (RN) workforce is white compared with approximately 72 percent of the total U.S. population (U.S. Department of Health and Human Services, 1996). By the year 2000 it is projected that the population will be comprised of about 224,818 thousand (42%) whites and, of that, minorities will comprise about 311,702 thousand (58%) of the total population (U.S. Department of Commerce, Bureau of the Census, 1997). Minorities in the United States can be categorized predominantly as Blacks, Hispanics, Asians, Pacific Islander Americans, American Indians, and Alaska Natives (U.S. Department of Health and Human Services, 1992). From 1983 to 1996, women, Blacks, and Hispanics in the workforce have increased by 8 percent (U.S. Department of Commerce, Bureau of the Census, 1997). As the minority population continues to increase one would expect that the minority workforce would increase as well.

In the area of health care these minority populations have been greatly underserved. The health status of minorities continues to be much lower than whites. With an ever-increasing minority population comes the need to match ethnic and cultural profiles of health care providers to those of the populations they serve. An increase in the number of minority health care providers can contribute to improving the overall health status of disadvantaged clients (Rosella, Regan-Kubinski, & Albrecht 1994; Steward, 1998). Within its own ranks nursing has not shaped a diverse workforce. This is alarming considering that affirmative action has been in place for 30 years.

Affirmative action policies and programs were initiated in the 1960's to ensure members of minority groups access to schools and positions formerly closed to them. Specifically, programs and policies were designed to increase employment and educational opportunities for minorities and women. The

Susan Cole, M.S.N., R.N., C.S., is assistant professor in the College of Nursing at Cardinal Stritch University in Milwaukee, WI. Lori Stutte, M.S.N., R.N., assistant professor of nursing, also teaches in the College of Nursing at Cardinal Stritch University.

Reprinted with permission from the *Journal of Cultural Diversity*, 5(2), 53–57, Summer, 1998.

belief was that adult white men made up the corporate world. The premise was that racial, ethnic, and sexual prejudices were barriers that kept out women and minorities and protected the corporate world from change. To overcome these barriers and facilitate change, legal and social mandates were necessary (Thomas, 1990).

In the thirty years since the inception of affirmative action, the debate has been whether it truly affords equal opportunities for minorities or is a form of reverse discrimination. Anti-affirmative action advocates argue that qualified whites are denied academic and job opportunities because they are not in a minority. The controversy over affirmative action has intensified across America. One result of this controversy is the passage of anti-affirmative action laws by California and Texas.

Chancellor Young of the University of California, Los Angeles (UCLA) raises the question of how to maintain diversity at UCLA without the benefit of affirmative action. In July 1995, the California Board of Regents, which governs nine state universities, voted to stop the practice of making hiring decisions and determining admissions based on race, sex, and ethnicity (Young, 1995). Two years later the California voters reaffirmed their commitment to anti-affirmative action by approving Proposition 209 which bans the use of racial and ethnic preferences in hiring and admission to all state institutions (Peterson, 1998). The question raised by Young, how to maintain diversity without affirmative action, is not just an issue at UCLA but at all institutions of higher learning.

Beverly Malone (1997), president of the American Nurses Association (ANA), notes that as the makeup of corporate organizations becomes more diverse, so too will that of students in higher education, requiring greater diversity among faculty and staff. However, in the past ten years representation of minorities in nursing has shown little growth. This is true in spite of grants and other funding to recruit, retain, and graduate minority nurses (Malone 1998). The 1996 National Sample Survey of Registered Nurses found that of the 2,558,874 RNs in this country, 246,363, or an estimated 10 percent, came from racial and ethnic minority backgrounds. The survey showed that although the number of minority nurses has doubled, the increase is not equivalent to that of the overall minority population (U.S. Department of Health and Human Service, 1996).

In spite of affirmative action, admission and graduation rates of minority nurses have not kept up with our counterparts in education. Enrollment in all RN programs has been down. Associate, diploma, and baccalaureate programs have all experienced a decline in applications (Brewer, 1997; Louden & Post, 1997). The enrollment of entry-level baccalaureate students has fallen for each of the past three years. From fall 1996 to fall 1997 there was a decline of more than six percent in the enrollment of entry-level baccalaureate students (American Association of Colleges of Nursing, 1998; Mezibov, 1998). This decrease in the number of students entering nursing programs is expected to be a continuing trend.

Louden and Post (1997) speculate that declining admissions may be in part due to changes in the job market for new graduates and the fall of hospital-based systems. In addition, budgetary constraints and the perception that there is a lack of employment opportunities for new nurses have prompted many nursing programs to reduce enrollments. This declining trend not only affects overall enrollments but also may seriously affect an already underrepresented minority nurse population. Nursing, as many other health care professions, faces the challenge of increasing the number of minority nurses to reflect the diversity of the American population as shown in Figure 14-1.

Higher education has recognized the cultural diversity of people in our society and the limited knowledge that many college graduates possess in understanding the relationship of culture and human experience (Yuen-Heung To Dutka, 1993). As the minority population increases, cultural diversity is commonplace and no longer the exception. Diversity should be a goal of all educational institutions.

Nursing recognizes and prioritizes the need to prepare students who are culturally sensitive. The nurse must be able to understand the cultural background of each client, including behaviors, beliefs and expectations. To promote optimal client outcomes, similarities between the nurse and the client must exist. It is crucial that nursing as a profession take a leadership role in developing culturally based care and becoming culturally competent (Rojas,

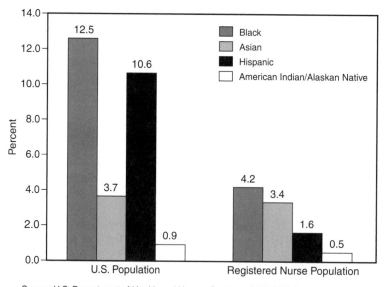

Source: U.S. Department of Health and Human Services, 1996; U.S. Department of Commerce, Bureau of the Census, 1997

FIGURE 14-1. Racial ethnic groups, 1996.

1994; Rosella, et al., 1994; Sims & Baldwin, 1995; Spicer, Repple, Louie, Baj, & Keating, 1994; Stewart, 1998).

Minorities are not only underrepresented in the health care professions but also in clinical research studies. Many research health-related studies and protocols have failed to sufficiently represent minority groups (Rosella, et al. 1994). It is essential that there be increased research into the health needs of minorities. Clinical and nursing research by minorities and about minorities can lead to an improvement of the delivery and health care of minorities (Huttlinger & Drevdahl, 1994; Rosella, et al., 1994).

Professional nursing organizations have addressed cultural and ethnic sensitivity in nursing education. The National League for Nursing (NLN) in 1983 recommended that nursing education incorporate diversity into nursing curricula (Caphinha-Bacote, 1998). The American Academy of Nursing's Expert Panel on Culturally Competent Nursing Care (1992) identified ten recommendations for nursing education. In 1986 the ANA published educational guidelines titled *Cultural diversity in the nursing curriculum: A guide for implementation*. These recommendations and guidelines were developed as a resource for faculty in preparing students to deliver culturally sensitive nursing care. In 1998 the ANA has made cultural diversity a high priority. A position statement by the ANA is soon to be released that addresses discrimination and racism in health care. In addition, an advisory council on cultural diversity is being established. The goals of this advisory council are to assure cultural competency in the current RN workforce, to increase the number of minorities in the RN workforce, and to attract minority students to nursing.

Despite the efforts to promote and integrate cultural awareness and diversity, nursing has not been able to achieve the results it anticipated. Grossman, et al. (1998) surveyed deans and directors of practical, associate, baccalaureate, and masters degree nursing programs in Florida. They were asked about the following: ethnic composition of students and faculty, importance of cultural diversity in the curriculum, critical issues related to cultural diversity, instructional activities on cultural diversity, barriers to recruitment of ethnically diverse faculty and students, strategies for recruitment of ethnically diverse faculty and students, and program needs related to cultural diversity. The results indicated that in Florida, one of the nation's most culturally diverse states, minorities were underrepresented in both faculty and student populations. The majority of the deans and directors indicated that cultural diversity is reflected in their program's mission statement, philosophy, and conceptual framework. Yet, one of the most critical issues identified in the survey relating to cultural diversity was the lack of cultural knowledge, sensitivity, and awareness.

The reason most often cited for a lack of diversity is the recruitment and retention of minority nursing students and nursing faculty. Many strategies used in the recruitment and retention of minority nursing students have been unsuccessful. One reason for this lack of success may be that these strategies are eurocentric and have not been thoroughly researched or looked at from a cultural perspective. Retention strategies should focus not only on the students' weaknesses but build on their strengths. Students should be encouraged to use and express their cultural attributes. These cultural attributes that make each student different will add to the profession of nursing (Campinha-Bacte, 1998).

July (1994) in a descriptive study examining marketing, recruiting, and retention of black nursing students found that high schools (78%) and community colleges (61%) were the main markets for recruiting black nursing students. Successful recruitment strategies included financial aid provisions, student housing, and other approaches unique to a school. Less successful were the traditional strategies of faculty visits, pre-nursing programs, and the use of recruiters. The reasons most frequently given for a school's ability to attract black nursing students was school reputation, black faculty role-models, and support programs which included peer tutoring and writing classes.

Sayles-Cross (1994) explored the issue of recruitment and retention of minority students, faculty, and staff. For minority candidates to be attracted to a school, the students must feel they belong in the school. She suggests a school with a welcoming environment that is sensitive and open to diversity with an atmosphere where minorities feel a sense of belonging. Another area of concern is the attrition rate of minority students. Minority student enrollment and graduations from basic baccalaureate programs in nursing are depicted in Figure 14-2. Sims and Baldwin (1995) cite the educational model as a source of high attrition rates for minorities. The predominant educational model focuses on teaching the exceptional and culturally different student but forces minority students into the mainstream so that they will acquire the knowledge, skills, and abilities valued by the dominant culture. Educational institutions need to design strategies that not only increase minority enrollments but also ensure success and graduation. America is a nation of culturally diverse people with culturally based health care needs. It is clear that nursing values and supports the teaching and practice of culturally sensitive nursing care. Nursing has implemented educational innovations to enhance cultural sensitivity and increase minority representation among nursing students and faculty. Yet there continues to be a shortage in the number of minority RNs to meet the health care needs of an increasing minority population.

Affirmative action has opened the door to opportunity for minorities and women. But it has not shaped a nursing workforce whose cultural profile reflects the diversity of the general population. Affirmative action alone is not the answer. Nursing as a profession and nurses as individuals need to take a leadership role in preparing future nurse leaders that respect and match the culturally diverse population.

Academia and the profession must be willing to give up what is not working and build on strategies that attract minorities into nursing. The literature shows that our traditional education environment and teaching methodolo-

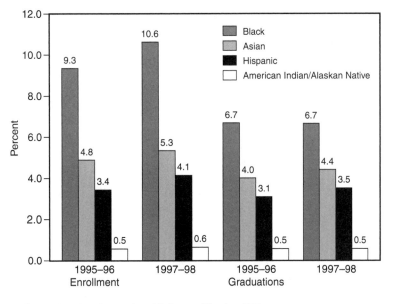

Source: American Association of Colleges of Nursing, 1998

FIGURE 14-2. Minority enrollment and graduations/basic baccalaureate programs in nursing.

gies have not fostered success in a diverse student population. We as nurses, educators, and leaders must look to ourselves in devising new ways to increase diversity in nursing.

References

American Academy of Nursing's Expert Panel on Culturally Competent Nursing Care. (1992). AAN expert panel report: Culturally competent health care. *Nursing Outlook, 40*(6), 277–283.

American Nurses Association, (1998). ANA addressing cultural diversity in profession. *The American Nurse, 30*(1), 25.

American Nurses Association. (1986). *Cultural diversity in the nursing curriculum: A guide for implementation.* Kansas City: Author.

Berlin, L.E., Bednash, G.D. & Scott, D.L. (1998). *1997–1998 Enrollment and graduations in Baccalaureate and graduate programs in nursing.* Washington D.C.: American Association of Colleges of Nursing.

Brewer, C.S. (1997). Through the looking glass: The labor market for registered nurses in the 21st century. *Nursing and Health Care Perspectives, 18*, 260–269.

Campinha-Bacote, J. (1998). Cultural diversity in nursing education: Issues and concerns. *Journal of Nursing Education, 37*, 3–4.

Grossman, D., Massey, P., Blais, K., Geiger, E., Lowe, J., Pereira, O., Stewart, A., Taylor, R., Filer, V., Nembhard, J., & Tally-Ross, N. (1998). Cultural diversity in

Florida nursing programs: A survey of deans and directors. *Journal of Nursing Education*, 37, 22–26.

Huttlinger, K., & Drevdahl, D. (1994). Increasing minority participation in biomedical and nursing research. *Journal of Professional Nursing*, 10, 13–21.

July, F.M. (1994). Marketing, recruiting and retaining African American baccalaureate nursing students. *The ABNF Journal*, 5, 164–167.

Louden, D., & Post, D. (1997). Decline in nursing school enrollment continues according to the latest NLN study. *N&HC: Perspectives on Community*, 18, 96.

Malone, B.L. (1998, January/February). Diversity, divisiveness and divinity. *The American Nurse*, 30, 5,27.

Malone, B.L. (1997). Why isn't nursing more diversified? In J.C. McCloskey, & H.K. Grace, (Eds.), *Current issues in nursing* (5th ed., pp. 574–579). New York: Mosby.

Mezibov, D. (1998, February). With demand for RNs climbing, and shortening supply, forecasters say what's ahead isn't typical "shortage cycle." *Issues Bulletin*, American Association of Colleges of Nursing.

Peterson, L.F. (1998). Affirmative action in education. Vista Magazine (on-line), Available: file http//www.vistamagazine.com/affirm.htm

Rojas, D. (1994). Leadership in a multicultural society: A case in role development. *Nursing & Health Care*, 15, 258–261.

Rosella, J.D., Regan-Kubinski, M.J., & Albrecht, S.A. (1994). The need for multicultural diversity among health professionals. *Nursing & Health Care*, 15, 242–246.

Sayles-Cross, S. (1994). Recruitment and retention of minority students, faculty and staff. *The ABNF Journal*, 5, 158–160.

Sims, G.P., & Baldwin, D. (1995). Race, class and gender considerations in nursing education. *N&HC: Perspectives on community*, 16, 316–321.

Spicer, J.G., Ripple, H.B., Louie, E., Baj, P., & Keating, S. (1994). Supporting ethnic and cultural diversity in nursing staff. *Nursing management*, 25, 38–40.

Stewart, M. (1998, January/February). Nurses need to strengthen cultural competence for next century to ensure quality patient care. *The American Nurse*, 30, 26–27.

Thomas, R., Jr. (1990). From affirmative action to affirming diversity. *Harvard Business Review*, 2, 107–117.

U.S. Department of Commerce, Bureau of the Census. (1997). Statistical abstract of the United States 1997. *The National Data Book*, (117th ed). Washington, D.C. (NTIS No. PB25–1130).

U.S. Department of Health and Human Services (1996). *The registered nurse population, findings from the national sample survey of registered nurses.* Washington, DC: U.S. Government Printing Office.

U.S. Department of Health and Human Services. (1992). *Healthy people 2000: National health promotion and disease prevention objectives: Summary.* Boston: Jones and Bartlett Publishers.

Young, C.E. (1995). *Maintaining diversity without affirmative action.* Higher Education & National Affairs "(On-line)", Available: http//www.acenet.edu/Programs/DGR/affaction/diversity.html

Yuen-Heung To Dutka. (1993). Institutionalizing multicultural education: Focus on the disciplines and the curriculum. *Proteus: A journal of ideas*, 10,11–15.

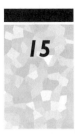

15 Promoting Cultural and Racial Diversity in Nursing: The Need for Political Activism

Mildred HB Roberson

INTRODUCTION

It has been predicted that early in the 21st century the current minority populations will account for 51% of the total U.S. population, and as many as one half of all students will be people of color. For some states in the U.S., such a change has already occurred (M. Andrews, 1997; Bednash, 1997, pp 140–141).

Thus we know that over the next few years there will be an increase in the cultural and ethnic diversity of client/patient populations, student bodies, the workforce, and community settings. In addition, it has become clear that more health care will be community-based in the future, thus requiring nurses to be skillful in functioning in the client's home base and on his/her terms. Such skills will require nurses to become more knowledgeable about acceptable and appropriate behavior in a variety of diverse settings.

For nurses to better serve such a changing population and to better prepare themselves, their students, and their staffs for the changes, nursing needs to more clearly identify what issues are involved in meeting the needs of a changing society. At present, there is considerable confusion in nursing over the concepts of culture, race and minority, which are often used as if they were interchangeable terms. The result is that nurses seek to address multicultural and multiracial issues utilizing the same principles, knowledge base and tactics for both. I am proposing a different approach.

CULTURE AND ITS IMPACT

First, the concept of culture needs to be clarified. Culture refers to the learned patterns of behavior shared widely by members of a particular social group. Culture includes customs, beliefs, values, communication systems and

Mildred HB Roberson, R.N., Ph.D., professor and chair, Department of Nursing, Albany State University, Albany, Georgia.

Reprinted with permission from the *Journal of Multicultural Nursing and Health*, 4(2) 11–15, Summer, 1998.

norms which serve to guide and sanction behavior of group members (Andrews in 1997; Cohen, 1998; Leininger, 1978). All of us are born into a cultural group, more if our ancestors are from different cultural backgrounds, and grow up under the influence of at least one culture. As time passes, we may become members of various sub-cultures which will also influence our values, beliefs and behaviors. Nursing can be considered an example of a sub-culture.

Culture has a major impact on the health beliefs and practices we have, such as: how we conceptualize physical and mental health or illness; what we believe about how to prevent illness or to promote health; what we think causes illness as well as what may have caused the specific symptoms or health problems a person is currently experiencing; what ideas we have about various healing modes, about self-care, about home remedies or about healers; what expectations we have of health providers; and how we express illness (pain, for instance). Culture influences what we perceive to be appropriate or acceptable behavior by ourselves and by others and how we communicate with others or expect others to communicate with us. Culture also influences beliefs about childbearing, child rearing, sexual behaviors, family roles, gender roles, dietary practices, religious practices, and a myriad of other beliefs and practices.

In order to be effective both in providing nursing care to clients and in interacting with co-workers, staff or students, nurses must gain sufficient knowledge and skills to develop a transcultural perspective (Leininger, 1996). Such a perspective requires conscious recognition of our own health beliefs and practices, an awareness that others may not share our health beliefs and practices, a minimal knowledge base about the range and variety of health cultural beliefs, a recognition of the importance of intracultural variation, and a willingness to strive to perceive a situation from the other person's perspective. Only then can a nurse hope to be able to mediate between differing perspectives. (DeSantis, 1991; Roberson, 1993).

It is neither realistic nor desirable for any one nurse to try to learn the multitude of diverse cultural beliefs in the health arena. It is unreasonable to expect any person to know all there is to know about even one culture. Even those nurses with specialized educational preparation in transcultural nursing or medical anthropology know only a few cultures in any depth, although they do have comprehensive knowledge of culture and transcultural principles. Rather than attempt a "recipe approach" of applying categories of customs and values of each ethnic or cultural group to individuals from that culture, it is more useful to learn how to handle cross-cultural situations involving diversity (DeSantis and Lowe, 1992; Kavanagh and Kennedy, 1992). Every nurse can incorporate transcultural principles into practice.

As Kavanagh and Kennedy (1992) suggest, general knowledge about cultural patterns and social organization provides a framework for cross-cultural communication and caregiving. It may be helpful to remember that in any health care encounter between nurses and clients or students there is "a minimum of three cultures involved" (DeSantis, 1990, p 6). One is the nurse's professional knowledge based on his/her education in combination with personal values, beliefs and practices. The second is the culture of the student or client which includes his/her interpretation of biomedicine based on personal experiences with health and illness, as well as the personal beliefs and values he/she brings to the situation. And last, there is the culture of the institution or community setting in which the encounter takes place (DeSantis, 1990).

■ RACE, RACISM AND NURSING

Let's look now at the concepts of race and minority. Race generally connotes genetic differences and is used to refer to persons sharing distinguishing physical characteristics. In the US, race is most often used to refer to skin tone (Barbee, 1993). It is a term becoming increasingly difficult to clarify in the United States both because of the evidence presented by biological anthropologists of extreme heterogeneity existing in supposed racial groups and also because of the fact that many Americans are multiracial (Dressler, 1993; Cohen, 1998). Indeed, almost 10 million Americans could not find an applicable racial category to check on the 1990 census. Minority is an even more elusive term. Although technically it refers to any group which is numerically smaller than a majority of a population, in practice, minority is more often used to refer to those persons lacking the power and/or status attributed to those holding majority status. So, even a group which is numerically larger than another, such as women in the US, may be referred to as a minority (Kavanagh & Kennedy, 1992; Roberson, 1994).

Neither race nor minority designations can or should be assumed to reveal cultural background to us (Kavanagh 1993; Roberson, 1993b). The US Census racial categories of Black; Native American/Eskimo/Aleut; Asian or Pacific Islander; Hispanic; and White each represent multiple cultures. While these cultures may share some elements in common, there are many elements not shared. In fact, some cultures which would be lumped together by the census categories, for instance Vietnamese and Chinese, may clash quite vigorously over beliefs and speak different languages (Galanti, 1991; Roberson, 1993b). Native Americans include several hundred tribes, each with its own culture. Similarly, Black Americans include the cultures of Jamaicans, Haitians, and specific African groups, in addition to that of American born Blacks. The category of Hispanic is perhaps the most confounding of all, since it can refer to persons of any race, as well as from a large variety of cultures.

As suggested by the preceding commentary, I do not believe that a transcultural perspective alone addresses the issues of a multiracial population which nursing must address to be effective in serving this population. What I am proposing is that nurses must also develop what I call a "transracial" perspective. Nursing needs to directly confront the problems of racism, prejudice, discrimination and race relations (Roberson, 1993b; Barbee, 1993;

Jackson, 1993). Racism entails a belief in the superiority of one's own race over others. Unlike ethnocentrism which is often associated with a knowledge deficit about other cultures, racism is more often associated with a prejudiced, sometimes irrational reaction to physical traits and assumptions about associated attitudes, behaviors and the like.

While education about race may help somewhat to reduce racism, education alone is not likely to overcome racism in nursing. Nursing values maintain homogeneity and avoid conflict (Barbee, 1993; Brink 1994; Kavanagh, 1993). Therefore, nurses are more comfortable in denying that racism exists in their world or avoiding racism by assuming a color-blind perspective and not using the term (Barbee, 1993). Moreover, recognizing that social action by nurses is a nursing role needed to address racism requires an understanding of political, economic and social influences at a population level, whereas nursing traditionally emphasizes an individual focus (Kavanagh, 1993). Nursing must examine and face the complex racial issues and problems existing in nursing and search more aggressively for solutions.

It is true that for both multicultural and multiracial issues, education of faculties, students, staff and administrators is needed. It is also true that nursing needs to more actively recruit and retain a more culturally and racially diverse nurse population. And it is true that for both issues nurses need to look at the impact of the larger society on beliefs and practices, such as the influence of political and economic factors on cultural and racial issues. But for racism, my sense is that nursing must tackle systems problems as well as individual beliefs, attitudes and knowledge. This action will require the "upstream thinking" described by Butterfield (1997), a focus on changing economic, political and societal factors impacting on a situation. Health care reform will need to include reform of nursing practices and mind sets of racism which interfere with meeting health care needs or with diversifying the nurse population.

▦ *NURSING READINESS TO CHANGE*

In sum, what I propose then is that nurses must become both transcultural and transracial in our perspective in order to adapt to our changing society. How ready are we for this challenge? As Brink (1994) has pointed out "the American belief system appears to view cultural diversity as a relatively unimportant subject for study. . . ." (p 658) and "American nurses know very little about cultural diversity. . . ." (p 659) "Cultural diversity does not happen peacefully, without struggle and strain. . . ." (p 664). Brink implies that attaining a nurse population with a transcultural perspective will not occur without "conflict or pain. . . ." (p 664).

And Barbee (1993) has commented on nursing readiness to address the challenges of race and racism: "The contradiction between caring, a principal part of the identity of nursing, and racism make it difficult for nurses to acknowledge racial prejudice in the profession" (p 346). She added that "race and racism remain taboo topics for most European Americans" (p 346). Moreover, because of the "profession's need to avoid conflict" (p 350) and maintain homogeneity, "certain types of racism have flourished" (p 350) in nursing, and the unwillingness of the profession "to recognize that racism is endemic in nursing and health care" (p 357) then leads to "a lack of discussion about racism. . . ." (p 357). Barbee believes that nursing can only move forward when we acknowledge racism in nursing and redirect the energy wasted in denying racism toward forming alliances and revising organizational goals that can change power relationships. Such action sounds like political activism to me.

■ *THE NEED FOR POLITICAL ACTIVISM*

I would like to now discuss how a transcultural and transracial perspective relates to the need for political activism by nurses focusing on the examples of migrant farm worker needs and human rights issues.

Migrant Farmworkers

Migrant farmworkers are, by government definition, people "whose principal employment has been in agriculture on a seasonal basis during the past 24 months and who established a temporary abode for employment" (United States Department of Health and Human Services [DHHS], 1990, p 3). Accurate statistics on this population are virtually impossible due to their transient status, but an estimate of between 2.7 and five million people annually has been made by the National Migrant Resource Program (NMRP) and the Migrant Clinicians Network for DHHS (1990). Migrant farmworkers are a multicultural and multiracial group with a variety of languages represented. They are a young group with close to 40% being under age 14 ("Accessing the Migrant", n.d.). Nearly one half of them have had less than a ninth grade education. Many speak and read little or no English (Sullivan, 1992). Their average family income in 1990 was estimated at less than $6000 per year. Ninety percent of migrant farm workers are thought to be below poverty level, yet only 10% receive any government assistance. Workers are also excluded from many benefits related to health needs such as insurance or paid sick days (Woodruff, 1990).

These demographics, however, tell only part of the health story. Migrant farmworker families live and work in very difficult environmental conditions both at their home bases and at their work sites. Access to hot water, to potable drinking water, to adequate refrigeration or to usable toilets may be limited. In addition, exposure to sun, to pesticides and other toxic chemicals, and to backbreaking work is an ongoing problem (Sullivan, 1992).

It is not surprising that the life expectancy for migrant farm workers is an appalling 49 years. They have TB and Hepatitis rates more often associated with a developing country. They have a rate of Diabetes 300 times higher than the general population and a rate of Parasitic infections 20 times higher (Sullivan, 1992). Their death rate from Pneumonia is 200% greater than the national average and the infant mortality rate is 25% greater ("Accessing the Migrant," n.d.).

Not only must migrant farm worker families face these and other health problems, but also they can expect to encounter major cultural, social, economic, racial, environmental and political barriers in trying to deal with these health problems. Nurses will likewise face similar barriers in trying to resolve this group's health needs. There is a tremendous need for nursing solutions and strategies for overcoming the barriers and meaningfully addressing the health needs. This is a clear case for political activism.

Human Rights Issues

Another way to look at how a transracial and transcultural perspective relates to the need for political activism is to consider human rights issues. There have been real battles on the international scene over what constitutes human rights, who sets or should set the standards and what practices are or should be considered violations of human rights. The US is accused of being ethnocentric in viewing its definition and standards as appropriate for everyone and for judging others ("Battle looms," 1993). Definitions and standards of human rights evolve in part from a group's cultural beliefs and practices. Thus even within the US, examples of human rights issues can be found, many of which relate to differences in cultural beliefs and customs.

Core American culture values individual rights and freedoms, equitable and just treatment of individuals, and respect for all humans. By our core cultural standards, women and ethnic minorities deserve equality, free speech should be permitted, health care should be a right, individuals' cultural beliefs should be respected and accepted, and violence used against another person should be seen as wrong (Roberson, 1993a).

However, some problems arise in the fulfillment of our core cultural ideals. Not only does it appear that some people are more equal than others and that money, power, race and gender all influence the exercising of one's rights, but also there are the questions of whose rights and values should prevail and whose should be protected?

For instance, what constitutes abuse within a family situation? The definition of abuse varies across cultures, because there are cultural differences as to what behaviors are deemed acceptable, what roles are appropriate, what child-rearing practices are permissible, how anger should be handled, when punishment is called for and what it may include. Religious beliefs within a segment of a cultural group may further define abuse. Actions which some nurses might label as abuse may be accepted as appropriate "discipline" within a given culture's view of spousal or parental roles in a family (Galanti, 1991).

There are multiple other examples of human rights issues that relate to differences in cultural beliefs and customs, such as in the area of reproductive rights, sexual harassment and end of life decisions. A basic human right is having one's cultural beliefs respected and addressed appropriately. A transcultural perspective requires that we recognize and understand the cultural beliefs and values relevant in a human rights situation and respond in a culturally competent manner.

Similarly a transracial perspective requires that we recognize and understand the racial factors relevant in a human rights situation and respond in a racially competent manner. A striking example came out several years ago in the stand taken by the US Congressional Black Caucus over the unequal treatment of African-American criminals. And both Barbee (1993) and Jackson (1993) provide nursing examples of race influencing human rights in the areas of nursing practice, education and research. For instance, Jackson (1993) points out the failure of nursing to consider the unequal access to and distribution of resources at the societal level as a prime contribution to the health status gap between races, and Barbee (1993) suggest that institutional racism is a factor in the lack of a more racially diverse nurse population and nursing student body.

To acknowledge race and culture in establishing human rights conventions requires a comprehensive knowledge of how culture and race impact human rights, and then a willingness to come to grips with our profession's belief system and stated values. It is relatively easy to say we believe in the core American values stated earlier, but infinitely more difficult to move beyond these abstract ideals to create a comprehensive definition of human rights standards and guidelines for nursing practice. I believe nursing needs a Human Rights Code for nurses that incorporates a transcultural and transracial perspective. Such an action by nurses would be one example of political activism in an area that calls out for nurses to exercise political influence.

■ STRATEGIES FOR CHANGE

To ensure incorporation of a transracial and transcultural perspective into health care reform, several strategies can be considered. It is helpful to be clear on the difference between local, state and national level laws and legislators, and the relationship between politics, policy and law. To influence state and national policy and laws, usually it is necessary to work through local contacts and with local constituents. We need to strategize regarding policy in agencies, schools of nursing and local communities, as well as at the state and national levels. To be effective in addressing transcultural and transracial concerns, we need to be knowledgeable about the issues, the demographics, specific problems and relevant laws or policies currently existing in our agencies, locales, states, and so forth. Then we need to assess the composition of the legislature or policy-making body for its commitment to a transracial/ transcultural perspective.

In the late 1990's, nurses ignore politics at their peril. If we wish to have our perspectives addressed when agendas are set and decisions are made, we need to be politically active. To do so means lobbying, networking, coalition-building and reaching out across disciplines, across ethnic groups, and across health care settings in both education and service to create a strong body of support for our issues.

We need to be willing to tackle specific problems relating to cultural and racial issues, such as those mentioned earlier. Minimal attention is paid by nurses to tracking migrant farmworker families to determine what their health needs and problems are and how or if these needs are being addressed. We can lobby to get these needs identified and met. We can educate others as to who migrant farmworkers are and why their health needs should be a concern to everyone. We can lobby for laws to protect migrant farmworkers.

They are probably the single most oppressed and overlooked group in the nation with some of the worst health problems. Nurses need to be politically active on their behalf.

Nurses must decide if we value cultural and racial diversity in nursing enough to take political action to achieve it. If so, we can seek to influence funding sources and allocation of resources at all levels that may assist in meeting the needs for recruitment and retention of a diverse group. Nurses can establish a policy requiring training and knowledge needed to gain transcultural and transracial competency in schools of nursing and in service agencies for staff, students, faculty and administration.

As for racism, nursing might consider Barbee's (1993) writings. She suggests that we acknowledge that racism in nursing exists, confront it, explore it, and form alliances to alter existing power relationships. Changing attitudes is never easy but cannot be accomplished at all if we do not make a start. It might also be helpful for nurses to conduct research on racism in nursing to more clearly identify what factors are contributing to its continued existence.

As indicated at the outset, nurses need to promote racial and cultural diversity in nursing and health care by developing a transcultural and transracial perspective and by being politically active. As the world changes around us, nursing needs to assure that these changes will be appropriately addressed. There is still an opportunity to be proactive in establishing nursing's role in meeting this challenge.

References

Accessing the Migrant Health Program (n.d.). *Bureau of Health Care Delivery and Assistance, Migrant Health Program,* Rockville, MD.

Andrews, MM (1997). Cultural diversity and community health nursing. In JM Swanson & MA Nies, *Community health nursing: Promoting the health of aggregates,* 2nd ed. (pp 435–475). Philadelphia: WB Saunders.

Barbee, EL (Guest Ed.). (1993). Racism, gender, class and health [special issue]. *Medical Anthropology Quarterly, 7* (4).

Barbee, EL (1993). Racism in US nursing. *Medical Anthropology Quarterly, 7* (4), 346–362.

Battle looms over definition of rights at Vienna meeting. (1993, June 14). *USA Today,* p. 10A.

Bednash, GP (1997). The changing pool of students. In JC McCloskey & HK Grace, Eds. *Current issues in nursing,* 5th ed. (pp 140–147). St. Louis: CV Mosby.

Brink, PJ (1994). Cultural diversity in nursing: How much can we tolerate? In JC McCloskey & HK Grace, Eds. *Current issues in nursing,* 4th ed. (pp 658–664). St. Louis: CV Mosby.

Butterfield, PG (1997). Thinking upstream: Conceptualizing health from a population perspective. In JM Swanson & MA Nies, *Community health nursing: Promoting the health of aggregates.* 2nd ed. Philadelphia: WB Saunders.

Cohen, MN (1998, April 17). Culture, not race, explains human diversity. *Chronicle of Higher Education, XLIV,* p. B4–5.

DeSantis, L. (1990, September). *Bridging the gap: Cultural diversity in nursing.* Paper presented at Florida Nurses Association Conference on Cultural Diversity, Marco Island, Florida.

DeSantis, L (1991). Developing faculty expertise in culturally focused care and research. *Journal of Professional Nursing, 7* (5), 300–309.

DeSantis, L & Lowe, J (1992, October 22). *Moving from cultural sensitivity to cultural competence.* Paper presented at the Eighteenth Annual Transcultural Nursing Society Conference, Miami, Florida.

Dressler, WW (1993). Health in the African-American community. *Medical Anthropology Quarterly, 7* (4), 325–345.

Galanti, GA (1991). *Caring for patients from different cultures.* Philadelphia: University of Pennsylvania Press.

Jackson, EM (1993). Whiting-out differences: Why US nursing research fails black families. *Medical Anthropology Quarterly, 7* (4), 363–385.

Kavanagh, KH (1993). Transcultural nursing: Facing the challenges of advocacy, and diversity/universality. *Journal of Transcultural Nursing, 5* (1), 4–13.

Kavanagh, KH & Kennedy, PH (1992). *Promoting cultural diversity.* Newbury Park, CA: Sage.

Leininger, MM (1978). *Transcultural nursing: Concepts, theories and practices.* New York: Wiley & Sons.

Leininger, MM (1996). Major directions for transcultural nursing: A journey into the 21st century. *Journal of Transcultural Nursing, 7* (2), 28–32.

Roberson, MHB (1993 a, Summer) Cultural aspects of human rights. Guest corner. *American Nurses Association Center for Ethics & Human Rights Communique, 2* (1), 4, 6.

Roberson, MHB (1993 b, September). Defining cultural and ethnic differences to adapt to a changing patient population. *The American Nurse, 25* (8): 6.

Roberson, MHB (1994, October 28). *Promoting cultural and racial diversity in health care: A case for political activism.* Paper presented at the plenary session, Oklahoma State Nurses Association Annual Convention.

Sullivan, LW (1992, First Quarter). Addressing the medical needs of the migrant population. *Texas Journal of Rural Health,* 1–5.

United States Department of Health and Human Services (1990). National Migrant Resource Program and the Migrant Clinicians Network. *Migrant and seasonal farmworker health objectives for the year 2000.* Rockville MD: DHHS.

United States Department of Health and Human Services (1991).

Migrant Health Program. *An Atlas of State profiles which estimate number of migrant and seasonal farmworkers and members of their families.* Rockville MD: DHHS.

Woodruff, J (1990). New harvest of shame. *Frontline.* Washington, DC: Public Broadcasting Service.

Acknowledgement: *This article is a revised version of an earlier article in* The American Nurse, 25*(8), with permission of the American Nurses Association.*

16

Alternative Medicine: Value and Risks

Wayne B. Jonas

Medical practices outside the mainstream of "official" medicine have always been an important part of the public's health care. Healers and herbalists, bonesetters and barbers, shamans and spiritualists have offered the public a multiplicity of ways to address the confusion and suffering that accompany disease. A century ago in the United States there was a period of "enchantment" with unorthodox medicine. Homeopaths, herbalists, psychic and magnetic healers, and "eclectics" proliferated—most with little to no training, regulation of practice, or standards for quality of care. The prominence and configuration of these "irregulars," as they were called, has waxed and waned, depending on the perceived value of orthodox medicine, the needs of the public, and the changing values of society. The prominence of these practices subsided with the development of scientific medicine in this century and its dramatic advances in the understanding and treatment of disease.

Historically, orthodox medicine fights these practices vigorously by denouncing and attacking them, restricting access to them, labeling them as antiscientific and quackery, and imposing penalties for practicing them. When these therapies persist and even rise in popularity despite this, mainstream medicine then turns more friendly, examining them, identifying similarities they have with the orthodox, and incorporating or "integrating" them into the routine practice of medicine. In the past, orthodox medicine has benefited from their selective integration by abandoning ineffective therapies such as bloodletting, adopting new drugs such as digitalis, and developing more rigorous scientific methods with which to test these practices, such as blinding and randomization.

Wayne B. Jonas, M.D., is Director of the National Center for Complementary and Alternative Medicine, National Institutes of Health.

Reprinted with permission from *Consumers' Research, 82* (1), 16–18, January, 1999.

A version of this article also ran in the November 11 issue of the *JAMA*, the journal of the American Medical Association.

The increasing popularity of complementary and alternative medicine (now used by more than 40% of the public) reflects changing needs and values in modern society in general. This includes a rise in prevalence of chronic disease, an increase in public access to worldwide health information, reduced tolerance for paternalism, an increased sense of entitlement to a quality life, declining faith that scientific breakthroughs will have relevance for the personal treatment of disease, and an increased interest in spiritualism. In addition, concern about the adverse effects and escalating costs of conventional health care are fueling the search for alternative approaches to the prevention and management of illness. As the public's use of healing practices outside conventional medicine accelerates, ignorance about these practices by physicians and scientists risks broadening the communication gap between the public and the profession that serves it.

Today, the overwhelming effort is toward attempts at "integrating" alternative practices into the mainstream. Sixty percent of medical schools have begun to teach about alternative medicine practices, hospitals are creating complementary and integrated medicine programs, health suppliers are offering expanded benefits packages that include the services of alternative practitioners, and biomedical research organizations are investing more substantial amounts toward the investigation of these practices. For example, the Office of Alternative Medicine at the National Institutes of Health has just become the National Center for Complementary and Alternative Medicine, with a budget of $50 million. The activities of the Office of Alternative Medicine and recent studies published in *JAMA* illustrate that quality scientific research can be conducted and published on alternative medicine topics. It appears that complementary and alternative medicine has again "come of age" in the United States. However, the rush to embrace a new integration of alternative and conventional medicine should be approached with great caution: Alternative medicine, like conventional medicine, has pros and cons, promotes bad ideas and good ones, and promises to hold both benefits and risks. Without critical assessment of what should be integrated and what should not, we risk developing a health care system that costs more, is less safe, and fails to address the management of chronic disease in a publicly responsible manner. the potential risks and benefits of alternative medicine must be examined carefully before heading into a new but not necessarily better health care world.

■ RISKS OF EMBRACING

Quality of Care. The formal components of medical physician licensure usually are not required of alternative medicine practitioners. These include the content and length of time of training, testing and certification, a defined scope of practice, review and audit, and professional liability with regulatory protection and statutory authorization complete with codified disciplinary action. All 50 states do provide licensure requirements for chiropractic practice, but only about half do so for acupuncture and massage therapy and fewer do for homeopathy and naturopathy. Many of these practitioners operate largely unmonitored.

Quality of Products. The "natural" products used by alternative medicine practitioners also are largely unmonitored and their quality is uncontrolled. These products are available on the market as dietary supplements and may be contaminated or vary tremendously in content, quality, and safety. Garlic, for example, claimed for many years to have cholesterol-lowering effects, may not produce such effects if processed in certain ways. Thus, even if one product is proven safe and effective, other similar products on the market may have quite different effects that preclude consistent dosing. Fifteen million Americans are taking high-dose vitamins or herbal preparations along with prescription drugs, thereby risking adverse effects from unknown interactions.

Quality of Science. The use of science for understanding alternative medicine is frequently missing from such practices. Most alternative medicine systems have been largely unchanged for hundreds or thousands of years. Often they begin from the teachings of a charismatic leader that are not advanced with new observations, hypothesis-driven testing, innovation, and peer-review. Claiming that their practices are too "individual" or "holistic" to study scientifically, many alternative medicine practices hide behind anecdote, case series, or "outcomes" research. To accept such views is falsely to label conventional medicine as nonholistic and reject the hard-fought gains made in the use of basic biological knowledge, the randomized, controlled clinical trial, and evidence-based medicine for health care decision-making.

To adopt alternative medicine without developing quality standards for its practices, products, and research is to return to a time in medicine when quackery and therapeutic confusion prevailed. Modern conventional medicine excels in the areas of quality health care and the use of science: alternative medicine must change to adopt similar standards. Conventional medicine is also the world's leader in the management of infectious, traumatic, and surgical diseases, in the study of pathology, and in biotechnology and drug development. All medical practices have the ethical obligation to retain these strengths for the benefit of patients.

■ RISKS OF CONVENTIONALIZING

Healing. Most alternative medicine systems carefully attend to the illness and suffering that accompany all disease. The time spent with each patient by an alternative medicine practitioner usually exceeds that spent by the average conventional physician, and patients are often more satisfied with their interactions with unorthodox than orthodox medical practitioners. Alternative medicine practitioners provide patients with understanding, meaning, and self-care methods for managing their condition. Empowerment, participation in the healing process, time, and personal attention are essential elements of all medicine. These elements are easily lost in the subspecialization, technology, and economics of modern medicine. Conventional medicine must develop a better language for managing illness and suffering or lose this essential message that alternative medicine provides.

Adverse Effects. In the last century, unconventional medicine increased in popularity because of the use of severe treatments such as bloodletting, purging, and toxic metals by conventional medicine. The popularity of alternative medicine in this century is also driven by the perception that conventional treatments are too harsh to use for chronic and non-life-threatening disease. Iatrogenic disease caused by conventional medicine is a major cause of death and hospitalization in the United States. While some alternative medicine practices have important toxicities, many have reduced potential for adverse effects when properly delivered. Conventional medicine can learn from alternative medicine how to "gentle" its approach by focusing on the patient's inherent capacity for self-healing.

Costs. Skyrocketing costs of conventional medicine also are driving the search for alternatives. Savings from managed care now are maximized and health care costs are predicted to double in the next 10 years. If low-cost interventions such as lifestyle changes, diet, supplement therapy, and behavioral medicine can be delivered as substitutes for high-cost drugs and technological interventions, true cost reductions and the compression of morbidity might be achieved.

If there is a single strength of alternative medicine that risks being lost in its "integration" with conventional care, it is an emphasis on self-healing as the lead approach for both improving wellness and for the treatment of disease. All the major alternative medicine systems approach illness first by trying to support and induce the self-healing processes of the person. If recovery can occur from this, the likelihood of adverse effects and the need for high-impact, high-cost interventions is reduced. It is this orientation toward self-healing and health promotion (salutogenesis rather than pathogenesis) that makes alternative medicine approaches to chronic disease especially attractive.

▦ THE FUTURE OF MEDICINE

The main "obstacles to discovery," writes Daniel Boorstin, are "the illusions of knowledge." Indeed, the capacity of humans to fool themselves by making claims of truth, postulating unfounded explanations, and denying the reality of observations they cannot explain is endless. Science has emerged as one of the few truly powerful approaches for mitigating this self-delusionary capacity. The clinical experimental method, in the form of the randomized, controlled trial, examines to what extent attributions and explanations of these therapies are accurate.

The goals of medicine, no matter what the label, are the same for all practices. Is the current trend toward "integrated" medicine a deluded temptation that will turn out to be a nightmare of unscientific practices? Or will these newfound tools of scientific medicine be used to look deeper into the processes of healing for their utility in treating disease and alleviating suffering? In the past 50 years, powerful social forces have transformed medicine. If a new evidence-based "integrated" medicine does emerge, it will likely be subject to the same forces shaping the future of medicine in general. This includes the continued takeover of medicine by managed care, a more refined ability to manipulate individual susceptibilities using nanotechnology, and the ability to track quality of care and individual patient outcomes with networks of information monitoring. Research in alternative medicine will help identify what is safe and effective and will further the understanding of biology by exploring, rather than marginalizing, unorthodox medical claims and findings. Alternative medicine is here to stay. It is no longer an option to ignore it or treat it as something outside the normal processes of science and medicine. The challenge is to move forward carefully, using both reason and wisdom, as we attempt to separate the pearls from the mud.

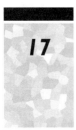

17

Alternative and Complementary Healing: Implications for Nursing

Joan Engebretson

The term "alternative therapy" has been used to describe therapeutic approaches that are unconventional, nontraditional, integral, and holistic. According to Micozzi, Kronenberg, and Jobst (1995), alternative therapies encompass healing paradigms and practices that are routine for much of the world but are not commonly embraced by Western allopathic or biomedical institutions. These authors estimate that 80 per cent of the world's population uses some form of what Western biomedicine considers alternative therapies. "Alternative" is a misleading term because in the United States and Europe, such therapies generally are used as a complement to rather than an alternative to biomedical therapy. Although a few patients may forsake biomedical treatment in favor of alternative therapies, the majority use these therapies in addition to biomedical treatment and/or for the promotion of health and prevention of disease.

Cassileth (1998) differentiated between unproven treatments that are used in lieu of biomedical treatment (alternative) and the noninvasive, gentle, pleasant, often natural, stress-reducing treatments (complementary) that are used in sickness and in health. Complimentary therapies can be defined as those therapies or modalities that are used adjunctively with biomedicine to augment healing, facilitate comfort, and promote health. Many of these therapies have their roots in cross-cultural or historical healing practices, and an investigation of the multicultural aspects of these practices, although fascinating, is beyond the scope of this article. Instead, this article will focus on the responses of the health care industry to complementary therapies; the similarities of these therapies to nursing practice; and the implications of these modalities for nursing research, practice, and education.

The popularity of complementary modalities, particularly among the well-educated middle class, has been well-documented (Engebretson, 1992; Hufford, 1986; McGuire, 1988). According to two large telephone surveys

Joan Engebretson, Dr. P.H., R.N., C.N.S., is an associate professor at the School of Nursing, Health Science Center, The University of Texas-Houston, Houston, TX.

Reprinted with permission from the *Journal of Professional Nursing, 15* (4), 214–223, July/August, 1999. Copyright © 1999, W.B. Saunders Company.

(Eisenberg et al. 1993; 1998), the use of alternative health care practices increased from 33.8 per cent in 1990 to 42.1 per cent in 1997, exceeding total visits to all US primary care physicians. Fewer than 40 per cent of participants discussed this use with their health care provider. This increase was attributable to an increase in the number of individuals seeking these therapies rather than an increase in the number of visits per patient. Estimated out-of-pocket expenditures for alternative therapies were $27 billion, which is comparable with projections for out-of-pocket expenditures for all US physician services. Another survey indicated that 42 per cent of participants reported using alternative therapies, and 67 per cent indicated that the availability of these therapies was important in choosing a health care plan (Landmark, 1998). A survey of more than 1,000 adults found that use of alternative therapies was associated with having a higher level of education and a more holistic orientation to health; having a chronic health problem or other recent illness; and having had a transformational experience that changed one's world view (Astin, 1998). These findings raise several questions about the social context that contributes to the current interest in healing modalities outside the biomedical establishment. Why are simple, nontechnical modalities gaining in popularity when technology and communication have become so advanced? The complementary healing community is responding to the public interest in healing and to these shifts in the social context. Many of these modalities are similar to autonomous nursing interventions, such as touch, massage, stress management, counseling, comfort measures, and activities to facilitate coping. The purpose and viability of any profession is to meet a public need. For the profession of nursing, it is therefore important to consider the implications of the popularity of complementary therapies.

■ CONTEMPORARY SOCIETAL CONTEXT

Health care, as a social institution, influences and is influenced by the social context in which it is practiced. A confluence of changes related to technology, economics, values, and philosophy in the United States contribute to the current increased interest in complementary healing modalities. Table 17-1 outlines some of the social factors that are changing in the transition from the Industrial to the Information Age and the concurrent response by complementary healers.

Technological Development

Science and technology have developed at an unprecedented pace, creating a different world of health care practice each decade. Electronic technology and microtechnologies challenge the limits of both time and space. Medical technology allows for diagnostic and treatment techniques that act at the cel-

TABLE 17-1. _Comparison of the Industrial and Information Ages With Responses of Complementary Healers_

Contextual Issues	Industrial Age	Information Age	Response of Complementary Healers
Technology			
Biotechnology	Technological promise	Human experience	High touch/low technology
Communication	Mass media	Individual access to universal data	Individualized care
Marketing of health information	Medical brokers	Direct access	Self-healing
Economics	Economic superpower	Global economy	Low-cost access
Politics	Centralized	Local	Personal locus of responsibility
Values			
Ecology	Control over nature	Harmony with nature	Connection with nature
Meaning	Materialism	Increased interest in meaning and spirituality	Spiritual is central
Philosophy	Logical positivism	Systems theory	Holism
Medical approach	Treatment	Prevention	Well-being
Metaphors	Military	Communications	Transformation

lular level or even at the level of DNA. Information technology allows communication from points around the globe to occur in seconds.

BIOTECHNOLOGY

Biotechnological methods of diagnosis and treatment have become so sophisticated that a subindustry has evolved to orient medical staff to appropriate equipment use. Reiser (1982) described the shift in medicine toward increased reliance on data obtained, analyzed, or interpreted by machines or laboratory tests rather than data gathered by provider–patient interaction. Science and technology have merged in the perception of the public, and the instrumental and secular claims of the scientific revolution have exerted an ideological dominance on the world at large (Tambiah, 1990). However, many people have become disenchanted with the limits of the technologized world. Despite the marvelous promise of these capabilities, people still get sick, die, and become unhappy, and babies are born imperfect. Although many people have become disillusioned with the limits of the technologized world, most people would not want to dispense with technological options.

The negative antiscience sentiments are more likely related to the public's unrealistic belief in the promise of science to solve all the problems of the human condition. Some diseases that have no known cure (eg, some cancers, acquired immunodeficiency syndrome [AIDS]), and some diseases previously thought to be under control (eg, tuberculosis and some infectious diseases) are re-emerging with great ferocity. Other diseases are emerging that previously were unknown (Ebola virus infection and chronic fatigue syndrome).

Reports of depersonalization and dehumanization are common to individuals' encounters with the health care system. Locsin (1995) reported that many nurses perceive that the emphasis on high technology has been at the expense of the human element in health care. One explanation for the popularity of alternative practices is that there has been an overreliance on science and technology to explain and solve the complex issues of human existence. Complementary therapies offer low-technology interventions that focus on some of the spiritual and comfort aspects of healing not generally addressed by high-tech medicine.

COMMUNICATION

Technological development has had great impact on communication. The Information Age is characterized by technology that allows for the diffusion of ideas at an unprecedented rate. This has expanded awareness of cultural pluralism in the United States and has exposed the general public to a diversity of ideas. Exposure to unfamiliar cultural ideas and practices challenges many accepted cultural beliefs and the assumptions on which those beliefs are founded. This exposure has made it clear to the public that biomedicine based in Western ideology is but one of many approaches to health. In response to this interest, bookstores often have entire sections devoted to self-help, new age topics, alternative health, and spirituality that contain a rich assortment of information on techniques for healing and/or promoting health.

Mass media, marketing, and delivery of services are typical of the Industrial Age and can be contrasted with the Information Age regarding the ability of providing individualized information. Negroponte (1995) described this shift from mass marketing and media to forecast an "audience the size of one" (p. 184). This "narrow casting" describes the electronic capacity of individuals to find information tailor-made to their unique and individual needs. This projection identifies the mass media/marketing age as typical of the Industrial Age and contrasts it with the impending Information Age as the age of mass demographic shrinks to a focus on the individual. Many alternative healers provide modalities specific to the complexities of the individual patient, not to specific diseases (Engebretson, 1996). This could be seen as an opportunity for nursing, which has, within its present constrictions, maintained the importance of the individual and individualizing patient care.

MARKETING HEALTH INFORMATION

More over-the-counter drugs and other treatments are being marketed directly to the public through advertising and media. The lay public can access books, films, television, the Internet, and other media that expand ideas on healing, treatment of disease, life-styles, and health-related practices. Many complementary therapies are marketed directly to the public without the intermediary input of health care providers or institutions. This direct marketing is evidenced by the plethora of books and workshops on alternative health services, health-promoting activities, stress reduction, and self-care programs. Over the past decade, this information has moved into mainstream stores across the United States. Many women's journals and Internet sites feature discussions about complementary therapies. Without a health care professional acting as broker and/or interpreter of health-related information, the consumer is an independent agent who seeks, finds, decides upon, and often uses various healing products and techniques. Use of these products and services often is independent of whatever biomedical treatment they may be receiving.

Economics

Economics, locally and globally, is a major factor influencing social institutions, including the health care industry. The growth of international trade and the lowering of trade barriers has accelerated the movement of manufacturing to second world countries and concentrated the science and technology industries in the United States. The resulting reorganization and disruption have led to economic insecurities even as the economy has become stronger. One immediate ramification of this shift is on workers' access to health care. Many families who recently enjoyed a middle-class life of comfort are now faced with unemployment or contract employment, conditions that often are without health care benefits. Alternative and complementary therapies may have the appeal of an affordable and readily accessible source of health care. Additionally, economic changes, insecurity, and the lowering of socioeconomic status create high levels of stress in families. A corpus of theory and research is developing in the health care field about the toxic effects of stress on individuals, families, and public health (Amick, Levine, Tarlov, & Walsh, 1995; Pincus & Callahan, 1995). Higher morbidity and mortality rates are associated with lower socioeconomic status (Evans, Barer, & Marmor, 1994). Many complementary modalities offer potential for promoting health and modulating stress. Many of them may have some efficacy in reducing the cardiovascular effects of stress, and some show promise of enhancing the immune system (Orth-Gomer & Schneiderman, 1996; Schneiderman, McCabe, & Baum, 1992).

Health care in the United States costs more per person and per unit of service, is provided at a more intense level, and offers comparatively poor gross outcomes. Health care costs grew at an annual rate of 11.6 per cent between 1970 and 1990, whereas income increased at a rate of 8.8 per cent as measured by the gross national product (Lee, Soffel, & Luft, 1997). Many health care institutions have joined businesses in re-engineering and attempting to cut overall costs of providing health care through managed care. Concern for health care costs and the impetus for health care reform have forced the health care community to begin looking at prevention and lower-cost interventions. Complementary therapies often offer low-cost, low-technology services aimed at promoting health.

Political and Social Change

Toffler and Toffler (1994) described "demassification" as a social force in the Information Age that returns decision-making to the local and personal level. This trend is reflected in programs that support communities and individuals to become more active participants in their own health and health care. It also is evidenced by the recent interest in community, family, and individual empowerment (McKnight, 1995). Community development, return to family values, and the reassertion of individual rights and responsibilities have become popular issues. This movement also may help address the high costs of government entitlement programs. Self-care currently is highly valued, and many complementary therapies are based on individual responsibility and stress the importance of relationships. Congruent with this, healers often incorporate personal empowerment and some include group support in clients' care.

Values

As the Industrial Age has shifted to the Information Age, American values concurrently have shifted away from modernism, which was characterized by a belief in progress, materialism, objectivism, and the control and exploitation of nature. These values are being expanded to include concern for quality-of-life, desire for personalization, and a reverence for nature. These new values are evident in the emphasis on the environment, a more overt interest in religion and spirituality, and an emergence of postmodern ideologies such as cultural relativism (Anderson, 1995; Borgmann, 1992).

ECOLOGY

Concern for the environment and ecology is now part of the public vocabulary. Increased public consciousness of our interactive relationship with nature and natural laws has challenged the attitude of overcoming and controlling nature. Despite some business and political moves to the contrary, contemporary society has been informed of the importance of the environment and our dependence on it. Many complementary therapies have the appeal of being natural, and many providers support a concern for the environment. Complementary healers often promote harmony with one's physical and social environment.

MOVE FROM MATERIALISM TO THE SEARCH FOR MEANING

A resurgence of interest in religion has taken the form of an increased interest in fundamentalist, charismatic, and other religious traditions. Many people are exploring nature-based and gnostic religions, and others are searching for truths in other cultures, eras, or esoteric writings (Lewis & Melton, 1992). There has been a recent growth of the ecstatic or experiential churches, which engage in spiritual healing throughout the United States and around the world (Cox, 1995). Other contemporary ideas include the reinvention of the soul, new-age mysticism, and the incorporation of Eastern and cross-cultural ideas in religion (Zukav, 1990). Evidence of the diffusion of ideas throughout a culture can be found in the popular media. An overview of the *New York Times* book section for several weeks in spring 1995 showed 10 books on the list related to the soul, spirituality, or inspiration. Seven of these sources had been on the list for more than 30 weeks. Gregorian chants and other sacred music are often on the best-seller list for musical tapes and compact discs. Many music stores now have entire sections devoted to medieval and other religious music. Even country, rock, and other forms of music often have religious or spiritual themes. A recent television show, "Touched by an Angel" is one of the most popular weekly series. Many of the providers of complementary therapies have strong spiritual underpinnings that stem from gnostic and nature religions as well as Buddhism and other Eastern religions (Engebretson, 1996). The centrality of spirituality in healing is a consistent theme in the practice of complementary modalities.

PHILOSOPHY

The philosophical emphasis on logical positivism prevalent during the Industrial Age has shifted toward a systems-theory emphasis on inter-relationships. The systems approach is reflected in the shift from sole reliance on linear causal models toward a more complex holistic systems perspective. Martin (1994) illustrated this shift in her study of the medical and public understanding of the immune system. She described the historical perspectives of understanding the immune system through the polio epidemic scare of the 1950s and that of AIDS in the 1990s. The linear causal metaphor in the 1950s was that of a mechanical fortress erected by the body to keep germs (the enemy) outside. Still in the same vein, this was replaced later with a military cellular metaphor of killer cells and "armies" that protect and defend the host. The shift to a systems perspective can be seen in the more contemporary metaphor of a sophisticated and dynamic communications that allows the host to survive in relationship with the environment. Healers often exemplify holistic ideologies of health and healing, believing that healing in any one human dimension may influence healing in other or all dimensions. Complementary healers often espouse a belief in holism. Thus, any given modality often has the universal ability to heal multiple ailments or to heal concurrently the biological, spiritual, and emotional dimensions.

■ CHANGES IN THE HEALTH CARE SYSTEM

External political and socioeconomic pressures have prompted a change in the health delivery system: it is moving away from a narrow, disease-focused perspective to a broader, more socially focused conception of health. This contrasts with the medical model wherein the physician makes the decisions for the patient or client, and the other providers follow these directives. This model is based on the belief that the patient is not responsible for the disease or its cure or prevention (Parsons, 1951). The medical model itself is being re-examined in light of the need for patient and client agency in chronic illness, disease prevention, and health promotion. Social influences and their relationship to health are gaining interest among public health professionals (Amick, et al. 1995). This interest coincides with the growing health movement, which promotes healthy eating, exercise, and avoidance of substance abuse, including smoking and drugs (Goldstein, 1992). Many complementary healers conceptualize the locus of responsibility as being with the client. They avoid blaming the victim for his or her illness as they remove the negative connotation of illness, thus allowing for a definition of health to encompass illness (Engebretson, 1996) rather than conceptualizing health and illness as binary opposites.

Complementary Therapies

Complementary therapies are often chosen as low-cost, low-risk options to enhance health. Although costs vary considerably—from a free-will donation to $150 per session for certain types of bodywork or energy healings to less than $10 for a book or tape on relaxation—on the whole these are small costs compared with those of biomedical treatment. Third-party reimbursement has been available for several alternative therapies (Malik, 1995). A survey conducted of the nation's largest health maintenance organizations (HMOs) found that 86 per cent covered some type of alternative therapy (Goodwin, 1997). According to Moore (1997a), chiropractic and acupuncture are the most likely modalities to be covered by insurance. In some cases, large corporations have circumvented insurance companies and contracted directly with providers, and a number of health care centers are providing comprehensive models of care, integrating complementary therapies with traditional biomedicine (Moore, 1997b).

In 1992, the US Congress, in response to public interest and the extensive use of alternative therapies, established the Office of Alternative Medicine (OAM) within the National Institutes of Health (NIH) (OAM, 1992), recently renamed the National Center for Complementary and Alternative Medicine (NCCAM). The purpose of this office is to conduct and support basic and applied research and training and to disseminate information about these therapies (NCCAM, 1998). This office has established several centers to study alternative and complementary therapies and to provide data bases of information about these therapies. A panel convened by NIH endorsed integrating behavioral and relaxation therapies—such as meditation, hypnosis, and biofeedback—into the medical management of chronic pain and insomnia (Chilton, 1996). Centers to study and disseminate information on alternative and complementary therapies also have been established in many European countries (Melchart, Linde, Weidenhammer, Worku, & Wagner, 1995; Rees, 1997; Tap & Goppel, 1995). *The Commission E System for Evaluating and Approving Herbs and Phytomedicines As Nonprescription Medicines in Germany*, a collection of studies of plant therapies with recommendations for safe and effective use, has been translated by the American Botanical Council and is available for clinical reference (Blumenthal, 1998).

Mind–Body Connection

Improved understanding of the mind–body mechanisms has validated many therapeutic techniques. Research on the effects of stress on physiology has led to an increased understanding of the interrelationships between thoughts, emotions, and physiology (Schneiderman et al. 1992). This understanding has been applied to many cardiovascular problems in which the psycho-neuro-hormonal link between stress, anger and hostility, has been explored. Many health care institutions now have cardiovascular programs that focus on stress reduction, relaxation, and coping with anger and hostility. These techniques for reducing stress are similar to strategies used by many complementary healers.

Many of the mechanisms involving neurotransmitters are now known; however, their link to specific diseases is still under investigation. Psychoneuroimmunology (PNI) has been investigated in relation to cancer, acquired immunodeficiency syndrome, multiple sclerosis, arthritis, and other health problems (Schwartz, 1994). Findings are intriguing although a complete theory linking mind to immunity has not yet been fully developed. This area of research has implications for healing, disease prevention, and health promotion. Although PNI is still under study, evidence is growing that many of the interventions currently used and labeled alternative or complementary may be effective as treatments as well as preventive measures. They may be health promoting in any case because they are often perceived as enhancing quality of life. Complementary treatments offer additional advantages of being economical, low-risk, and noninvasive methods of alleviating pain and symptoms.

Sources of Additional Information and Recommendations

Several refereed journals about alternative and complementary therapies are currently on the market. Examples include *Alternative Therapies in Health and Medicine, Journal of Alternative and Complementary Medicine,* and *Complementary Medicine Advances: The Journal of Mind–Body Medicine.* The Hastings Center, in a special supplement on establishing new priorities for the goals of medicine, addressed calls for more research on the effects of alternative therapies (Callahan, 1996). The Robert Wood Johnson Foundation (RWJ) and the Pew Charitable Trust have established commissions to study health professions and make recommendations to the educational institutions related to educating health care workers to meet the changing needs of the health care system. Among the recommendations from RWJ are to increase interdisciplinary education, place more attention on community and health, and promote the transition of the patient from a passive object to active partner (Marston & Jones, 1992). The Pew report (1995) makes similar recommendations and identifies a focus on accountability to populations served and a concern for cost-containment. It also emphasizes health promotion with innovative and diverse provisions for health care. All professional schools are advised to enlarge the scientific bases of their educational programs to include the psychosocial–behavioral sciences. In addition to the academic centers established around the country to research alternative approaches, several medical schools have established courses in alternative therapies (Laken & Cosovic, 1995). The Institute for Alternative Futures (1998) predicts the continual growth of complementary and alternative aspects of health care with an emphasis on health-promotion activities. They also predict a changing paradigm that encompasses more self-care activities, and increased prevention and individualized or personalized care. Increasingly, complementary approaches are being integrated into conventional medical protocols and are becoming major tools for health promotion and disease prevention.

■ IMPLICATIONS FOR PROFESSIONAL NURSING

The confluence of social factors outlined above make changes in nursing inevitable. Complementary healers are responding to public demands for humanized, individualized, and holistic approaches that reduce stress and address the emotional, social, and spiritual aspects of health in a low-cost manner. Many of these complementary therapies are being investigated and incorporated into mainstream medicine to enhance the delivery of health care.

Nursing has been divided in response to this trend. Many nurses have distanced themselves from the complementary movement because of lack of knowledge or because they are skeptical about complementary therapies. Other nurses have embraced the complementary healing movement and integrated the unified holistic approach of the alternative healers with nursing. Nursing theorists, such as Rogers, Watson, Newman, Parse and others, have laid a holistic foundation for nursing to view health and illness from a broader perspective than a biomedical one. These holistic approaches lay the groundwork for incorporating interventions to promote comfort, encourage self-healing, and enhance and promote health. A number of these nursing interventions are similar to therapies provided by the complementary healing community (Engebretson, 1997). Snyder and Lindquist (1998), in a revised edition of a book on independent nursing interventions, discussed therapeutic touch, massage, relaxation techniques, meditation, and imagery. All of these modalities are commonly found in the complementary therapy lexicon.

Watson (1995) described nursing's evolving system of caring and healing within a unitary-transformative context as an exemplar for incorporating complementary practices into health care. Interest in complementary therapies is rapidly expanding in nursing, as evidenced by the expanding membership of the American Holistic Nurses Association (AHNA), which has been growing at the rate of approximately 100 members each month (AHNA, 1995). Many of these therapeutic techniques are congruent with autonomous nursing interventions to facilitate coping, reduce stress and discomfort, and put the patient in the best possible position for natural healing to occur.

Research

Many nurses are skeptical of therapies that lack hard scientific research or do not have physician endorsement. The spiritual and nonmaterial nature of many of the complementary modalities may require different research approaches than double-blinded, randomized, controlled clinical trials (Dossey, 1995; Pincus, 1997; Vickers, 1995). Because many of these modalities are grounded in cultural constructs of health and the human condition that differ from biomedical constructs, a thorough understanding of these constructs is necessary to select an appropriate research approach. Determining outcomes for measurement may be premature because basic science studies have not addressed many of the physiological and experimental effects of these modalities. Cassidy (1996) suggested using social science methodologies such as observation and naturalistic studies as a more appropriate approach. Such studies are systematic, allow for accurate data gathering and give the researcher expanded freedom to ask questions, study contextual issues, and ultimately to provide broader understanding of these modalities. For example, a recent study on therapeutic touch (Rosa, Rosa, Sarner, & Barrett, 1998) would have benefited from a better understanding of the modality and the impact of therapeutic touch on the recipients. Nurses who write about these interventions must ground their commentary in research and tested hypothesis whenever possible and identify clinical phenomena that do not fit existing theories and thus require more basic research.

Information regarding existing research and recommended approaches also can be found in the Chantilly Report (OAM, 1992). An opportunity currently exists for nurses to identify many autonomous nursing actions that parallel these approaches and to begin studying the effects of these actions. Nurses must be engaged in conducting the research on autonomous nursing actions. Incorporating other disciplines may be necessary to enhance the research methods and understanding, but nursing must take the lead in researching generic nursing actions.

The most common use of these therapies is to complement biomedicine rather than replace it. This understanding must be incorporated into the selection of research outcomes. Much research is modeled on drug studies, with the medical outcome of cure as the goal. If these modalities are used adjunctively, rather than alternatively, outcomes should reflect that purposeful use and include responses that impact the illness experience, not just the ones that cure the disease.

Practice

Many nurses are incorporating aspects of complementary therapies into their practice, either by establishing a healing practice using the Holistic Nurse Certification (Andrus & Lunt, 1997) or by using one or more techniques in their regular practice in acute, primary, or tertiary settings. Others may not actively practice any of the modalities, but they may refer clients to other healers in the community. Whether or not the nurse uses complementary healing modalities, he or she should be cognizant of therapeutic treatments the client may be undergoing.

To be credible to clients who wish to discuss health issues and to maximize health promotion, nurses must have some familiarity with information available to the public to assess a patient's use of self-help techniques. Knowledge also allows the nurse to be alert for side effects or synergistic effects. In addition, nurses in clinical practice must consider individual client preferences. Many clients seek these therapies because they reflect a holistic philosophy that the client has embraced, and others may be dissatisfied with biomedicine for a variety of reasons and seek out these approaches with a similar "magic bullet" expectation. Some will recognize the spiritual or natural aspects of these therapies as compatible with their belief system whereas others may find the mention of these therapies offensive, frightening, or superfluous. A thorough assessment is necessary to ensure appropriate care.

The issue of the growing number of therapies approved for third-party reimbursement, either directly or with physician referral, must be examined by the nursing profession because many of these modalities are similar to autonomous interventions nurses have historically used in providing comprehensive patient care. For example, in a survey of the nation's largest HMOs, 86 per cent covered some type of alternative therapy, the most prevalent being nutritional programs, wellness counseling, massage, therapeutic touch, and stress reduction (Goodwin, 1997). The nursing profession has a history of unclear domain boundaries wherein traditional nursing activities have been assumed by another profession that has articulated a particular expertise to meet a societal need. Many traditional nursing activities involve stress management, an area rapidly being developed by psychology. Traditional nursing activities also involve activities to promote comfort, coping, symptom relief, and other measures to help patients deal with the illness experience. It would be ironic if massage, touch, and other long-standing nursing activities became the domain of healers who receive direct third-party payment but nurses were deemed no longer qualified to perform them or to receive reimbursement.

Education

Most nursing curricula do not address complementary therapies although many medical schools are adding courses on alternative therapies to their curricula (Daly, 1995). Because these modalities are more closely related to nursing theoretical frameworks than to those of biomedicine, it would be disappointing indeed if biomedicine were to take the lead in incorporating this information into curricula. However, some nursing schools are including holistic nursing theories into their curricula, and complementary therapies that already exist as autonomous nursing interventions could easily be added.

■ CONCLUSION

Science and technology are insufficient to explain and solve complex issues of human existence and dimensions of the health–illness experience. The emphasis on science and technology without the balance of the art of healing, which includes touch, caring, and spirituality, has become a concern of both health providers and the public. Complementary therapies embrace low technology and center on spirituality, love, touch, wellness, relationships, personal growth, and other aspects of the healing arts. The growing popularity and use of these therapies is evidence of the deficit of these elements in traditional biomedical services. The nursing profession should take careful note of this trend because many of the healing components delivered by complementary healers—such as care, touch, comfort, and a focus on health—are presently identified in nursing theories and nursing literature as autonomous actions of professional nursing.

To restrict the development of nursing scholarship and research along only the biomedical framework does a grave disservice to the profession. At a time when biomedicine and others in the health care industry are beginning to incorporate these approaches, nursing should not move backwards by restricting its paradigm to that which is derivative of traditional biomedicine. Changes in technology, economics, and politics—with the concurrent shift in social values, philosophy, and health care—have created a window of opportunity for nursing. The shift in health care to health promotion, individualized care, personal empowerment, and search for meaning have traditionally been within nursing's scope of practice. Nursing can take the lead in investigating and incorporating those elements into an integrated practice that meets the public's need and promotes the profession.

References

Amick III, B. C., Levine, S., Tarlov, A. R., & Walsh, D. C. (1995). *Society and health.* New York: Oxford University Press.

Anderson, W. T. (1995). *The truth about the truth.* New York: Putnam.

Andrus, V., & Lunt, J. Y. (1997). Bringing holistic nursing into the new millennium. *Alternative and Complementary Therapies, 3* (2), 24–28.

Astin, J. A. (1998). Why patients use alternative medicine. *Journal of the American Medical Association, 279* (19), 1548–1553.

American Holistic Nurses Association. (1995). Happy 14th birthday AHNA. *Beginnings, 15* (3), 1–2.

Callahan, D. (1996). The goals of medicine. *Hastings Center Report—Special Supplement.* November-December, S1–26.

Blumenthal, M. (1998). Commission E progress. *Herbalgram, 42,* 6.

Borgmann, A. (1992). *Crossing the postmodern divide.* Chicago: The University of Chicago Press.

Cassidy, C. M. (1996). Cultural context of complementary and alternative medicine systems. In M. S. Micozzi (Ed.), *Fundamental of complementary and alternative medicine* (pp. 9–34). New York: Churchill Livingstone.

Cassileth, B. R. (1998). *The alternative medicine handbook: The complete guide to alternative and complementary therapies.* New York: Norton.

Chilton, M. (1996). Panel recommends integrating behavioral and relaxation approaches into medical treatment of chronic pain, insomnia. *Alternative Therapies in Health and Medicine, 2* (1), 18–28.

Cox, H. (1995). *Fire from heaven.* Boston: Addison-Wesley.

Daly, D. (1995). Alternative medicine courses taught at U.S. medical schools: An ongoing listing. *The Journal of Alternative and Complementary Medicine, 1* (2), 205–207.

Dossey, L. (1995). How should alternative therapies be evaluated? *Alternative Therapies in Health and Medicine, 1* (2), 6–10, 79–85.

Eisenberg, D. M., Davis, R. B., Ettner, S. L., Appel, S., Wilkey, S., Van Rompay, M., & Kessler, R. C. (1998). Trends in alternative medicine use in the United States, 1990–1997: Results of a follow up national survey. *Journal of the American Medical Association, 280* (180), 1569–1575.

Eisenberg, D. M., Kessler, R. C., Foster, C., Norlock, F. E., Calkins, D. R., & Delbanco, T. L. (1993). Unconventional medicine in the United States: Prevalence, costs, and patterns of use. *The New England Journal of Medicine, 328* (4), 252–256.

Engebretson, J. (1992). *Cultural models of healing and health: An ethnography of professional nurses and healers.* (Doctoral dissertation, The University of Texas Health

Science Center at Houston School of Public Health, 1992). *Dissertation Abstracts International* 9302792.

Engebretson, J. (1996). Comparison of nurses and alternative nurses. *Image—The Journal of Nursing Scholarship, 28* (2), 95–99.

Engebretson, J. (1997). A metaparadigm approach to nursing. *Advances in Nursing Science, 20* (1), 21–33.

Evans, R. G., Barer, M. L., & Marmor, T. R. (1994). *Why are some people healthy and others not? The determinants of health populations.* New York: de Gruyter.

Goldstein, M. (1992). *The health movement—Promoting fitness in America.* New York: Twayne.

Goodwin, M. (1997). A health insurance revolution. *New Age Journal: 1997–1998 Special Edition,* 66–69.

Hufford, D. J. (1986). Contemporary folk medicine. In N. Gevitz (Ed.), *Other healers.* Baltimore: John Hopkins University Press.

Institute for Alternative Futures. (1998). *The future of complementary and alternative approaches (CAAs) in US health care.* Alexandria, VA: NCMIC Insurance Co.

Laken, M., & Cosovic, S. (1995). Introducing alternative/complementary healing to allopathic medical students. *The Journal of Alternative and Complementary Medicine. 1* (1), 93–98.

Landmark Report on Public Perceptions of Alternative Care. (1998). *Landmark healthcare.* Available at: http://www.landmarkhealthcare.com.

Lee, D. R., Soffel, D., & Luft, H. S. (1997). Costs and coverage: Pressures toward health care reform. In P. Conrad (Ed.), *The sociology of health and illness* (pp. 281–292). New York: St. Martin's.

Lewis, J., & Melton, J. (Eds.) (1992). *Perspectives on the new age.* Albany, NY: New York State University.

Locsin, R. C. (1995). Machine technologies and caring in nursing. *Image—The Journal of Nursing Scholarship, 27* (3), 201–203.

Malik, T. (1995). Health care insurers opening up to alternatives. *Alternative Therapies in Health and Medicine, 1* (1), 12–13.

Marston, R. Q., & Jones, R. M. (Eds.). (1992). *Medical education in transition.* Princeton: The Robert Wood Johnson Foundation.

Martin, E. (1994). *Flexible bodies—Tracking immunity in American culture from the days of Polio to the age of AIDS.* Boston: Beacon Press.

Mason, J. O. (1992). *Healthy people 2000—National health promotion and disease prevention objectives.* Boston: Jones and Bartlett.

McKnight, J. (1995). *The careless society, community, and its counterfeits.* New York: Basic.

McGuire, M. B. (1988). *Ritual healing in suburban American.* New Brunswick, NJ: Rutgers University Press.

Melchart, D., Linde, K., Weidenhammer, W., Worku, F., & Wagner, H. (1995). The integration of natural healing procedures into research and teaching at German universities. *Alternative Therapies in Health and Medicine, 1* (1), 30–33.

Micozzi, M. S., Kronenberg, F., & Jobst, K. A. (1995). Introducing the *Journal of Alternative and Complementary Medicine:* Research on paradigm, practice, and policy. *The Journal of Alternative and Complementary Medicine, 1* (1), 1–5.

Moore, N. G. (1997a). A review of reimbursement policies for alternative and complementary therapies. *Alternative Therapies in Health and Medicine, 3* (1), 26–29.

Moore, N. G. (1997b). The Columbia-Presbyterian Complementary Care Center: Comprehensive care of the mind, body, and spirit. *Alternative Therapies in Health and Medicine, 3* (10), 30–32.

National Center for Complementary and Alternative Medicine. Information available at http://altmed.ood.nih.gov.

Negroponte, N. (1995). *Being digital.* New York: Knopf.

Office of Alternative Medicine. (1992). *Alternative medicine: Expanding medical horizons—A report to the National Institutes of Health on Alternative Medical Systems and Practices in the United States* (DHHS Publication no. 017-040-00537-7). Washington, DC: US Government Printing Office.

Orth-Gomer, K., & Schneiderman, N. (1996). *Behavioral medicine approaches to cardiovascular disease prevention.* Hillsdale, NJ: Erlbaum.

Parsons, T. (1951). *The social system.* New York: Free Press.

Pew Health Professions Commission. (1995). *Critical challenges: Revitalizing the health profession for the twenty-first century.* San Francisco: Author.

Pincus, T. (1997). Are randomized clinical trials always the best answer? *Advances: The Journal of Mind–Body Medicine, 13* (2), 3–66.

Pincus, T., & Callahan, L. F. (1995). What explains the association between socioeconomic status and health: Primarily access to medical care or mind–body variables? *Advances: The Journal of Mind–Body Health, 11* (1), 4–36.

Rosa, L., Rosa, E., Sarner, L., & Barrett, S. (1998). A close look at therapeutic touch. *Journal of the American Medical Association, 279* (13), 1005–1010.

Rees, R. (1997). A review of complementary medicine in Europe. *Alternative Therapies in Health and Medicine, 3* (1), 82–83, 90.

Reiser, S. J. (1978). *Medicine and the reign of technology.* New York: Cambridge University Press.

Schneiderman, N., McCabe, P., & Baum, A. (1992). *Perspectives in behavioral medicine—Stress and disease processes.* Hillsdale, NJ: Erlbaum.

Schwartz, G. E. (1994). Introduction: Old methodological challenges and new mindbody links in psychoneuroimmunology. *Advance: The Journal of Mind-Body Medicine, 10* (4), 4–7.

Snyder, M., & Lindquist, R. (1998). *Complementary/alternative therapies in nursing* (ed. 3). New York: Springer.

Tambiah, S. J. (1995). Magic, science, religion, and the scope of rationality. *Lewis Henry Morgan lectures.* Cambridge, MA: Cambridge University Press.

Tap, V., & Goppel, M. (1995). Summary of a report by the Health Council of the Netherlands on alternative modes of treatment under scientific investigation. *Alternative Therapies in Health and Medicine, 1* (2), 58–63.

Toffler, A., & Toffler, A. (1994). *Creating a new civilization: The politics of the third wave.* Atlanta, GA: Turner.

Vickers, A. (1995). The NIH methodology conference: The methodology debate in the United Kingdom during the past ten years. *The Journal of Alternative and Complementary Medicine, 1* (2), 209–212.

Watson, J. (1995). Nursing's caring-healing paradigm as exemplar for alternative medicine. *Alternative Therapies in Health and Medicine, 1* (3), 64–69.

Zukav, G. (1990). *The seat of the soul.* New York: Fireside.

Discussion Questions

1. What events in Carnegie's history of black nurses (Article 13) were significant for you? Explain.

2. Have the efforts of black nurses to achieve parity with white nurses succeeded? Explain your conclusion.

3. What is the minority representation in your school? In your practice setting?

4. In your opinion, what problems do minority students have in your nursing program? How are these problems being addressed in your school?

5. What difficulties (if any) have you experienced with students of color? How were they resolved?

6. Is there racism in nursing? Justify your explanation.

7. How culturally competent are you? Cite examples.

8. Compare and contrast transcultural and transracial nursing as discussed in Roberson (Article 15).

9. To what extent do you think nurses are transracial in their practice setting?

10. Assess the extent to which you are culturally sensitive. What areas need further development?

11. What do you see as the biggest danger in the use of alternative and complementary medicine? Elaborate.

12. Evaluate the merits of marketing alternative and complementary over-the-counter drugs.

13. How would you counsel a person who is interested in using alternative and/or complementary healing?

14. To what extent, if at all, should hospitals incorporate alternative and complementary medicine into their services?

Further Readings

Baldanaro, A.A. (1996). Transcending the barriers of cultural diversity in health care. *Journal of Cultural Diversity, 3* (1), 20–22.

Davidhizar, R., Dowd, S., & Newman, S. (1999). Managing diversity in the health care workplace. *Health Care Manager, 17* (3), 51–62.

Evans, B. M. (1999). Complementary therapies and HIV infection. *American Journal of Nursing, 99* (2), 42–45.

Hodge, P. & Ullrich S. (1999). Does your assessment include alternative therapies? *RN, 62* (6), 47–49.

Jackson, B. S. (1998). Subtle and not-so-subtle insensitivity to ethnic diversity. *Journal of Nursing Administration, 28* (12), 11–14.

Yearwood, E. L. (1998). "We value cultural diversity"—the schizophrenic message in health care. *Journal of Child and Adolescent Psychiatric Nursing, 11* (3), 85–86.

Web Site Resources for Cultural Diversity

Alternative/Complementary Medicine—Wellness Web   http://www.wellweb.com

Ask NOAH about: Alternative (Complementary) Medicine   http://www.noah.cuny.edu

Consumer Lab   www.consumerlab.com

Diversity Rx   http://www.diversityrx.org

Fraud   www.ncahf.org

Health Care Reality Check   www.ncrhi.org

Indian Health Service   http://www.ihs.gov

Museum of Questionable Medical Devices   www.mtn.org/quack

National Center for Complimentary and Alternative Medicine   http://nccam.nih.gov/

National Forum on People's Differences   http://www.yforum.com

Office of Minority Health Resource Center   http://www.omhrc.gov

Quackwatch   www.quackwatch.com

General Search Engine Web Sites

Excite   www.excite.com

Lycos   www.lycos.com

Health Web Sites

Black Health   www.blackhealthnet.com

Life Matters   www.lifematters.com

Professional Journal Web Sites

Holistic Nursing Practice   www.aspenpub.com

Journal of Alternative & Complementary Medicine   www.liebertpub.com

Journal of Cultural Diversity   www.tuckerpub.com

Journal of Holistic Nursing   www.sagepub.com

PART TWO

ISSUES OF ACCESS AND BOUNDARIES

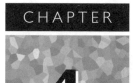

CHAPTER

4

The Legal Responsibilities of Practice

Years ago, when George Orwell wrote his futuristic novel *1984*, no one could imagine living in a society where an individual's rights were nonexistent, where free speech was punished, and privacy was an impossibility. In Orwell's futuristic society, signs were posted everywhere reminding people that "Big Brother is watching you." The notion that "someone" could be watching and monitoring a person's every move was both laughable and unbelievable. No one is laughing now, and the unbelievable has become more real with each passing day.

As the 21st century begins, individual rights are in the forefront of a growing and heated national debate. Is it still possible to have individual rights in this computer age? Is there a clear distinction between a person's individual rights and the pervasive use of computer technology intruding upon those rights? Are a person's individual rights an illusion, some hoax perpetrated by this nation's founding fathers? Are we in danger of becoming a society where the rights of the masses supersede an individual's rights? How do people maintain their individual rights in the face of new and proliferating technology? These questions, and many others, are firing our national debate. They have yet to be answered fully or clearly. Increasingly, the emerging problems they generate are being addressed by our legal and legislative systems. But their attempts are slow, cumbersome, and politically charged.

In the meantime, information technology marches on, identifying, isolating, and transferring personal data from one source to another many times over without our knowledge or permission. Every day, bits and pieces of our personal data are snatched away, eroding whatever remains of our privacy. How can we complain, argues the technology industry, when they are only trying, through their database warehouses, to meet our every need and want? Isn't profiling our likes, dislikes, purchases, and preferences an affirmation of our individual rights? Shouldn't they get some credit for improving our lives? Don't we want progress? Don't we think progress is good? Some people think that giving up a few individual rights is the price of progress; others think that it's progress at a price.

Increasingly, patients are becoming wary about sharing information related to their medical problems in health care settings. Their caution is understandable. It is surprisingly easy to access patient data. Nurses, physicians, ancillary health workers, business office personnel, and quality assurance staff are, among others, people who have access to patient records. Others, who have vested interests in the information, can access data without ever being in the patient's health care setting. The easier it becomes (and it's getting easier each month), the easier information can be shared, making it all the harder to monitor how the information is being used and by whom. No wonder patients are reluctant to share certain aspects of their health history. The need to protect themselves becomes so great that self-incrimination seems like a viable alternative, especially if patients think that their banks, credit card companies, insurers and loan agencies, and others have access to their medical records. The problem is not easily solved. Is it possible that a person will no longer be able to have secrets? Is this the end of privacy as we understand it? So many questions. So few answers.

The right to privacy is the focus of this chapter. The chapter begins on an historical note with an article written in 1900 by an early pioneer in the evolution of the nursing profession, Lavinia Dock. In her article, Miss Dock delineates what nurses may expect from the law. Her insights are as sound today as they were in 1900. The readings that follow explore patients' rights, each proposing what should be included, and the problems that continue, in making these rights a legal reality. Articles on confidentiality between nurse and patient and other health care workers follow next, all of which have legal implications for professional nurses. Suggestions on how medical records can be kept private in this information age conclude the focus of this chapter.

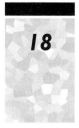

18

What We May Expect From the Law

Lavinia L. Dock

Many of us have an indistinct impression that the "law" is something of the nature of a finished product, of which certain ready-made quantities may be procured as one orders household goods. One often hears the words, "There ought to be a law to compel" thus and so, or, "Such a thing ought to be forbidden by law." It is the natural attitude of the mind toward something unfamiliar. Let us realize that laws are public agreements which people just like us make and which we can also make. To have laws passed regulating our profession is only to do on a large scale what we now do in a small way in our voluntary constitutions and by-laws. We must first decide what we want to do, then find out what others who are of different opinions want, and finally by mutual agreement decide on concessions which we can get a good working majority to support. Even as to compulsory power, which is the essential characteristic of law, the difference is only one of degree: our voluntary constitutions have the germ of the compulsory idea, the difference being that this compulsion cannot reach outside of the association, whereas in state law the compulsion reaches throughout the state.

To be effective, a compulsory law must not only provide the penalty for disobedience, but must make provision for enforcing this penalty and for defraying costs.

Many laws, especially such as are meant to regulate the conditions of labor of, let us say, women and children, fail entirely to effect the desired changes because they have been so constructed that the method of endorsing the penalty has been left out. This point needs emphasis; so many people imagine that law is like an automatically working machine; that once passed it will keep on going of its own accord, protecting the good and restraining the bad. On the contrary, unless some one is enough interested to be responsible for seeing that it is obeyed, it will stand on the books forever as harmlessly as a verse from "Mother Goose." If the mere passage of restraining acts were sufficient to keep men from crime, or even in any great measure to limit it, there would be no such thing as theft, for there are enough laws against it."[1] Who then is responsible for seeing that law is obeyed? Whoever is injuriously affected by its being disobeyed must see to it. If the state is injured, the state will see to it. But if we make laws for our benefit, the state will not concern itself further than by providing courts of justice. Thus we find that in the best medical laws, the county medical societies are designed as being the bodies who shall bring prosecution for violations of law, and the expenses they incur are to be repaid from the fines.

We, if we wish to secure laws, will have to do the same. The only alternative would be to allow some other body of persons to take this trouble off our hands, in return for which service we would place ourselves under their control. This would be slavery, of which not even the shadow can be tolerated.

So it comes down to this: not, What can we expect from the law? but, What can we expect from ourselves and from the people all about us? They will not willingly allow us an advantage which they think will disadvantage themselves, and we may not disregard their interests in considering our own, but should rather seek to safeguard both, and so go amicably on together.

What, then, do we want to do? To establish a recognized standard of professional education. There will be a disappointment here to many, for we cannot establish by law our *highest* professional standards, only the medium,—only the fair general average, at any rate, at first. The secretary of the University of the State of New York writes: "It would be wise, in a movement for licensing trained nurses, to establish a state society and then to determine *minimum* qualifications to be exacted in preliminary and professional training. The object of the law will be defeated if the requirements are fixed too high at first."

Restrictive legislation affecting the professions, then, is not to be gained once and forever; this is another point for us to remember. It does not mean just one effort, but continuous efforts for the rest of time.

The American Medical Association has been working at legislation for fifty years, and the secretary writes: "The laws are *gradually becoming more stringent* (italics are ours) in the states which have adopted medical laws." Our highest present standards are the result of special intelligence and special advantages; all have not the same, and it would be no more reasonable to expect all to suddenly conform to the highest, than it would be to expect the bread to bake without being long enough in the oven. We must first have the higher education, and then the law to protect it. The secretary of a certain national association writes: "We have secured laws in several states; . . . while these are not such as we would like to have them, yet they are as an entering wedge; . . . the one thing that is needed first is good technical education before we can expect good legislation." And another: "It is worse than folly to hope to make men ethical by the law, just as it is supreme inanity to expect legislation to make them intelligent or learned; . . . we urge the abandonment

---

[1]Proceedings, Sixteenth Annual Convention, National Association of Dental Faculties, 1899.

of professional strife, the burying of personal differences, and the union of all in one common purpose to raise our professional standards as fast as, and no faster than, they can be firmly maintained."[2]

We have, as nurses, a fair average standard of two-years' general training, sanctioned by public consent during thirty years. We are developing a three-years' general training through the individual initiative and mutual agreement of those who have grown to this stage of progress.

We may safely trust this element to go on distributing the leaven. It is instinct with the spirit of growth and needs only to be let alone. But we can *not* trust those who, from mistaken motives or from imperfect intelligence, attack our two-years' minimum. These are they against whom we must defend ourselves by laws which will forbid them to chip away a bit here and a bit there, like thieves at a cellar-wall.

Such encroachment on fair standards as a *six-weeks' theoretical course* in nursing, concluded by the giving of a diploma, which is now in existence in one of our large cities (not conducted, one is glad to say, by nurses), could be put an end to by a state association of nurses by passing a simple law requiring a stated time-limit, just as similar medical swindles, bogus colleges, and the like have been put an end to by the state medical societies.

Another sorely needed protection, toward which the "time-limit" of study, which is considered essential by all the professions, would not help us, is against the multiplication of training-schools in specialty hospitals and those of limited clinical material. To obviate this it would be necessary to specify in the law the variety of subjects in which a nurse applying for state registration would be required to pass examination. This is done in the best medical laws, but we would hardly secure such provision at law for some time to come, as it would naturally meet with great opposition at first.

The dental profession has successfully limited the numbers of dental colleges through its Association of Dental Faculties, and so maintains their standards: needless, however, to point out the difference between their circumstances and ours. Hospitals not only ought not to be limited, but ought to be multiplied, of every kind, special as well as general, and the training-school is usually a part of the hospital, not a separate entity like a college. However, that it might be made more so than it is has been repeatedly urged by nurses who consider these things, for the past six years or more. A system of paid graduates for private hospitals, postgraduate courses in large specialty hospitals, and a rotation of pupils from some large central school for the small general and specialty hospitals has been urged by nurses at private duty and in hospital work, by the American Society of Superintendents, and by the English Matrons in Council in print and in public discussions over and over again. It is satisfactory to see that members of the medical profession are now adopting our views and advising hospital managers to work out the plan, "First the blade, then the ear, then the full corn in the year."

---

[2]*Ibid.*

The secretary of the University of the State of New York writes, again: "It would probably be impossible to effect direct legislation to prevent training-schools from being established in small or specialty hospitals, from the innate American desire for personal liberty, and legislators hesitate to enact such laws. The indirect method would doubtless receive wider support."

As to how legislation would affect nurses already practising, a study of the medical laws of the different states shows that reputable practitioners already established were in no case taken by surprise in their disadvantage, but were treated with extreme consideration. In some states they were not required to pass the newly established examinations, but received the state certificate for registration simply on the strength of their diplomas or from five to ten years' practice. Other states gave two or three years' time in which they might prepare for examination. The newly made laws usually provided that such steps as extending the course or amplifying the subjects for examination should not take place immediately, but at a given date from two to five years after the passage of the law. This gave time for accommodation to take place, and worked no immediate hardship. Such questions as moving one's residence are easily arranged for on common-sense principles.

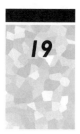

19

Why We Need a Patients' Bill of Rights

Richard Sorian and Judith Feder

■ BACKGROUND

Over the last ten years, Americans have experienced a substantial change in the way they receive health care. Not surprisingly, that shift has generated popular discontent. Also not surprisingly, that discontent has generated heated political debate about the need for greater consumer protections in the health care marketplace. The nature of that debate—particularly its partisanship at the national level—has called into question its basis in policy.

Some argue that there really is no problem in terms of the quality of care; that change, while disruptive, is constructive in bringing cost concerns into play in decisions about the delivery of medical care. From this perspective, the only significant threat managed care poses is to provider incomes. If that's the case, then action to mitigate that threat represents at best political pandering and at worst a costly caving to the interests of a well-paid few. In other words, the market is working and politicians should leave it alone.

Although pandering and caving are undoubtedly a part of the political process, this argument ignores the fundamental problem that underlies the current debate: a lack of accountability in the health care market. Since the demise of the Clinton health plan, the United States has followed a market-based approach to health care cost containment. The more we rely on market forces in health care, the more important it is that the market is held to the kind of accountability provided in other markets. In fact, considering the potential impact of poor quality health care on people's lives, it is even more important. While we certainly agree that intervention can go overboard, to fail to balance market forces with accountability is to leave people at unaccept-

Richard Sorian, senior advisor for health policy at the U.S. Department of Health & Human Services, Washington, DC. Judith Feder, Institute for Health Care Research & Policy, Georgetown University, Washington, DC.

able risk and undermine the basic trust that is essential to a well-working system of care.

■ TOO MUCH CHANGE, TOO LITTLE CHOICE

The roots of the consumer protection debate can be found in the rapid transformation of the health insurance market from fee-for-service coverage to managed care. Between 1988 and 1998, the percentage of privately insured Americans in managed care plans skyrocketed from 14 percent to 71 percent (KFF: 18). For most Americans, the decision to move from fee-for-service coverage to managed care was made by their employer. Such an involuntary shift was bound to breed distrust among consumers, and it has. A series of public opinion polls indicates a strong and abiding discontent with many of the common traits of managed care plans:

- a July 1997 ABC News/*Washington Post* survey[1] found that 52 percent of Americans had an "unfavorable" opinion of managed care plans compared with 30 percent who had a "favorable" view;
- a September 1998 poll by the Kaiser Family Foundation (KFF) and the Harvard School of Public Health (KFF and Harvard 1998) found that 64 percent of Americans blamed managed care for allowing them less time with their doctors while 62 percent said plans made it harder for sick patients to see specialists; and,
- a February 1999 Associated Press poll[2] found that 34 percent of Americans believe the quality of their care was "worse" than it was five years ago.

■ WHO PUT THE BASH INTO MANAGED CARE?

A central question is whether this opinion is based on personal experience or is simply a reflection of the intense media coverage of the political debate. Certainly consumers are hearing much more negative news about managed care and not all of it is based on hard evidence. Between 1990 and 1997, news coverage of the managed care industry took a turn for the worse. While earlier coverage tended to portray HMOs as the health system's "savior," later coverage was significantly more negative, often featuring vivid examples of consumers injured by health plans (Brodie, Brady, and Altman 1998). The question is, Did consumer unhappiness drive news coverage or did the media foment the discontent?

---

[1] The poll was conducted 9–12 July 1998. It surveyed 1,515 adults and had a margin of error of plus or minus 3.1 percent.

[2] The poll was conducted 29 January–2 February 1999. It surveyed 1,008 adults and margin of error of plus or minus 3 percent.

In the Kaiser/Harvard poll, 77 percent of those who disliked HMOs said they were influenced by their personal experiences or the experiences of their friends and families; only 17 percent cited negative media coverage. While news editors and reporters admit there often is a "pack approach" to covering national news, they argue strongly that the public's interest drove the coverage. As one national news editor put it, "If we didn't think people would read it, we wouldn't publish it."

Consumer discontent alone is unlikely to drive a national debate. In the case of managed care reform, consumer dissatisfaction was effectively harnessed to one of the nation's more influential lobbies—the medical profession. Physicians who saw their income and their autonomy reduced by the growing power of such plans were among the first to complain about managed care and seek reform.

■ THE STATES RESPOND: FROM PANDERING TO DUE PROCESS

Public and professional unrest with managed care was bound to create a governmental response. As is usually the case, this response began first in the states and later spread to the national scene. State lawmakers were clearly torn about what to do about managed care. On the one hand, they recognized that health plans were serving an important role in controlling the rate of growth in health costs—a job that government had abandoned in the wake of the 1994 defeat of the Clinton health reform plan. Legislators were loathe to interfere with what seemed to be a welcome respite in health care inflation. At the same time, there was a clear feeling that many HMOs had gone too far in their zeal to cut costs and compete for market share.

The first wave of state efforts in 1994–1995 was driven primarily by providers. Unhappy with the strictures imposed by tight provider networks, the American Medical Association and state medical societies pressed for legislation to force open those networks and require plans to accept "any willing provider" into their midst. While most states rejected that approach, fearing that it would destroy the basic tenets of managed care, many did adopt laws requiring plans to provide direct access to specific types of providers (e.g., chiropractors, acupuncturists, optometrists, and dermatologists).

The second wave of state legislation, in 1995–1996, focused more on consumer concerns but still tended to added the symptoms (e.g., drive-through deliveries and mastectomies) rather than the underlying causes. States enacted 245 managed care laws in that period, most taking a "body-part" approach. For example, thirty states mandated minimum maternity hospital stays and fourteen states took the same approach to care after a mastectomy. Others mandated coverage of specific procedures (e.g., infertility services, bone mass measurement, and bone marrow transplants).

State policy makers grew uncomfortable with the body-part approach to managed care reform and began searching for a more traditional consumer protection approach. In most other markets, government tends to establish basic ground rules that outlaw egregious practices, mandate information disclosure, and establish due process standards for accountability. In 1996, New York became the first state to take this approach to managed care reform.

The New York law included minimum standards for the adequacy of provider networks, greater access to specialists for the severely ill, direct access to pediatricians and obstetrician/gynecologists, utilization review standards, easier access to emergency care, internal quality assurance standards, information disclosure, and standards for appeals (PPEFNY 1995).

New York's success shifted the state debate away from micromanagement and toward accountability and due process. In 1997–1998, states passed another four hundred managed care laws, including twenty-eight comprehensive packages. Two states—Texas and Missouri—took the debate further by voting to allow consumers to sue their health plans in state courts for damages caused by a denial or delay in coverage of needed care.

While final figures aren't in yet for 1999, it appears certain that the number of state laws will continue to rise. A survey of state legislators at the beginning of the year found that every state was planning to debate managed care reform with twenty-two states planning to consider adopting external appeal systems (Dixon, Rothouse, and Stauffer 1998). It is likely that by the end of this year, states will have enacted upward of one thousand managed care laws in only six years, a remarkable record.

A surprising element of the state debate has been the minimal level of partisanship. Most state laws were enacted with strong bipartisan support. In fact, many of the leading states (New York, New Jersey, and Connecticut) were run by Republican governors with Democratic legislatures. While the insurance industry was active in opposing provisions that it felt went too far, it did not run the kind of high-priced lobbying and ad campaigns for which it has become famous. The industry's quiescence may have lulled national policy makers into a false sense of confidence.

◼ THE FEDS RESPOND: POLITICS AND PARTISANSHIP

Policy makers in Washington had stayed on the sidelines for most of the initial phase of debate over managed care reform. In 1996, however, with a presidential and congressional election looming, federal lawmakers looked for ways to jump on the anti–managed care bandwagon. In August, Congress enacted modest legislation requiring all plans to provide a minimum of forty-eight hours of hospitalization for women and their newborns—the same body-part approach that many states had followed.

Perhaps more significant was the enactment of the Health Insurance Portability and Accountability Act (HIPAA) of 1996, which set federal rules for the sale and renewal of individual and group insurance. This expansion of federal regulation of insurance marked a sea change in the tradition of leaving insurance regulation to the states.

Beyond the political attractiveness of the issue, a significant factor in the passage of the maternity stay mandate and HIPAA was the inability of states to regulate much of the insurance market. The Employee Retirement Income Security Act (ERISA) of 1974 exempts self-funded health plans from all state regulations and protects fully insured plans from many state rules. ERISA also prohibits consumers from suing HMOs in state courts for damages associated with a plan's wrongful denial of coverage. Consumers who are injured must go to federal court and damages are effectively limited to the cost of the service denied. An estimated 124 million Americans are in ERISA-regulated plans, including about 48 million in self-funded plans.

There were some signs of bipartisan interest in HMO reform early in 1997 with major proposals by Representative Charlie Norwood (R-GA), Senator Alfonse D' Amato (R-NY), Representative John Dingell (D-MI), and Senator Edward Kennedy (D-MA). Ironically, it was the GOP plan that was the most invasive bill. Norwood's "Patients' Access to Responsible Care Act" (PARCA) would make sweeping changes in managed care regulation, requiring plans to allow certain providers to participate in their networks and establishing due process protections for consumers. Norwood's bill also would allow consumers to sue their health plans in state courts. PARCA was surprisingly popular with House members of both parties, eventually garnering nearly two hundred cosponsors, a clear sign of the viability of managed care reform as a political issue.

Democrats were less certain how to proceed. Burned by health reform, the White House was reluctant to take the lead on managed care reform. Instead, President Clinton created the thirty-four-member Advisory Commission on Consumer Protection and Quality in the Health Care Industry and asked it to advise him "on changes occurring in the health care system and recommend such measures as may be necessary to promote and assure health care quality and value, and protect consumers and workers in the health care system Executive Order # 13017, dated 5 September 1996." With its broad representation (including consumer advocates, physicians, nurses, HMO executives, large and small employers), the Commission also was an attempt to find a political middle ground. In November, the Commission recommended the Consumer Bill of Rights and Responsibilities, which hewed closely to the states' model of due process and accountability.

In early 1998, the Democratic leadership of both houses of Congress introduced a new managed care bill that added several provisions recommended by the Commission—most notably a requirement for external review of plans' decisions to deny or curtail coverage—and adopted Norwood's proposal to allow consumers to sue health plans in state courts.

While the Republican rank-in-file was embracing reform, Republican leaders were adamantly opposed. House Majority Leader Dick Armey (R-Texas) dubbed the various proposals "Clinton Care II," saying they were an incremental attempt to enact the defeated Clinton health reform plan of 1993–1994. Senate Majority Leader Trent Lott (R-MS) urged the insurance and employer lobbies to fight a "real war" against reform and the industry heeded that call with a campaign that would eventually cost more than $60 million (Salant 1998).

In mid-1998, GOP leaders abruptly abandoned their "just say no" approach to reform when pollsters reported that public support for managed care reform was strong and growing and that the party risked losing its majority in the House of Representatives. In June, House and Senate Republicans introduced their own versions of a Patients' Bill of Rights, which resembled the Democratic bill in its broad outline, but differed dramatically in the details.

In the end, Congress failed to enact any meaningful managed care reform legislation in 1998. Ironically, the single piece of legislation to pass was a return to the body-part approach mandating plan coverage of breast reconstruction after a mastectomy.

■ WHAT'S AT STAKE?

Continuing public demand for change still makes it likely that Congress will eventually adopt a managed care reform package. The question remains: What form will it take? Will it pander to the medical profession and undermine the legitimate role of HMOs in containing health care costs? Will it promise consumers real protections but deliver only pabulum? Or will it provide patients with a system that makes decisions out in the open and is held accountable when it makes the wrong decision?

The answer is likely to be a combination of all three. Any political process demands trade-offs and managed care is no different. But some issues are more important than others. Take, for example, the question of medical necessity as a major sticking point in the current congressional debate. Health plan contracts typically include a list of covered services but condition that coverage on the service being "medically necessary." There is, however, a growing trend among health plans to define medical necessity arbitrarily as a means to control costs through claim denials. In a small number of cases, such denials lead to irreversible damage or even death. In a larger number of cases, it results in unnecessary delays in needed care.

Legislative action is needed to create a better balance between HMOs' desire to control costs and patients' desire to get appropriate medical care. External review is an effort to accomplish that balance but it can only reach that goal if external review panels can take a fresh look at each case and base their decision on the relevant evidence and expertise. State experience shows that such a process will result in better decisions by health plans at a modest cost.

A next step would be to allow consumers who are dissatisfied with the results to seek review in court as a means to assure that the process is honest. Use of the courts is highly controversial and vulnerable to misinterpretation. No one is advocating that courts should be used to make medical decisions. The legal system is far too costly and cumbersome for that. Rather, courts are needed to provide the entire system with legitimacy. By punishing the miscreants, courts are a powerful deterrent for bad behavior. In all other markets, the ultimate consumer protection is the ability to go to court and be made whole. As long as health plans are shielded from liability, consumers will continue to believe that the deck is stacked against them.

Enactment of a federal Patients' Bill of Rights is a vital step toward restoring the appropriate balance between cost and access. And it is a crucial part of restoring public trust in a market-based health care system. Six years of debate have refined the approach to managed care reform to the point where we can confidently move forward and complete the job at hand.

References

Brodie, M., L. A. Brady, and D. Altman. 1998. Media Coverage of Managed Care: Is There Negative Bias? *Health Affairs* 17(1):9–25.

Dixon, L., M. Rothouse, and M. Stauffer. 1998. *1999 State Health Care Priorities: Health Policy Tracking Service.* Washington, DC: National Conference of State Legislatures, December.

Kaiser Family Foundation (KFF). 1998. *Trends and Indicators in the Changing Health Care Marketplace.* Menlo Park, CA: Kaiser Family Foundation.

Kaiser Family Foundation (KFF) and Harvard University School of Public Health. 1998. *Survey of Americans' Views on the Consumer Protection Debate.* Storrs, CT: Roper Center, 17 September.

Public Policy and Education Fund of New York (PPEFNY). 1995. *The Managed Care Consumers' Bill of Rights: A Health Policy Guide for Consumer Advocates.* 1995. New York: PPEFNY, October.

Salant, J. 1998. Foes of New HMO Rules Spent $60 Million for Lobbying in Six Months. *Philadelphia Inquirer,* 28 November, A10.

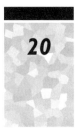

20

The Wrong Rights

Barry R. Bloom

*T*he patriotically named "Patients' Bill of Rights" is making its way through Congress. It would put into law sound medical practice—requiring insurance companies to cover care that doctors believe is "medically necessary" and allow subscribers easier access to emergency rooms and to care from obstetricians and other specialists.

There's only one problem: the Patients' Bill of Rights would affect only a minority of Americans—even of those who are insured. And it will do very little to improve the nation's health.

The real issue is not how to make group health plans pay more, but how to keep Americans from getting critically ill in the first place. Of the 2 million deaths that occur in the United States each year, half are preventable. While the top killers appear to be heart disease (one third of all deaths), cancer (one fourth), stroke (7 percent) and injuries (14 percent), the real culprits are the underlying causes of these conditions—tobacco use (leading to 19 percent of all deaths), unhealthy diet and inactivity (14 percent), alcohol (5 percent), infectious disease (5 percent), firearms (about 2 percent) and accidents (1 percent). These figures represent a million lives that could be saved by an investment of only a few cents of each health dollar into what we call public health.

Public health differs from clinical medicine in two respects: it focuses on prevention rather than cure, and it works on broad measures to protect large populations and communities, not just individual patients. In this century, life expectancy has risen by more than 30 years, due largely to public health, not medical interventions.

But Americans are not getting the modern public-health care they deserve. They need a national defense against the risks of illness and accidents, not just payment for high-tech procedures and emergency care after the fact. We need, in short, a Public Health Bill of Rights. It would include:

Reprinted with permission of Barry R. Bloom, dean, Harvard School of Public Health, in *Newsweek*, October 11, 1999, p. 92.

The right to information. Citizens deserve the most accurate information medical science can provide on how to promote health and prevent illness. Although we have perhaps the world's best doctors and hospitals, Americans in some regions live 25 years less than those in others. We should use our new information technologies to analyze the disparities in health status and disease risk in various areas of the country, and then erase them.

A right to information also means being vigilant about emerging resistant infections and local threats to the environment. We need federal support for state and local public-health authorities and population experts who first notice trends and sound the alarms.

The right to mother and infant care. We must enable every woman to plan for her family and, when pregnant, to protect her unborn baby's health as well as her own. Despite this century's 90 percent drop in infant and maternal mortality, America ranks only 25th worldwide in preventing infant mortality. We need a national strategy to reduce the disparities among ethnic and low-income groups. It can be done. Over the past 14 years, for example, the state of Massachusetts lowered its infant-mortality rate from 10.1 per 1,000 births to 6.2 deaths per 1,000 births, the best in the country. The state guaranteed all pregnant women payment for prenatal care and created community programs to reach vulnerable "at-risk" women. That is public health.

The right to childhood immunization. American children are free from diseases like polio and diphtheria because of immunization. We must ensure that all newborns receive their vaccines. For every dollar spent on immunization against measles, mumps and rubella, for example, we save more than $13 in medical expenses, amounting to about $4 billion a year.

The right to teenage counseling. There are no vaccines against sexually transmitted diseases and access to addictive substances. Teenagers should have the right to counseling about AIDS—which has killed 14 million people worldwide and 410,000 in this country—and how to protect themselves from other STDs. In addition, we should sharply reduce portrayals of tobacco and alcohol use in entertainment media: think of the impact on teens of Leonardo DiCaprio's smoking cigarettes in scene after scene of "Titanic."

The right to health screening. Simple and inexpensive tests can detect cancers of the breast, cervix, colon and prostate in early stages when further spread can be prevented. Routine screening reduces the risk of dying from colon cancer, for example, by at least 33 percent. We also need screening tests for high blood pressure—the major risk factor for heart attacks and strokes.

The right to a healthy environment. The dramatic gains in longevity over this century resulted largely from improvements in environmental health. Malnutrition and specific dietary deficiencies were reduced, housing was improved, and air and water quality became a concern of government and the public. We need more investment in infrastructure such as municipal water systems and tighter controls on air pollution. We must also make indoor environments healthier, especially schools and workplaces, thereby reducing the incidence of illnesses like asthma.

Individual rights imply collective responsibilities. Investing just a minuscule percentage of the trillion dollars we now spend on medical care could result in a dramatic improvement in the well-being of our entire citizenry. It would also save billions of dollars in medical costs for everyone involved. The Patients' Bill of Rights now before the House is one answer to our health-care problems. But it's an incomplete one.

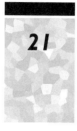

21

Seeking Confidentiality
of Medical Records

Linda L. Kloss

*E*very American, from the beginning of life to its end, enjoys a fundamental, but not absolute, right to privacy that is deeply rooted in both tradition and law. In no area is this right more cherished, or more unsettled, than in protecting the confidentiality of identifiable personal health information, as lawmakers, judges, and health care professionals struggle to balance individual privacy interests against other strong societal concerns.

Personal health information is maintained not only by physicians, but in the records and/or databases of hospitals and clinics that provide treatment or diagnostic services, laboratories that perform tests, pharmacies, and insurance companies and managed care organizations to which claims are submitted or that provide coverage. In addition, personal health data frequently is shared with universities and pharmaceutical companies for research purposes.

Certain medical information, by law, must be reported to state and local governments, where it is maintained in databases. For instance, U.S. jurisdictions typically require the reporting of venereal disease to public health agencies, of child abuse to child welfare agencies, and of injuries caused by firearms to law enforcement agencies.

The flow of medical information carries numerous personal and societal benefits. The ability to access medical records has saved the lives of unconscious patients brought into hospital emergency rooms. Pharmacists have detected dangerous, sometimes potentially lethal, drug combinations. In the public health arena, computerized records have made possible the prompt detection of infectious disease epidemics and enabled health authorities to take emergency action. Researchers have used databases to analyze the causes of a illness, a process that, for example, established the connection between smoking and lung cancer. On the other hand, the vast accumulation of

Linda L. Kloss is executive vice president and CEO, American Health Information and Management Association, Chicago, IL.

personal medical data gives rise to serious privacy concerns because of the potential for misuse.

Breaches of confidentiality have been widespread. In some instances, they occur within the parameters of present law. Pharmacies in some states legally sell individual prescription records to pharmaceutical companies for use in marketing campaigns.

Other breaches have been illegal. The medical records of a candidate for Congress, indicating that she once had attempted suicide, were sent to the *New York Post* on the eve of her primary election. A Colorado medical student sold patient records to lawyers soliciting malpractice plaintiffs. In Florida, the names of 4,000 HIV-positive patients was carelessly released to two newspapers.

The collateral social consequences of improper or illegal dissemination of personal health information are far more devastating than solicitations from drug companies and malpractice lawyers. They include the denial of such basic social rights as employment, insurance, health care, housing, and education. The consequences of HIV/AIDS stigmatization have been particularly catastrophic. The confidentiality issue has become so serious that President Clinton went before the nation late in 1999 with a speech calling for legislation to protect patient privacy.

As genetic testing becomes more common and as the potential dangers lurking in DNA become better understood, the danger of illegal discrimination against persons at risk of developing serious conditions is likely to increase. A May, 1997, article in the *Journal of the American Medical Association* advised: "Participants in genetic testing should be informed that the genetic testing for cancer susceptibility may limit their ability to obtain health, life, or disability insurance; may lead to limitations in health insurance coverage; or may result in higher premiums for insurance products. Participants also should be informed that genetic testing may pose a risk to their present or future employment."

The confidentiality of personal health information is an issue that profoundly affects every American. The fundamental question, maintains Secretary of Health and Human Services Donna Shalala, is: "Will our health records be used to heal us or reveal us?"

On Sept. 11, 1997, Shalala presented recommendations for Federal legislation to the Senate Committee on Labor and Human Resources and testified that "The computer revolution means that our deepest and darkest secrets no longer exist in one place and can no longer be protected by simply locking up the office doors each night.

"And, revolutions in biology mean that a whole new world of genetic tests have the potential to help either prevent disease or reveal our families' most personal secrets. Because without safeguards that assure citizens that getting tested won't endanger their families' privacy or health insurance or jobs, we could, in turn, endanger one of the most promising areas of research our nation has ever seen.

"We are at a decision point. Depending on what we do . . . these revolutions in health care, communications, and biology could bring us great promise or even greater peril. The choice is ours. For example, will health care information flow safely to improve care, cut fraud, ensure quality, and reach citizens in underserved areas? Or will it flow recklessly into the wrong hands?"

Current legal protections of the privacy of health information are fragmented and uncertain. All 50 states provide statutory protection for personal health data maintained by public agencies, but permit disclosure for one or more purposes, the most common of which are statistical evaluation, contact tracing of persons diagnosed to have sexually transmitted and infectious diseases, epidemiological investigations, and use in court pursuant to subpoena or court order. However, just 42 states provide either criminal or civil penalties for improper disclosure.

On the Federal level, the Privacy Act of 1974 provides limited protection against the disclosure by the government of individual health records maintained by government agencies such as the Veterans Administration and the Department of Defense. The act contains a "routine use" exception, though, that privacy advocates complain guts the protection. The Americans with Disabilities Act of 1990 prohibits discrimination on the basis of a disability, including HIV or AIDS, but does not directly protect privacy. Rather, it merely provides a remedy for discrimination based on breaches of confidentiality.

In 1977, the Supreme Court, in its sole major encounter with the constitutional risks arising from the storage of health information in government data banks, unanimously recognized a qualified constitutional right to privacy of personal information that could reflect unfavorably on an individual. At the same time, the unanimous Court upheld the constitutionality of a New York statute requiring physicians to forward to the State Health Department the name, age, and address of every patient obtaining certain dangerous, yet legitimate, drugs.

The constitutional protection of private information, such as it is, applies just to violations by the government—not by private parties, who sometimes are responsible for the most intrusive invasions of privacy. The majority of states protects privately held medical information to at least some extent. Thirty-six impose a general duty upon physicians to maintain patient confidentiality, and 26 of those extend that duty to other health care providers. A mere four states have legislation specifically extending the duty to insurers, and nine impose restrictions on employers. This patchwork of state and Federal laws obviously falls far short of delivering consistent, comprehensive protection of the privacy of health information nationwide.

Aside from legal shortcomings in regulating what information is available to whom and for what purposes, as well as protecting the security of databases containing personal health information, there is no standard legal mechanism allowing consumers to verify the accuracy of their personal health information. Accuracy is a huge issue. For example, the

Massachusetts-based Medical Information Bureau, a clearinghouse for about 750 insurers, has acknowledged that as many as 3.5% of its approximately 15,000,000 individual files contain inaccurate data. Because the information relates to life expectancy—blood pressure, weight, and cholesterol level—and is used by the insurers for underwriting purposes, inaccuracies may result in a decision to deny coverage or charge higher rates.

Yet, until the insurance industry reached a voluntary agreement with the Federal Trade Commission in 1995 to inform applicants when a report plays a role in the denial or rating of insurance, few consumers knew that such reports existed. Those who might have known could not find out what their reports said. Under the agreement, applicants receive notices that they are entitled to a free copy of their reports and have 30 days to request and verify that the information is correct.

Employers, though, have no obligation to inform present or prospective employees when medical information is used in making employment decisions. Because most Fortune 500 companies are self-insured and, therefore, have access to employees' prescription and other health records, unreliable data may have serious consequences. Yet, there presently is no mechanism to allow employees or job applicants to review or correct the information.

▨ SETTING STANDARDS

To address the various health privacy issues, the Department of Health and Human Services has developed proposed standards, to "strike a balance between the privacy needs of our citizens and the critical needs of our health care system." The proposed standards embody five principles that the American Health Information Management Association (AHIMA), representing 38,000 health information management professionals, believes "comprise the exact formula necessary to protect the privacy of Americans [and] place the needs of individuals ahead of powerful commercial interests that use health information for purposes well outside the boundaries of patient care."

The first principle set forth by Shalala is that, "With very few exceptions, health care information about a consumer should be disclosed for health purposes and health purposes only. It should be easy to use it for those purposes, and very difficult to use it for other purposes." The legislation must include requirements that persons who legally receive individual health information take "real and reasonable steps" to safeguard it, ensuring that it is not used improperly by those who have access and is not obtained by "hackers and others on the outside." The steps should include administrative and management techniques, education of employees, and disciplinary sanctions against those who use individual health information improperly.

The second principle is that the legislation must contain technical security safeguards for computerized data. These would include audit trails showing who accessed data, facilitating the identification of—and thereby the prosecution or other appropriate action against—anyone who may have used health records for illegal or improper purposes.

The third principle is consumer access, an area where state laws are inconsistent. All patients should be able to access their medical records. They should be able to find out who has access to them and how to inspect, copy, and, if necessary, correct them. Patients should have access to information about the laws, regulations, or policies that protect their information. In testimony before the Senate Committee on Labor and Human Resources, Shalala cited the example of a California woman who was denied disability and life insurance. The woman discovered that the Medical Information Bureau had provided her prospective insurers with information falsely indicating she suffered from heart problems and Alzheimer's disease. "What if she hadn't requested her records?," Shalala asked rhetorically.

Accountability, the fourth principle, is closely linked to security and consumer control. Shalala has called for criminal penalties (fines and imprisonment) against those who breach security of personal health information and civil remedies (actual and punitive monetary damage recoveries) for injured parties. The penalties, she says, should be higher when violations are committed for monetary gain.

The fifth and final principle is public responsibility. The legislation must balance personal privacy interests against the national priorities of public health, research, and law enforcement. The free flow of information, without patient authorization, is essential to prompt discovery, investigation, and intervention in public health crises, such as the 1997 outbreak of *E. coli* in ground beef that resulted in the largest recall of meat products in history. Patient consent should not be required for the discrimination of personal health information for research purposes, provided that the disclosures will not adversely affect their rights or welfare and that the research would not be practical if consent were required.

These five principles, of course, are but a broad outline of a sensible public policy that, if codified, would reasonably balance personal privacy interests and other important social interests. The remaining task is to resolve such issues as whether national privacy standards should preempt existing state legislation and whether genetic information should be treated differently than other personal health information for research purposes.

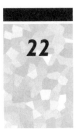

22

The Real Meaning
of Patient–Nurse Confidentiality

Maureen Cochran

". . . Grant that my patients have confidence in me and my art . . ."
—Prayer of Maimonides

Neither the giving of trust nor the gaining of confidence is always easy, but gaining a patient's trust and confidence is essential to the nurse-patient relationship. If patients were to be secretive with their health care providers, all concerned could be at a serious disadvantage. For a nurse to gain a patient's trust and then reveal that patient's private matters would be disrespectful, unprofessional, and in many cases, illegal. The issue of confidentiality is not always easily resolved, however. The right to privacy has assumed new meaning in the computer age and policies and customs have not always kept pace. In addition, there are situations in which a patient's privacy must be balanced against both public safety and justice.

This article examines the critical care nurse's legal, ethical, and professional obligations related to issues of patient confidentiality and privacy. In three case study scenarios, the questions of disclosure of medical information and disclosure of communication are addressed.

■ SCENARIO ONE

Joe is a 33-year-old intensive care unit (ICU) patient who was admitted following a large intentional overdose of Tylenol #3, phenobarbital, and other unspecified, over-the-counter (OTC) drugs. A note he left stated that he could not face an upcoming criminal arrest for stalking and sexually assaulting a former girlfriend. He also has been accused of workplace sexual harassment of the same woman. Joe is currently unconscious and mechanically ventilated, but before he became unresponsive, he made some incriminating re-

Maureen Cochran, Ph.D., R.N., is an instructor, Critical Care Nursing, University of Massachusetts and adjunct faculty, College of Management, Suffolk University, Boston, Massachusetts.

Reprinted from *Critical Care Nurse Quarterly*, 22(1) 42–51, 1999, with permission of Aspen Publishers, Inc. © 1999.

marks about these matters in the presence of both his nurse and his physician. Since Joe became unconscious, there have been two requests for review of his medical record, one from his insurance company and the other from the District Attorney's (DA) office. In addition, an investigator from the DA's office has asked both Joe's nurse and his physician what, if anything, Joe said to them about his legal problems while he could still speak. Before the nurse can deal with any of these issues, she receives a telephone call from a man identifying himself as Joe's brother. He wants to know what happened and what Joe's condition and prognosis are.

This scenario poses a host of legal, ethical, and professional problems related to Joe's privacy and the nurse's obligations of confidentiality. The problems encompass three major areas: access to Joe's medical record, doctor-patient and nurse-patient communication, and disclosure of information to a member of Joe's family.

Confidentiality of Medical Records

The medical record is the property of the hospital. The purpose of a record for each patient is to document assessments, treatments, and progress of that patient. It is expected that the documentation be accurate, complete, and timely and that it be held in a confidential and secure manner.[1]

In reality, most medical records are available for legitimate review by many people despite the fact that they often contain very personal information. It has been estimated that in a teaching hospital, more than 60 individuals may have access to any one patient's record during an average hospital stay.[2] Consent for in-house use of patient information is implied when the patient agrees to treatment. In addition to review by people directly involved in the care of any individual patient, records may be reviewed legitimately for utilization review purposes, for quality assurance purposes, and for research purposes. Review of all or part of a record by third-party payers, managed care organizations (MCOs), and even self-insured employers is both common and legitimate,[3] with consent for review either contractually agreed to or presumably agreed to as condition for payment of bills. Courts have allowed access to medical records by insurers for several years (for example, Pyramid Life Insurance Company v. Masonic Hospital Association[4]). Thus, the first medical records problem is a nonproblem. Joe's insurance provider is entitled to review his record.

The DA's office, on the other hand, is not entitled to review Joe's medical record at this time without his expressed consent or a court order. At first glance, it is unclear what this office would want with the record because Joe's medical condition and treatment would appear to offer no unique evidentiary issues in the case pending against him. The matter should be referred to the hospital's legal department, which automatically will refuse the DA's request, at least at this time.

There are several federal and state statutes that protect the confidentiality of medical information, such as The Federal Privacy Act of 1974. Unauthorized or improper disclosure can be a legal misdemeanor or felony, with punishment ranging from fine to imprisonment. In states that allow civil suits, patients may be entitled to collect both compensatory and punitive damages. Any professional health care provider who improperly disclosed information would be subject to institutional sanctions including suspension from or loss of a job. Revocation of a professional license could occur.

Patients may give permission to have their medical records disclosed to whomever they wish. They also may waive their right to confidentiality under certain conditions; for example, if their mental or physical condition is at issue in a legal proceeding such as a malpractice suit or a workmen's compensation claim, among other conditions.

Twenty-two states mandate compliance with a subpoena or court order for medical records and most states expect, if not mandate, compliance with any type of court order. If the DA's office were to obtain a court order for Joe's records, then the hospital would no doubt comply. In order to obtain such an order, however, the DA would have to show that there was probable cause to believe that the records would be helpful in the legal case against Joe, which relates to the investigator's question to both Joe's nurse and physician. The question could be no more than a simple fishing expedition or the investigator could suspect, or even know, that Joe spoke to his nurse and physician. After the question is asked, there are only three choices for answers: Joe didn't say anything; no comment; or yes, Joe spoke about it. Each answer carries its own risks.

Although the nurse is not being asked for any medical information about Joe, he or she is being asked about his or her communication with Joe and the question of confidentiality is at stake. It is a question that may not be resolved easily. If the nurse says that Joe did not say anything, he or she will not have violated any confidentiality principles but he or she will have lied. If it is later discovered that the nurse lied, he or she could be charged with obstruction of justice. If the nurse answers honestly and says yes, Joe did speak to him or her, the nurse may or may not have violated Joe's privacy. Even if the nurse does not tell the investigator what Joe said, he or she has given that investigator probable cause to get a court order for Joe's medical record on the assumption that the communication would have been documented.

The best course for both the nurse and the physician at this time would be to refuse to answer the investigator until each has consulted with his or her respective supervisors and possibly the hospital's legal counsel. The nurse's concern is not what eventually happens to Joe legally or even what eventually happens to his medical record. The nurse's concern is how the issue of confidentiality should be handled.

Privileged Communication

The privilege of confidentiality belongs to patients, not to their health care providers. Patients are under no obligation to keep their medical conditions private or to keep their conversations with their caregivers confidential. It is their caregivers that have that obligation. Patients expect that what they say to their physicians will be held in confidence and this expectation is supported in common law, in statutory law, in professional codes, and in institutional policy and practice. In all probability, patients also expect that what they say to their nurses will be held in confidence, but although support for this expectation is present in professional codes and institutional policies, it is not universally present in common law or statutory law. In fact, there is no law enacted in any state mandating nurse-patient confidentiality.

The only absolute confidentiality privilege accepted in all 50 states is that between penitent and clergy. Attorney-client privilege is recognized in all 50 states as well, but there are instances specified state by state that override that privilege; for example, in some states, an attorney must report a client's expressed intent to break the law. Forty-two states recognize the doctor-patient confidentiality privilege[5] but most have specific exceptions in which that privilege does not apply. In 1966, New York State[6] found in People v. Capra that the privilege did not extend to the discovery of drugs on the defendant by the physician during a physical examination. In California, if the patient is involved in criminal proceedings, the privilege does not apply.[7]

The scope of the doctor-patient privilege varies from state to state as well. In some states, the privilege is limited to doctor-patient only. In other states, mainly through case law rather than enacted law, psychotherapists are included in the privilege (e.g., in Oklahoma), and in other states, nurses are included (e.g., in Colorado). Most of the specified privileged relationships include various exceptions. Although it often is assumed that doctor-patient confidentiality extends to health care institutions and their employees, this most often is expressed in institutional policy. It may or may not apply in a court of law.

Because Joe's expectations of confidentiality will be mitigated by whatever exceptions are specified under individual state laws, it is imperative that the nurse seek guidance before officially speaking to the DA's office. Because this is a criminal matter, it is more likely than unlikely that there will be a confidentiality exception that applies. After a court orders a health care provider to speak, there is no confidentiality privilege that enables that person to refuse to answer without risking contempt charges. The health care provider becomes the same as any other citizen. It will be left to the attorneys prosecuting Joe and those defending him to argue the various legal points around Joe's statements such as whether Joe was mentally impaired when he made his statements, whether his Fifth Amendment rights against self incrimination were violated, whether he thought he was making a dying declaration, whether a confession to a non-law enforcement person is valid, and so on.

Although there probably will be legal guidelines that govern the nurse's actions in Joe's case, the ethical and professional obligations related to confidentiality must also be examined. The American Nurses Association (ANA) Code for Nurses states:

"The nurse safeguards the client's right to privacy by judiciously protecting information of a confidential nature. With some exceptions, only information pertinent to a client's treatment and welfare is disclosed, and it is disclosed only to those directly concerned with the client's care."[8]

At first glance, this would seem to argue against revealing the type of information asked for, but the "with some exceptions" clause takes the absolutes out of the argument. If Joe had told the nurse that he has committed the crimes for which he is being investigated, the ethics of justice and fairness would argue for revealing the information. Confidentiality guidelines and laws exist to protect patients, but exceptions that have been judged beneficial to society also exist. Professional codes have been given weight in courts of law, but if a nurse were to cite this code as a prohibition against telling what he or she knew, the nurse should expect that the exceptions clause would apply. In the eyes of the law, Joe has committed crimes against society and he has admitted his guilt to the nurse. Justice, both legal and ethical, probably would outweigh Joe's right to privacy.

Information to Patients' Families

The last problem related to Joe's scenario is what to say to his brother on the telephone without violating Joe's privacy. The first consideration is whether the person really is Joe's brother or if Joe even has a brother. The person on the phone could be anyone. Even if it is Joe's brother, the nurse does not know whether Joe would want him to receive the information he is seeking. The only one entitled to the type of information that the person on the telephone is asking for is Joe himself. Because Joe obviously is now unable to competently speak for himself, it is his proxy and/or the person that he designated on his admission as next of kin who is entitled to the information.

Many hospitals have adopted policies governing the dissemination of information to patient's families to cover situations such as this. In some institutions, code words or numbers are being given to those people authorized by the patient or next of kin to receive information. Others give no information to anyone except the patient or next of kin, with those people being solely responsible for any dissemination of the information. Privacy exists within families and must be respected. Family relationships and dynamics, both open and subtle, usually are not evident when patients are admitted, often stay hidden through discharge, and unless they directly affect the care of the patient, are not the business of health care providers anyway. Although nursing's efforts to involve families in the care of patients is laudable, there may be a fine line between revealing too little and revealing too much. In the interest of maintaining Joe's privacy, information should not be given to this caller.

■ *SCENARIO TWO*

John is a 22-year-old man who is a first-time admission to the emergency department. He was brought in by ambulance with a gunshot wound to his right shoulder. He was not accompanied by the police. As the nurse is assessing him, he is very angry and states "This is payback for what I did" and "He is not going to get away with this. When I get out of here, it won't be his shoulder I'm after." As the nurse is folding his clothes, a gun falls to the floor.

Safety in the Emergency Department

John's possession of a gun may or may not be illegal depending on the licensing or registration laws of the state he is in. Either way, there are three unfortunate problems for the nurse in this scenario. The first problem is that the nurse is alone with an armed person and could be in danger. The second problem is that the gun, which could be incriminating evidence, is now on the floor and not in John's possession. Even if the nurse called for someone to come into the room immediately (which he or she should do for safety reasons), the gun is now "tainted evidence." No one but the nurse and John saw it fall from his clothing, and John can very easily deny that it is his. The third problem is what John said. Not only has John implied that he did something to bring on the attack against himself, he also has threatened serious physical retaliation against a person who is known to him. The nurse also knows he has a gun.

Patient Privacy Versus Harm to Society

This scenario demonstrates the conflict between the nurse's duty to maintain John's confidentiality and his or her ethical, moral, and legal duty to prevent harm to another person. If the nurse were to decide that John's right to privacy were paramount, he or she could say nothing about what happened, not chart it, and simply put John's gun in the bag with the rest of his possessions, knowing that the entire bag will be returned to him when he leaves the hospital.

There are definite risks to this course of action because both the nurse and John know what happened. If John does later shoot and possibly kill the person who shot him and then states that the nurse knew he was going to do it, the nurse could be in some serious legal trouble. By simply keeping quiet, the nurse could have aided and abetted John's past, present, and future criminal actions and could be civilly liable, at least in part, for a preventable death. Even if John never told anyone the nurse knew what he was going to do, the nurse will know it and will have to live with his or her own personal emotional and moral aftermath.

Although the requirements of confidentiality would support this action, the wiser course of action, both legally and ethically, would be to take seriously what John said, to take his gun possession seriously, and to take some action. Although John's privacy is important, there are other matters of equal or greater importance. In many states, health care providers have a legal obligation, imposed either through statute or through case law, to disclose confidential information when the welfare or safety of a third party is in jeopardy. This is carried out most often when reporting suspected child abuse, elder abuse, or certain communicable diseases, but the threat of harm to a third party is a valid exception to the confidentiality privilege in many states. Many states also require that suspicious wounds, including any gunshot wounds, be reported.

As in the previous case, it is important for the nurse to seek guidance when determining how to handle what John said. However, before the nurse does this, he or she needs to look to his or her own safety and those of others and to establish John's ownership of the gun on the floor. If feasible, the nurse should leave the gun where it fell and quickly have someone witness its existence and listen to the patient's version of its source. Hospital police or security is the best option both for safety and verification purposes. Removal of the gun is then in everyone's best interest. When safety is assured, the nurse can move forward with the next problem.

The nurse should try to get John to repeat his statements in front of someone else. In the absence of a police officer, hospital police or security would be the most ideal, but any other witness would suffice. Uncorroborated hearsay evidence is worth far less than that which may be corroborated. However, regardless of whatever John says to whom, the nurse has an affirmative obligation to do something with the information he or she has. As in Joe's situation, the nurse received the information during the course of providing care. Theoretically, this wraps it in confidentiality, but unlike Joe's situation, the content of the information poses a threat to the safety of a third party. Disclosing confidential information in order to protect a third party is both legally and morally correct.

The leading court case that dealt with the duty of a health care provider to warn a third party of danger is California's Tarasoff v. Regents of the University of California case.[9] In this case, a patient of a psychotherapist at the University of California made explicit threats to his former girlfriend during therapy, including threats to kill her. The therapist did not warn the woman and the patient carried out his threats. The California Supreme Court held the therapist and his superiors liable in the death of Tarasoff, stating that the relationship between the therapist and the patient was such that there was a duty to protect a third party.

In applying the Tarasoff case to John's situation, there are two key points to be considered. The first is what may be termed "psychiatric dangerousness;"[7(p.244)] the second is that a specific individual has been identified as being in danger. The latter speaks for itself, the former gives the nurse an avenue of recourse. In light of John's anger and the presumed emotional trauma of being shot, the nurse would not be remiss in believing that John is emotionally upset. If John were to repeat his threats to a psychiatric consultant, the burden of disclosure would be on that consultant, with the nurse being the corroborator rather than the primary reporter. Because much of the "psychiatric dangerousness" case law regarding a duty to warn relates to mental health situations, there could be little question as to the appropriateness of the disclosure.

Even if John chose not to speak to the psychiatrist, the "psychiatric dangerousness" issue and the fact that John identified a specific individual who was in danger could cover the nurse's own disclosure. However, as with Joe's case, the nurse needs to be aware of the laws in his or her own state related to the disclosure issue, both in scope and in substance. Some courts have limited the duty to warn to situations that parallel the Tarasoff case (e.g., in Colorado); others have expanded it to cover many other types of third-party peril situations (e.g., in Michigan); while others have rejected it altogether (e.g., in Delaware).[7(p.244)] Other states have statutes that spell out specific third parties who must be warned such as Arizona and Kentucky.

Emergency department patients expect information about themselves to be kept confidential. Unfortunately, emergency department staff may be put at physical, legal, and ethical risk by the very people they are trying to help. In order to minimize these risks, it is unwise to be alone with a patient who has been either a victim or a perpetrator of violence. In some institutions, if the police have accompanied a patient to the emergency department for whatever reason, the police officer stays with the patient while he or she is being undressed and witnesses what is being listed under belongings. In the absence of the police, a member of the hospital police or security force does this. If these or similar policies were in place in John's scenario, many of the nurse's problems could have been avoided.

■ *SCENARIO THREE*

Mary is a 40-year-old woman who has been a patient in the ICU for two days. She was admitted with an esophogeal bleed secondary to cirrhosis secondary to long-time alcoholism. She is also Human Immunodeficiency Virus (HIV) positive with exposure believed to be due to her 20 years as a prostitute. On day three of her stay, Tom, the brother of another patient, comes to the charge nurse and complains about his relative being cared for by the same nurse who is caring for Mary. He tells her he knows that Mary is "infectious and immoral."

There is not enough information in the scenario as presented to know if Mary is or is not "infectious." The use of standard universal precautions by all those involved in her direct care should preclude any threat to Tom's brother. Whether or not Mary is "immoral" is a judgment beyond the scope of this article and should have no bearing whatsoever on her care. There are two main issues for the nurse in this scenario: how to respond to Tom and how to find out where Tom got his information and then close off that source of information for Tom and everyone else in the future, if at all possible.

Responding to an Apparent Confidentiality Breach

Because Tom has a legitimate concern about his brother, the nurse must respond to him, but her duty to maintain Mary's confidentiality also is paramount. She can neither validate the information Tom apparently has about Mary nor can she add to it in any way. A suggested response might be: "You must realize that I cannot discuss Mary or any other patient with you, but I also realize that you are very concerned about your brother. I can assure you that your brother is not at risk from any nursing care assignments that are made." In such a response, the nurse has acknowledged Tom's right to be concerned, has offered assurance that his brother is safe, and has indicated that Mary and every other patient has a right to confidentiality. If Tom were to go on to reiterate his concerns and to spell out knowledge of specifics about Mary, the nurse's answers must stay within the boundaries of her initial response.

Possible Sources of Confidentiality Breach

When Tom's fears have been allayed, it is time for the charge nurse to start her detective work. The best way to find out how Tom received any information about Mary is to ask him directly and go on from there. Hopefully, the answer the nurse receives will not indicate that any health care provider has discussed Mary with Tom. If that is the case, then whoever was at fault is subject to, and deserves, any and all institutional and professional sanctions for violation of a patient's privacy.

It is always possible that one of Mary's visitors and Tom have shared information, a situation over which nurses have no control. If this turns out to be the case, the boundaries of the nurse's initial response still apply.

Regardless of what Tom answers, if anything, the more likely source or sources of Tom's information are myriad and troublesome. Overheard informal conversations may be immediately suspect, but hospital systems and routines themselves often lend to confidentiality violations. Just as nursing has been more forthcoming with information for patients' families, so too have visiting hours been liberalized in many ICUs. Overheard change of shift reports and overheard physicians' rounds offer opportunities for visitor information that must be considered. Bedside charts, any unattended paperwork, including an entire medical record, may be scrutinized by visitors.

Computers and Privacy

During the past decade, the shift from paper medical records to electronically generated permanent records and clinical information systems has been rapid. Electronically transferred information through fax and computer also has become common. These changes have opened up new avenues for unauthorized access to information that must be considered both in Mary's case and in general. Unattended faxes left in sight may provide information for those who should not have it, but unattended computers, or even attended computers, also may be an excellent source. User habits of leaving information visible on an unattended screen, turning a screen so that it is visible to passersby, sharing passwords, or logging on in a manner that makes passwords obvious speak for themselves as careless and ill-advised practices. Not logging off if called away is another ill-advised practice. Even if a screen saver blocks visible information, one push of a button provides any user, authorized or unauthorized, with whatever is available. It would be naive to assume that no ICU visitors have any knowledge of computers and equally naive to assume that at least some of them would not hesitate to use that knowledge.

Computers without sufficient privacy controls also are an enticement. As society has become computer literate, it has become essential that layered security programs be in place to ensure that only authorized personnel have access to information. Layered security also would help to prevent any unauthorized users with their own modems from hacking into clinical information systems from their own remote terminals.

Concern for computer security of medical information goes beyond the scenario presented in this article. Medical information is sent not only between departments in the same institution but also from one institution or agency to another, which enhances the opportunity for it to go astray. The Office of Technology Assessment found that existing laws neither provide consistent or comprehensive protection for medical information nor do they adequately guide the health care industry in its obligations to protect the privacy of information in a computerized environment.[10(p.15)] Unauthorized access to, and use of, private information is an ongoing concern and still needs to be addressed more fully, both technically and legally.

▦ CONCLUSION

When drafting the U.S. Constitution, the founding fathers of this country did not provide for any right to privacy except for a poorly defined right to be free from government intrusion into private affairs. Laws related to confidentiality in medicine have been promulgated by the individual states and these are noteworthy for their differences in scope and content. Although there is no state that mandates nurse-patient confidentiality, the confidentiality laws that apply to medical professionals in each state are imperative sources of guidance when a nurse is faced with a confidentiality dilemma. Professional codes and institutional policies also will be helpful. It is important for nurses to respect patients and their expectations of confidentiality. It also is important for nurses to realize that there are ethical, professional, and legal exceptions to the patient's confidentiality privilege.

References

1. Joint Commission on Accreditation of Healthcare Organizations. *Accreditation Manual for Hospitals.* Oakbrook Terrace, IL: Joint Commission on Accreditation of Healthcare Organizations; 1994.
2. Waller A, Fulton D. The electronic chart: Keeping it confidential and secure. *J Health Hosp Law.* 1993;4:463.
3. Hiller M. Computers, medical records and the right to privacy. *J Health Policy, Politics Law.* 1981;(6):163.
4. *Pyramid Life Insurance Company v. Masonic Hospital Association of Payne County, Oklahoma.* 191 F. Supp. 51 (1961).
5. Gostin L. *Legislative Survey of State Confidentiality Laws, with Specific Emphasis on HIV and Immunizations.* Electronic Privacy Information Center; 1997.
6. *People v. Capra,* 269 N.Y.S.2d 411, 216 N.E.2d 610 (1966).
7. Furrow B, Greaney T, Johnson S, Jost T, Schwartz R. *Health Law.* Vol. I. St. Paul, MN: West Publishing Company; 1995.
8. American Nurses Association. *Code For Nurses with Interpretations.* Washington, D.C.: American Nurses Association; 1976.
9. *Tarasoff v. Regents of the University of California,* 17 Cal.3d 425, 551 P.2d 334, 131 Cal. Repr. 14 (1976).
10. U.S. Office of Technology Assessment. *Protecting Privacy in Computerized Medical Information.* Washington, D.C.: U.S. Government Printing Office; 1996.

Suggested Readings

Goldstein B. Confidentiality and dissemination of personal information: An examination of state laws governing data protection. *Emory Law J.* 1992;41:1185.

Harshbarger S. Patient confidentiality: A legal overview. *Health Data News.* August 1998:1–2.

King J, ed. (1991). *Legalines: Criminal Procedure.* Chicago: Harcourt, Brace, Jovanovich Legal and Professional Publications; 1998.

Legal Questions. *Nursing 98.* 1998;1:66.

www.senate.gov/leahy/s971028.html.

23

Medical Records: Enhancing Privacy, Preserving the Common Good

Amitai Etzioni

*T*he privacy of medical records, which contain highly intimate information that people legitimately are keen to keep from others, often is violated. Some of these violations are random, while others are systematic and are said to serve the common good, including quality control, cost reduction, medical research, public health, and public safety. Yet *these goods can be served to a considerable extent* even if medical privacy is enhanced in ways discussed below. And *to the extent that common goods must be sacrificed to better respect medical privacy, these intrusions can be minimized.* This, I shall show, requires a shift from relying largely on individualistic doctrines reflected in the notions of informed consent to relying much more on communitarian institutions. These institutions provide a special bonus: because they primarily are proactive and preventive, they mainly rely not on new legislation, prohibitions, and penalties for violators, but on arrangements that render violations of privacy less likely.

■ UNAUTHORIZED USE OF MEDICAL INFORMATION

The notion that one's personal medical information could be obtained by others not involved in the person's care and not authorized to receive it, and used to harm the person, is frightening. A few examples of the many that could be given: a database created by the state of Maryland in 1993 to keep the medical records of all its residents for cost-containment purposes was used by state employees to sell confidential information on Medicaid recipients to health maintenance organizations, and was accessed by a banker who employed the information to call in the loans of customers who he discovered had cancer.[1] A medical student in Colorado sold the medical records of patients to mal-

Dr. Amitai Etzioni is a university professor, The George Washington University, Washington, DC.

Reprinted with permission of A. Etzioni from *The Limits of Privacy* (New York: Basic Books) 1999.

practice lawyers.[2] In Newton, Massachusetts, a convicted child rapist working at a local hospital used a former employee's computer password to access nearly 1,000 patient files to make obscene phone calls to young girls.[3] In Florida, a state health department worker used state computers to compile a list of 4,000 people who tested positive for HIV and forwarded it to two newspapers, the *St. Petersburg Times* and the *Tampa Tribune*.[4]

All such incidents have several attributes in common: they typically are isolated acts, often committed by a single person; they are as a rule in violation of the policies and ethical codes of the institutions in which they take place; and in some occasions they violate federal or state laws. Hence I refer to them as "unauthorized uses." As troubling as some of these incidents are, the scope of their ill consequences pales in comparison to what might be called "authorized abuses." However, before I can turn to the latter, massive form of abuse, I must digress briefly to discuss recent developments that make these abuses possible.

■ PRIVACY-DIMINISHING DEVELOPMENTS

There has been a trend in recent years to gather and record greater and more detailed information in medical records, including genetic information and lifestyle details.[5] And the health insurance industry now collects much larger amounts of information from physicians than it gathered in the past, amassing large databases of personal information.

Also, until recently insurance companies usually received *only* an abstract of a patient's record, containing information on diagnoses, tests performed, and treatment provided. Nowadays, it is not uncommon for insurers to gain a patient's *entire* record.[6] The shift to managed care programs, especially, has generated considerable additional demand for detailed patient information by groups other than the treating personnel.[7] For instance, representatives of managed care companies have required psychiatrists, as a condition for payment, to reveal considerable details about their patients to verify that treatment was necessary.[8]

Equally important are technological developments, especially a switch by health care organizations from traditional paper-based files to computerized records that are stored in online databases.[9] Retrieval and access is much easier from electronic records than from paper records.

Increasing linkages are formed among various health care databases. These, in effect, turn numerous databases into one. A report issued by the Congressional Office of Technology Assessment states that "as a result of the linkage of computers, patient information will no longer be maintained, be accessed, or even necessarily originate with a single institution, but will instead travel among a myriad of facilities. As a result, the limited protection to privacy of health care information now in place will be further strained."[10]

Additional concerns are raised by the fact that once online, health information can be linked with nonhealth data sets, such as an individual's credit report, to create still more encompassing personal dossiers (p. 11). In 1995 Equifax, the giant consumer credit reporting agency, announced it would supply computerized medical records systems in addition to consumer credit reports.[11] Information brokers obtain and sell individual, personal data: $400 will buy ten years' medical history; $40 to $80 will uncover stock, bond, and mutual fund holdings; $450 will reveal a credit card number; $80 to $200 will bring telephone records; and between $10 and $20 will buy a divorce search, death claim search, fictitious name search, or bankruptcy search.[12]

> The Institute of Medicine concluded that these developments raised numerous issues, including (1) worries on the part of health care providers and clinicians about use or misuse of the information health database organizations will compile and release, and (2) alarm on the part of consumers, patients, and their physicians about how well the privacy and confidentiality of personal health information will be guarded.[13]

The main issue that these developments raise, though, is not an explosion of unauthorized use, but a much more widespread and systematic violation of privacy via what might be called "authorized abuse."

■ *AUTHORIZED ABUSE*

Most violations of medical privacy seem due to the legally sanctioned, or at least tolerated, unconcealed, systematic flow of medical information from the orbit of the physician-patient-health insurer and health management corporations to other, non-health-care parties, including employers, marketers, and the media. Reference is not to the occasional slip-up or the work of a rogue employee, but to daily, continuous, and numerous disclosures and usages that are quite legal but of questionable ethical value and intent.

One major problem is the disclosure by some health insurance companies to employers of information that employers then use to the detriment of prospective or current employees.[14] In 1996, 35 percent of the Fortune 500 companies acknowledged that they draw on personal health information in making employment decisions.[15]

Also, corporations that self-insure draw on their personnel departments or medical claims divisions for privacy-violating data. A 1991 survey by the OTA found that one-third of employers used their personnel departments to examine the medical records of their employees, without notifying the employees.[16]

In addition, there is, as Kathleen A. Frawley, vice president of the American Health Information Management Association, puts it, "a whole market of people buying and selling medical information."[17] Indeed there are firms that specialize in collecting and selling medical information about many millions of people, including IMS America, the Medical Information Bureau, and MetroMail.[18]

The medical information obtained in this way is used in hiring and firing and other employment decisions, including information about the person's genetic attributes, mental illness, drug abuse, and other conditions,[19] even if these conditions have not affected the person's work performance.

Medical information is also sought by marketers to hawk their wares. Pharmaceutical companies have obtained medical records to discover which prescription drugs individuals use and which physicians prescribe them, allowing these companies to solicit physicians to prescribe different drugs sold by the company.[20] For about $.30 per name, large drug companies pitch their products directly to angina sufferers, diabetics, or arthritics.[21]

Given such facts, the National Committee on Vital and Health Statistics, a committee of health care experts not given to hyperbole, concluded that the "United States is in the midst of a health privacy crisis" and urged the Administration to "assign the highest priority" to dealing with the matter.[22]

Large proportions of patients are troubled by the matter as well. For instance, a 1993 Harris/Equifax survey on the privacy of medical records found that half of respondents were concerned about the effects of computers used by health care providers; 60 percent were worried that the use of computerized medical records would result in mistaken information regarding medical conditions being placed in patient records; and 75 percent said they were concerned that a computerized health information system will be used for many nonhealth-care purposes.[23] Eighty-five percent of those surveyed said that protecting the confidentiality of medical records was "absolutely essential" or "very important."[24]

▉ *BIG BROTHER OR BIG BUCKS?*

While the concern for privacy is widespread, the same cannot be said about people's understanding of the source of the new threats. The evidence about the nature of privacy violations suggests that Americans now need protection against the abuses and intrusions of private enterprises as much or more than from government agencies. Still, leading libertarians persist in their focus on the government as the greatest enemy to individual privacy. Writing about this issue (although without specific reference to medical records) in the libetarian publication *Reason*, Brian Taylor states, "While private-sector surveillance is commonplace and widely accepted . . . the trends of placing cameras in public areas for use by law enforcement is a new and disconcerting variation on the established practice."[25] Solveig Singleton stakes out this anachronistic position more starkly in a Cato Institute report.

> We have no good reason to create new privacy rights. Most private-sector firms that collect information about consumers do so only in order to sell

more merchandise. That hardly constitutes a sinister motive. There is little reason to fear the growth of private-sector databases. What we should fear is the growth of government databases.[26]

Fortunately, we shall see that the tension between the competing concerns of privacy and the common good in this area can be sharply curtailed, allowing us to avoid the full brunt of the political opposition that so far has sidetracked several efforts to protect privacy in this area. To put it in the terms followed here: privacy violations of medical records constitute a significant problem. The next question is, are these violations justified by some major service to the common good, and can this service be rendered even if these abuses are greatly curtailed? These questions are examined next in relation to four particular common goods.

■ THE COMMON GOODS SERVED
BY ELECTRONIC MEDICAL RECORDS

Public Safety. In 1997 the Clinton Administration suggested legislation that would allow law enforcement authorities "quick, confidential, unhindered"[27] access to medical records; that is, access without prior consent of the patient whose records are being combed and without notifying the patient that his or her records are being examined. Two main reasons are given to support this stance: first, it would facilitate the investigation of time-sensitive cases, such as when law enforcement officers may need to search emergency room records to look for someone who has just fled a crime scene. Second, such examination would allow the government to scan records to curb medical and financial fraud.[28] Hence, Health and Human Services Secretary Donna Shalala recommends that actions taken to better protect the privacy of medical records impose no new hindrances on law enforcement access to medical records.

Two different relevant situations need to be considered. One occurs when there is a specific indication that a crime has been committed. Here the American legal tradition already allows the search of records if a reasonable case can be made. Currently if the FBI or a local police force seeks to examine any private records, say a person's or a corporation's financial files, they must provide evidence to a magistrate that there is reasonable suspicion that a crime has been or is being committed. There seems to be no reason that medical records, correctly considered more intimate and hence having a higher claim for privacy, should be accessed more easily. Here too, if there is a legitimate need, a warrant can be obtained.

The second situation arises under some special conditions when there is no time to gain a warrant. For instance, the police may be looking for a killer on the loose who is believed to have been stabbed and treated in an emergency room and the police are anxious to comb records before he disappears.

The law, however, already provides for such instances and allows such "hot pursuit" searches to be justified after the fact.

A rather different situation arises when law enforcers need to comb a large number of records to determine whether fraud has been committed. Because the "suspects" in these cases typically are not the patients but the health care providers, law enforcement authorities can be limited in the scope of their search so that they can obtain the facts they need without violating the privacy of patients, as I will show below. If patients are suspected of having committed or participated in committing the crime, say by having conspired with a physician to defraud an insurance company, the rules of specific suspicion would apply. In short, there seems to be no reason to conclude that better protection of the privacy of medical records would significantly undercut public safety. The mechanisms for setting it aside—when justified—are already in place.

Quality Control, Cost Control, and Research. Three related but far from identical health care goods are served by accessing medical records. *Quality control* seeks to ensure that care is given in line with established practices. Hospitals typically maintain internal mechanisms to ensure quality of care. For instance, committees routinely review patients' charts to determine whether the surgery performed was required, whether the correct procedure was performed, and whether the proper aftercare was provided. Some outside agencies, such as accreditation organizations and some HMOs, review data for the same purpose.

Cost control seeks to curb waste and fraudulent use and to promote the utilization of effective and efficient products and procedures. Such "utilization reviews" are conducted routinely by HMOs, health insurance companies, and federal and state government agencies and encompass numerous items of information, from the costs and nature of drugs prescribed to the number of days a patient stayed in a hospital, from the specialists the patients were assigned to the number of X-rays conducted.

Medical records research also enables researchers to monitor a population's health, identify populations at high risk for disease, determine the effectiveness of treatments, assess the usefulness of diagnostic tests and screening programs, conduct cost-effectiveness analysis, support administrative functions, and monitor the general adequacy of care.[29]

The fact that these three health care goals benefit greatly from access to medical records of individual patients is self-evident. One point, though, should be emphasized: all three goals stand to gain a great deal from precisely the same technological and organizational developments that constitute a major source of the new threats to privacy. Instead of laboriously piecing together information from thousands of paper records maintained in physicians' private offices or in numerous hospitals and clinics, new electronic databases in principle provide a much more expeditious and efficient resource to those who seek to evaluate care, control cost, and advance knowledge. One area of benefit, quality of care, will stand for all the others.

The quality of medical care has long suffered from grossly deficient evaluations of the efforts of its practitioners.[30] Medical treatments still often rely on notions transmitted from masters to apprentices (during medical training), but the effectiveness of these notions has been poorly evaluated, if at all. Medical history, including within the most recent decades, is rich with accounts of interventions used on a mass scale and for long periods that later have been discovered to be useless, if not harmful, while other procedures, tools, or medications are more effective. The Rand Corporation estimated in 1991 that as much as one-third of the financial resources devoted to health care are being spent on providing ineffective or unproductive care.[31] Many of the interventions take place in physicians' offices in which small numbers of people are treated, and hence it is often impossible statistically to assess the outcomes of the interventions.

Medical evaluators long have sought to collect information from numerous private practices and hospitals to determine which interventions are effective, in order to foster improvements in the quality of care. This often has proven rather difficult because of access and other problems. In the new electronic world, such outcome studies are becoming much easier, promising great advances in the quality of care.[32]

All this seems to suggest that ready access to medical records is essential for the advancement of major health care goals, and that privacy may have to yield if these important common goods are to be better served. However, to a large extent these health care goals can be achieved and privacy can be better protected at one and the same time.

▪ INFORMED CONSENT
OR INSTITUTIONALIZED REFORMS?

Oddly, both the prevailing suggestions for dealing with the tension between privacy and health care goals and a major source of the tension itself are based on the same legal-ethical doctrine, that of informed consent. While it is rarely explicitly stated as such, the prevailing doctrine implies that if a person is informed and then voluntarily consents to release information from his or her medical records, privacy is not violated and the tension between privacy and the common good has been resolved.

I am hardly the first one to observe that the agreements patients routinely endorse are neither voluntary nor informed. Very often, for an individual to receive health insurance or join a HMO plan, the person is required to sign a form that authorizes the provider of health care[33] to disclose any medical information that is requested for the payment of the individual's claims.[34]

As the OTA report notes, "usually no restriction is placed on the amount of information that may be released, the use to which these parties may put the information, or the length of time for which the consent form is valid."[35] Once an individual has signed a payment provider's blanket consent/authorization form, the floodgates have been opened. From this point on, the individual exercises no control over how much health information may be disclosed from his or her records to other parties—parties that do not come to mind when consent forms are endorsed—and loses control over what these parties do with that information once they receive it.[36] This may take the form of sharing an individual's medical records with different departments of a single organization (for example, the health and life insurance divisions of a single company) or between different organizations (for example, between the insurance company and an employer that provides the insurance). Moreover, once in the hands of external parties, the information may be redisclosed again (say, from an individual's current employer to a potential new one).[37] Given such blanket and open-ended consent forms, as the Institute of Medicine correctly points out, "consent cannot be truly voluntary or informed . . . because the patient cannot know in advance what information will be in the record, who will subsequently have access to it, or how it will be used" (p. 150).[38]

Furthermore, redisclosures to external parties "are [also] rationalized as being conducted by consent of the patient or a patient representative."[39] Because "many patients are neither granted access to their medical records, nor apprised of which portions of the record are accessible to others, most patients are ill equipped to make intelligent choices about authorizing disclosures."[40]

Theoretically, one can refuse to endorse a consent form, and, as the libertarians say, live with the consequence, which is to forgo health care insurance. However, as an OTA report confirms, "individuals for the most part are not in a position to forego such benefits, so that they really have no choice whether or not to consent to disclose their medical information" (p. 60). The Institute of Medicine similarly notes that in the final analysis, "consent [to disclosure of medical information] is so often not informed or is given under economic compulsion that it does not provide sufficient protection to patients."[41] As the OTA report put it, the idea of informed consent is "largely a myth and the mechanism of informed consent has no force."[42]

As a solution, civil libertarians have suggested a remedy, which is also based on the consent theory, that would require patients to grant a *specific consent* for each use of information about themselves. The National Academy of Science advocates the development of authorization forms that make it clear to patients the organizations to which their medical information will be released and that limit the time period for which the authorization is valid. The 1973 Code of Fair Information Practices and legislation based on it already require that when the federal government collects information of any kind in a database, specific consent must be given for every usage of information (not for every item of information, but for every purpose for which information is used). The privacy act proposed by the Clinton Administration in 1997 seeks to apply the same notion to collection of information by private agencies. American people strongly support this version of consent. Most

Americans (87 percent) believe patients should be asked for permission every time any information about them is used.[43]

The difficulties in relying on this approach are rather evident. When medical researchers are expected to gain consent for each specific use of medical records, they have found that a significant segment of the population does not return the needed forms. The researchers, such as those at the Mayo Clinic who have undertaken such an effort, then need to spend considerable resources contacting those who did not respond. Some remain hidden or refuse to participate, which distorts the database. The difficulties multiply when one needs to deal with old data (to find people who have moved, for example) and with data about deceased patients. Obtaining needed consent "would be impossible to accomplish in the retrospective studies that are so vital for assessing trends in disease over time and the long-term outcomes of treatment; such studies often involve thousands of subjects who may have last been seen many years ago."[44] In addition, studies conducted using only live patients (because the deceased cannot consent, or their living kin may not consent or may be unreachable) may produce distorted results, reflecting outcomes primarily among the younger and living population (pp. 1467–68).

Alarmed by the damages specific consent imposes upon health care goals, medical authorities have advanced a third notion of consent, that of *implied, presumed, or constructed* consent. According to this doctrine, anyone who comes to a physician's office or health care facility is treated as if he or she gave consent for the data generated to be used and released, without a need for explicit consent. Some versions of this concept at least sound rather nonthreatening to privacy and autonomy. For instance, Arnold J. Rosoff defines the concept of implied consent as "that which arises by reasonable inference from the conduct of the patient."[45] A physician at the health sciences research department of the Mayo Clinic suggests that "since the vast majority of patients agree to the broad use of their medical-records data for research . . . the overwhelming preponderance of agreement is consistent with the notion of 'constructed consent' from the whole patient population."[46]

While a widespread introduction of concepts such as presumed consent would serve various health care goals, they may not so much diminish or redefine privacy as abolish it. While some may not abuse the privilege these concepts grant, others may convince themselves all too readily that whatever they seek to do with the data is something the patients would have consented to. Still others would simply build on such concepts to conduct experiments and introduce interventions to which they know patients would be unlikely to consent if they were asked.

None of these forms of consent—old-fashioned, specific, and presumed— are likely to provide the desired balance between health care goals and privacy. Before I turn to what might be done, I should stress that I am *not* calling for an end to consent forms; they can serve as a limited, secondary source for protection of privacy. I merely argue that the mainstay of medical privacy is to be found elsewhere.

▨ *INSTITUTIONAL REFORMS*

The communitarian approach I favor here is based on the concept that people, far from being freestanding agents able to form and follow their own preferences at will, are profoundly affected by social institutions that prevail in the societies in which they are situated.[47] As Robert Bellah and his colleagues note,

> Institutions form individuals by making possible or impossible certain ways of behaving and relating to others. They shape character by assigning responsibility, demanding accountability, and providing the standards in terms of which each person recognizes the excellence of his or her achievements. Each individual's possibilities depend on the opportunities opened up within the institutional contexts to which that person has access.[48]

When these institutions affect people in ways that offend our values or raise considerable resentment or opposition, often the most effective way to treat such an ethical or sociopolitical problem is to modify or recast institutions rather than to rely solely or even chiefly upon the aggregation of millions of actions by newly informed individuals. To provide but one example of this general principle from a non-health-related area, if the savings rate of a nation must be raised, and this has been agreed upon following a proper societal dialogue and by the proper elective institutions, it is much more effective to reduce the public deficits (or to run a budgetary surplus) than to convince or create an incentive for millions of individuals to change their behavior to save more.[49]

Another of the grand advantages of drawing on institutional changes is that they tend to be preventive. American individualism favors a cop-and-robber approach to social issues, in which the culture prescribes waiting for individuals to transgress and then trying to catch them and penalize them. In contrast, institutional changes seek to encourage people to do what is right in the first place.

I provide next an elementary outline of institutional reforms that could produce more effective protection of the medical privacy without significantly setting back desired health care goals. This is a highly complex matter, one that is affected by numerous technical, economic, and political considerations that I cannot examine here. Moreover, all such suggestions should be subject to experimentation and further development before they can be adopted. I should note, though, that the suggested arrangements are based on at least some current practice.

Throughout the ensuing discussion, I refer to the *inner circle* as all those who are directly involved in the treatment of the patient. These people obviously require ready access to medical records, although some layering of access is called for even in this circle. (Already, this often is done regarding HIV tests, which are treated as more confidential than other information even in the inner circle.[50]) While these inner circle personnel are far from immune to financial considerations, they share a culture that respects confidentiality and is sensitive to privacy issues.

The *intermediate circle* includes health insurance and managed care corporations. They are much more driven by profit considerations and much less imbued with the medical culture of confidentiality. However, unless the current reimbursement system is changed radically, those in the intermediate circle need detailed and specific information about individual patients.

The *outer circle* includes parties not directly involved in health care, such as life insurers, employers, marketers, and the media, whose access to medical records may be legal but raises grave concerns because such access, as a rule, does not advance the health care goals either of the patients or of society.

Drawing on these distinctions among the three circles, the following remedies are suggested:

(1) *Layered Records and Graduated Release.* In the past, a typical paper record, or "chart," included medical history, records of treatment, and lab results. Similar records are kept in hospitals, where they are typically centrally filed. When a patient is moved from department to department, the whole chart typically accompanies the patient.

The implicit assumption reflected in this highly institutionalized arrangement is that this inner circle is an extension of the personal physician and is bound by the same legal, ethical, and socially enforced mores of confidentiality. Violations of privacy by the inner circle seem to be few and largely of the unauthorized kind. However, the setup, which has not changed for generations, does little to prevent curious members of the medical staff from rummaging through patient charts.

The introduction of electronic medical records into the inner circle makes it possible to enhance the privacy within this circle by layering the records. Various segments of the records could be assigned different passwords, with the understanding that certain segments would be open only to the treating physician(s) while others might be more accessible to people such as rehabilitation workers or dietitians.

(2) *Audit Trails.* Audit trails are computer technologies that record all efforts to access a record, including information identifying the person gaining access. For instance, to access information the user would have to log his or her unique password.[51] Some suggest that patients should be able to review these audit trails in addition to the privacy committees of the medical facilities involved. This would provide a built-in, privacy-protecting enforcement mechanism.

In general, passwords and audit trails constitute a fine example of how privacy can be protected, especially from unauthorized use, with minimal losses to the common good—and without waiting for each patient to act, consent, or even be involved personally.

(3) *Smart Cards.* Smart cards are credit-card-sized devices that can store health information and/or serve as the key to accessing personal health infor-

mation stored in a computer network. Thus if a patient visits a physician, clinic, or emergency room, the patient would hand the card to the treating personnel, who would display the information on their computer screens and encode in the card additional information—say, new test results. As the technologies improve, visuals such as X-rays, EKGs, and sonograms also could be included and encoded. If such a card remains in the possession of the person whose medical record is encoded in or accessed by the card, the card has the potential to greatly enhance privacy by affording patients effective control over who has access to their medical information.[52] Access by those other than the patient can be made only with the active collaboration of the individual to whom the information pertains. Further enhancing privacy, the card itself can be layered so that the patient can determine which segments to open to whom.

In emergency situations, of course, difficulties might arise if the patient is not carrying the card or is unable to provide the needed passwords for some of the segments. (One would expect patients not to password-protect elementary information.) This should not prove to be too detrimental, however; after all, patients today typically do not carry with them their charts when they are rolled into the ER. And a person may share key passwords with a next of kin or a friend, whose names and phone numbers would be noted on the card's open segment.

A serious consideration is the very likely need for a backup database, which would be accessible without the card and thus subject to many of the privacy considerations raised for linked online databases (p. 6). Such backup databases could be well sequestered, however. Another significant consideration is that smart cards may severely curtail researchers' and health care professionals' ability to serve the common goods of quality and cost control as well as medical research, because of limitations on access to the data. They are hence less desirable than audit trails.

(4) *Interface and Unique Patient Identifiers.* Probably the most encompassing measure would be the introduction of an interface that turns most of the information in medical records into "unidentifiable" information at the point it is transmitted beyond the inner circle. This would greatly enhance privacy but would not curtail most services to several albeit not all common goods at issue.

An "interface" refers to processes and individuals that transmit information contained in medical records to users other than members of the inner circle by conducting various coding procedures, in the process removing patients' names, addresses, phone and Social Security numbers, and a few other such items that could enable outsiders to identify the individuals. The information that is transmitted is coded instead by unique patient identifiers (UPIs).

Unidentifiable information may at first seem useless, but for many purposes this type of information is all that is needed. For instance, for many medical research purposes it is sufficient to know from a patient's record that the individual scored x on variable y, what the same person scored on a certain number of other variables, and so on. True, many of the personal attributes may need to be known, such as race, gender, age, but not the individual's identity—the name, address, and other details that identify a specific person.

In the rare cases in which information contained in the address of the patient or other highly personal details are critical to the research, those who provide the interface could "code" these details as well. Thus instead of including the person's address as, say, 240 Central Park West, New York City, the person could be coded as living in a highly affluent, urban neighborhood in the northeastern United States. Instead of providing birthdays, the month and year of birth would suffice. It should be noted, though, that if the interface leaves out names and personal numbers such as the Social Security number, it will be difficult, although far from impossible, to correlate these databases with data from non–healthcare databases

To the extent that such correlations are legitimately called for, special provisions would need to be made to allow interdatabase analyses by computers, releasing only the correlations and not individuals' identities. Special bonded interdatabank agents could be employed to carry out such correlations.

The information needs of quality control often are similar. A typical question is: If the patient's condition was x, y, and z, were proper procedures a, b, and c undertaken in the correct sequence, given the patient's age, gender, and so on? To address these questions, still no personal identification is needed. The same can be said about several cost control procedures. For a patient with condition x and other attributes including y and z, was a less costly or more costly procedure used? Most often, one would seek to establish a rate or identify a pattern of diagnoses, procedures, and referrals (how often does the particular physician or hospital err in the direction of expensive and unneeded procedures, for example), rather than try to second-guess every case.

A major concern might be that if a patient is treated at different medical facilities, data could not be collated if personal identifiers are removed. However, this issue largely can be resolved by giving each patient a unique identifying number that he or she would provide in all encounters with medical personnel. When the same patient is seen by different professionals or hospitals and the data are aggregated by researchers or quality assurance programs, it will be known that the information is about one and the same person—but not who he or she is.

One may suggest that it will be all too easy for those who command considerable financial and technical resources, and who have access to the data that contain only information without individual identifiers, to correlate the UPIs with data from other databases that contain individual identifiers and thus establish who the persons are whose medical privacy is being protected. This may well be true. Still, UPIs will limit many kinds of unauthorized use because they will prevent casual perusal of records.

Moreover, the introduction of an interface of the kind suggested establishes a new, clear line between legal and (what from then on will be) illegal uses of the data. Members of the intermediate and especially outer circles can no longer simply use (commit authorized abuse of) data that is legally generated by tapping into existing databases. If they persist, under the new arrangements they will have to engage in an activity whose one and only purpose will be to violate the confidentiality built into the data—in effect, to engage in codebreaking. Granted, even after such activities are defined as a violation of the law, abuse will not cease; completely airtight databases cannot be created. But the introduction of the interface will largely halt such illicit penetrations.

(5) *Capping as an Option.* UPIs will not work for those reimbursement programs that pay providers on the basis of procedures performed, time spent with the patient, and drugs or equipment handed out to the patient. The simple reason is that these programs work by linking the identity of the person who purchased the insurance policy, is enrolled in the particular HMO, or is entitled to Medicare or Medicaid, and the one for whom the said measures were taken. As a result, in the currently prevailing system, payment to providers is often conditioned on delivering highly detailed, specific, and individually identified medical information to members of the intermediate circle. Indeed, precisely because reimbursement differs according to the nature of the intervention, payers engage in the cumbersome and costly procedure of either seeking to approve before the fact the coverage specific patients have for specific interventions, or haggling with the provider over how much of the intervention will be reimbursed.

However, the particularly costly reimbursement arrangements of the American medical care system are not one of the common goods that have been identified. Indeed, they are a major reason the United States spends a much greater proportion of its health care dollars on administration than most other developed nations. Many would regard a simplification and streamlining of these arrangements to be a service to the common good. It should be noted, though, that within the existing medical care system there is a way to protect privacy much more effectively while still relying on the existing reimbursement system.

Unique Patient Identifiers can be employed in those reimbursement schemes that use "capitation," that is, that provide a fixed payment per member per month to a health provider or plan for each member, regardless of the amount or type of care that person receives. In capitated systems there is no need to report the specifics of care given to each individual.

Whatever its other advantages or disadvantages, in principle, capping is much more compatible with privacy than other prevailing payment systems for medical care. Hence a privacy-minded polity could enact a law requiring that whenever people are provided by an employer or government program (such as Medicare) with a menu of alternative forms of health care insurance, the capped option must be included. It then would be up to the patients, who could draw on advice from different sources (such as consumer unions, health care newsletters, or their labor union) to decide if they prefer a program that provides more privacy but is capped or one that is leakier but not capped. One might suggest that here we are falling back on the individualistic model of choice. In effect, though, what is proposed is a change in the institutionalized options the public is offered, which will significantly restructure the choices available to it.

For those reimbursement schemes that are uncapped, one can imagine an approach that would minimize the potential for authorized abuse, but one must acknowledge that it flies in the face of the currently dominant approach of setting up leaky systems and then trying to ferret out abuses after the fact. In the envisioned system, whenever a group is insured and all its members pay the same premium for the same kind of insurance (or are given the same benefit by their employers), the reimbursable services provided to them would not be traced to a person but to a UPI. The insurance company would still be able to check whether service was excessive or inappropriate, given the attributes of the case on file. True, insurance companies would not be able to draw on data from other sources about the same person (unless coded by the UPI) to get information given to the companies by the treating professionals, who often take the side of the patient. This might be handled by indicating conditions under which the veil of UPIs might be partially lifted, or better yet, by mandating that a third, neutral body investigate such matters. In any case, insurance companies' cost controls would be set back only to a limited extent, if at all, under such a system. However, insurers would no longer be able to sell these data to members of the outer circle, who would find it useless without personal identifiers.

All this is not to suggest that changes in the laws governing medical privacy should not be considered. Some such changes are needed to back up the suggested institutional reforms. And new legal limitations might be set on commercial trafficking in personal medical information. However, reliance on law is best activated when social arrangements do not suffice, and the needed legislation faces great political difficulties. This further points to the merits of building primarily on technological changes and institutional reforms.[53]

References

1. Booth Gunter, "It's No Secret: What You Tell Your Doctor—and What Medical Documents Reveal About You—May Be Open to the Scrutiny of Insurers, Employers, Lenders, Credit Bureaus, and Others," *Tampa Tribune*, 6 October 1996.
2. Donna E. Shalala, U.S. Secretary of Health and Human Services, speech delivered at National Press Club, Washington, D.C., 31 July 1997.
3. Matthew Brelis, "Patients' Files Allegedly Used for Obscene Calls," *Boston Globe*, 11 April 1995.

4. Bill Siwicki, "Health Data Security: A New Priority," *Health Data Management,* September 1997; Doug Stanley and Craig S. Palosky, "HIV Tracked on Unauthorized Lists," *Tampa Tribune,* 35 October 1996.

5. Institute of Medicine, *Health Data in the Information Age: Use, Disclosure, and Privacy* (Washington, D.C.: National Academy Press, 1994), p. 140.

6. A.G. Breitenstein, J.D., Director, JRI Health law Institute, Statement to the Senate Committee on Labor and Human Resources, 28 October 1997; Patrick J. Leahy, Testimony before the Senate Labor and Human Resources Committee on Confidential Medical Information.

7. National Academy of Sciences, *For the Record: Protecting Electronic Health Information* (Washington, D.C.: National Academy Press, 1997), pp. 22–23.

8. Carol Hymowitz, "Psychotherapy Patients Pay a Price for Privacy," *Wall Street Journal,* 22 January 1998; John Riley, "When You Can't Keep a Secret/Insurers' Cost-Cutters Demand Your Medical Details," *Newsday,* 1 April 1996.

9. National Academy of Sciences, *For the Record.*

10. Office of Technology Assessment, *Protecting Privacy in Computerized Medical Records* (Washington, D.C.: U.S. Government Printing Office, 1993), p. 6.

11. John Riley, "Know and Tell: Sharing Medical Data Becomes Prescription for Profit," *Newsday,* 2 April 1996.

12. International Research Bureau, Inc., http://www.irb-online.com/services.html; Nina Bernstein, "On Line, High-Tech Sleuths Find Private Facts," *New York Times,* 15 September 1997.

13. Institute of Medicine, *Health Data,* p. 3.

14. Workgroup for Electronic Data Interchange, "Appendix 4: Confidentiality and Antitrust Issues," in *Report to Secretary of U.S. Department of Health and Human Services* (Washington, D.C.: U.S. Government Printing Office, 1992), p. 19.

15. David F. Linowes, "A Research Survey of Privacy in the Workplace," unpublished white paper available from University of Illinois at Urbana-Champaign. Available at: http://www.taff.uiuc.edu/~dlinowes/survey.htm.

16. Office of Technology Assessment, *Medical Monitoring and Screening in the Workplace: Results of a Survey* (Washington, D.C.: U.S. Government Printing Office, 1991).

17. "New Medical Privacy Law to be Proposed," *Medical Industry Today,* 12 August 1997. Also cited in Robert Pear, "Clinton to Back a Law on Patient Privacy," *New York Times,* 10 August 1997.

18. Gina Kolata, "When Patients' Records Are Commodities for Sale," *New York Times,* 15 November 1995; National Academy of Sciences, *For the Record,* p. 32.

19. See, for example, L. N. Geller, J. S. Alper, P. R. Billings et al., "Individual, Family, and Societal Dimensions of Genetic Discrimination: A Case Study Analysis," *Science and Engineering Ethics* 2 (1996): 71–88, cited in National Academy of Sciences, *For the Record,* p. 77; Samuel Greengard, "Genetic Testing; Should You Be Afraid?" *Workforce* (July 1997); Suzanne E. Stipe, "Genetic Testing Battle Pits Insurers Against Consumers," *Best's Review-Life/Health Insurance Edition* (August 1996); Olympia Snowe Testimony before the Senate Labor and Human Resources Committee, 21 May 1998.

20. National Academy of Sciences, *For the Record,* p. 77; "Who's Reading Your Medical Records?" *Consumer Reports* (October 1994): 628–32. Reprinted in Robert Emmet Long, *Rights to Privacy* (New York: H.W. Wilson Company, 1997), pp. 71–80.

21. "Who's Reading Your Medical Records?" p. 631.

22. National Committee on Vital and Health Statistics, "Health Privacy and Confidentiality Recommendations," 25 June 1997. Available at: http://aspe.os.hhs.gov/nchvs/privrecs.htm.

23. "Health Care Information Privacy," Louis Harris and Associates poll conducted for Equifax (1993).

24. "Who's Reading Your Medical Records?"

25. Brian J. Taylor, "The Screening of America: Crime, Cops, and Cameras," *Reason* (May 1997): 44–46, at 44.

26. Solveig Singleton, "Privacy as Censorship: A Skeptical View of Proposals to Regulate Privacy in the Private Sector," *Cato Policy Analysis No. 295* (Washington, D.C.: Cato Institute, 1998), p. 1.

27. Robert Pear, "Plan Would Broaden Access of Police to Medical Records," *New York Times*, 10 September 1997.

28. Both recommendations are outlined in "Confidentiality of Individually-Identifiable Health Information," Recommendations of the Secretary of Health and Human Services to the Committee on Labor and Human Resources and the Committee on Finance of the Senate and the Committee on Commerce and the Committee on Ways and Means of the House of Representatives, 11 September 1997. Available http://aspe.os.dhhs.gov/admnsimp/pvcrecO.htm.

29. L. Joseph Melton III, "The Threat to Medical-Records Research," *NEJM* 337 (1997): 1468.

30. Robert H. Brook and Kathleen N. Lohr, "Will We Need to Ration Effective Health Care?" *Issues in Science and Technology* 3 (1986): 68–77; Barry Meier, "Rx for a System in Crisis," *New York Times*, 6 October 1991; Stephen C. Schoenbaum, "Toward Fewer Procedures and Better Outcomes," *JAMA* 269 (1993): 794–96. Schoenbaum states: "It should be disturbing to us as a profession that we have so few outcomes data and use so few in our practices. Most of us do not learn enough in our training to collect or analyze our own data or to interpret consistently the work of others."

31. Brook and Lohr, "Will We Need to Ration Effective Health Care?" Reprinted as RAND Report N-3375-HHS.

32. See, for example, Richard S. Dick and Elaine B. Steen, eds., *The Computer-Based Patient Record: Essential Technology for Health Care* (Washington, D.C.: National Academy Press, 1991): 13–19, 24; S.L. Yenney, "Solving the Health Data Management Puzzle," *Business Health* (September 1990): 41–49, cited in Lawrence O. Gostin et al., "Privacy and Security of Personal Information in a New Health Care System," *JAMA* 270 (1993): 2488, 2493.

33. Office of Technology Assessment, *Protecting Privacy*, p. 59.

34. Workgroup for Electronic Data Interchange, "Appendix 4," p. 1.

35. Office of Technology Assessment, *Protecting Privacy*, p. 59.

36. Janlori Goldman and Deirdre Mulligan, *Privacy and Health Information Systems: A Guide to Protecting Patient Confidentiality* (Washington, D.C.: Center for Democracy and Technology, 1996), pp. 5–6.

37. Institute of Medicine, *Health Data*, p. 158.

38. See also Glenn McGee, "Subject to Payments? Cash and Informed Consent," *Penn Bioethics* 3 (1997): 3, 5.

39. Institute of Medicine, *Health Data*, p. 150. Emphasis added.

40. Office of Technology Assessment, *Protecting Privacy*, p. 56.

41. Institute of Medicine, *Health Data*, p. 150.

42. Office of Technology Assessment, *Protecting Privacy*, p. 60.

43. Christine Gorman, "Who's Looking at Your Files?" *Time* (6 May 1996): 60–62. Reprinted in Robert Emmet Long, ed., *Rights to Privacy* (New York: H.W. Wilson Company, 1997), pp. 81–84, at 82–83.

44. Melton, "The Threat to Medical-Records Research," p. 1467.

45. Arnold J. Rosoff, *Informed Consent: A Guide for Health Care Providers* (Rockville, Md.: Aspen Systems Corporation, 1991), p. 5.

46. Melton, "The Threat to Medical-Records Research," p. 1467.

47. Robert Bellah, Richard Madsen, William M. Sullivan et al., *The Good Society* (New York: Alfred A. Knopf, 1991); Michael J. Sandel, *Liberalism and the Limits of Justice* (Cambridge: Cambridge University Press, 1982); Amitai Etzioni, *The New Golden Rule: Community and Morality in a Democratic Society* (New York: Basic Books, 1996).

48. Bellah et al., *The Good Society*, p. 40.

49. On the features of the requisite societal dialogue, see Etzioni, *The New Golden Rule*, pp. 93ff.

50. Yank D. Coble, Jr., M.D. for the American Medical Association, statement to the House Committee on Commerce Task Force on Health Records and Genetic Privacy, Subject: Privacy, Confidentiality and Discrimination in Genetics. Dr. Coble states: "(P)hysicians and other entities regularly deal with categories of extra-sensitive information which have been afforded specific legislative projections above and beyond that applicable to more generalized records (e.g., HIV/AIDS information . . .)."

51. National Academy of Sciences, *For the Record*, pp. 8, 93–97.

52. Office of Technology Assessment, *Protecting Privacy*, pp. 48–49.

53. For documentation see Amitai Etzioni, *The Limits of Privacy* (New York: Basic Books, 1999), forthcoming.

Discussion Questions

1. In 1900, Lavinia Dock spoke of the need for a recognized standard of professional education. Does nursing today have one professional standard for nursing education? If not, what are some of the problems preventing standardization?

2. What are the major arguments for and against a patient's bill of rights? Which side do you support? Elaborate.

3. In Article 20, "The Wrong Rights," Bloom lists six additional rights he feels should be included in a patient's bill of rights. If you were given the opportunity to include two of the six, which two would they be? Explain your reasoning.

4. Prioritize Bloom's six rights in order of their importance (in your view) to your community's health care needs.

5. How do you personally define confidentiality? To what extent does your definition correspond to what you have been taught about confidentiality?

6. What would you say is the most difficult aspect of maintaining patient confidentiality?

7. What personal information would you want kept confidential if you were a patient? or a consumer? as a nursing student?

8. What breaches in computer security have you observed in your practice setting?

9. If you were given the authority, what would you do to protect patient privacy?

10. Kloss (Article 21) lists five principles of proposed standards to protect patient information. One of them is accountability. What suggestions other than legal recourse would you employ to insure accountability in your health care setting?

11. What course of action would you take if a patient revealed something of a confidential nature to you that was illegal or violated the safety of others? Discuss the legal implications for your decision.

12. In Etzioni's article (Article 23), several institutional reforms are suggested to protect patients' medical records. Which of the suggested reforms would have the most direct and feasible effect on you and your patients?

13. Etzioni asserts that the common good can be best served by communtarian institutions rather than on individualistic doctrines. How feasible do you think this assertion is? Explain your rationale.

Further Readings

Badzek, L., & Gross, L. (1999). Confidentiality & privacy: At the forefront for nurses. *American Journal of Nursing, 99*(6), 52–54.

Curtin, L. & Simpson, R. (1999). Privacy in the information age? *Health Management Technology*, August 1999, 32–33.

Garfinkel, S. (2000). Privacy and the new technology: What they do know can hurt you. *The Nation, 270*(8), 11–15.

Serafini, M.W. (1999). Open secrets. *The National Journal, 31*(41), 2878–2881.

Ventura, M.J. (1999). When information must be revealed. *RN, 62*(2) 61–64.

Wakefield, M.K. (1999). Legislating patient privacy, *Nursing Economics, 17*(4) 222–226.

Web Site Resources for Legal Responsibilities

American Civil Liberties Union   www.aclu.org/privacy
Find Law   www.findlaw.com
Identity Theft   www.consumer.gov/idtheft
Lectric Law Library   www.lectlaw.com
Nolo Press Self-Help Law Center   www.nolo.com
The Nurse Advocate   www.nurseadvocate.org
Privacy Net   www.privacy.net
Privacy Ratings   www.privacyratings.org
U.S. Department of Justice   www.usdoj.gov

General Search Engine Web Sites

Ask Jeeves   www.askjeeves.com
GoTo   www.goto.com
Net Center   www.netcenter.com

Health Web Sites

Go Ask Alice   http://www.alice.columbia.edu
Health Central   www.healthcentral.com
Mayo Clinic   www.mayohealth.org

Professional Journal Web Sites

MedWebPlus   www.medwebplus.com

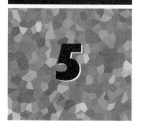

Ethics: The Moral Boundaries of Practice

Ours is a world of choices. We make them every day. From buying a new car, taking a holiday, or choosing a flavor of ice cream, making choices is generally no big deal. We know how to make choices because we know what the "rules" are, how far we can stretch them, and what will happen when we stretch them too much.

Then, along came Dolly. And when the novelty of cloning sheep wore off, somehow choices that seemed easy before don't seem as easy anymore. The rules are changing, the boundaries are fuzzy, and the consequences less clear and more ominous. Other hard choices followed, and the debate between science and ethics has begun in earnest. Scientists point to their progress in ridding us of disease and insist that by mapping our genetic profiles they can not only predict what will happen to us in the future, but they can take steps to eliminate its negative impact on us. Ethicists are alarmed at the suggestion that in tinkering with human genes, science alone may determine our genetic destiny. They insist that guidelines must be in place before anyone gets on the genetic roller coaster and that others, including scientists, contribute to this process. They argue that while science has the tools for this endeavor, it lacks the predictability and sense of direction that using these tools require. Without boundaries within which to guide the direction of these scientific efforts, the moral consequences could be hazardous to our health.

The same concerns are present in the issue of who gets health care. The major premise of public policy is that it serves the common good of all citizens. How ethical is it then that extraordinary amounts of money are spent on the health care of the few rather than the many? Does the health care of one individual supersede those for whom society is obligated to care? The "no expense is too great" notion of caring for individual patients misses the point. The expense *is* too great when society fails in its obligations to all its citizens. What then are the boundaries and limits of health care in our society? Who determines which people get health care? Is it unethical not to consider cost? The ethical dilemmas of these two issues are complex and perhaps extend beyond the ethical principles upon which we make choices about the human condition. But we will have to make those choices sooner than we think and sooner than we like.

The historical context for this chapter begins with an account of the evolution of nursing ethics. The remaining readings selected for this chapter focus on the problems and ethical dilemmas posed by genetic engineering and health care rationing. They offer no concrete solutions—only concerns and questions about the morality of the messages being communicated about the value of human life. Some of the viewpoints expressed in the readings selected for this chapter see only positive outcomes, while others differ strenuously. Both viewpoints, however, require that we become engaged in a dialogue about choices. The choices are not easy. In this case, they are not meant to be.

24 Manners, Morals, and Nurses: An Historical Overview of Nursing Ethics

Eleanor Crowder

Seventeen years prior to the opening of the Nightingale School of Nursing in 1860, at St. Thomas Hospital, in London, Charles Dickens introduced the character of a "sick nurse" in his serialized story, *The Adventures of Martin Chuzzlewit* (1). She appeared in the person of Sairey Gamp. Dickens claimed that she was not an inaccurate image of what "sick nurses" were at the time (5: 3–4). Supposedly, Sairey Gamp personified the nurse of the day who hired out to work in private homes. The addition of Betsy Prig, who typified "hospital nurses" of the day, compounded the wretched image of nurses and nursing. Dickens made the statement: "I mean to make my mark with her (5: X1)." That he did—to the detriment of future nurses. Thus, those who chose to try to raise nursing from the depths of degradation, as characterized by Sairey and her friend Betsy, had to overcome the image of port-sipping, morbid, unkempt, scheming women—a difficult task to say the least!

The women of the mid-19th century who dared to dream of pulling nursing out of the dark ages were working against almost insurmountable odds. To get the public to view nurses as possessing some degree of respectability was no small chore, and to elevate nursing to the status of a profession was another matter. Women who nursed for a livelihood were not held in high esteem. Their dubious reputation was characterized and reinforced in the minds of the general public by the fictional Sairey Gamp.

When Florence Nightingale founded the first formal school of nursing, one of her greatest problems was combating the existing image of the nurse. She deliberately set out to attract women of the highest caliber and good breeding to be students in her school. She then cloistered them in a nurses residence to be certain that no ill would come to their gentle status while they were entrusted to her school. A Mrs. Wardroper was hired to supervise the students in the school, and a sister was in charge of the nurses' home. Miss Nightingale supervised the school, home, and students with a critical eye (15, pp. 236–239).

Eleanor Crowder was an instructor, University of Texas School of Nursing at Austin, Texas.

Reprinted from *Texas Reports on Biology and Medicine, 32*(1), Spring, 1974, pp. 173–180, with permission by University of Texas, Austin.

Many of the "ethical" issues of early nursing came from the deliberate effort to overcome the image left by Sairey Gamp, and the fact that bedside nursing, for a fee, had been a task relegated to those of the servant class, or lower.

It is difficult to ascertain to what extent ethical considerations were pursued in the earliest days of modern nursing education. Johns and Pfefferkorn mention that the students of the Johns Hopkins Hospital School of Nursing were taught ethical issues soon after the opening of the school in 1889. Unfortunately, the authors do not say what issues were taught, or to what extent (8, pp. 76–78).

Isabel Hampton Robb published a book entitled *Nursing Ethics* in 1900. In it she defined ethics as:

> ". . . the science that treats of human actions from a standpoint of right and wrong. It teaches men the practice of duties of human life and the reasons for what they do and for what they should leave undone (13, p. 13)."

Mrs. Robb appears to have discussed anything and everything touching on manners and morals deemed necessary for a woman to possess or acquire in order to become a successful nurse. She lists the necessary qualifications of a nurse as health, education and culture (13, pp. 47–49). Some of the topics discussed are underwear, posture, table manners, strength, and what kind of wardrobe a nurse should possess. At the end of the book, Mrs. Robb laments:

> ". . . outside the hospital the trained nurse is still regarded as a not altogether unmixed blessing, and the public will need several more years of education in which perhaps proper legislation, defining more precisely the standard requirements for members of the profession, will be of no little assistance—before they can be brought to thoroughly appreciate her position or the relative value of the services of the trained nurse and those of the untrained attendant or the well-meaning, enthusiastic, but untaught amateur. Nor would it be reasonable for us to look upon legal registration or other legislative enactments as a panacea for the present unsatisfactory conditions of affairs, for always, as now, it will largely rest with ourselves what status we and our work are to hold in the eyes of the public at large. The trained nurse then should teach those with whom she is brought into contact to expect of her the same high order of services, though of a different nature, as is demanded of the physician, and her instruction must take the form not of words but of thorough work and the most exemplary personal conduct (13: 262)."

Mrs. Robb was one of the outstanding nurses of the time and a strong motivating force in all phases of nursing and nursing education. She had been instrumental in forming two national nurses associations and in initiating the publication of an official journal for nurses in the United States. It was no wonder that the appearance of her book on ethics was heralded by many nurses as a great step toward professionalism in nursing. Although it had been 27 years since the founding of the first training school for nurses in the United States, textbooks for nurses were still relatively scarce. Robb herself considered the book to be suitable as a textbook in ethics or as a hand-book for graduate nurses.

With the initiation of the *American Journal of Nursing* in October, 1900, American nurses had a sounding board in which to explore matters of in-terest and concern. In this journal we have readily available evidence of the considerable concern about the ethics of a fledging profession. Ethical considerations, as we perceive them today, were nonexistent. Rather, the ethi-cal code was one which this writer chooses to call a "manners and morals" code.

The themes of articles written early in the century on ethics have many of the same ideas. The desirable qualities of the nurse were stated as dogma, with very little rebuttal by anyone. The most prevailing desirable trait was that of *unquestioning obedience.* In speaking of obedience, one nurse said: "It is expected of all in training to do what they are told; no more, no less (12, p. 452)." On this same subject Robb said:

> "Implicit, unquestioning obedience is one of the first lessons a probationer must learn, for this is a quality that will be expected from her in her profes-sional capacity for all future use (13, p. 57)."

As late as 1917 Sarah Dock was echoing the cry. In an article published in the *American Journal of Nursing,* she stated:

> "In my estimation obedience is the first law and the very cornerstone of good nursing. And here is the first stumbling block for the beginner. No matter how gifted she may be, she will never become a reliable nurse until she can obey without question. The first and most helpful criticism I ever received from a doctor was when he told me that I was supposed to be simply an intel-ligent machine for the purpose of carrying out his orders (6, p. 394)."

Perhaps the point of unquestioning obedience was not so unusual a de-mand. The whole culture, at that time, was permeated with relatively strict lines of authority. The adage, "Children should be seen and not heard," was an oft-quoted one.

Helen Scott Hay was the first nurse to break out of the pattern of "man-ners and morals" ethics. In 1910 at the 13th Annual Convention of the Nurses Associated Alumnae of the United States, she gave an address entitled "Con-cerning our Ethics." In that speech she said:

> ". . . ethics is not a question of law but of living; of practice not of precept; . . . the value of any ethical system is dependent not on moral rules but on moral qualities (7: 896)."

Not once did she speak of the necessity for tidiness of one's uniform, unques-tioning obedience, or manners, but rather of the more intangible qualities that nurses should possess. Mrs. Hay divided ethics into lessons. The first she called the "Lesson of Correct Discrimination," where she implores the nurse to have a ". . . correct evaluation of things for the good of humanity." The examples she uses is that the comfort of a patient should not be jeopardized for the sake of straightening out a ward. The second lesson she called the "Lesson of Magnanimity" and the third the "Lesson of Unremitting Helpfulness." Mrs. Hays challenged nurses ". . . to hunt up ways of being serviceable." Her admonishments were a far cry from the unquestioning obedience theme so prominent at the time. Women who felt as Hays did were definitely in the minority, and manners and morals continued to be taught under the guise of ethics for many years to come (7, pp. 897–902).

Although what the nurses of the early 20th century called ethics was completely different from our present code, Mary Adelaide Nutting gave an extremely logical reason for its evolution:

> "We can train women as nurses but we can not change the character. We may not be able to discover the faults in character early; they may come out afterwards to our great regret and grief, and we should be very careful about signing our names to diplomas, even after pupils have reached the degree required by the school and have come to the last months of their career there. We do not stand in the position of colleges and universities. They do not vouch for character but only for a certain degree of training or schooling. We stand in a different and peculiar position. We assume a moral responsibility for the character of the nurses we send out (10, pp. 89–90)."

Paralleling ethical concern was the question of whether nursing was a profession. One argument to the contrary was the simple fact that it did not have a formal code of ethics. In 1902, Dr. S. Weir Mitchell published an article in the *American Journal of Nursing* concerned primarily with reforms in the education of nurses, yet he also mentioned the ethical question. His point of contention was that when physicians cared for other physicians no fee was involved but this was not the case when nurses cared for other nurses (11, pp. 899–907). Though the article was well-intended, one nurse took exception to its ethical aspect and offered a rebuttal in the *Journal* several months later, True, nursing did not have a formal code of ethics, but she felt that:

> "When our code (of ethics) is finally evolved there can be little doubt of our ability to maintain it, when for so long we have lived up to our watchword 'faithful to the doctor' (14, pp. 41–42)."

Relative to Dr. Mitchell's point regarding charging fellow professionals, she then stated: "Doctors give at most a few hours of their time where nurses give days or weeks (14, pp. 41–42)."

The adoption of an ethical code for nurses was bandied about for years without any tangible results. Robb's book was still a standby for teaching ethics to student nurses. Other books were published on the subject but were not really different in their approach. In 1926, an Ethical Code was presented to the membership of the American Nurses Association for consideration and discussion; it was to be ruled on at the next biennial convention in 1928 (3, pp. 599–601). Nothing came of it.

In 1932, Paul Limbert, Ph.D., admonished the nursing profession for not adopting a code of ethics. He claimed that ". . . nurses confuse professional ethics with personal morality," which indeed had been the case. He further stated:

> "The purpose of such a code is not to provide rules of conduct covering specific types of situations arising in the practice of a profession, but rather to create a sensitiveness to ethical situations and to formulate general principles which, rooted in conviction and supported with enthusiasm, create the individual habit of forming conscious and critical judgments resulting in action in specific situations (9, pp. 1257–1263)."

Increasing interest concerning an ethical code stimulated the Committee on Ethical Standards of the American Nurses Association to issue "A Tentative Code for the Nursing Profession" in 1940. This lengthy document deals with the nurse's responsibilities to the profession, her relationship to the patient, to other nurses, to her employer, to the public and to others, as well as her responsibilities to herself. The code is comprehensive and extremely cumbersome; it attempted to give explicit instructions for specific situations rather than a broad framework that could be applied to a variety of situations (4, pp. 977–980). The Committee on Ethical Standards solicited reaction to the code before it was to be put into final form. That final form never materialized.

Undoubtedly the problems brought about by the entry of the United States into World War II contributed to the continued absence of a code of ethics. Perhaps the pragmatism necessary to cope with immediate and pressing problems did not allow time for the necessary introspection. One can only speculate.

The House of Delegates of the American Nurses Association did at last adopt a code of ethics at their convention in San Francisco in 1950, the first ever adopted by a national nursing organization. Even then, 77 years after the opening of the first school of nursing in the United States, the code still reflected some adherence to the manners and morals ethics of yesteryear. One should not be too critical of that code, though, for it came many years prior to the social upheavals of the 1960's and the "new morality." Of the 17 basic tenets, only three fall into a morality framework. They are:

> "12. The Golden Rule should guide the nurse in relationships with members of other professions and with nursing associates.
> "13. The nurses in private life adhere to standards of personal ethics which reflect credit upon the profession.
> "14. The personal conduct nurses should not knowingly disregard the pattern of behavior of the community in which they live and work (2: 1247)."

Adoption of that Code of Ethics was a major step for the profession, and put on record what the members of the profession, at least those in the American Nurses Association, could agree to adhere to.

The social upheaval, including controversial social legislation of the 1960's coupled with monumental improvements in the capabilities and delivery of health care, forced nurses to re-evaluate what nurses and nursing stood for. At least the unquestioning obedience thesis of former years was a thing of the past. Perhaps for the first time nurses looked at situations and asked "Why?" "Why should I be forced to help with abortions when I'm violently opposed to them?" "Why should so much energy be expended to care for a client who could not possibly live if the life-sustaining machines were turned off?" "Why is one person chosen over another to be allowed to use expensive but lifesaving renal dialysis machines?" "What are the ethical considerations of transplants of any kind?"

Nurses now feel free to express their philosophies on the vital issues with which they are concerned. The American Nurses Association's Code of Ethics, which was revised in 1968, gives nurses an ethical framework within which to practice their profession. It is a sophisticated, but concise, document nearly free of manners and morals ethics. At least one nurse who violated the code has been censured (16, p. 2).

It has been 100 years since the founding of the first school of nursing in the United States. Hopefully, the end of professional growth will never be seen. Undoubtedly, the present Code of Ethics will have to be changed, but now nurses can say—to paraphrase the professor in *My Fair Lady*—"By jove—we've made it."

References

1. Charles, Edwin: *Some Dickens Women.* London, 1926.
2. Committee on Ethical Standards of the American Nurses Association: A code for professional nurses. *Am. J. Nurs.* 52, #10, 1952.
3. ———: A suggested code. *Am. J. Nurs.* 26, #8, 1926.
4. ———: A tentative code. *Am J. Nurs.* 40, #9, 1940.
5. Dickens, Charles: *Mrs. Gamp.* New York, 1956.
6. Dock, Sarah: The relation of the nurse to the doctor and the doctor to the nurse. *Am. J. Nurs.* 17, #5, 1917.
7. Hay, Helen Scott: Concerning our ethics. *Am. J. Nurs.* 10, #6, 1910.
8. Johns, Ethel and Blanche Pfefferkorn: *The Johns Hopkins Hospital School of Nursing, 1889–1949.* Baltimore, 1954.
9. Limbert, Paul: Developing a code of ethics for the nursing profession. *Am. J. Nurs.* 32, #12, 1932.
10. Marshall, Helen E.: *Mary Adelaide Nutting.* Baltimore, 1972.
11. Mitchell, S. Weir: Nurses and their education. *Am. J. Nurs.* 11, #11, 1932.
12. Perry, Charlotte M.: Nursing ethics and etiquette. *Am. J. Nurs.* 6, #7, 1906.
13. Robb, Isabel Hampton: *Nursing Ethics.* Cleveland, 1915.
14. Ross, Annie: A few points of ethics. *Am. J. Nurs.* 3, #1, 1902.
15. Woodham-Smith, Cecil: *Florence Nightingale.* New York, 1951.
16. Unknown: A.N.A. cites R.N. for violation of nurses code. *Tex. Nurs.* 47, #8, 1973.

25

Genetic Engineering: Is It Morally Acceptable?

Bernard Gert

Genetic engineering involves directly altering the genetic structure of an organism to provide it with traits deemed useful or desirable by those doing the altering. Genetic engineering of plants and animals has been going on since the 1970s, though attempts to introduce such traits through selective breeding has been going on for centuries.

The most straightforward use of genetic engineering involves producing a plant or animal with "improved" characteristics. In the case of agriculture, for example, genetic engineering has produced crop plants resistant to lower temperatures, herbicides, and insect attack, as well as tomatoes with a longer shelf life. A completely different type of genetic engineering involves transplanting a gene, usually human, from one species to another in order to produce a useful product. A patent already has been applied for to mix human embryo cells with those from a monkey or ape to create an animal that might have kidneys or a liver more suitable for transplantation to human beings. There seem to be no limits to the creatures made possible by genetic engineering—*e.g.*, creating edible birds and mammals with minimal brain functions, including no consciousness, so as to avoid protests about the cruelty involved in raising and killing conscious animals for food.

Although particular instances of genetic engineering of plants and animals have caused some controversy, mostly because of environmental or health concerns, genetic engineering is a generally accepted practice. The major moral controversy concerns whether to allow directly altering the genetic structure of human beings. Genetic engineering done by altering the somatic cells of an individual in order to cure genetic and non-genetic diseases has not been controversial. Indeed, what is known as somatic cell gene therapy is becoming a standard method for treating both kinds of diseases. Unlike the genetic engineering used in plants and animals, somatic cell gene therapy alters only the genetic structure of the individual who receives it; the altered

Dr. Gert is the Eunice and Julian Cohen Professor for the Study of Ethics and Human Values, Dartmouth College, Hanover, N.H.

Reprinted from *USA Today* magazine, January © 1999 by the Society for the Advancement of Education Inc., pp. 28–30.

genetic structure is not passed on to that individual's offspring. However, now that large mammals such as cows and sheep can be cloned, it may be possible that genetic engineering done by altering somatic cells in human beings may be passed on to future generations of human beings.

Presently, somatic cell genetic engineering is limited to therapy—there has not even been a proposal to use it for enhancement. Clinical trials using human patients have demonstrated the feasibility of somatic cell gene therapy in humans, successfully correcting genetic defects in a large number of cell types. In principle, there is no important moral distinction between injecting insulin into a diabetic's leg and injecting the insulin gene into a diabetic's cells.

The most serious moral controversy concerns the application to human beings of the kind of genetic engineering used on plants and animals. This type of human genetic engineering, usually referred to as germ line gene therapy, is regarded by some as the best means to correct severe hereditary defects such as thalassemia, severe combined immune deficiency, or cystic fibrosis. Many believe, though, that genetic engineering to treat or eliminate serious genetic disorders—the practice of negative eugenics—will lead to the process being directed toward enhancing or improving humans, or positive eugenics. This slippery slope argument presupposes that there is something morally unacceptable about positive eugenics, but that has not been shown. No one yet has provided a strong theoretical argument demonstrating that genetic engineering to produce enhanced size, strength, intelligence, or increased resistance to toxic substances is morally problematic.

Eugenics properly has a bad connotation because, prior to the possibility of genetic engineering, eugenics only could be practiced by preventing those who were regarded as having undesirable traits from reproducing. Genetic engineering allows for positive eugenics without limiting the freedom of anyone. The moral force of the objection that genetic engineering, especially positive eugenics or genetic enhancement, is "playing God" is that we do not know that there are no risks. A proper humility and recognition of limited human knowledge and fallibility is required for reliable moral behavior. A strong argument for concluding that genetic enhancement and perhaps even genetic therapy is morally unacceptable is that it risks great harm for many in future generations in order to provide benefits for a few in this one.

■ ARGUMENTS AGAINST EUGENICS

Two standard arguments have been put forward that even negative eugenics should not be practiced. The first is that it will result in the elimination of those deleterious alleles (alternate forms of a gene) which may be of some future benefit to the species. The argument is that the genetic variation of a species affords evolutionary plasticity or potential for subsequent adaptation to new and perhaps unforeseen conditions. To eliminate a deleterious mutant allele, like those responsible for cystic fibrosis or sickle cell anemia, could have some risk. It generally is agreed that the recessive gene responsible for sickle cell anemia evolved as an adaptive response to malaria.

This argument is false for two different reasons. The first concerns the nature of genetic maladies. For those based on the inheritance of recessive alleles, it is not the presence of two mutant alleles that causes the malady, but the absence of a normal allele. As long as a normal allele is present, the mutant ones do not cause a genetic disorder. In the case of sickle cell anemia, gene therapy for recessive disorders will work, even though the mutant and non-functional alleles remain. When it is possible not merely to add a gene, but to replace a non-functional mutant allele, the latter no longer will remain. No evolutionary problem is caused by eliminating dominant genes that cause serious genetic disorders such as Huntington's disease.

Almost all genetic disorders are caused by recessive genes, and it seems quite unlikely that there will be any serious attempt to eradicate these genes from the human gene pool, even if it becomes possible and desirable. The technology required must be applied on an individual basis with rather limited accessibility. Because it is a surgical procedure, germ line gene therapy would be done in a medical setting and on a voluntary basis. Although many couples might qualify for gene therapy, just a small number likely would elect to participate. For example, if germ line gene therapy involving gene replacement could be developed for Tay Sachs and was used to treat all embryos showing the disease, the frequency of the Tay Sachs allele in the entire population merely would decrease from 0.0100 to 0.0099 over a generation.

The second argument is an iatrogenic (produced inadvertently in a medical procedure) one. The claim is that, since it is impossible to draw a non-arbitrary line that distinguishes positive from negative eugenics by defining what a genetic disorder is, genetic therapy may cause more serious maladies in future generations than it prevents for the present one. However, genetic conditions like hemophilia, cystic fibrosis, and muscular dystrophy all share features common to other serious diseases or disorders, such as cancer. An objective and culture-free distinction can be made between genetic conditions that everyone counts as diseases or disorders and those that no one does. Even if there are some borderline conditions, it is theoretically possible to limit genetic engineering to those conditions about which there is no disagreement. The topic of what counts as a malady—in particular, what counts as a genetic malady—is important for it may affect not only what conditions will be covered by medical insurance, but which ones are suitable for gene therapy. If genetic engineering is used just to cure serious genetic maladies such as Tay Sachs, it is extremely unlikely that more serious genetic maladies will be created in the future.

While there is no theoretical reason for not using germ line gene therapy, there is a persuasive argument which concludes that all forms of germ line genetic engineering involving humans should be prohibited. This argument, similar to the one against genetic enhancement, claims that even genetic therapy risks great harm for many in future generations, and that there is not sufficient harm prevented to justify these risks. Genetic therapy, like genetic enhancement, not only is permanent during the entire lifetime of the affected individual, the transgene becomes inheritably transmitted to countless members of future generations.

New facts about basic genetic phenomena are being discovered—*e.g.*, five human genetic disorders have been found that are based on mutations involving expandable and contractible trinucleotide repeats. This baffling and novel mechanism for producing mutations was unpredicted, and there currently is no complete explanation for its cause. Similarly, geneticists have discovered another novel and unpredicted phenomenon—genetic imprinting. For a small, but significant, fraction of genes, in humans and other species, the expression of the gene during early embryonic development varies according to its paternal or maternal origin. The biological role of imprinting and the molecular mechanism responsible for selective gene expression remain mysteries. Nevertheless, the effect of genetic imprinting and trinucleotide expansion may be critical in terms of carrying out germ line gene therapy. Problems might not be discovered until the third or fourth generation. Moreover, it seems likely that unpredicted future facts about basic genetic phenomena will be discovered which carry similar risks.

Given even this small possibility of significant harm to many, an analysis of risks and benefits indicates that germ line gene therapy would be justified just in cases of severe maladies, and then only if there were no less radical way of preventing them from occurring. Pre-implantation genetic screening, whereby embryos first are produced by *in vitro* fertilization, does provide such an alternative. At an early blastocyst stage of development, when the embryo is at the eight- or 16-cell stage, a single embryonic cell is removed and screened, genetically, for the presence of defective alleles. If analysis reveals that the fetus would develop a severe genetic malady, the embryo would not be implanted. If the embryo has no severe genetic malady, uterine implantation would be carried out so that normal development could occur.

Pre-implantation screening can eliminate essentially all severe genetic maladies that could be eliminated by genetic engineering. For those with religious or metaphysical beliefs that prohibit destroying any fertilized human egg, it should be pointed out that genetic engineering usually involves creating more fertilized eggs than one plans to use, since implanting of any fertilized egg, including a genetically altered one, often is not successful.

Consequently, pre-implantation screening eliminates the need for germ line gene therapy. The number of cases whereby both parents carry the genes for a rare deleterious recessive allele, such as cystic fibrosis, are microscopically small. Genetic engineering, then, is necessary only for improving or enhancing people by adding new genes for strength, intelligence, or resistance to pathogens or toxins. Genetic engineering to add improvements, rather than to eliminate defects, may give rise to serious social and political problems.

Moreover, gene therapy will be, for the foreseeable future, a very expensive procedure, so only the wealthy will be able to afford it. Germ line gene therapy probably comes as close as is humanly possible to guaranteeing that those families who can afford it will be able to perpetuate their social and political dominance. Thus, together with cloning, it may give rise to a genetically stratified society, as envisioned in Aldous Huxley's novel, *Brave New World*. Once this technology is well-developed, it can be used by societies in which those in power are not governed by ethical restraints. Individuals may be genetically engineered to provide various tasks—*e.g.*, as warriors. Imagine a group of people engineered to be resistant to various poisonous gases. Still, these concerns, although genuine, are speculative.

On the other hand, scientists know from experience that cutting-edge technology generates pressures for its use. Consequently, it is likely that, if genetic engineering were permitted, the technology would be utilized inappropriately, employed even when a comparable outcome could be accomplished using a less risky method. There is justified concern that genetic engineering advocates will make claims that the risks are less than they really are and the benefits are greater than will be realized. It is at least disconcerting that proponents of germ line gene therapy do not talk at all of the far less risky alternative of pre-implantation screening.

If every scientist, administrator, and venture capitalist involved in applying and commercializing genetic engineering were appropriately thoughtful, there would be much less reason to prohibit development and application for those rare cases in which it could be the therapy of choice. However, based on the cited risks, there is insufficient potential benefit to justify any human genetic engineering. Until certain knowledge of the real risks and benefits associated with human genetic engineering has been obtained, the potential risks to all of the future descendants of the patient outweigh any benefit to a very small number of persons who might benefit. In the event of an unanticipated harmful outcome of genetic engineering using mice or corn, the transgenic organisms can be killed, but clearly this option can not be used with humans.

It takes just a few scientists who have convinced themselves that they know the risks are imaginary and the benefits are real for human genetic engineering to become a field in which researchers compete to be first. National and international recognition, prizes, awards, patents, grants, and other measures of status, wealth, and power are potent incentives to overstate successes and benefits, take unacceptable risks, and dismiss valid objections. The extraordinary loyalty of scientists to one another, resulting in their reluctance to interfere with any research project that their colleagues wish to pursue, makes it very likely that some misguided projects will be carried out.

Technology can not justifiably be used to provide benefits to only a few, even if such benefits are great. In cases where no great harm is being prevented and a large number of people may be put as significant risk, caution must prevail. Even if there is no chance of completely stopping germ line gene therapy, it may be possible to delay it long enough that the technology is developed that enables scientists to repair a gene, rather than replace it. Similarly, it might have been better if the building of nuclear power plants had been delayed until they were designed so that there would be virtually no chance of a nuclear explosion. Indeed, it might have been better to postpone building them until acceptable plans for disposing of nuclear wastes had been developed.

The Human Genome Project involves mapping the entire genome—that is, showing where each gene is located, not only which chromosome it is on, but where on that chromosome. This project was sold to Congress in a somewhat misleading way, its proponents claiming that, by finding the genes responsible for major genetic maladies like cystic fibrosis, as well as those that provide dispositions for standard maladies like cancer and heart disease, scientists better would be able to prevent and cure these conditions. That was true, but the whole Human Genome Project was not needed for this purpose. Most scientists were not so optimistic about it, and there was difficulty in lobbying Congress to appropriate all that money. The solution was to pick just those scientists who were on the optimistic fringe to testify before Congress.

The Human Genome Project also involves sequencing each gene—that is, showing how it is built up out of the base pairs that make up a gene. Most defective genes involve a change in a few of these base pairs, often merely one. Gene repair involves changing the base pair causing the problem. This form of genetic engineering has far less potential for disaster or misuse than the kind being considered. Further, the concept of gene repair reinforces the difference between gene therapy and gene enhancement. It would be inappropriate to regard making any change in a gene as repairing it unless that gene is both different from the standard form and results in some genetic malady. Limiting human genetic engineering to the repairing of genes dramatically would lessen the risks of such engineering while not preventing any of its therapeutic benefits.

Application of common moral reasoning to the question of human genetic engineering—both gene therapy and genetic enhancement—thus seems to lead to a natural solution. The present lack of knowledge should restrict genetic engineering to genetic repair. Such a limitation allows the prevention of all the evils of more expansive forms of genetic engineering while not incurring any of the risks. Given this alternative, allowing any more expansive form of genetic therapy or genetic enhancement does not seem morally acceptable.

26

Fountain of Youth

Mortimer B. Zuckerman

On the edge of the millennium, this is the prospect: A child born in 2000-plus may have more than a 1-in-3 chance of living in good health beyond the age of 100. At the beginning of the 20th century, the average life expectancy was about 46 years for the male, 48 for the female. There has been a convergence of discoveries of the most thrilling nature, and they will benefit lots of us who may not be around for 2050. Last week, for instance, researchers announced that they had grown complete heart valves in the lab, a dramatic example of the explosion in tissue engineering. Researchers are already cultivating cells to create new blood vessels, new skin. Within the next few years, we'll be able to replace bones and cartilage and some aspects of joints, tendons, and ligaments.

Bionic man must genuflect to a variety of brilliant minds, men and women who had the nerve to reject the conventional wisdom handed down from before the Renaissance. Health, until then, had been a mysterious process, wholly in the hands of God; mortal intervention was permitted only through religion or obscure herbs. Think of the Frenchman Louis Pasteur, outraging medicine with the preposterous notion that there were invisible microbes that infected our bodies and killed us. We owe the doubling of the life span directly to that man, to the doctors who pushed for antiseptic procedures in surgery and childbirth, to the politicians like Theodore Roosevelt and Cleveland Mayor Tom Johnson who insisted on protecting our food and water.

Visionaries. Consider the forces that, even today, urge specious excuses to resist clean air and water for all the people. Then contrast them with the visionaries like Jonas Salk, who devoted their lives to developing vaccines to prevent epidemics of polio, smallpox, diphtheria, and typhoid, a predominantly American disease. Today, few of us will die from the microbes Pasteur discovered.

Mortimer B. Zuckerman is editor-in-chief of U.S. News and World Report.

The second medical revolution began when chemistry and science exploded. Disease was now seen as internal chemistry gone awry, the remedy the addition of new ingredients to the body to combat microbes from without while righting the chemical imbalance within. The result was a great pharmaceutical revolution, an age of biochemical medicine, its principles applied to internal killers, i.e., cancer, diabetes, cardiovascular disease, asthma, arthritis, etc. Examples were drugs that cut cholesterol, reduced blood pressure, and, more recently, improved quality of life.

Now we are on the threshold of yet a third revolution, this one based on James Watson and Francis Crick's discovery of the structure of DNA in the 1950s. Amazingly, we may be able to use genes and their products to rebuild and restore damage to our bodies wrought by the trinity of disease, trauma, and time. Researchers will be able to reset the rheostat, the clock that tells the cell the age of the host body. This opens up the prospect of chemically inducing the manufacture of a stem cell that can be cultured indefinitely so that we may rebuild damaged organs, tissues, and cells. When we're young, our bodies maintain good working order by systematic and orderly replacement of worn cells and tissues. As we come to understand these repair processes better, we may be able to maintain the health and youthfulness of our bodies for much longer. This new gene-based medicine will do far more than patching the punctures of workaday life.

Transplants of organs will give way to organ regeneration by the regrowth of healthy tissues as younger cells are introduced and integrated. Such genetic intervention will enable us to cure cardiovascular disease affecting 50 percent of men and 30 percent of women over 40. In fact, we will be able to extend human life in a spectacular way. The Fountain of Youth lies within us all!

We have barely begun to ponder the profound implications of this third revolution. Industrial countries now devote more than 10 percent of their GDP to health care. With expenditures devoted primarily to the chronically ill and the really old, health care costs will fall sharply. It is the social equivalent of the Big Bang, changing the economy, retirement, relationships and politics. A brave new world indeed.

27

A World of Immortal Men

Edward O. Wilson

We're on the verge of becoming the first species to decide its own evolution. Scientists are within five years of getting a complete readout of the 5.6 billion genetic letters in the human genome, and soon after, they'll have a complete genetic map of the eighty thousand or so genes these letters compose. So genetic engineering to increase longevity is on the near horizon. Right now we're in a narrow window of concern where the aim is to eliminate genetic disease, to correct the thousands of genes that cause hereditary defects. That should be the first goal of biomedical science, because it will eliminate an immense amount of suffering. But keep in mind that the possibility to enhance genetic traits in normal genes comes quickly behind.

These gene therapies will add up, statistically, to longer life spans. Take, for example, one of the main causes of death in America: heart disease. We know a certain percentage of heart disease is due to hereditary elevation of blood cholesterol to abnormal levels. A whole class of genes that cause increased lipids and imbalances of various kinds, low and high, of lipodensity are under continuous study. Ultimately, we'll get significant life extension simply by spotting and treating certain genotypes: You recognize a tendency, you correct it through gene therapy, either at the level of early genetic regulation or with changes in the genes themselves, and you wind up adding—statistically, at least—decades of longevity.

We'll be able to extend life by working at two levels. One, of course, is the phenotypic—you jog, you avoid bad foods, and that gives you maybe five years—and then there is the genotypic, correcting your genetic tendency toward building up plaques or having weak arterial walls or whatever. That's the way longevity is likely to increase. There won't be any magic change in one or a small number of genes. Progress will be a gradual advance by better lifestyle and small genetic changes to correct serious genetic defects.

If life expectancies wind up being significantly extended—say, by twenty or fifty or a hundred years—the consequences will be enormous. The first

---

Dr. Wilson is professor emeritus, Harvard University, Cambridge, Massachusetts.

Reprinted with permission of Edward O. Wilson from *Esquire, 131*(5) p. 84, May 1999.

thing people will have to do is virtually stop having children. In order to keep the population from exploding, people will have to cut down drastically on the number of children they have or face the severe effects of space and resource depletion. Who will be allowed to have babies? If you extend life to 150 or more years, and especially if you expand the reproductive period of women, then society will have some very hard choices to make. There will have to be some kind of policy to prevent explosive population growth. The old taboos will have to be discarded in favor of realism. We're already approaching the Malthusian wall in terms of how much life the planet can sustain. Arable-land and water supplies per capita are dropping worldwide in what appear to be irreversible trajectories. So the ecological implications of extended life expectancy are quite serious and will need to be addressed precisely as individual health is improved. We may reach a point when it becomes a high privilege to be able to have a child or to provide the DNA for a new child. And rarely would you be able to participate in that lottery or win it, because everyone would be of comparable age, in the early decades at least.

The species is likely to end up with people who have the physical capabilities of teenagers but who are culturally, educationally, and emotionally aged. It's likely to be a very conservative culture, one in which those who have survived and enjoyed longevity extension have a very high level of security guaranteed by their own activities. They won't be revolutionaries. They won't be bold entrepreneurs or explorers who risk their lives. They're not going to throw away any intimation of physical immortality. It's too precious a gift. What would it mean to have healthy, physically young bodies—and aging minds? With certainty, at the very least, a very different civilization.

Harvard would probably stop giving tenure.

28

Redrawing the Ethics Map

Richard D. Lamm

Medical ethics, as it is usually understood, is a map to a world I am not familiar with and cannot follow. It describes a very different world from the world of public budgets. The ethics of delivering health care is a different "moral universe" from the ethics of funding health care. Because of this, the existing map is leading to increasingly unethical public policy results. Medical ethics needs to be revised if it is to provide meaningful guides to future health policy. We need a new ethics map.

You cannot build an ethical code for a publicly funded system around the assumptions that "cost is never a consideration" and that the focus of moral concern must be solely on the individual. Most health care is paid for with pooled funds, either taxpayer or insurance, and you cannot distribute pooled funds by focusing on one patient at a time. Pooled funds must maximize the health of the pool. Cost is *always* a consideration. Most medical ethics, however, assume that resources are unlimited and that the sole issue is the interest of the individual patient. Indeed, some ethicists claim that "medical ethics becomes interesting and relevant only when it abandons the ephemeral realm of theory and abstract speculations and gets down to practical questions raised by real, everyday problems of health and illness . . . It is real-life, flesh-and-blood cases which raise fundamental questions."[1]

Laudatory words, but not the language of public policy. Such a view, highlighting individual needs and ignoring costs, violates the first rule of public policy, which is to maximize the general good using limited funds. Constructing a public budget is a process of trade-offs and priority setting, and it would be public policy malpractice to ignore costs. Indeed, Rudolph Klein suggests from the British perspective that "It is unethical to ignore costs."[2] As Allan Williams has perceptively remarked, "anyone who says that no account should be paid to costs is really saying that no account should be paid to the sacrifices imposed on others."[3]

Richard D. Lamm, LL.B., is the former Governor of Colorado and is now at The Center for Public Policy, University of Denver, Denver, CO.

Reproduced by permission of the Hastings Center from the *Hastings Report* 29(2) 28–29, 1999.

The "moral unit" of a physician is the patient, while the moral unit of public policy is *all* citizens. It took John Kitzhaber, a physician-politician, to point out to a disbelieving nation that as an office holder he was responsible both for those *covered* and for those *not covered*, and he had to consider not only Coby Howard's need for a transplant, but also the state's duty to all of the medically indigent. He was not arguing for a two-tiered system; he was trying to maximize limited public funds in the only health care program for the medically indigent that the state had legislated. It made more ethical sense to him as a public policymaker to cover all the medically indigent and ration *what* was subsidized, not *who* was subsidized. "Last dollar" rationing was preferable to leaving medically indigent people outside of Medicaid.

Additionally, public policy doesn't have the luxury of focusing on one policy area (or funding one program) at a time. Everything is on the table, all the time. As General George Marshall said during World War II, "When deciding what to do one is also deciding what not to do." I cannot express my frustration at sitting in a hospital ethics meeting, agonizing over whether to recognize a living will and knowing that within blocks there are medically indigent citizens with very restricted access to *any* health care. Doctors on their way to work drive on streets filled with potholes. They drive past crumbling schools in an inadequately policed part of the city while sanctimoniously telling themselves that they will never let cost be a consideration in health care. How do I justify $150,000 for each year of life gained by CPR in the hospital, knowing that in my world $150,000 funds five school teachers for a year? Should I be proud of a system that kept Rita Green alive but comatose for forty-two years in Washington, D.C., which has the nation's highest infant mortality rate? Can you give me the password to the moral code that maintained Karen Ann Quinlan on life support in a state that doesn't bother to cover 14 percent of its citizens with basic health care? How can a government with inadequate infrastructure and kids without vaccinations use public funds to maintain anencephalic infants?

For fifty years the medical profession has ignored the World Health Organization definition of health as "the complete physical, mental, and social well-being, and not merely the absence of disease or injury."[4] Should public policy also ignore it? Perhaps a doctor, as a patient advocate, cannot make such a definition work, but public policy has a duty to maximize health, not health care. At least public policy has more comprehensive tools to follow such a definition. We know now that health care is not the only way, or even the best way, to keep a population healthy.

In short, everything we do in a budget prevents us from doing something else we also care about. No sane governor would hire Mother Teresa to run a state's health care system, for we cannot "wipe every tear from every eye," however lofty the goal. If there is a conflict between the total social good and the good of an individual, public policy is sworn to uphold the public interest. Public policy has to place the one-way streets, the fire stations, the television towers, and the garbage dumps somewhere. Choices and trade-offs must be made. It is not a "do no harm" world and cannot be. There is no "cloistered virtue" in public policy.

Achieving this broad view of the good requires deep change in our moral outlook. To begin with, as Haavi Morreim has pointed out, because the common resource pool depends on individual contributions, justice demands that individuals not make unreasonable demands on collective funds.[5] Americans must develop the civic maturity to understand that they cannot have unlimited health care with limited premiums and limited taxes. One person overuses at the expense of others. Likewise, "generous compassion for one is inevitably bought at the expense of many whose contributions create and who in turn rely on the common resource pool" (p. 256).

We must adopt a similar holism when we turn to the theory behind our choices. Medical ethics cannot be constructed in an ethical vacuum. Taxpayers now fund approximately 50 percent of the nation's health care. Publicly funded health care must be weighed against the other health needs of the community, and also against public needs other than health. But most contemporary ethical theories are built around individuals and do not take into consideration the cumulative impact of those ethics. Such individual-centered ethics are incompatible with maximization of the social good. Unavoidably, there is a conflict between individual goods and societal goods. All "a priori" thinking developed around individual cases and assuming unlimited resources must be rethought.

What public policy demands is some sort of public interest imperative, analogous to Kant's "categorical imperative," whereby we could test actions relating to specific individuals against an ethical whole. Currently, the sum of our ethical choices in "real life, flesh-and-blood cases" has given us an unethical system that ignores forty-three million uninsured. But our moral universe ought to encompass both forest and trees. Barney Clark and his artificial heart did not exist in a vacuum, but as a member of a society with a myriad of public needs. We cannot optimize his care and also deal ethically with the whole of society. While he is entitled to his "rights" as an American citizen, these rights do not include publicly subsidized longevity at all costs. To advance such a right is to endorse an ethical code built around a standard of conduct that cumulatively will destroy the system.

The view I am affirming is not as harsh as patient advocates might think. It reflects, not an absence of caring, but a broader definition of caring. Public policy is compassionate, not an individual at a time, but in view of total unmet social needs. Public policy is a different world from the world of the bedside, and making optimum social policy is "terra incognito" that must be mapped anew.

References

1. Robert M. Veatch, *Case Studies in Medical Ethics* (Cambridge, Mass.: Harvard University Press, 1979), p. 1.

2. Rudolph Klein et al., *Managing Scarcity* (Buckingham, England: Open University Press, 1996), p. 31.

3. Alan Williams, "Cost-Effectiveness Analysis: Is It Ethical?," *Journal of Medical Ethics* 18, no. 1 (1992): 7–11, at 7.

4. World Health Organization, *The First Ten Years of the World Health Organization* (Geneva: World Health Organization, 1958).

5. Haavi E. Morreim, "Moral Justice and Legal Justice in Managed Care: The Ascent of Contributive Justice," *Journal of Law, Medicine & Ethics* 23, no. 3 (1995): 247–65.

29

Health Care Rationing in the Aged

Edmund G. Howe and Christopher J. Lettieri

Medical resources are limited, especially in the 1990s. These limitations pose new ethical questions in all areas of medicine. For example, in regard to critical care, Lanken[1] states, 'As 1994 begins, the nature of critical care medicine stands at another crossroads where new economic constraints intersect with the patient-based ethics of current ICU [intensive care unit] practice'.

It is particularly important that these new ethical questions be analysed now in regard to aged people, not only in the US but in other countries, for several reasons. In the US, business ethics are increasingly coming into competition with medical ethics because of the emergence of managed care.[2] How these different ethical perspectives should be integrated is currently controversial. In addition, resources are staying the same but the number of aged people is increasing. Medicare, a system of government funding for the elderly and disabled, spent $US154 billion dollars in 1993. This represented 19.3% of the total health care spending. Some predict that Medicare will be bankrupt by the year 2001.[3] If this occurs, it will have been mostly the result of the increasing number of people over the age of 65 years.[4] Finally, the prevalence of Alzheimer's disease (AD) increases markedly with age. Its prevalence doubles approximately every 5 years.[5] In the US, the cost of treating these patients now ranks behind only that of treating patients with heart disease and cancer.[6] Moreover, this cost has increased 2-fold in less than a decade.[7]

However, in all countries, the need to address questions regarding the allegation of resources to the aged is comparably urgent not because of financial or demographic developments, but because of humane considerations transcending these and other national circumstances. That is, empirical findings recently published suggest that the mental deterioration which has been

Edmund G. Howe and Christopher J. Lettieri, Uniformed Services University of the Health Sciences, Bethesda, MD.

Reprinted from *Drugs and Aging*, 1999; *15*(1):37–47 with permission. Copyright © Adis International Inc.

assumed most patients with AD inevitably undergo may not be inevitable.[8,9] New drugs, such as tacrine, donepezil and tocopherol (vitamin E), may slow the progression of AD and, thus, make it possible for these patients to live longer at home without having to be institutionalised.[10,11] This itself would be cost-effective.[12]

However, the beneficial effects of these drugs may be dwarfed by new findings of more pronounced effects with psychosocial interventions. These data suggests that progression of AD may not only be slowed, but possibly reversed to some extent by an enriched interpersonal environment. For instance, Kitwood and Bredin,[13] citing behavioral studies in patients with AD, state '[S]ome individuals who had seriously deteriorated . . . including some who had been written off as hopelessly demented, show considerable reversal . . . when their conditions of life, and especially their social relationships, are changed.'

Laboratory data obtained from animal research also support claims of both the slowing of progression and reversal of AD. This research[14] indicates that adverse psychological influences can destroy neurons within the hippocampus, the part of the brain most associated with memory and most severely affected in AD.[15] Thus, if these adverse influences can be eliminated by providing a more supportive interpersonal environment, it may be possible to retard the rate of progression of this disease. In addition, data from animal studies show that an enriched environment can bring about the formation of new neurons within the hippocampus and that this can occur not only in newborns, but adults.[9] These new neurons may, at least to some extent, like fetal tissue in Parkinson's disease, reverse the effects of AD.

The significance of these new findings for the clinical treatment of AD are no less than profound. They are well summarised by Kitwood:[16] 'We do not yet know what the course of the main dementing conditions will be when care is of excellent quality!'. No wonder a leading authority in treating these patients with psychosocial interventions describes this discovery as a 'breakthrough'.[17] The ethical implications of this awareness would seem unequivocal. The outcome for these patients and their families is devastating. Thus, if it conceivably could be postponed or even avoided altogether, it would seem mandatory that these possibilities be pursued, at once.

Yet, patients with other illnesses have urgent needs as well. Obviously, healthcare is a precious commodity in short supply.[18] Age-based rationing might be more justifiable as a means of containing costs than most other approaches because, in response to receiving the same medical interventions, the aged will gain less healthy, not to mention productive, years to enjoy. In addition, age-based rationing could result in substantial economic savings.[19]

Should, then, the aged be singled out and be denied access to at least certain kinds of medical care on the basis of this utilitarian rationale? Or should the needs of the aged or of one or more subgroups, such as those with AD, be given some priority or, perhaps, even greatest priority for receiving limited health care resources?

These inquiries will be the focus of the subsequent discussion. Initially, this article will review some of the predominant approaches now put forward for allocating treatment among the aged. It will then discuss an approach we believe is most warranted and why. Finally, obstacles that could arise in societies instituting this approach will be enumerated.

▪ *I. CONTEMPORARY ETHICAL APPROACHES TO ALLOCATING CARE AMONG THE AGED*

In bioethics, there are 2 different kinds of values. The first kind are deontological values. These values are not based on consequences but on respecting a person's dignity and treating them equally.[20] Individuals can be treated equally or, according to the principle of justice, in several different ways. One way is to treat individuals equally according to their needs. This approach gives priority on the basis of the degree to which people are worst off.

When people are treated according to this approach, they are treated equally in that they receive treatment proportionate to their needs. We shall argue in this article that this value, and this particular application of justice, should prevail over all other values. We shall argue that patients with AD, and some other aged patients not mentally impaired, are worse off relative to other patients and, accordingly, that their treatment warrants greater priority.

The second kind of values are utilitarian values. We have already referred to this category of values implicitly when relating the possible significance of aged patients enjoying reduced benefits, relative to younger patients, when receiving the same medical interventions. Utilitarian values involve only consequences. When a utilitarian approach is used exclusively an attempt is made, in one way or another, to achieve the greatest good for the greatest number. Consequently, approaches which give priority to utilitarian values give greater moral weight to the needs of the many than to the needs of the few, even if the few are much worse off. The common exception to this is, of course, when giving priority to the needs of the few will ultimately benefit the many.

Generally, when economic resources are allocated, this allocation is based much more on utilitarian than deontological values. Since the aged generally gain less in terms of healthy and productive years, they are disadvantaged from the start because public policy, whether for better or worse, tends to give exceptional moral weight to utilitarian values. Yet, in some contexts, deontological values receive priority and, in their own right, not just because this furthers utility. In some contexts, they even receive absolute priority.

The absolute priority of deontological values is exemplified in current practices regarding research. Research cannot be conducted on competent patients without their consent, even if the results of this research could benefit future patients immensely. To do otherwise would violate the autonomy of research patients, and violate their dignity because it would use them as a means to others' ends rather than ends in themselves.

We shall argue that even though when public policymakers allocate economic resources they customarily prioritise utilitarian values, the treatment of patients with AD, and of another group of aged patients yet to be discussed, should be an exception. We shall argue that decisions regarding the allocation of treatments for these individuals, like decisions regarding research individuals, should be based absolutely on deontological values and, specifically, on justice which requires treating people equally and according to their needs.

What approaches for allocating limited resources among the aged have others recently proposed? One approach, theoretically plausible but rarely suggested because it would be too expensive, is to give total priority to the principle of justice applied in a different way, namely, valuing the lives of old and young equally. This approach is illustrated by imagining 2 individuals who require a liver transplant to survive. One is aged and the other is young. This approach would require flipping a coin. This approach is rarely applied since, as alluded to, it totally ignores considerations of utility.

The approach most commonly applied in one form or another is to allow both deontological and utilitarian values, and to balance them. Both deontological and utilitarian values are taken into account, for example, when patients are selected for organ transplantation. For example, in the US the criteria initially used are medical. Patients who have untreatable illnesses, such as cancer, may be ineligible. This exclusion is based solely on utilitarian concerns. However, once a patient is medically eligible, the criteria for selection change so that deontological values become included. The criteria then depend on many factors. For example, kidneys are allocated on the basis of points assigned. Some points are given for utilitarian reasons, such as the degree to which antigens are matched because the degree of matching increases the likelihood that a kidney will not be rejected. Points are also given for time on the waiting list. This criterion is based on the deontological principle of justice. It treats patients equally, because the time they have been on the waiting list functions essentially as a means of random selection. Thus, all patients are treated the same. To some extent, of course, who gets on a waiting list first may reflect the extent to which a patient is socio-economically well off, as opposed to a matter of chance.

When this deontological value is given moral weight in organ transplantation, the value of maximising utility is sacrificed to some extent. This is true when any allocation scheme involves both these kinds of values. Thus, if priority is given to even only some aged patients, this will necessitate sacrificing utility.

However, justice may be applied in several different ways. Another application of justice is to see the ultimate goal to be to provide all patients with the same opportunity to live a full life. Veatch,[21] for example, proposes that the priority of health care be inversely proportionate to age because older people have had the opportunity to live longer. Applying justice in this way, Veatch sees younger people as worse off than older people because they have lived less of their lives. He argues that they deserve a greater proportion of limited medical resources. This application of justice would favour giving the liver to the 20-year-old rather than to the 90-year-old on deontological as well as utilitarian grounds.[22]

On the other hand, Callahan[23] argues that people have a 'natural life span' which generally extends into the eighties. Similarly to Veatch, he contends that age is an appropriate criteria for prioritising care, but for a different reason. Calllahan argues that although palliative care should be given to the aged, great amounts of money should not be spent to extend their natural lifespan. Preferably, he believes, the aged should attempt to find meaning in other ways, such as by their passing on the wisdom they have acquired to the young. This wisdom might include, for example, their accepting that the time must come to die.

Daniels[24] applies the principle of justice in still a different way. He would allow the aged to receive proportionately less resources than younger people, like Veatch and Callahan, but for different reasons. He argues that age differs from other characteristics, such as gender and race. He points out that while no one can change their gender or race, all will age. Consequently, if people at different ages receive different amounts of health care, as he believes they should, this will not violate justice because, unless people die early, all will age in time and, thus, be subject to these same differences over time. He argues then that it only makes sense to make distinctions among people in different age groups. Unless sufficient resources are given to patients in earlier years, for instance, they may not reach older ages at all.

Another aspect of Daniels' argument is essential to what we are arguing here. That is that being in good health is critical because it is a prerequisite for having important opportunities. He states, '. . . [N]ormal functioning has a central effect on the opportunity open to an individual'.[25] This insight, although essential to our argument as well, does not go far enough. That is, it provides an absolute ground for prioritising some ends over others, namely, these ends being a prerequisite to individuals having something else which is important. However, Daniels' formulation is at the same time too limited in that to too great an extent he views all 'normal functions' as the same and, thus, fails to identify how some 'normal functions' are exponentially more important than the rest.

This is where the argument in this article begins and this is what it contributes to the argument of Daniels. We contend that the normal function that people need and want, which far exceeds all others, is the capacity to enjoy meaningful relationships with other people. This capacity to relate meaningfully is what is lost in AD as it progresses. Consequently, if psychosocial interventions could, indeed, help preserve or enhance this capacity, limited resources should be prioritised for these patients more than for other patient groups.

However, the capacity to enjoy meaningful relationships may be lost in another way in people who do not have dementia and whose brains have not become impaired. These people may lose this capacity because of external events. For example, physical disability may result in aged people losing proximity to others whom they have known their whole lives. This can occur, for example, if they must be sent to a nursing home far away from those they love. It is implausible to believe that in the nursing homes to which they are sent, they could form comparably meaningful relationships with staff or with other patients.

Thus, once this normal function is delineated and recognised accurately to be as all-overriding as it is, it is apparent that people worse off because they lack this capacity include groups such as the one just considered who do not have AD or other dementia. Recognising these groups is comparably important because in some instances, their loss may be eliminated to a far greater extent and at a far lesser cost.

Home healthcare could enable some of these patients, for example, to remain at home and close to those they love.[26] Allocating this resource to these patients could enable them to maintain meaningful relationships, albeit in a totally different way. As we shall discuss in section 3, the needs of this second group should also be considered when deciding how resources should be allocated to the aged because, relative to those who experience dementia, those who do not may experience more emotional pain since they remain aware of the isolation they endure. It may be, then, that antidementia drugs which slow these patients' cognitive decline actually increase their suffering.[27]

▓ 2. APPROACHES WHICH SHOULD BE PRIORITISED

Societies tend to ignore their worst off, particularly when this group is a disadvantaged population that lacks power. Bell[28] asserts that since women live longer than men and, therefore, there are more women among the aged than men, discrimination against the elderly disproportionately discriminates against women as well. Jecker[29] agrees and she asserts that this inherent discrimination against women is more ethically problematic than discrimination merely against the aged.

The views of Bell and Jecker are open to challenge on the ground that since men live shorter life spans, they may be seen as having a stronger claim than women on limited health resources. This claim would be based on the rationale regarding the aged and young put forth by Veatch, as presented in section 1.[21] Yet, women may live longer for a variety of reasons. They may live longer, for instance, in spite of having been subject to discrimination. The relative paucity of research on women's health problems until recently, supports this possibility.[30] It may be that women live longer despite being subject to discrimination in their younger years. Consequently, if the aged are allowed now to be subject to discrimination when this could be readily prevented, women would be doubly subject to discrimination in their aged years. If women were doubly subject to discrimination, Veatch's view still could be considered valid and, thus, held to prevail.

Yet, since discrimination against women singularly, as with any other group, violates their dignity, allowing discrimination doubly could approach being unconscionable. Consequently, at the very least, when the aged are considered, Bell and Jecker's concerns should be accorded additional moral weight.

However, others are concerned with another subgroup disproportionately affected by discrimination against the aged, namely, the poor.[31] This group, like women, would be doubly disadvantaged if policies allowing discrimination against the aged were enacted. Thus, this consideration also warrants additional moral weight.

Notwithstanding their being disproportionately women and/or poor and/or the subjects of discrimination doubly in some other way, we contend that the aged are worse off than at least most other patient populations (whether as a result of dementia or external factors) because they have lost their capacity to enjoy meaningful interactions with others. This judgment, that this loss is worse than many or all others, is supported by many considerations. It is consistent, for example, with what innumerable people say when they enunciate advance directives. These people indicate that they would rather not live than live without the capacity to relate meaningfully with others.

They do not say that they would not want to live if they remain mentally intact but unable to see those they love as a result of external factors. However, we would argue, that their not saying this is not because it is untrue but because they have not considered this or, if they have, could not anticipate this outcome accurately. Paradoxically, it well may be that it is not patients such as those with AD who have lost this capacity because of their disease whose suffering is greatest. Aged patients who remain mentally intact may be those who suffer most profoundly because they remain aware of what they could have but have lost.

The loss of personal identity which occurs with severe dementia is unequivocally tragic. Brock[32] argues, for instance, that since this identity is so important, when individuals lose it as a result of dementia, only palliative, not life-sustaining health care should be provided. Yet, since people with intact cognition remain wholly aware of their circumstances, their suffering may be much greater even though they retain their identity. The following 2 examples are illustrative.

A patient had a stroke and was placed in a nursing care facility several hours away from her family. She lived in a small room and lay flat on her bed, unable to move without assistance. After conversing with a relative during a rare visit, she said. 'You know I really would like to die'. When her relative left, her eyes returned to the position at which they had been when this relative first arrived. The patient stared at a point directly above her on the ceiling. This was the way she spent most of her waking hours. A second patient had also experienced a stroke. She too was imprisoned in her body and unable to move. Her husband was in a different room. He too had a stroke and could not recognise her. A staff person asked her, 'Is there anything I can do for you?'. She replied, not facetiously but genuinely, 'What could you do?'.

This second patient's suffering, unlike the first, may be beyond anyone's help. However, the nature of their suffering was the same. Each thought that their careproviders could show them the greatest compassion by helping them to die.

This preference, like that of patients who express this same thought in advance directives, could be taken as a rough barometer of the degree to which patients regard different conditions as causing them suffering. If so, the relative rarity of patients expressing this preference to die in contexts other than these when they are not 'suicidal' is, perhaps, the clearest basis of any for inferring that these patients are among the worst off.

■ 3. GUIDELINES FOR MAKING ECONOMIC DECISIONS

How should resources for both these groups be prioritised? It is most useful, when deciding what economic decisions should be made, to divide these patients into the 2 groups delineated above: those whose cognition is intact and those whose cognition is impaired.

3.1 Patients Who Are Cognitively Intact

As a result of economic decisions, society may benefit some of these patients immensely. As suggested, if resources are given to mentally intact aged patients for home health care so that they can remain at home with their families, this may be enough to give their lives meaning, even in the face of grave physical illness.

However, achieving this and comparable ends may require significant attitudinal changes within society. Allowing aged patients to remain in their own homes may, for example, require not only a shift in the use of financial resources but an openness to allowing them to live at an increased risk of injury to themselves. Allowing this risk is not as discrepant from present value priorities as it may appear. In fact, it is more consistent. That is, patients now retain the capacity to decline life preserving treatment on a hospital ward, but they are often deemed to lack the capacity to choose to stay at home even though the danger to them is only slightly increased. The latter practice, unlike the decision-making capacity afforded these patients in hospitals, disrespects aged patients' autonomy. Even according to contemporary ethical standards, this is unjustifiable.

When patients are cognitively intact, caregivers may, with society's economic support, also help patients acquire or reacquire meaning in their lives in other ways. Patients may, for example, find that recording stories of their lives on tape or making a journal for their grandchildren gives unprecedented renewed meaning to their lives. Surprisingly, even after they have concluded this activity, they may retain not only the cognitive sense that their life has meaning but the emotional ebullience they experienced while engaging in this activity. To do this, caregivers first have to establish a trusting interpersonal relationship. Only then can they help patients find meaning.

For physicians and other people to make such attempts, economic resources are necessary. Caregivers must be reimbursed if they are to be expected to provide this care. It may, in addition, require special training.

3.2 Patients with Alzheimer's Disease

Research is needed to find additional biological treatments to prevent and alleviate such illnesses as AD.[33] This research requires economic resources. This need is, of course, not new. What is new is our awareness of the degree to which patients with dementia may respond to interpersonal interventions.[34,35] This potential responsivity is alleged to exist whether the patients' dementia is mild or severe. In regard to patients whose dementia is milder such that they can still make choices, Folsom[36] states 'Only by spending the time and energy needed to help the demented resident remain in control of such personal choices can the staff avert the confusion, disorientation, and disengagement that result when all decision-making responsibility is removed from the person in the process of providing total institutional care'. In patients much more severely demented, Butler and Lewis[37] report, 'Smiles, hugs, handholding, and a warm supportive manner are forms of non-verbal communication to which even the most severely demented person may respond'.

A paradigmatic example of the exceptional benefits interpersonal support can offer, even when less expensive interventions will 'suffice', is the patient with dementia who habitually loses control. For these patients, there are 3 options: restraints, drugs and interpersonal interventions.

Restraints may be less expensive, but patients may experience mental anguish from being restrained. Moreover, the act of restraining patients may be so painful for those who care for these patients that their applying restraints impairs their relationship with them.[38] That is, the careproviders may have to distance themselves emotionally from the patients when they apply restraints, and this may reduce the comfort they could provide at other times.

Drugs, such as benzodiazepines and small doses of antipsychotics,[39,40] may reduce the patients' emotional pain and aggressive outbursts and, as a result, increase their capacity to relate more intimately with others. Yet, these drugs may also result in patients becoming less interpersonally responsive.[41-43] If drugs impair patients' ability to relate to others, this may reduce the degree to which they can respond to interpersonal interventions.

This third option is for careproviders to give patients optimal interpersonal attention, caring and support. This approach presupposes that the patients' inability to control themselves can be diminished and even curtailed by these interventions alone. This presupposition seems to be true. The extent to which interpersonal interventions can benefit these patients is, as stated, unknown. However, patients' possibly benefit far more than previously imagined.

Naomi Feil[17] gives examples suggesting the possible extent to which these patients may gain. If, for instance, these patients have a capacity to verbalise, careproviders can understand what these verbalisations mean in the light of their prior experiences. With this understanding, the patients' otherwise incoherent ramblings may become coherent. If the patients cannot communicate, such actions as touching and using a gentle tone of voice still may be significantly effective. They may induce not only serenity but an unprecedented, greater capacity to relate to others.

The availability of this option also presupposes that with proper training, staff can learn these interventions and, clearly, this is so. Rango[44] states, for example, 'If trained to tolerate potentially bothersome or disruptive behaviours such as incoherent verbalisation, repetitive demands, and harmless wandering, the staff will refrain from using physical or chemical restraint except as a last resort'. These skills and the dedication required to help these patients optimally, demand much more than these careproviders learning greater toleration. Kitwood[45] states that to maximise the patients' gains, caregivers must become engaged with the 'sufferer's psychology'. He also relates that the qualities required to do this 'are remarkably lacking in the everyday world, and they do not feature strongly in the training of . . . professionals'.[34]

Economic support is obviously needed so that careproviders can learn and be sufficiently motivated to engage patients in this way. The present use of restraints and drugs may be due, in part, to insufficient economic support for careproviders' to be trained to and then make the desirable interpersonal interventions.

■ 4. WHO SHOULD DECIDE

However, even if the above findings were proved valid, would the majority of people choose to bring these changes about? There are 2 reasons to think they would not: attitudes which devalue aging and bias against those who are aged.

4.1 Attitudes Which Devalue Aging

Different attitudes among the general population to aging make it more difficult to achieve an informed consensus on how economic resources should be allocated for this population. This difficulty is also experienced when another approach, attempting to provide precise measures of utility, is used to allocate resources: attempting to quantify the relative value of different medical interventions so that they can be selected on the basis of this comparison.[46] We use the following example to illustrate this difficulty.

Under this approach, one might try to compare how patients value living a 'normal' life with living while receiving kidney dialysis.[47] Problems in making this quantitative determination are that different people have different views on what makes life worth living and, as stated, people of different ages are likely to value medical interventions differently. Younger people may think the last years of life worth little, but those at the end of these years may value each second. Both physicians and the greater population may project to these patients feelings they believe they would have if they were aged, had these patients' illnesses and were receiving such treatments as kidney dialysis. In addition, aged people may remind them of their own impending death. As Kitwood and Bredin[13] state, 'Professionals and informal caregivers are vulnerable people too, bearing their own anxiety and dread concerning frailty, dependence, madness, ageing, dying, and death'.

Becker[48] describes the psychological mechanism which states how this vulnerability we all possess may work against aged patients: 'We have an ever-present fear of death, but, due to our instinct for self-preservation, tend to be utterly oblivious to this fear in our conscious life'. Oblivious of these negative emotions, we do not feel them, but instead may act them out. These emotions may take the form of believing that their situation is hopeless, and either communicating these feelings to these patients directly or by enacting policies which deny them care. In either case, aged people experiencing themselves as hopeless may be the result of a self-fulfilling prophecy.

Accordingly, if aged people are asked to place values on interventions for themselves, they may value them less. This judgement, as opposed to reflecting unchangeable subjective realities, may also reflect circumstances they presently face. This may include, for instance, the external factors enumerated in sections 1 and 2, which result in their losing the capacity to continue to enjoy meaningful relationships with others.

4.2 Bias Against Those Who Are Aged

Deciding who should make decisions about the aged is additionally problematic because younger people may feel bias against the aged and, knowingly or unknowingly, express this bias when they make these judgements. Youth in the US, relative to people in many other countries may have a negative bias toward the aged. In 'Is dying young worse than dying old', Jecker and Schneiderman[49] discuss the bias in Western societies. They assert that in these societies, many people view the deaths of younger and older people differently. The death of younger people produces greater feelings of sorrow, anger, despair and bitterness. Furthermore, they assert that the relative lack of such responses toward the aged stem, in part, from false stereotypes younger people hold toward them. As a result of these stereotypes, younger people may devalue the aged and more easily accept their dying.

Callahan[23] asserts that people in the US respond similarly. Typically, he claims, people respond to the death of young people with sharp regret, but to the death of older people only with sadness. His holding this view is particularly credible and telling, because, unlike Jecker and Schneiderman, he is not arguing that this is an unwarranted prejudice based on a false stereotype. Rather, he believes, this is how it should be.

Post,[50] in contrast, is concerned with not only people having this negative bias but with how they could express it. He asserts that if age is used as a criteria for rationing health care, this runs an undue risk of discrimination against the elderly. Therefore, he argues that decisions for patients to not receive care should be voluntary, at least to the degree that this can be achieved.

This view may accord with what most people believe. A national survey of public opinion in the US, for instance, indicates that although the people responding would withhold life-prolonging care from critically ill elderly patients when they had little chance of survival, they would not withhold it solely on account of a patient's age.[51]

Who, then, would act as advocates for those who are aged? Who would act to promote interventions which would maintain and enhance their capacity to enjoy meaningful relationships with others? Aged people who must go to nursing homes because they lack home care and patients who have AD are themselves essentially voiceless. Their most devoted advocates, no doubt, would be members of their families. However, their families' views might be seen as not objective, because they are exceptionally emotionally biased, by the rest of society, such that these families exaggerate the true extent of these patients' despair.[52]

■ 5. CONCLUSION

Should societies provide the economic support so that physicians and other careproviders can provide both these 'worse off' groups of aged patients (those who are isolated and those with AD) the treatments they need? Their allocating resources in this manner would operate, of course, against the pursuit of utility. Why, then, should resources be prioritised to meet the needs of the aged patients described in section 3, as isolated and demented.

Both patients who are mentally intact but isolated from others and those who experience dementia share the same loss—the loss of meaningful interactions with others. These interactions are to most people what makes life worthwhile. The need for these interactions may be seen as being close to that of their need for food and shelter. Accordingly, when this loss occurs, it is substantially greater than that which may result from even extensive physical illness alone.

The loss of the capacity for meaningful interactions similarly may be validly considered more profound than most illness in younger patients. Disproportionate resources may be justified, therefore, solely on the ground of reducing the extent to which aged patients in these 2 groups are worst off, thus furthering towards them this application of the principle of justice.

Yet, paradoxically, 2 other arguments may also favour this disproportionate allocation. The first involves Daniels' concept that all of us age. He uses this to justify withholding some degree of resources to the aged, but it could be used to support the very opposite. We are all subject to losing this capacity for meaningful interactions as we age. Thus, as we would want to give any infant, regardless of the extent of special needs, the minimal resources to experience a meaningful life, we would want to do no less for those who are aged.

Secondly, what would be the effect of all of us as we age knowing that society has established a priority of enabling us to continue to enjoy meaningful relationships with others if there is some way that we can. All people, young and aged, may feel more valued. This disproportionate allocation may then be valued if not on other grounds, on the basis of utility.

References

1. Lanken PN. Critical care medicine at a new crossroads: the intersection of economies and ethics in the intensive care unit. Am J Respir Crit Care Med 1994: 149: 3–5.
2. Ruskin A. Capitation: the legal implications of using capitation to affect physician decision-making processes. J Contemp Health Law Policy 1997; 13: 391–21.
3. King G. Health care reform and the Medicare program. Health Aff 1994; 3: 39–45.
4. Lubitz J, Beech J, Baker C. Longevity and Medicare expenditures. N Engl J Med 1995; 332: 999–1003.
5. Evans DA, Funkenstein HH, Albert MS, et al. Prevalence of Alzheimer's disease in a community population of older persons; higher than previously reported. JAMA 1989; 262: 2551–6.
6. Snow C. Medicare HMOs develop plan for future of Alzheimer's programming. Mod Healthc 1996; 23: 66–70.
7. Ernst RL, Hay JW. The US economic and social costs of Alzheimer's disease revisited. Am J Public Health 1994; 84: 1261–4.
8. Karlsson I, Mandahl N, Brane G, et al. Effects of environmental stimulation on biochemical and psychological variables in dementia. Acta Psychiatr Scand 1988; 77 (2): 207–13.
9. Kempermann HG, Kuhn HG, Gage FH. More hippocampal neurons in adult mice living in an enriched environment. Nature 1997; 356: 493–5.
10. Knopman D, Schneider L, Davis K. et al. Long-term tacrine (Cognex) treatment: effects on nursing home placement and mortality. Neurology 1996; 47: 166–77.
11. Karlawish JHT, Whitehouse PJ. Is the placebo obsolete in a world after donepezil and vitamin E? Arch Neurol 1998; 55: 1420–4.

12. Knapp M, Wilkinson D, Wigglesworth R. The economic consequences of Alzheimer's disease in the context of new drug developments. Int J Geriatr Psychiatry 1998; 13: 531–43.

13. Kitwood T, Bredin K. Towards a theory of dementia care: personhood and well-being. Ageing Soc 1992; 12: 269–87.

14. Sapolsky RM, Uno H, Rebert CS, et al. Hippocampal damage associated with prolonged glucocorticoid exposure in primates. J Neurosci 1990; 10 (9): 2897–902.

15. Damasio AR. Alzheimer's disease and related dementias. In: Wyngaarden JB, Smith Jr LH, Bennett JC, editors. Cecil textbook of medicine. 19th ed. Philadelphia: Saunders, 1992: 2075–9.

16. Kitwood T. Toward a theory of dementia care: ethics and interaction. J Clin Ethics 1998; 9: 23–34.

17. Feil N. The validation breakthrough. Baltimore (MD): Health Professions Press, Inc., 1993.

18. Shaw AB. In defence of ageism. J Med Ethics 1994; 20: 188–91.

19. Hunt R. A critique of using age to ration care. J Med Ethics 1993; 19 (1): 19–23.

20. Sulmasy DP. Physicians, cost control, and ethics. Ann Intern Med 1992; 116 (11): 920–6.

21. Veatch R. Justice and the economics of terminal illness. Hastings Cent Rep 1988; 18 (4): 34–40.

22. Kilner JF. Age as a basis for allocating life-saving medical resources: an ethical analysis. J Health Polit Policy Law 1988; 13 (3): 405–23.

23. Callahan D. Setting limits. New York: Simon and Schuster, 1987.

24. Daniels N. Am I my parents keeper? An essay on justice between the young and old. New York: Oxford University Press, 1988.

25. Daniels N. A lifespan approach to health care. In: Jecker N, editor. Aging and health care. Clifton (NJ): Humana Press, 1991: 227–246.

26. Colombo M, Vitali S, Molla G, et al. The home environment modification program in the care of demented elderly: some examples. Arch Gerontol Geriatr 1998; Suppl. 6: 83–90.

27. Post SG, Whitehouse PJ. Emerging antidementia drugs: a preliminary ethical view. J Am Geriatr Soc 1998; 46: 787–7.

28. Bell NK. What setting limits may mean: a feminist critique of Daniel Callahan's setting limits. Hypatia 1989; 4 (2): 168–78.

29. Jecker NS. Age-based rationing and women. JAMA 1991; 266 (21): 3012–5.

30. Bennett JC. Special reports/inclusion of women in clinical trials: policies for population subgroups. N Engl J Med 1993; 329: 288–92.

31. Levinsky NG. Age as a criterion for rationing health care. N Engl J Med 1990; 322 (25): 1813–5.

32. Brock DW. Justice and the severely demented. J Med Philos 1988; 13 (1): 73–99.

33. Kumar V, Cantillon M. Update on the development of medication for memory and cognition in Alzheimer's disease. Psychiatr Ann 1996; 26 (5): 280–8.

34. Kitwood T. The dialectics of dementia: with particular reference to Alzheimer's disease. Ageing Soc 1990; 10: 177–96.

35. Barnes T, Sack J, Shore J. Guidelines to treatment approaches. Gerontologist 1973; 13: 513–27.

36. Folsom JC. Reality orientation. In: Reisberg B, editor. Alzheimer's disease. New York: The Free Press, 1983: 449–54.

37. Butler RN, Lewis MI. Aging and mental health. 3rd ed. St Louis: Mosby Company, 1982: 366.

38. Evans LK, Strumpf NE. Tying down the elderly. J Am Geriatr Soc 1989; 37: 65–74.

39. Beardsley RS, Larson DB, Burns BJ, et al. Prescribing of psychotropics in elderly nursing home patients. J Am Geriatr Soc 1989; 37: 327–30.

40. Svarstad BL, Mount JK. Nursing home resources and tranquilizer use among the institutionalized elderly. J Am Geriatr Soc 1991; 39: 869–75.

41. Garrard J, Makris L, Dunham T, et al. Evaluation of neuroleptic drug use by nursing home elderly under proposed Medicare and Medicaid regulations. JAMA 1991; 265: 463–7.

42. Sloane PD, Matthew LJ, Scarborough M, et al. Physical and pharmacological restraint of nursing home patients with dementia: impact of specialized unit. JAMA 1991; 265: 1278–82.

43. Beers M, Avorn J, Scarborough M, et al. Psychoactive medication use in intermediate-care facility residents. JAMA 1988; 260: 3016–20.

44. Rango N. The nursing home resident with dementia. Ann Intern Med 1985; 102: 835–41.

45. Kitwood T. Brain, mind and dementia: with particular reference to Alzheimer's disease. Ageing Soc 1989; 9: 1–15.

46. Avorn J. Benefit and cost analysis in geriatric care: turning age discrimination into health policy. N Engl J Med 1984; 310 (20): 1294–301.

47. Sackett DC, Torrance GW. The utility of different health states as perceived by the general public. J Chronic Dis 1978; 31: 697–704.

48. Becker E. The denial of death. New York: The Free Press, 1973.

49. Jecker N, Schneiderman L. Is dying young worse than dying old? Gerontologist 1994; 34 (1): 66–73.

50. Post S. Technology and the aging society: ethics and public policy. In: Blank RH, Mills MK, editors. Biomedical technology and public policy. New York: Greenwood Press, 1989: 201–22.

51. Zweibel N, Cassel C, Karrison T. Public attitudes about the use of chronological age as a criterion for allocating health care resources. Gerontologist 1993; 33 (1): 74–80.

52. Jecker N. The role of intimate others in medical decision making. In: Jecker N, editor. Aging and ethics. Clifton (NJ): Humana Press, 1991: 199–216.

Discussion Questions

1. Crowder (Article 24) states that ethics in the early years of nursing dealt primarily with manners and morals. The most prevailing and desirable trait for nurses to have was unquestioning obedience. In today's world, would unquestioning obedience be a violation of ethical principles? Explain.

2. What are your views on genetic profiling?

3. If you were given the opportunity, would you want to know your medical future? Discuss your reasons.

4. What would you do if you found you had a predisposition to Alzheimer's disease, schizophrenia, or other serious or untreatable diseases?

5. Is self-knowledge about our genetic future too much knowledge? Discuss.

6. The Zuckerman and Wilson readings (Articles 27 and 28) have differing views of genetic engineering. Discuss the merits of both points of view. Which is more realistic?

7. If you had the opportunity, would you like to have some parts of your body genetically engineered? Elaborate.

8. How can a government with an inadequate infrastructure and children without vaccinations use public funds to maintain anencephalic infants? Apply ethical principles to both sides of this question.

9. In Article 28, Lamm asserts that most contemporary ethical theories are built around individuals and that as such, these theories are incompatible with maximization of the social good. Using your knowledge of ethical principles, discuss whether this apparent conflict has merit.

10. Imagine you are the governor of your state. You are asked to sign a bill that would continue state funding for the care of a woman who was alive but comatose for 20 years. At the same time, 15% of the residents of your state continue to go without health coverage. What choices are open to you? Discuss your reasoning.

11. What ethical principles would apply in this statement: "Health care rationing should be initiated for all people over 75 years of age."?

12. To what extent have you noticed bias against the aged or a devaluing of people who are old in your health care setting?

Further Readings

Anderson, C.E. (2000). Genetic engineering: Dangers and opportunities. *The Futurist, 34*(2), 20–26.

Caplan, A. (1999). Silence = Disease. *Forbes, 163*(11), 82–84.

Johns, C. (1999). Unravelling the dilemmas within everyday nursing practice. *Nursing Ethics, 6*(4), 287–298.

Kass, L.R. (1999). The moral meaning of genetic technology. *Commentary, 105*(2), 32–38.

Kraft, M.R. (1999). Refusal of treatment: An ethical dilemma. *SCI Nursing, 16*(1), 9–13; 20.

Viens, D. C. (1989). A History of Nursing's Code of Ethics, *Nursing Outlook,* (37)1, 45–49.

Web Site Resources for Ethics

American Bioethics Advisory Commission   www.all.org/abac
Center for Bioethics and Human Dignity   www.cbhd.org
Center for Bioethics—University of Pennsylvania   www.med.upenn.edu/~bioethic
The Ethics Library   www.acusd.edu
Law, Ethics, and End of Life Issues   www.jtgrafx.com/nurselink/law.html
Nursing Ethics Network   www.bc.edu/bc_org/avp/son/nen/nen.html

General Search Engine Web Sites

Google   www.google.com
Savvy Search   www.savvysearch.com

Health Web Sites

Center Watch   www.centerwatch.com/main.htm
Clinical Trials   www.clinicaltrials.com
Discovery Health   www.discoveryhealth.com

Professional Journal Web Sites

MedWebPlus   www.medwebplus.com
National Reference Center for Bioethics Literature
    www.georgetown.edu/research/nrcbl
Nursing Ethics   www.arnoldpublishers.com
The On-Line Journal of Ethics   http://condor.depaul.edu/ethics/ethgl.html

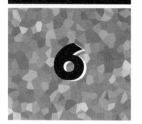

6

Computers, the Internet, and Nursing: Riding the Information Wave

The information revolution began slowly and in stages. Like most revolutions, unrelated events converged, setting into motion an unstoppable force. So it was that ink, paper, and blocks of wood, all discovered at different times and in different countries during the Middle Ages, were brought together in 1457, when Johannes Gutenberg invented the printing press. With the printing of the first Bible, the written word spread beyond monastic libraries and royal palaces. Words became public. And, in the age once darkened by ignorance, fear, and illiteracy, access to information became a reality, knowledge expanded, communication extended, and ideas took flight.

In the centuries that followed, other events propelled the information revolution forward. Typewriters became each person's printing press. Electricity made the radio, telephone, and television possible, and with the click of a switch, information about the world and its events were brought into our homes. Each home became connected to other homes, each community became linked with others, and each country became a lifeline to another.

Now we are in the next stage of the information revolution, one in which the computer and the Internet are major players. The way we think, live, and work are being transformed by a technology whose uses and possibilities are infinite in ways that most of us do not fully comprehend. We are moving along the information superhighway at warp speed, collecting information of astounding proportions. It took Gutenberg months and months of painstaking work to set the type and print the first Bible. Today, we can access it on the computer in seconds, and with e-books, we can hold it in our hands to read. Library research, games, general information, languages, world events, and more are ours with the click of the "mouse."

But the freedom to access and disseminate information through computer technology is not limitless. How it is used is the challenge before us. Issues of privacy, breaches in security, the limits of free speech, the promotion and distribution of violent computer games, and the downloading of unauthorized copyrighted material are already undergoing intense scrutiny and discussion. What are the responsibilities and parameters of this freedom? Where will this unbridled freedom lead us? Will computer and information technology fall prey to anarchy, where anything goes and nothing is sacred? The euphoria of technological innovation must be tempered by our responses to these challenges.

The issues involving the application of computer technology to health care are no less a concern. The timesaving features of technology, the ability to access and coordinate health care data, and the participation of the health care consumer are considerable improvements from past efforts in health care. But while these technological advances have facilitated health care, they provoke other concerns. Of these, one stands out. Are we substituting technological care, in the form of monitoring and surveillance mechanisms, for person-to-person care?

In this chapter, the evolution and use of technology in nursing provides an overview of nurses' adaptation to technological change and the innovations nurses have made in the face of these changes. At the same time, a cautionary note expressing concern is voiced. By using the very technology that has facilitated nursing care, are we running the risk of physically distancing ourselves from our patients? With this overview of how we have adapted to and used technology in the past, the concluding readings offer a sense of what health care technology may be like in the future and how those changes will affect our system of health care. The ride on the information superhighway continues. It will not be dull.

30

"Making the Best of Things": Technology in American Nursing, 1870–1940

Margarete Sandelowski

*I*t has become commonplace in contemporary nursing literature to describe, laud, or lament the impact of technology on nursing.[1] Whether appearing as the main subject matter of a text or only in a passing reference, *technology* is usually depicted as a critical and explanatory event in nursing history. The effect of this is to divide nursing history into two periods: (1) before World War II and (2) after, with the incorporation of "high" or "modern" technology, such as vital function monitoring and assisted ventilation systems. The implication here is either that there was no technology in nursing before the advent of critical or intensive care nursing, or that the impact on nursing of whatever technology existed before the 1960s was essentially unremarkable. Julie Fairman found that nurses who worked in the first special care units in the late 1950s did not think of familiar equipment, such as sphygmomanometers, chest tubes, tracheotomy tubes, and catheters as technology, but rather reserved this term for such new devices as dialysis machines and cardiac monitors.[2] Feminist critics of technology studies have noted a Western and masculinist cultural tendency to think of only the most modern, spectacular, and dramatic equipment (often of primary interest to men) as technology or as significant technology.[3]

The technology that nurses began to incorporate into their practice after World War II was, in many respects, very different from the technology that prevailed in nursing before that time, and it engendered problems, especially ethical dilemmas, for nurses who had not previously encountered it. But there are also important technology issues that have not changed in American nursing history. Nursing concerns about the nature and use of devices and about what devices mean for the care of patients and for the advancement of nursing have not been confined to encounters with "high" technol-

Margarete Sandelowski, Ph.D., R.N., F.A.A.N., is professor and chair, Department of Women's and Children's Health, School of Nursing, University of North Carolina at Chapel Hill, 7460 Carrington Hall, Chapel Hill, North Carolina.

Reprinted with permission of *Nursing History Review*, Official Journal of the American Association for the History of Nursing, 5(1997) 3–22.

ogy. Nurses have always sought to understand and to make the best of the things that have increasingly and paradoxically both defined and blurred the definition of their practice. They have advised and admonished each other about the use and abuse of devices and the problems of simultaneously "nursing the equipment" and nursing the patient.[4] They have also been concerned about how the use of these things has contributed to or detracted from the image of nursing as an academic and caring profession involving intellectual and empathic skills. Indeed, devices have always been central to debates concerning the relationship between the hands and the mind and spirit of the nurse and whether nursing is best understood as primarily an art, a science, or a craft.[5]

In this article, I describe the technology of American nursing and some of the issues and problems nurses encountered around this technology, from the appearance of the first trained nurses in the 1870s to the beginning of World War II. I use the term "technology" to refer primarily to the use of material objects to achieve practical human ends. Although the meaning of technology is historically and culturally "context dependent" and encompasses much more than things,[6] the essence of technology can nevertheless be said to lie in things. The means, ends, and expressions of technology are physical or material.[7] Accordingly, I only allude here to such issues of critical importance in nursing history as the transformation of nursing work and thought and the altered social relations and division of labor resulting from the delegation, or transfer, of technology from medicine to nursing.

Between the 1870s and the 1940s, craft (as opposed to machine or automated) technology prevailed in nursing practice. Craft technology may be differentiated from other technology by the individualized (as opposed to standardized) use of implements that require human energy and direction (as opposed to external sources of energy and direction).[8] Although medical practice in this same time period was transformed by devices such as the thermometer, stethoscope, microscope, and X-ray and electrocardiograph machines, which placed a new emphasis on diagnosis and served to distance physicians from patients,[9] nursing practice (or those techniques nurses performed themselves on their own initiative or under orders from physicians) remained focused on patient comfort and continued to be characterized by techniques and devices that maintained intimate physical contact with patients.[10]

The primary sources I used included advice and instructional literature for nurses (i.e., textbooks and professional journal articles), hospital and training school procedure manuals, medical trade and advertising ephemera, photographs and drawings, and a miscellaneous collection of materials, such as hospital correspondence and student lecture notes. I also had the opportunity to see and handle in museum collections certain implements used in practice in the late nineteenth and early twentieth centuries, such as glass cups and metal scarifiers for wet cupping. Many of the devices used then (e.g., glass thermometers, enema cans with rubber tubing, manually operated beds) were still in use when I began to practice as a nurse in the late 1960s. The secondary sources I used were in the history of nursing and medical technology. Together, these sources offer a basis for understanding continuity and change in the history of technology in nursing, a story that remains largely untold.

■ "COMMON UTENSILS AND APPLIANCES"

From the appearance of the first trained nurses in the 1870s through the 1930s, American nursing practice was largely concerned with providing for the physical needs and comfort of, administering physical therapies to, and managing the physical environment of ailing patients and childbearing women.[11] Nursing work comprised two large categories of techniques. The first category included "in-the-flesh" techniques,[12] such as observation, positioning, and lifting, which involved only (or primarily) nurses' "trained" senses of sight, hearing, smell, and touch; deft and gentle hands; and strong back and limbs. Nurses were taught to cultivate their senses for the close observation that made nursing a scientific profession, as opposed to a merely mechanical practice. Yet their hands were singled out for the development of the manual dexterity and sure, swift, and sensitive touch that made trained nursing indispensable to patients and physicians.[13] Although nurses were cautioned to "use [their] eyes and ears, but not the tongue,"[14] they were to use their voices to soothe patients. Indeed, one of the reasons nurses were initially viewed as ideal to give anesthesia was because the feminine voice calmed the patient for an easier induction; nurse anesthesia was often referred to as "vocal anesthesia."[15] Nursing practice was also physically arduous, requiring nurses to push, pull, lift, and carry heavy patients and objects. In short, the body of the nurse was the critical element in ministering to the body of the patient.

The second category of techniques included the device-mediated procedures, such as medication administration, the application of poultices, catheterization, and purgation, which involved or required the use of a variety of appliances, utensils, implements, and other material objects. Even with the increasing availability of utilities such as electricity and central plumbing, which reduced physical labor, these objects relied for their use largely on the manipulations and muscle power of the nurse. The physical world of the nurse typically involved familiar and everyday objects, or "common utensils and appliances,"[16] generally found in the home and not at all exclusive to nursing or medical care. Indeed, nursing practice included a wide range of household and domestic work and therefore included cooking, housekeeping, and child care crafts.[17] Examples of such everyday objects were the materials, implements, and chemical solutions used for bed-making, bathing, bandaging, feeding, cleaning, and the implementation of various water and mechanical therapies. Watches, safety pins, needles and threads, ice picks, and matches were included among the "equipment of the nurse's bag."[18] Early anesthesia, for which nurses were often largely responsible, involved no more than a "bottle and rag."[19]

The bed, in particular, was portrayed as an object demanding the painstaking attention of the nurse: the "greatest part of her work is around, about, and with the bed,"[20] and patients were often "condemned to weeks of imprisonment in bed."[21] Dozens of kinds of beds were differentiated in instructional texts for nurses according to cases (e.g., surgical versus obstetric), therapeutic intent or purpose (e.g., for resting versus a pelvic examination), and the primary therapeutic modality employed (e.g., air versus water beds).[22] Nurses expressed preferences for what they viewed as the best materials out of which to construct beds (e.g., brass, iron, or wood) and bedding (e.g., linen, straw, rubber) to achieve the various purposes for which they were used and to facilitate maintenance and hygiene. Dozens of kinds of bandages, poultices, and other external remedies, as well as cleansing and therapeutic baths, were also important foci of didactic literature for nurses, with instruction including the materials and containers needed to make, apply, or provide the most functional, effective, and aesthetically pleasing treatment.[23]

Fewer of the objects that nurses used in practice, such as the hypodermic syringe and the urinary catheter, distinctively signaled nursing, or a kind of specialized work. Nurses shared the use of these objects with physicians. Even in the many cases where nurses were the primary and probably (by virtue of greater use) more proficient users of these things and in the better position to determine when and under what conditions they should be used, they were viewed as medical (as opposed to nursing) objects, to be used only by order or under the direction of physicians. In theory, if not actually, nurses worked as agents for physicians. Indeed, physicians viewed nursing care as a kind of medical therapy and increasingly became dependent on nurses to harness the benefits of technological advances in diagnosis, medical therapeutics, anesthesia, and surgery.[24]

The devices nurses typically used in their practice generally extended their (and, nominally, physicians') reach over and into the patient's body. Most nursing practice through the 1930s involved ministrations to the outside of the body, including applications of heat and cold, poultices and dressings, and splints and bandages. Typical courses of training included the application of cups and leeches, dressing bedsores and wounds, and applying friction, fomentations, and other irritants and counterirritants.

Fewer techniques involved the use of devices to enter body orifices, but those that did increasingly characterized nursing as opposed to medical practice. Nurses instilled and removed air and gases, fluids, and substances for various cleansing, nutritional, and other therapeutic purposes. They used inhalers and tents for various kinds of respiratory and oxygen therapies, rubber or glass tubing to suction, gavage, lavage, administer enemas, douche, irrigate, and catheterize. These kinds of bodily entries emphasized the viscerality and "dirty work" of everyday nursing practice,[25] which involved handling human excrement and waste and bound nurses and patients in the most intimate and often embarrassing of human contacts.

Even fewer nursing procedures involved needles, such as the hypodermic injection and hypodermoclysis. Although nurses gave hypodermic injections in the nineteenth century and hypodermoclysis injections in the early twentieth century (both involving insertion of needles in tissue just beneath the skin), it was not until well into the 1930s that it was considered appropriate for a nurse to administer intramuscular injections.[26] Intravenous instillations of substances and the removal of blood remained controversial as nursing functions until well into the 1960s.[27] Many activities that involved deep piercing of the body with a needle or other implement were seen as exclusively in the physician's domain, with nurses only assisting. Yet assistance here typically meant doing everything involved in the procedure except the discrete act of piercing the skin. That is, whether assisting physicians to perform a paracentesis or lumbar puncture or surgery, nurses were expected to have the knowledge to prepare and set up the equipment, prepare the patient and the room, and care for the patient and equipment after the procedure, which included watching for untoward treatment effects and cleaning up. This kind of division of labor, in which nurses did "everything but" (in the case of needle therapies, everything but the act of penetration), often characterized the process by which the use of devices was delegated to nurses. That is, the transfer of technology from medicine to nursing was controlled to maintain a line between medicine and nursing and even the dominance and authority of physicians over nurses.

Because of the design and purposes of the devices nurses commonly used, the kinds of devices available, and the strict controls placed on nurses by physicians, few devices extended either the senses or interpretive capacities of the nurse. That is, few devices entailed an embodiment relationship between nurse and machine,[28] helping them see, hear, or feel better or differently. Nurses did not routinely use such sense extenders as microscopes and stethoscopes. Taking the blood pressure with a sphygmomanometer and stethoscope did not become part of routine nursing practice until the 1930s.[29]

Moreover, few devices entailed hermeneutic relationships with devices.[30] That is, few devices demanded that nurses interpret the texts produced by instruments or machines. When the thermometer first made its way into nursing practice in the late nineteenth century, nurses were only responsible for reading and recording the number registered at the top of the column of mercury. Only physicians were obligated and even deemed capable of interpreting the meaning of that number and initiating clinical action on the basis of that interpretation. Indeed, an argument apparently offered for why it might be acceptable to delegate the use of the thermometer, a medical "instrument of precision,"[31] to nurses was that they would not be distracted by everything physicians knew about the science of clinical thermometry and thus make mistakes in reading it.[32]

■ *"A MANIA FOR ADAPTING AND INVENTING"*

In addition to using familiar household objects and objects exclusive to nursing or medical care, nurses also transformed everyday objects into implements for comfort and healing. They used bedside tables to relieve dyspnea,[33] and they fashioned bed supports out of broom handles.[34] The innovative use of the broom handle not only provided comfort to the patient, but it was also labor-saving; it saved nurses from the physical exertions of tugging and lifting patients who were constantly sliding down in their beds. Moreover, as exemplified by the bedside table and the broom handle, relatively few of the objects nurses used in practice had, or were restricted because of their design to, only one purpose. In the hands of nurses, everyday objects often became "technological objects" in the domain of nursing.[35]

Indeed, a prevailing theme in instructional and advice literature for nurses was the need to improvise and to use their ingenuity in using, fashioning, and transforming existing objects to provide nursing care.[36] Private duty nurses in the home, who were faced with "a deficient supply of things" available to hospital nurses for whom "everything is at hand,"[37] were especially encouraged to improvise and were counseled on how to use the implements they had for a variety of purposes. A 1935 photograph, taken in the home of a Maternity Center Association patient, shows the nurse how to set up a room for a home delivery by making good use of articles normally found there. This improvised room, which featured a soft bed, newspapers, linens, jars, and basins, stood in sharp aesthetic contrast to the hard metal furnishings and equipment shown in a photograph on the next page of a delivery room at New York Hospital.[38] But it demonstrated how nurses could "imitate hospital conditions in the home" by using the "utensils and materials . . . at hand."[39]

Nurses were repeatedly admonished not to waste the resources nor add to the expenses of their patients, no matter whether their patients were economically advantaged or disadvantaged, by having them buy unnecessary implements. Public health nurses, who also had limited access to the latest hospital equipment and for whom "tools [were] as necessary for doing a good piece of public health work as [were] the hundred and one mechanical appliances in a machinist's kit,"[40] were similarly encouraged to use their ingenuity in making and adapting devices in the home.

As one nurse summarized it, nursing involved "making the best of things."[41] With "fire, water, salt, and newspapers, [the nurse] will seldom be embarrassed in any emergency."[42] Instead of a fountain syringe, a nurse could use a funnel and rubber tubing.[43] Instead of forceps, a nurse could use a clothespin. Nurses could refashion teapots and flower sprinklers into enema cans.[44] They could turn miners' pails into stupe kettles.[45] They could use paper bags as inhalers.[46] The "nursing appliances" exhibited at the 1903 meeting of the American Society of Superintendents of Training Schools for Nursing demonstrated the interest nurses had in devices,[47] the value they placed on ingenuity, and even somewhat of "a mania for adapting and inventing."[48] Nurses were encouraged to see the things around them in new ways and not be easily or unnecessarily taken in by the latest inventions. Indeed, it was easy to be seduced by new appliances. One student nurse, on a tour of her hospital in 1930, wrote in her log that the instruments in a sterilization room "took my eye immediately." She found the infant respirator, one of only four such machines in the country, "the most interesting part of the whole trip."[49]

Nurses were encouraged to be inventive by adapting ready-to-hand objects, but they were also, if not as frequently, cautioned not to ignore the inventions that were not so ready to hand and even to invent these kinds of devices themselves. Nurses were invited to publicize their improvisations and inventions. Professional nursing journals, such as the *Trained Nurse* (and later the *Trained Nurse and Hospital Review*) and the *American Journal of Nursing*, regularly featured articles about, photographs and drawings of, and brief written descriptions on the latest "remedies and appliances" either invented for use by nurses or invented by nurses themselves.[50]

Although improvisation constituted an important and often unrecognized kind of invention, nurses were encouraged to move beyond simply making do with what they had and to collaborate with manufacturers to place new inventions of primary usefulness to nurses on the market. The invention and manufacture of the Good Samaritan Infusion Radiator, featured in a 1931 *American Journal of Nursing* article, was offered as an example of the successful collaboration possible between a nurse inventor and manufacturer.[51] The New York City Board of Health adopted another nurse's invention of a new plug for infant bottles.[52]

As one nurse argued, instead of "grumbling" about the inadequacies of hospital furniture, nurses needed to study this furniture with a view toward "chanc[ing] on a remunerative invention."[53] Nurses were intimately concerned with hospital furnishings and were therefore in the best position to create equipment that conserved the time and energy of the nurses (and others) who had to use it. Patients could not be well served if the people around them were struggling with poorly designed equipment. Nurses were advised of the opportunities and even the obligation they had to participate in "original work in the improvement of hospital appliances."[54] There were no persons better suited to this work than the women who daily struggled with the problems and impediments to patient care the poorly designed appliances presented. Indeed, one nurse lamented that, even in hospitals boasting complete operating rooms, X-ray departments, laboratories, and the latest equipment for hydrotherapy and electrotherapy, there was no satisfactory equipment for nursing. Using the same object for different purposes could actually harm patients and impede efficient practice, as when infectious organisms were transferred on basins used for both clean and dirty procedures and when the overuse of devices contributed to their early destruction.[55]

Nurses applauded labor-saving products and utilities, such as the electric pad that warmed solutions to be administered internally to patients, beds and carts with rubber wheels, and a central water supply to fill bathtubs. Much of the nurses' work obliged them to carry heavy objects to and from designated areas while maintaining the proper temperature and cleanliness of these items. As one nurse noted about the electric warming pad, "only nurses who have, quite literally, spent hours in filling and carrying hot water bags intended to keep solutions warm, can appreciate fully the simplicity of this carefully worked-out device."[56]

Although "necessity [was] the mother of invention," nurses had to anticipate needs, rather than wait for "dire necessity" to occur.[57] Not only might nursing invention be impeded by too much improvisation (or too great a readiness to make do), it was also thwarted by the lack of recognition of nurses' contributions to the design of equipment. The "individuality of the inventor [was often] totally lost."[58] Either nurses were unaware of the commercial opportunities available to them or manufacturers deliberately contributed to their ignorance by preferring that "royalties never [be] considered."[59]

■ *"BUY THE BEST"*

Instructional texts for nurses emphasized improvisation, or *making the best of things*, and, less frequently, invention, or *making the best things*. Yet a third emphasis was on *buying the best things*. Instructional, but primarily promotional, literature advised nurses that the effectiveness of their work and their reputation in the eyes of physicians depended, in part, on buying the best equipment. Indeed, as one text addressing the "ethics of nursing" promised: "The doctor will see at a glance if your instruments are just what they should be, that you know how to keep them, and the inference will be that you know how to use them."[60] One physician encouraged nurses in private practice to always buy the best thermometers, scissors, forceps, and dressing instruments. He also suggested adding to nurses' instrument collection manometers (to determine the specific gravity of urine), litmus paper, and an 8-ounce graduated glass measure, since physicians could not carry all of these items from house to house, and it was easier for the nurse to include them as part of her outfit.[61]

Attention was given in didactic literature to the devices that should be included in the nurse's outfit, nursing bag, or pocket case.[62] Advertising literature also featured such containers. For example, the Chicago Nurse's Case (made of the "best Morocco leather" and selling for $10), shown in a 1918 catalog of surgical instruments and supplies, included vials, glass syringes and needles, forceps, thermometer, scissors, knife, probes and directors, baby scales, metal and rubber catheters, a scarifier, and razor.[63] Outfits including such items were promoted as suitable gifts for nurses.[64]

Promotional literature also included testimonials by nurses on behalf of the thermometers and other implements they favored. In 1914, in the third edition of her popular nursing text, Clara Weeks-Shaw described the clinical thermometer as "this now familiar instrument [that] is indispensable to every nurse."[65] Becton, Dickinson, and Company (B-D) featured the B-D Clinical Thermometer as the one having "found much favor among the Nursing Profession."[66] Judson Pin Company advertised the Capsheaf Safety Pin as "highly endorsed by trained nurses."[67] Meinecke and Company printed a nurse's testimonial for their Ideal Douche Pan.[68] The Lister Surgical Company claimed that nurses who used Lister's Towels preferred them to any other pads for women.[69] These advertisements, placed in nursing journals, made nurses aware of products to buy (or to recommend to physicians and hospitals for purchasing). A note from the "Publisher's Desk" of the *Trained Nurse and Hospital Review* encouraged nurses to send for samples of the products they saw advertised in the journal. Assured that the journal permitted only advertisements of reputable products, nurses were encouraged to see these ads as being as "valuable" as the other reading matter in the journal.[70]

The advertisements also appealed directly to nurses by emphasizing the value of their products for both patient comfort and safety and nursing efficiency. Moreover, they offer clues about the problems devices themselves may have posed for nurses in practice. For example, a B-D ad for clinical thermometers suggested problems with reading the markings, resetting the mercury, and preventing breakage.[71] A Taylor Instrument Companies ad, showing a drawing of a nurse with a thermometer in a Tycos Safety Case pinned to her apron, suggested that nurses often lost thermometers.[72] Judson Pin Company promised nurses a safety pin that "cannot catch in the fabric."[73] The Lister Surgical Company promised a gynecological towel that was more absorbent, did not need to be washed, and, in general, saved "time, money, and annoyance."[74] Meinecke and Company's douche pan was "ideal" because (by virtue of being "anatomically correct in shape") it did "not hurt," had a "capacious interior," and was easy to maintain "in a sanitary condition."[75]

Medical trade catalogs, although largely oriented toward the physician consumer, promoted products that solved problems nurses had in promoting patient comfort and safety and that promised to make practice safer, less laborious, and even more aesthetically pleasing. Becton, Dickinson, and Company, in their 1918 *Physician Catalog*, advertised the HY-JEN-IC thermometer as filling the requirements of nurses (and others) whenever "economy is a factor," and the Olympian thermometer as popular with nurses (and others) "preferring strength, legibility, and 'easy shakers' to quick registration."[76] Greeley Laboratories promised to meet and conquer common objections to administering medicines via hypodermic injection. These objections were caused by poorly designed syringes and needles that became clogged, stuck, slipped, leaked, and permitted breaks in aseptic technique.[77] In the Hospital Supply Company of New York 1913 *Catalogue of Sterilizers,* ad copy acknowledged the "unjustifiably disagreeable duty on nurses" to make do with the "obnoxious prevailing method of emptying bed pans into open sinks." The Climax Combined Bedpan Sterilizer and Washer made this job less disagreeable and reduced hospital odors.[78] The same company advertised the Climax Dressing Sterilizer as preventing injury to the nurse because of poor design. As pictured and described in the ad, the nurse used to be forced to "pass her arm past a hot Sterilizer and manipulate the valves in the constricted space between the apparatus and the wall."[79] A new design feature eliminated this potential hazard.

■ *"NURSING THE EQUIPMENT"*

Nurses regularly discussed the problems they encountered in using devices, whether they were as simply constructed as rubber tubing or as complex an apparatus as an oxygen tent. A procedure involving as ostensibly simple a device as the rubber tube used for an enema or colonic irrigation could be hazardous to patients and a problem for nurses; hard tips could puncture delicate membranes and rubber goods were difficult to clean and preserve.[80]

Nurses described the many nursing problems, ignored in the medical literature, that oxygen therapy caused. Physicians might order this therapy, but nurses had to administer it. That is, they had to find ways to maintain the appropriate dose or concentration of oxygen in a tent or chamber while simultaneously providing other kinds of care that allowed oxygen to escape, as when nurses bathed patients.[81] Although many of the objects nurses used routinely in practice were simply constructed, they were not necessarily simple to use and did not produce simple outcomes. As one prominent nurse author observed, applying a compress to the eyes might appear simple, but the patients' eyesight was still at stake.[82] An ostensibly simple device such as a glass thermometer was much more complicated than it seemed. Formal analyses of nursing tasks, which became increasingly common in the 1920s and 1930s, showed the complexity of even the most "elementary nursing procedures."[83]

Devices were increasingly central components of these procedures, making "nursing the equipment" as important in practice as nursing the patient.[84] Didactic texts typically emphasized the articles required for procedures both the nurse and physician performed, including the increasingly equipment-embodied domains of physical and laboratory diagnosis, surgery, anesthesia, and orthopedics. They also emphasized the before and after care of equipment, which involved selecting and then arranging devices on trays; cleaning, disinfecting, or sterilizing equipment; mending and otherwise maintaining the integrity of equipment; and preventing their destruction. A key feature of instructional literature and visual displays was the variety of specialized "trays" of equipment for the procedures nurses performed themselves or for those they assisted physicians to perform.[85] Nurses also held positions as keepers of equipment in central supply rooms in hospitals.

Nurses were evaluated not only on their technical abilities, but also on their "appreciation of equipment."[86] A nurse could be judged as extravagant and as misusing equipment. The breaking of glass syringes required a written incident report. The need to preserve glass thermometers inspired friendly rivalry among wards as to which ward had the lowest incidence of breakage.[87] In an effort to "teach care of hospital equipment," some hospitals had bulletin boards displaying the number of various devices used and destroyed in a year, how they were ruined, and the cost to replace them.[88] In the era before the widespread use of disposable devices, nurses had to develop a reverence for the things they used, if only for the sake of economy.

Nurses were also to use devices in ways that contributed to their professional mission of creating an environment most conducive to patient recovery. For example, one nurse advised that medical and surgical appliances ought not to be visible in the sick room.[89] Nurses were also concerned with the noise caused by handling the glass- and enamelware that constituted many of the devices they used.[90]

■ CONCLUSION: THE "WORLD OF THE TOOL"

Technological devices are a source of information about both the empirical and aesthetical dimensions, or content and form, of nursing practice.[91] These devices also entail different kinds of human engagements with and experiences of the world.[92] Indeed, the diversity of the devices used by nurses over time has in part shaped the world in which nurses practice.

The "world of the tool" in which nurses practiced prior to World War II seems to have entailed a very different engagement with technology than the "world of the screen" in which nurses now practice.[93] In the older world of the tool, nurses were typically preoccupied with the manual complexities and even physical labor of manipulating simply constructed yet often unyielding, fragile, and hard-to-clean items. They were also concerned with the artful and scientifically principled integration of these devices into nursing care. Yet for all the difficulties they encountered in bending sometimes unpliable items to their will, nurses seemed to have a close and, by necessity, hands-on relationship with the tools of their trade, which, in turn, kept them in close physical contact with their patients. While physicians were increasingly looking at their patients through microscopes and X rays, listening to them through stethoscopes, and interpreting their conditions via laboratory assays and electrocardiograms, nurses continued to maintain more direct sensory and other physical contact with their patients.

In contrast, in the contemporary world of the screen, nurses appear more physically removed from both patient and machine. They are increasingly preoccupied with the hermeneutic complexity of interpreting machine-generated texts (such as rhythm strips on monitor screens or numerical data in digital displays and computer printouts). Instead of problems of hand manipulation, the technology making up the world of the screen poses largely interpretive problems of distinguishing true representations from artifactual misrepresentations of patient conditions. Instead of the tool-world problem of too much physical manipulation or touching, screen technology seems to have created the new problem of not literally and figuratively touching patients enough or in the right way. Technology no longer seems to incorporate the touch of the nurse so much as it stands in physical and even paradigmatic opposition to it.[94] Although more detailed investigation is needed in the history of technology in nursing to warrant any conclusions about continuity and change, in the world of the screen, devices appear heavy because of the epistemological and even moral freight they carry. Technology now often appears at odds with the mission and ethic of nursing care. In the world of the tool, devices often seemed to be just plain heavy or hard to handle.

The renewed call for nurses to invent equipment, to forge relationships with engineers, and to be better educated concerning the making and using of devices evokes the earlier call for nurses to adapt, invent, and reinvent the world to promote nursing goals.[95] There is still the concern that nurses, because of knowledge deficits in the engineering, physical, and other scientific and technological principles and theories underlying the operations of devices, are leaving the design and development of the material world of practice to others less equipped to understand that world. In the modern calls for technological expertise, we can still hear the invitation to nurses to make the best of things, for themselves and for the patients in their care.

This study was supported by a Lillian Sholtis Brunner Fellowship from the Center for the Study of the History of Nursing at the University of Pennsylvania in Philadelphia. I am especially grateful to Joan Lynaugh, director of the center, for her astute advice and gentle counsel, and to Margo Szabunia, curator, and Betsy Weiss, administrative assistant, at the center for facilitating access to relevant collections. I also gratefully acknowledge the assistance of Gretchen Worden, curator at the Mutter Museum, and John Parker, reference assistant, Charles Greifenstein, reference librarian, and Keven Crawford, manuscript curator, at the Historical Services Division of the Library of the College of Physicians of Philadelphia.

Notes

1. See, for example, Carolyn Cooper, "The Intersection of Technology and Care in the ICU," *Advances in Nursing Sciences* 15, no. 3 (1993): 23–32; Sally Gadow, "Touch and Technology: Two Paradigms of Patient Care," *Journal of Religion and Health* 23, no. 1 (1984): 63–69; Virginia Henderson, "The Essence of Nursing in High Technology," *Nursing Administration Quarterly* 9, no. 4 (1985): 1–9; G. Laing, "The Impact of Technology on Nursing," *Medical Instrumentation* 16, no. 5 (1982):

241–42; Margarete Sandelowski, "A Case of Conflicting Paradigms: Nursing and Reproductive Technology," *Advances in Nursing Science* 10, no. 3 (1988): 34–45; J. K. Schultz, "Nursing and Technology," *Medical Instrumentation* 14, no. 4 (1980): 211–14; and Sallie Tisdale, "Swept Away by Technology," *American Journal of Nursing* 86, no. 4 (1986): 429–30 (hereafter cited as *AJN*).

2. Julie Fairman, "Watchful Vigilance: Nursing Care, Technology, and the Development of Intensive Care Units," *Nursing Research* 41, no. 1 (1992): 56–60.

3. Autumn Stanley, *Mothers and Daughters of Invention: Notes for a Revised History of Technology* (New Brunswick, N.J.: Rutgers University Press, 1995), xxxi-xxxii, and Judy Wajcman, *Feminism Confronts Technology* (University Park: Pennsylvania State University, 1991), 16–17, 137.

4. M. R. Smith, "What Are We Doing to Improve Nursing Practice, II: Through Improvement of Nursing Methods," *AJN* 32, no. 6 (1932): 685–88. Quote on p. 687.

5. See, for example, Mary M. Roberts, "Modification of Nursing Procedures as Demanded by Progress in Medicine," *Hospital Progress* 12, no. 9 (1931): 390–93, and Isabel M. Stewart, "The Science and Art of Nursing," *The Nursing Education Bulletin* 2, no. 1 (1929): 1–4.

6. Carl Mitcham, *Thinking Through Technology: The Path Between Engineering and Philosophy* (Chicago: University of Chicago Press, 1994), 152.

7. Brooke Hindle, "The Exhilaration of Early American Technology: An Essay," in *Early American Technology: Making and Doing Things from the Colonial Era to 1850*, ed. Judith A. McGraw (1966: reprint, Chapel Hill: University of North Carolina Press, 1994), 40–48.

8. Mitcham, 162, and I. R. McWhinney, "Medical Knowledge and the Rise of Technology," *The Journal of Medicine and Philosophy* 3, no. 4 (1978): 293–304.

9. See Audrey B. Davis, *Medicine and Its Technology: An Introduction to the History of Medical Instrumentation* (Westport, Conn.: Greenwood Press, 1981); Joel D. Howell, ed., *Technology and American Medical Practice, 1880–1930: Anthology of Sources* (New York: Garland Press, 1988); Stanley J. Reiser, *Medicine Reign of Technology* (Cambridge, U.K.: Cambridge University Press, 1978).

10. As itemized in Ethel Johns and Blanche Pfefferkorn, *An Activity Analysis of Nursing* (New York: Committee on the Grading of Nursing Schools, 1934) 150–66, even with the increasing use of electric power, the vast majority of devices nurses used in this period were nurse powered. See also Theodore J. Berry, *The Bryn Mawr Hospital, 1893–1968* (Bryn Mawr, Pa.: Bryn Mawr Hospital, 1969), 132–42; Kathleen H. McIlveen and Janice M. Morse, "The Role of Comfort in Nursing Care: 1900–1980," *Clinical Nursing Research* 4, no. 2 (1995): 127–48; and Ruth Sleeper, "The Two Inseparables: Nursing Service and Nursing Education," *AJN* 48, no. 11 (1948): 678–81.

11. See, for example, *A Handbook of Nursing for Family and General Use* (New Haven: Connecticut Training School for Nurses, 1878); *A Manual of Nursing Prepared for the Training School for Nurses Attached to Bellevue Hospital* (New York: Putnam, 1878); Annual Report, January 1878, Records of Woman's Hospital of Philadelphia, Center for the Study of the History of Nursing, University of Pennsylvania School of Nursing (hereafter cited as CSHN); Carolyn V. Van Blarcom, *Obstetrical Nursing*, 1st–3d eds. (New York: Macmillan, 1922, 1928, and 1936); Joseph B. DeLee, *Obstetrics for Nurses*, 5th and 10th eds. (Philadelphia: W. B. Saunders, 1917 and 1933); Joseph B. DeLee and Mabel C. Carmon, *Obstetrics for Nurses*, 11th ed. (Philadelphia: W. B. Saunders, 1937); Minnie Goodnow, *The Technic of Nursing*

(Philadelphia: W. B. Saunders, 1928); Isabel A. Hampton, *Nursing: Its Principles and Practice*, 2d ed. (Cleveland: E. C. Koeckert, 1903); Bertha Harmer, *Textbook of the Principles and Practice of Nursing*, 1st–3d eds. (New York: Macmillan, 1922, 1928, 1934); Bertha Harmer and Virginia Henderson, *Textbook of the Principles and Practice of Nursing*, 4th ed. (New York: Macmillan, 1939); Anna C. Maxwell and Amy E. Pope, *Practical Nursing: A Textbook for Nurses*, 2d ed., rev. (New York: Putnam, 1910); Clara S. Weeks-Shaw, *A Textbook of Nursing: For the Use of Training Schools, Families, and Private Students*, 3d ed. (New York: D. Appleton and Company, 1914); and Henry L. Woodard and Bernice Gardner, *Obstetric Management and Nursing* (Philadelphia: F. A. Davis, 1936).

12. I borrowed this phrase from Don Ihde, *Technics and Praxis* (Boston: Dordrecht, 1979), 18.

13. See, for example, Harmer (1922), 7, 45; *Nursing Procedures*, Philadelphia General Hospital School of Nursing, 1924, p. 120, CSHN; Lecture no. 1, 1902, p. 4, Chautauqua School of Nursing Lecture Notes, CSHN.

14. Lecture, 17 November 1887, Mary U. Clymer Papers, CSHN.

15. Maurine Ligon, "Psychology and Suggestive Therapy in Anesthesia," *Trained Nurse and Hospital Review* 96, no. 3 (1936): 260–62. Quote on p. 260.

16. Marie Koeneke, *Nursing Procedures: The Lankenau Hospital*, 1927, Lankenau Hospital School of Nursing Records, CSHN.

17. As noted on p. 470 in the editorial "Anybody Can Nurse!" *Trained Nurse and Hospital Review* 105, no. 6 (1940): 470–72, nursing practice did not lend itself to definite lines of demarcation, with some tasks bordering on housework while others absorbed the latest medical techniques, such as blood transfusions.

18. Emily A. M. Stoney, *Practical Points in Nursing for Nurses in Private Practice*, 2d ed. (Philadelphia: W. B. Saunders, 1897), 25.

19. Martin S. Pernick, *A Calculus of Suffering: Pain, Professionalism, and Anesthesia in Nineteenth-Century America* (New York: Columbia University Press, 1985), 223.

20. Harmer (1922), 33.

21. Lecture no. 13, circa 1904, p. 4, Chautauqua School of Nursing Lecture Notes, CSHN.

22. Forty-three varieties of beds and bed-making were listed in an unpublished study referred to in Johns and Pfefferkorn, 25.

23. See, for example, citations listed in note 11 above and K. L. Milligan, "Bandaging," *Trained Nurse and Hospital Review* 41, no. 5 (1908): 299–302; E. M. Simpson, "The Bath as a Healing Agent," *AJN* 3, no. 5 (1903): 333–37.

24. William R. Houston, *The Art of Treatment* (New York: Macmillan, 1937). See also Jo Ann Ashley, *Hospitals, Paternalism, and the Role of the Nurse* (New York: Teachers College Press, 1976); Joan E. Lynaugh and Claire M. Fagin, "Nursing Comes of Age," *Image: Journal of Nursing Scholarship* 20, no. 4 (1988): 184–90; and Barbara Melosh, *"The Physician's Hand": Work Culture and Conflict in American Nursing* (Philadelphia: Temple University Press, 1982).

25. Nurses do "dirty work" in the literal and sociological sense, as introduced in Everett C. Hughes, *Men and Their Work* (Glencoe, Ill.: Free Press, 1958), 49–53.

26. See, for example, Harmer (1928), 448–68; Harmer and Henderson (1939), 565–97; and Bertha Harmer and Virginia Henderson, *Textbook of the Principles and Practice of Nursing*, 5th ed. (New York: Macmillan, 1955), 712–65.

27. See, for example, J. R. Anderzon, "Emerging Nursing Techniques: Venipuncture," *Nursing Clinics of North America*, 3, no. 1 (1968): 165–78; Jules K. Joseph, "Should

We Permit Qualified Nurses to Administer Intravenous Therapy?" *Hospital Management* 64, no. 1 (1947): 65–68; "Nursing Practice and Intravenous Therapy," *AJN* 56, no. 5 (1956): 572–73; "Should Nurses Do Venipunctures?" *AJN* 51, no. 10 (1951): 603–4; J. A. Willan, "How the States Stand on IV Administration by Nurses," *Hospital Topics* 40, no. 7 (1962): 41–45.

28. For a fuller explanation of embodied human-machine relations, see Ihde (1979) and Don Ihde, *Existential Technics* (Albany: State University of New York Press, 1983) and *Technology and the Lifeworld: From Garden to Earth* (Bloomington: Indiana University Press, 1990).

29. See the Harmer and the Harmer and Henderson series of textbooks cited above in note 11. The Philadelphia General Hospital School of Nursing included this technique for the first time in their 1948 procedure book. See *Nursing Procedures*, 1948, p. 40, Philadelphia General Hospital School of Nursing, CSHN.

30. For a fuller explanation of hermeneutic human-machine relations, see Ihde (1979, 1983, 1990).

31. S. Weir Mitchell, *The Early History of Instrumental Precision in Medicine*, an address before the Second Congress of the American College of Physicians and Surgeons, 23 September 1891 (New Haven, Conn.: Tuttle, Morehouse, and Taylor, 1892).

32. Reiser, 117.

33. Harmer (1922), 59.

34. "A Practical Point," *Trained Nurse and Hospital Review* 40, no. 1 (1908): 17.

35. Ihde (1990), 70.

36. See, for example, Lyla M. Olson, *Improvised Equipment: In the Home Care of the Sick*, 1st–3d eds. (Philadelphia: W. B. Saunders, 1928, 1933, 1939); A. H. Ross, "Ingenuity and Private Nursing," *AJN* 5, no. 12 (1905): 873–75; Emma V. Skillman, "Improvisations in Private Duty Nursing," *AJN* 26, no. 4 (1926): 269–70; and Stoney.

37. Lecture, 17 November 1887, Mary U. Clymer Papers, CSHN.

38. Louise Zabriskie, *Mother and Baby Care in Pictures* (Philadelphia: J. B. Lippincott, 1935), 64–65.

39. DeLee and Carmon, 19.

40. Louise B. Nichols, "For the Limited Budget," *Public Health Nurse* 20, no. 8 (1928): 416–18.

41. E. M. Rice, "Making the Best of Things," *Trained Nurse and Hospital Review* 41, no. 1 (1908): 22–24.

42. Ibid., 24.

43. Ross, 874.

44. Olson (1939), 100.

45. Pauline Carlson, "The Evolution of a Stupe Kettle," *AJN* 37, no. 6 (1937): 584–85.

46. As shown in *AJN* 26, no. 11 (1926): 846.

47. Carolyn C. Van Blarcom, "Appliances Exhibited at the Meeting of the American Society of Superintendents of Training Schools for Nurses in Pittsburgh," *AJN* 4, nos. 6 and 9 (1904): 436–37, 681–84.

48. Ross, 875.

49. Log, 4 November 1930, Charlotte Tyson Rath Papers, CSHN.

50. See, for example, the picture of a practical croup tent, shown on p. 472, *AJN* 26, no. 6 (1926); E. Berends, "An Improvised Funnel," *Trained Nurse and Hospital Review* 96, no. 3 (1936): 223; and, N. E. Cadmus, "Some Hospital Devices and Procedures," *AJN* 16, no. 7 (1916): 589–605.

51. M. Theodore, "The Good Samaritan Infusion Radiator," *AJN* 31, no. 11 (1931): 1267–68.

52. "An Interesting Device," *AJN* 26, no. 4 (1926): 280.

53. Martha M. Russell, "Hospital Furnishings," *AJN* 26, no. 11 (1926): 841–46. Quote on p. 841.

54. Nancy P. Ellicott, "Opportunities for Original Work in the Improvement of Hospital Appliances," *AJN* 14, no. 10 (1914): 843–45.

55. Amy M. Hilliard, "Equipment for Nursing Procedures," *AJN* 21, no. 7 (1921): 728–31.

56. Mary L. Duchesne, "A Labor-Saving Device," *AJN* 23, no. 3 (1923): 470–71. Quote on p. 472.

57. Ellicott, 845.

58. Ibid., 844.

59. Ibid., 843.

60. "Ethics of Nursing, No. IV: The Doctor," *The Trained Nurse* 3, no. 1 (1889): 80–85. Quote on p. 85.

61. P. C. Remondino, "The Trained Nurse in Private Practice," *The Trained Nurse* 32, no. 2 (1904): 77–82.

62. See, for example, "Bag Equipment for Rural Nursing," *Public Health Nurse* 21, no. 7 (1929): 352; J. E. Hitchcock, "The Story of Our Bag," *Public Health Nursing* 27, no. 1 (1935): 29–31; Ruth W. Hubbard, "Bag Technic and the Hourly Nurse," *AJN* 28, no. 6 (1928): 557–59.

63. Frank S. Betz Company, *Surgical Instruments and Supplies*, 1918, p. 37, Medical Trade Ephemera Collection, College of Physicians of Philadelphia (hereafter cited as MTEC).

64. See the ad for a "nurse's outfit" on the back of the March 1929 table of contents in *AJN* 29, nos. 1–6 (1929).

65. Weeks-Shaw, 58.

66. See the ad for B-D Clinical Thermometers in *Trained Nurse and Hospital Review* 66, no. 1 (1921): 73.

67. See the ad for Capsheaf Safety Pin in *Trained Nurse and Hospital Review* 35, no. 6 (1905).

68. See the ad for the "Ideal" Douche Pan, *Trained Nurse and Hospital Review* 32 (1904).

69. See the ad for Lister's Towels, *Trained Nurse and Hospital Review* 33, no. 6 (1904).

70. "Publisher's Desk," *Trained Nurse and Hospital Review* 32, no. 2 (1904): 152.

71. See note 66 above.

72. See the ad for Tycos Fever Thermometer, *Trained Nurse and Hospital Review* (1915).

73. See note 67 above.

74. See note 69 above.

75. See note 68 above.

76. Becton, Dickinson, and Company, *Physician Catalog*, 1918, p. 14, MTEC.

77. Greeley Laboratories, *Greeley Hypodermic Unit*, circa 1906, p. 8, MTEC.

78. Hospital Supply Company of New York, *Catalogue of Sterilizers*, 1913, p. 41, MTEC.

79. Ibid., 10.

80. See, for example, G. W. Aurt, "Perforation of the Rectum With Enema Tips," *Transactions—American Proctologic Society* 40 (1 September 1939): 203–13; and

H. H. Rayner, "Injury of the Rectum Caused by the Faulty Administration of an Enema," *British Medical Journal* 1 (5 March 1932): 419–21.

81. See, for example, Harmer and Henderson (1939), 603, and Margaret J. Hawthorne et al., "Oxygen Therapy: A Study in Some Nursing Aspects of the Operation of an Oxygen Tent," *AJN* 38, no. 11 (1938): 1203–16.

82. Harmer (1928), vi.

83. See, for example, Martha E. Erdmann and Margaret Welsh, "Studies in Thermometer Technique," *Nursing Education Bulletin* 2, no. 1 (1929): 8–33; S. M. Therese, "Why the Nurse Needs Sound Education: Analysis of Elementary Nursing Procedures," *Trained Nurse and Hospital Review* 95, no. 6 (1935): 557–62.

84. Smith, 687.

85. See, for example, the Harmer and the Harmer and Henderson textbooks cited in note 11 above; "Comparative Nursing Methods: Lumbar Puncture, Hypodermoclysis, and Intravenous Infusion Trays," *AJN* 30, no. 3 (1930): 253–60; Photo Collection of Equipment Trays and *Procedure Books,* 1924–1954, Philadelphia General Hospital School of Nursing, CSHN; "Student Experience Record of Central Surgical Service," 1935, Albert Einstein Medical Center (formerly Jewish Hospital) School of Nursing Records, CSHN.

86. "Evaluation of Nursing Care," 1935, Albert Einstein Medical Center School of Nursing Records, CSHN.

87. Harriet M. Gillette, "A Practical Thermometer Tray," *AJN* 26, no. 11 (1926): 840.

88. Charlotte J. Garrison, "Teaching Care of Hospital Equipment," *AJN* 27, no. 10 (1927): 823–26.

89. Weeks-Shaw, 16.

90. See, for example, "Bulletin," 1936, Albert Einstein Medical Center School of Nursing Records, CSHN, and the note on "noisiness," *The Trained Nurse* 2, no. 1 (1888): 27.

91. I. Katims, "Nursing as Aesthetic Experience and the Notion of Practice," *Scholarly Inquiry for Nursing Practice* 7, no. 4 (1993): 269–78; and H. Schnadelbach, "Is Technology Ethically Neutral?" in *Ethics in an Age of Pervasive Technology,* ed. Melvin Kranzberg (Boulder, Colo.: Westview Press, 1980), 28–30.

92. Ihde (1979, 1983, 1990).

93. Mitcham, 191.

94. See, for example, Leah L. Curtin, "Nursing: High-Touch in a High-Tech World," *Nursing Management* 15, no. 7 (1984): 7–8, and Sally Gadow, "Touch and Technology: Two Paradigms of Patient Care," *Journal of Religion and Health* 23, no. 1 (1984): 63–69.

95. See, for example, June C. Abbey and Marvin D. Shepherd, "Nursing and Technology: Moving into the 21st Century," *Dean's Notes* 10, no. 3 (1989): 1–2; Marianne Neighbors and Evelyn E. Eldred, "Technology and Nursing Education," *Nursing and Health Care* 14, no. 2 (1993): 96–99; and "Nursing and Technology: Redefining Relationships," *Biomedical Instrumentation and Technology* 25, no. 2 (1991): 89–98.

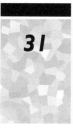

31

Looking to Care or Caring to Look?
Technology and the Rise
of Spectacular Nursing

Margarete Sandelowski

It is she who watches over the sick. . . . It is she who stands watch while the sick sleep.[1(p31)]

Ever since Florence Nightingale[2] established observation as the habit and faculty that legitimize the need for trained nurses, nursing has been synonymous with watchful care,[3] that is, with looking for signs of improvement or decline in patient health and with looking after patient safety, comfort, and well-being. Nightingale promoted nursing observation as the artful corrective to the scientific "averages,"[2] which threatened to seduce physicians into believing that they knew their patients. Arguably, the most enduring and evocative image of nursing is the "lady with the lamp," an eternally and quintessentially nurturing woman who, with the illumination from a candle, watches out for her patients against the encroaching shadows of sickness and the permanent darkness of death.

This lady (and her gentleman nursing counterpart) now have devices other than the candle to help them see the patients in their charge. Owing largely to technologies such as ultrasonography, cardiac and fetal monitoring, and the critical care unit, which offer humans new ways to look and new things to see, the nature of this watchful care has changed considerably over the years and, with it, the caring practices of the nurse. Nursing care is now more spectacular. In this article, I consider the nature of the intersection of these visualist technologies and care in the rise of spectacular nursing, a new kind of "hands-off"[4] nursing practice dominated by instrumentally mediated watchful care. I also consider the implications of spectacular nursing for holistic practice, that is, for a kind of nursing that unites biology and biography in the interests of "rounded understandings"[5] and treatments of patients.

Margarete Sandelowski, Ph.D., R.N., F.A.A.N., is professor and chair, Department of Women's and Children's Health, School of Nursing, University of North Carolina at Chapel Hill, Chapel Hill, North Carolina.

Reprinted with permission from *Holistic Nursing Practice*, *12*(4) 1–11, 1998, Aspen Publishers, Inc. © 1998.

■ *NEW VISUALITIES*

Like other members of their culture, Western nurses live in a "society of the spectacle," a time and place where images increasingly rule and their referents increasingly fade from view.[6] Indeed, contemporary culture "consists in the images [that] make the imagination possible [and] in the media [that] mediate experience."[7(p33)] Spectacular technologies, such as ultrasonography, cardiac and fetal monitoring, computed tomography (CT), and mammography, are not simply tools for diagnosis and screening but also mass media, which, like television, movies, and print advertising, re-present, create, and advertise realities for the viewing public. These media technologies do not enable viewers to see an objective reality so much as change what and how viewers see; they also require humans to learn to see in new ways as they produce images unnatural to the eye.[8] These technologies do not reveal or reflect a fixed nature but rather render a new nature, especially for the human eye. Philosopher Ihde[9] described the "instrumental reality" produced by visualist technologies that Westerners now take to be more real than the directly sensed reality they have replaced.

In the case of fetal ultrasonography, what viewers make out of the sonogram includes meanings as diverse as the viewers themselves. To obstetric clinicians, what is imaged is the fetal patient. To researchers, what is imaged is the source of fetal tissue for experimentation. To expectant parents, what is imaged is their "ultrasound baby."[10] To antiabortion proponents, what is imaged is human life.[11,12] Sonographic viewers must be taught to see the animate in the inanimate; more ominously, they must be programmed to see a yawning fetus in an ultrasound image even though it more closely resembles a grinning skeleton than a sleepy baby.[13]

Indeed, nurses are often unaware of the full extent to which they are bombarded by simulations and representations of the real and to which their knowing is informed by postmodern "visualities."[13] These technologies are themselves a way of knowing in nursing and part of a new nursing informatics.[14]

■ *FROM FLESH TO TEXT: A BRIEF HISTORY OF NURSING OBSERVATION*

For most of American-trained nursing, from 1873 and the opening of the first training schools for nursing in the United States to the 1950s, nursing observation was largely an embodied relation with patients in which nurses relied on their trained senses, principally sight, touch, and smell.[15] Indeed, the trained nurse (typically conceived as female) was characterized by the "trained senses" she directed toward the "close observation" that elevated nursing above "mechanical, routine, nonintelligent practice and place[d] it upon a scientific, professional basis."[16(p45)] "Knowing the patient"[17] (now a watchword in nursing often used to support nursing claims to uniqueness in perspective and value and to holistic practice) used to mean, in large part, knowing the patient in the flesh. Nursing was primarily an intimate, corporeal relation involving the physical bodies of patients and the senses and physical exertions of nurses. Listening to patients, in the sense of making space for their stories and knowing them "by heart" as well as "by sight,"[18] had yet to become an integral part of the rhetoric or fabric of the nurse-patient relationship.[19] Indeed, Nightingale[2] viewed too much talking on the part of patients as physically taxing and, therefore, an indication of poor nursing practice.

If nurses used any devices at all to observe their patients before the 1960s, they were more likely to use them in the service of physician observation and medical intervention than nursing care per se. Sharp lines were still drawn between nursing care and medical cure,[20] with nursing care being conceived as, or in the service of, medical cure.[21] When thermometers were first introduced into clinical practice in the latter half of the 19th century, nurses were charged with taking and recording patient temperature, not with interpreting it.[15] When nurses began to use stethoscopes and sphygmomanometers regularly in the 1930s to ascertain blood pressure, they were delegated the use of these devices largely to serve physician diagnosis. Nurses were seen, and largely saw themselves, as the eyes and ears of physically absent physicians. Nurses performed much of the labor associated with new technologies for observing patients, but physicians acquired most of the cultural prestige because these technologies were seen to represent advances in scientific medicine and to legitimize physicians' captaincy of the health care ship.[22,23]

Beginning in the 1960s, with the advent of machine monitoring in clinical nursing practice, nursing observation increasingly included what Ihde[24,25] described as hermeneutic relations with devices. Hermeneutic human-machine relations entail that humans "read," or interpret, device-generated "texts," such as rhythm strips and digital displays, as opposed to gathering information directly from the senses. Knowing the patient, whether in the critical care unit, the labor room, or the home, increasingly meant reading, and then acting on, the conclusions drawn from machine-generated texts. This kind of knowing entailed a new kind of "hands-off"[4] care, in contrast to the classic hands-on contact with the physical body.[26] (The traditional mercury thermometer also entails a hermeneutic human-machine relation in that inferences about temperature are drawn from reading the number linked to the height of a column of mercury as opposed to touching a patient's brow to ascertain fever.)

Whether nurses after 1960 engaged in hermeneutic or any other kind of relations with the "new machinery"[27] for nurse purposes is still a debatable point. Indeed, some scholars have argued that technologic innovations in medicine expanded the sphere of influence and elevated the status of nursing. In contrast, others have argued that these same innovations only expanded the sphere of responsibility of nursing[28] and offered what Parker called a "vicarious status"[29] no different from the subordinate one nursing had always held vis-à-vis medicine. Instead of being handmaidens, or extensions of the physical capacities of physicians, nurses became physicians' assistants, or human extensions of their technology. Nurses were still the eyes and ears of physicians, albeit at the end of devices.

■ SHE'S GOT THE LOOK: SURVEILLANCE AS NURSING INTERVENTION

No matter whether nurses were using new diagnostic and screening technologies for nursing or medical purposes, after 1960 knowing patients increasingly meant monitoring them or keeping them under technologic surveillance. (I do not consider here other kinds of non–device-mediated extensions of nursing observation into the inner life of patients as private subjects involving the mind, emotions, spirit, and overall personhood of the patient.[19,30] This kind of watching is not referred to as surveillance in nursing literature, although it is so designated in critical studies of medicine and health care.[31]) *Surveillance* is a relatively new term in nursing that implies a kind of watchful nursing care very different from the embodied observation that characterized much of the history of American-training nursing. Indeed, before being imported into medical and nursing language and practice, the term was used largely in connection with deviant behavior and espionage. Surveillance in these contexts is ostensibly for the common good, not for the good of the individual persons under surveillance, and it implies an intervention of social control as opposed to benign assessment.[32,33]

The surveillance of individuals and the new medi(c)a(l) technologies that now permit more frequent intrusion have been the subject of increasing concern and scholarly critique in the sciences, humanities, and arts, most notably in philosophies and cultural studies of science, technology, and medicine; in film, media, and communication studies; and in feminist criticism. Indeed, much of what ties these disparate fields together is their concern with the experiences of looking and being looked at, spectator and spectacle, or the looking subject and the watched object. Scholars, social critics, and political activists have variously expressed a postmodern angst with modern Enlightenment visualist epistemology, in which what is taken in by the eye is tied to objective truth.[34-41] More committed to the notion that believing is seeing (as opposed to the idea that seeing is believing), they have been eager to examine the complex relations and to expose the confusion between representation and reality in the images we see.

Theoretically fueling much of the concern about the new surveillance in health care is Foucault's frequently cited work emphasizing the power-in-knowledge derived from watching and, therefore, the control that surveillance disciplines, such as criminal justice, psychiatry, and medicine, exert by virtue of their authority to look.[42] Foucault used the image of the panopticon, as envisioned by Jeremy Bentham, to problematize the Western equation of seeing with knowing and to propose the new equation of seeing with power. The panopticon is a prison constructed so that all inmates are in view of a single guard who, in turn, is in view of the prison warden. Because neither prisoners nor guards know when they are actually being watched, the effect is to make them compliant. Foucault conceived of the hospital as a kind of panopticon and of medicine as a disciplinary practice wielding power via surveillance techniques directed toward detecting deviations from normality.

In Foucauldian terms, nurses may be conceived as bodies made docile by gender and class socialization and the cultural authority vested in medicine and as the guards who deploy surveillance technologies on behalf of physicians and medicalized notions of normality. Parker and Wiltshire[43] labeled this kind of nursing observation "savoir" or "the nursing gaze," which, like the "medical gaze" it mimics, is organized around scientific abstractions that function to normalize, control, and contain. They contrasted this medicallike gaze with "reconnoitre" or "the nursing scan," which nurses use to survey the terrain of their work and the "spatial organization" and "features of the environment [that] constrain or facilitate effective nursing,"[43(p157)] and with "connaissance" or "the nursing look," which involves concrete knowledge of actual persons. Connaissance is the "embodied situated caring attentiveness"[43(pp163–164)] often heralded as exemplifying the casuistry of expert nursing practice.

Parker and Wiltshire[43] concluded that nursing reconnaissance is the "reflective integration" of these three kinds of observation, although connaissance is still seen (if seen at all) as a less valuable kind of observation. Their analysis of nursing observation, to which they referred as the nursing practice knowledge exhibited in the hand-over (or change of shift reporting), calls into question nurses' use of technologies for monitoring, diagnosing, and screening patients. That is, do nurses use these technologies in the holistic context of an integrative reconnaissance or in the more fragmented service of the nursing gaze, scan, or look? Do nurses look to care and/or care to look?

Scholars describing the successful synthesis or integration of technology with nursing care have argued that expert nurses can and/or actually do use technologies in the holistic manner of an integrative reconnaissance. Such nurses never simply rely on the nursing gaze to know their patients but rather readily employ the nursing look, which involves maintaining an embodied relation with patients. For example, Ray[44] equated caring with technology in her model of technologic caring in critical care. Technologic caring involves a hermeneutic nurse-machine relation because it entails interpreting "the meaning of the monitors, the numbers, the tubes, and the lines"[44(p168)] and acting on that interpretation with right judgment. Technologic caring also involves an embodied nurse-patient relation because it entails looking beyond the technical to "touch"[44] patients. Jones and Alexander[45] proposed definitions of both technology and caring that permitted nurses to see how they could be synthesized for humanistic nursing administration. For these writers, caring ought to be conceived as a nursing technology. Similarly, Locsin argued that machine technologies and caring are harmonious features of nursing practice whereby nurses use technology to "know a patient more fully as a person."[46(p202)]

In contrast, critics of nursing deployment of monitoring or surveillance technologies see nurses as using these technologies primarily in the service of the nursing (read medical) gaze. Such nurses show the kind of nursing "attending" that Bottorff and Morse referred to as "doing tasks,"[47(p58)] where the focus of the nurse is technology and the technical features of practice, not patients. Several scholars have noted nurses' uncritical deployment of medical technologies, which they see as expressing and consolidating male/medical values and power. In their view, nurses are seduced by technology and deceived into believing that technology will empower nursing.[48–50]

■ THE "SONOGENIC" FETUS AND THE RISE OF FETAL NURSING

An especially fruitful domain to explore in the rise of spectacular nursing is the field of perinatal, or fetal–maternal, nursing. Indeed, no other facet and symbol of visualist technology has been more generally fascinating[51] to viewing professionals and the public than the fetus. No other patient has garnered so much attention in recent years as the fetal patient. No other patient has been so spectacular. Yet what is most fascinating and most ominous about the new discovery of the fetus is that this fetus had to be made before it was found. Arguably, both the fetus and the fetal patient are "carpentered"[9] entities that are wholly products of the visualist technologies that created them. Indeed, the fetus is constructed as itself a technology in discourses on fetal surgery and fetal tissue research.[52] Historian Duden[53] observed that the fetus we know today (beginning with the photographic displays of life before birth that appeared in *Life* magazine in 1965 and continuing with the ubiquitous sonographic displays that followed) is completely unlike the unseen entity contained in the flesh of women that prevailed for most of human history. The fetus that is the object of nursing assessment, monitoring, and evaluation—that is, surveillance—never existed before the visualist technologies that caused it to appear. The examined fetus is an "engineered construct . . . [and] synthesis . . . of modern society."[53(p4)]

Feminist scholars, in particular, have been concerned with how visualist technologies, such as fetoscopy, electronic fetal monitoring, amniocentesis, and especially ultrasonography, have changed the iconography and experience of pregnancy from a private, embodied state emphasizing the "carnal knowledge"[53] of women to a public spectacle symbolizing scientific knowledge and technologic progress, promulgating human life, and advertising cars.[11,36,41,51,54–57] Especially ominous to these scholars is the "fetishizing" of the fetus at the expanse of the personhood of women. In photographic, sonographic, and other visual displays, the fetus "floats disembodied in its amnesiac ahistorical representational space."[58(p170)] Visualist technologies have created the discourse of fetal autonomy and, paradoxically, of both maternal insignificance and maternal culpability. Fetuses are visually and "ideologically amputated"[59] from the female bodies in which they are housed and on which they depend for life, which creates the fiction of the independently viable and amaternal fetus. Women are cut away in displays of the fetus. Yet, although women are technologically erased as the beings in whom fetuses reside, they are made to reappear as the agents responsible for, and even at odds with, fetal well-being, which thereby justifies the transformation of professional caregivers into "technological voyeurs"[50] and keeps childbearing women under technologic (and other kinds of) surveillance.

As targets of obstetric surveillance, fetuses, but not women, are the "privileged objects of medical concern."[60(p22)] In the public health media campaign against tuberculosis from the late 1930s to the mid-1950s, women were prominent as objects of X-ray surveillance, but their prominence was in inverse relationship to the regard for women and their health. Contemporary visualist technologies for obstetric surveillance continue and reinforce a historical trend of looking at and through women on behalf of others—whether society as a whole or the fetus—and of implicating nurses in the deployment of technologies that often serve the interests of neither women's health nor nursing. Cartwright noted that nurses were key players in promoting X-ray surveillance as a safe and even pleasurable experience. In the 1950 General Electric film "Target TB," which Cartwright described, a female nurse is shown obtaining a chest radiograph from a woman who declares that it was "as easy as having your picture taken."[60(p29)] The nurse reinforces the analogy between the radiograph and an everyday and familiar snapshot by replying that radiographs are "simpler" and that the person being radiographed does not have to worry about the "sun in your eyes."[60(p29)] According to Cartwright, this exchange "undercuts the view" that radiographs are a special form of "technical looking." Moreover, radiographs are "naively" consented to by both nurses and female patients, who do not see that their participation with this technology is not really authorized by their consent but rather by a "public (gazing) culture."[60(p29)]

Fetal ultrasonography has emerged as a similar occasion for minimizing the uniqueness of a new kind of technical looking, whereby the sonogram of a fetus is made out to be equal to a photograph or movie of a baby. Arguably, nurses today, like the nurse in "Target TB," also participate in a naive equalization of very different modes of looking, of intrauterine fetus with out-of-womb baby, or parent–child encounter with clinician–patient encounter, and of pleasurable viewing with technologic investigation whenever they liken the fetus to the baby yet to be born and invite expectant parents to "bond" with this baby. Moreover, nurses undermine the informed consent process whenever they permit expectant couples to understand fetal ultrasonography solely as a Kodak moment with their baby. By virtue of this naive equalization, nurses may also contribute to the suffering of couples with perinatal losses. As one couple once intimated to me, losing a fetus is a more scientific affair than losing a baby.

■ STILL LIFE: ON FETAL LIFE, DEATH, AND DISPLAY

Visual displays of fetuses and referents to fetuses are also increasingly integral to prenatal diagnosis and genetic counseling.[61] Displays of one's own fetus or other fetuses, fetal parts, and fetal karyotypes provide evidence for and dramatize fetal (ab)normality and fetal life or death. Yet these same visual displays also confuse. While looking over data I had collected from couples who learned of fetal impairments during pregnancy, I was struck by the array of visual representations of fetus/baby they encountered and how these displays blurred the lines between fetus/baby and alive/dead. Casper described the fetus as "at the margins of humanity,"[52(p307)] not as "either" human or nonhuman but rather in the "spaces between . . . this conceptual dualism."[52(p308)] Technologic displays contribute to fetal marginality. Indeed, several scholars have noted the irony that the fetuses shown to the public as "life" are often actually dead. For example, the pictorial narrative of life before birth that appeared in *Life* was constructed from photographic renderings of fetuses obtained from pregnancy terminations.[13,56,62] Couples are shown, or offered to keep as a record of the beginning of a life or proof of a life after death, ultrasonic or photographic pictures (often ultrasonic pictures) of fetuses and fetal parts, photographs or schematic drawings of normal and abnormal karyotypes, pictures of anomalous or dead fetuses made to look as if they are alive but sleeping, and/or actual pieces or traces of their fetus' body, such as hair, fingernails, and footprints. Women now often keep the strip from the home pregnancy test indicating that they are pregnant as the first sign of a baby. Infertile couples often view eggs, sperm, follicles, and embryos in various stages of development under a microscope or in photographs of microscopic displays.

In short, never before have the questions of what is a pregnancy versus what is once- or never-pregnant, what is a baby versus what stands for a baby, and what is life versus what stands for life been harder to answer.[63–68] Never before has showing played a role at least as important as telling/talking in prenatal/genetic counseling encounters and discourse. Never before have patients been shown so much visual data that are more than meet the eye. That is, never before have expectant couples been asked to interpret representations of babies at so many levels of abstraction and visibility. What is visible in one medium may be invisible in another; what is visible to the naked eye may be invisible to the instrumental eye.

New visual modes of representing patients and their health conditions are reshaping the esthetics, politics, and ethics of nursing practice. They give nurse–patient relations a different look, offer nurses the power to look, and confront nurses with all the practical and ethical dilemmas of looking. Whether they notice it or not, nurses participate in a visual culture, deploying images in the service of knowing the patient that "constitute privileged medical knowledge and power."[60(p49)] I am not suggesting, following Cartwright,[60] that nurses should resist being imaging subjects (or that women patients should resist being imaged objects); rather, I am suggesting that nurses "actively reconfigure imaging technologies"[60(p49)] for nursing purposes. Indeed, nurses must provide a "countersurveillance"[60] to the surveillance technologies that are now part of the nursing landscape. Nurses must "reconnoitre,"[43] or employ the nursing scan, to ensure appropriate nursing use of these technologies.

Nurses have a special "angle of vision"[69] by virtue of their distinctive epistemologic, social, and even moral position on the front lines and at the point of impact of technologies on patient care. Because of this unique vantage point, nurses have an important contribution to make to the understanding and the critical assessment and informed use of technology. Nevertheless, nurses must recognize that technologies are desired, not needed. As Van Dyck observed, the need for technology is never simply "there" but rather is created via a complex process of "image-building and storytelling."[70(p11)] Technologies need stories to sell themselves and to justify their expense. Nurses must re-vision themselves as critical players in the selling, justification, and storying of technologies, deploying images of persons and health that re-create both.

References

1. The nurse. In: *The Nightingale* (Annual of Rex Hospital Training School for Nursing). Raleigh, NC: Rex Hospital Library/Archives; 1923.
2. Nightingale F. *Notes on Nursing: What It Is and What It Is Not.* New York: Dover; 1969.
3. Bankert M. *Watchful Care: A History of America's Nurse Anesthetists.* New York: Continuum; 1989.
4. Symonds A. Angels and interfering busybodies: The social construction of two occupations. *Soc Health Illness.* 1991;13:249–264.
5. Mason J. *Qualitative Researching.* London: Sage; 1996.
6. Walters SD. *Material Girls: Making Sense of Feminist Cultural Theory.* Berkeley: University California Press; 1995.
7. Strathern M. *Reproducing the Future: Anthropology, Kinship, and the New Reproductive Technologies.* Manchester, England: Manchester University Press; 1992.
8. Lerner BH. The perils of "x-ray vision": How radiographic images have historically influenced perception. *Perspect Biol Med.* 1992;35:382–397.

9. Ihde D. *Instrumental Realism: The Interface Between Philosophy of Science and Philosophy of Technology.* Bloomington: Indiana University Press; 1991.
10. Sandelowski M. Channel of desire: Fetal ultrasonography in two use-contexts. *Qual Health Res.* 1994; 4:262–280.
11. Petchesky RP. Fetal images: The power of visual culture in the politics of reproduction. In: Stanworth M, ed. *Reproductive Technologies: Gender, Motherhood, and Medicine.* Minneapolis: University of Minnesota Press; 1987.
12. Ginsburg F. The "word-made" flesh: The disembodiment of gender in the abortion debate. In: Ginsburg F, Tsing AL, eds. *Uncertain Terms: Negotiating Gender in American Culture.* Boston: Beacon; 1990.
13. Newman K. *Fetal Positions: Individualism, Science, Visuality.* Stanford, CA: Stanford University Press; 1996.
14. Sandelowski M. Knowing and forgetting: The challenge of technology for a reflexive practice science of nursing. In: Thorne S, Hayes J, eds. *Nursing Praxis: Knowledge and Action.* Thousand Oaks, CA: Sage; 1997.
15. Sandelowski M. "Making the best of things": Technology in American nursing, 1870–1940. *Nurs Hist Rev.* 1997;5:3–22.
16. Harmer B. *Textbook of the Principles and Practice of Nursing.* New York: Macmillan; 1922.
17. Tanner CA, Benner P, Chesla C, Gordon DR. The phenomenology of knowing the patient. *Image.* 1993; 25:273–280.
18. Rafferty A. Decorous didactics: Early explorations in the art and science of caring, circa 1860–90. In: Kitson A, ed. *Nursing: Art and Science.* London: Chapman & Hall; 1993.
19. Armstrong D. The fabrication of nurse-patient relationships. *Soc Sci Med.* 1983;17:457–460.
20. Jecker NS, Self DJ. Separating care and cure: An analysis of historical and contemporary images of nursing and medicine. *J Med Phil.* 1991;16:285–306.
21. Houston WR. *The Art of Treatment.* New York: Macmillan; 1937.
22. Reverby SM. A legitimate relationship: Nursing, hospitals, and science in the twentieth century. In: Long DE, Golden J, eds. *The American General Hospital: Communities and Social Contexts.* Ithaca, NY: Cornell University Press; 1989.
23. Lynaugh J. Narrow passageways: Nurses and physicians in conflict and concert since 1875. In: King NM, Churchill LR, Cross AW, eds. *The Physician as Captain of the Ship: A Critical Reappraisal.* Dordrecht, Holland: Reidel; 1988.
24. Ihde D. *Technology and the Lifeworld: From Garden to Earth.* Bloomington: Indiana University Press; 1990.
25. Ihde D. *Technics and Praxis.* Boston: Dordrecht; 1979.
26. Treichler PA, Cartwright L. Introduction: Imaging technologies, inscribing science. *Camera Obscura* 1992;28:5–18.
27. Harris FM. Symposium on the nurse and the new machinery. *Nurs Clin North Am.* 1966;1:535–536.
28. Sandelowski M. (Ir)Reconcilable differences? The debate concerning nursing and technology. *Image.* 1997;29:169–174.
29. Parker J. Searching for the body in nursing. In: Gray G, Pratt R, eds. *Scholarship in the Discipline of Nursing.* Melbourne, Australia: Churchill Livingstone; 1995.
30. May C. Nursing work, nurses' knowledge, and the subjectification of the patient. *Soc Health Illness.* 1992;14:472–487.

31. Arney WR. *Power and the Profession of Obstetrics.* Chicago: University of Chicago Press; 1982.
32. Dougherty CM. Surveillance. In: Bulechek GM, McCloskey JC, eds. *Nursing Intervention: Essential Nursing Treatments.* 2nd ed. Philadelphia: Saunders; 1992.
33. Titler MG: Interventions related to surveillance. *Nurs Clin North Am.* 1992; 27:495–515.
34. Armstrong D. The rise of surveillance medicine. *Soc Health Illness.* 1995; 17:393–404.
35. Cartwright L. *Screening the Body: Tracing Medicine's Visual Culture.* Minneapolis: University of Minnesota Press; 1995.
36. Hartouni V. Fetal exposures: Abortion politics and the optics of allusion. *Camera Obscura.* 1992;29:130–149.
37. Kember S. Medical diagnostic imaging: The geometry of chaos. *New Formations.* 1991;15:55–66.
38. Lynch M, Woolgar S. *Representation in Scientific Practice.* Dordrecht, Netherlands: Kluwer Academic; 1988.
39. Pasveer B. Knowledge of shadows: The introduction of X-ray images in medicine. *Soc Health Illness.* 1989;11:360–381.
40. Stafford BM. Voyeur or observer? Enlightenment thoughts on the dilemmas of display. *Configurations.* 1993;1:95–128.
41. Treichler PA, Cartwright L, eds. Imaging technologies, inscribing science. *Camera Obscura.* 1992;28–29. Special issues.
42. Cheek J, Ridge T. The panopticon revisited? An exploration of the social and political dimensions of contemporary health care and nursing practice. *Int J Nurs Stud.* 1994;31:583–591.
43. Parker J, Wiltshire J. The handover: Three modes of nursing practice knowledge. In: Gray G, Pratt R, eds. *Scholarship in the Discipline of Nursing.* Melbourne, Australia: Churchill Livingstone; 1995.
44. Ray MA. Technological caring: A new model in critical care. *Dimens Crit Care Nurs.* 1987;6:166–173.
45. Jones CB, Alexander JW. The technology of caring: A synthesis of technology and caring for nursing administration. *Nurs Adm Q.* 1993;17:11–20.
46. Locsin RC. Machine technologies and caring in nursing. *Image.* 1995;27:201–204.
47. Bottorff JL, Morse JM. Identifying types of attending: Patterns of nurses' work. *Image.* 1994;26:53–60.
48. Allan JD, Hall BA. Challenging the focus on technology: A critique of the medical model. *Adv Nurs Sci.* 1988;10:22–33.
49. Lovell M. The politics of medical deception: Challenging the trajectory of history. *Adv Nurs Sci.* 1980;2:73–86.
50. Sandelowski M. A. case of conflicting paradigms: Nursing and reproductive technology. *Adv Nurs Sci.* 1988;10:35–45.
51. Franklin S. Fetal fascinations: New dimensions to the medical-scientific construction of fetal personhood. In: Franklin S, Lury C, Stacey J, eds. *Off-Centre: Feminism and Cultural Studies.* New York: Harper-Collins; 1991.
52. Casper MJ. At the margins of humanity: Fetal positions in science and medicine. *Sci Technol Hum Values.* 1994;19:307–323.
53. Duden B. *Disembodying Women: Perspectives on Pregnancy and the Unborn.* Cambridge, MA: Harvard University Press; 1993.

54. Adams A. Out of the womb: The future of the uterine metaphor. *Femin Stud.* 1993;19:269–289.
55. Duden B. Visualizing "life." *Sci Cult.* 1993;17:562–600.
56. Farquhar D. *The Other Machine: Discourse and Reproductive Technologies.* New York: Routledge; 1996.
57. Lor JS. The public fetus and the family car: From abortion politics to a Volvo advertisement. *Public Cult.* 1992;4:67–80.
58. Biddick K. Stranded histories: Feminist allegories of artificial life. *Res Phil Technol.* 1993;13:165–182.
59. Stabile CA. Shooting the mother: Fetal photography and the politics of disappearance. *Camera Obscura.* 1992;28:179–205.
60. Cartwright L. Women, X-rays, and the public culture of prophylactic imaging. *Camera Obscura.* 1992;29:18–54.
61. Bosk CL. *All God's Mistakes: Genetic Counseling in a Pediatric Hospital.* Chicago: University of Chicago Press; 1992.
62. Adams AE. *Reproducing the Womb: Images of Childbirth in Science, Feminist Theory, and Literature.* Ithaca, NY: Cornell University Press; 1994.
63. Kovit L. Babies as social products: The social determinants of classification. *Soc Sci Med.* 1978;12:347–351.
64. Layne LL. Of fetuses and angels: Fragmentation and integration in narratives of pregnancy loss. *Knowledge Soc.* 1992;9:29–58.
65. Lovell A. Some questions of identity: Late miscarriage, stillbirth and perinatal loss. *Soc Sci Med.* 1983;17:755–761.
66. Primeau MR, Recht CK. Professional bereavement photographs: One aspect of a perinatal bereavement program. *J Obstet Gynecol Neonat Nurs.* 1994;23:22–25.
67. Reddin SK. The photography of stillborn children and neonatal deaths. *J Audiovisual Media Med.* 1987;10:49–51.
68. Sandelowski M, Harris BG, Holditch-Davis D. Pregnant moments: The process of conception in infertile couples. *Res Nurs Health.* 1990;13:273–282.
69. Kim HS. *The Nature of Theoretical Thinking in Nursing.* Norwalk, CT: Appleton-Century-Crofts; 1983.
70. Van Dyck J. *Manufacturing Babies and Public Consent: Debating the New Reproductive Technologies.* New York: New York University Press; 1995.

32

Healthcare: Technology in the New Millennium

Russell C. Coile, Jr. and Brett E. Trusko

When you pump your own gas at the filling station are you working for the gas station or yourself? When you take a pregnancy test at home are you a savvy self-helper or part of the HMO's plan to cut costs? Outsiders act as employees, employees act as outsiders. New relationships blur the roles of employees and customers to the point of unity.

> —*Kevin Kelly, "New Rules for the New Economy"*

*T*he most pervasive change in the new millennium will be the way technology empowers patients to take control of their healthcare. Internet-informed patients will become partners in the promotion of their health, using physicians and other providers as consultants rather than managers. Information technology will allow patients to access the health system on a "7×24" basis, at their convenience.

Language is often the precursor to change. The word coined for this kind of patient involvement has been called prosumption. In his 1996 book, "Digital Economy," Don Tapscott describes the increasing role of the consumer in functions formerly performed by the producer. For example, "prosumers" might receive custom newspapers over the Internet, with only the stories and subjects that are of interest to them. When the consumer defines, then receives this type of newspaper, he or she has assumed the role of publisher (producer) and consumer. The same might be said for home pregnancy tests (doctor and patient), and pumping your own gasoline (mechanic and driver).

So, over the next 20 years, the adoption and embracing of technology in healthcare will increase at an accelerating pace. The process of healthcare will become substantially digitized and electronically enabled. Managed care

Russell C. Coile, Jr. is vice president/national strategy advisor, and Brett E. Trusko is an executive director, both with Superior Consultant Company, Southfield, MI.

From *Health Management Technology*, December 1999, *20*(11) 44–48. Reprinted with permission of Nelson Publishing, 2500 N. Tamiami Tr. Nokomis, FL. 34275, (941) 966-9521, *www.healthmgttech.com.*

will switch from a gatekeeper concept to one of highly automated care management.

■ *DREAM COME TRUE*

The wired world of healthcare in 2020 isn't just a dream. Recent breakthroughs in remote surgery, gene manipulation, cloning, and molecularization of microchips have opened a world of possibilities. Questions of morality, government intervention, and the cost-benefit tradeoff between health and illness are the issues facing the nation in the new millennium of healthcare.

There is a concern that technology will accelerate the emergence of a two-tier health system. Uniquely personalized high-tech treatments such as gene therapy may not be covered by health insurance. These services will be available at a cost. Some patients will have the discretionary resources to pay these costs, but others will not.

A public policy debate on high-cost technology is likely in the next two decades (see October issue of HMT). Over time, the debate may ease as the technology have-nots eventually reap many of the benefits of those who pay, since the technology cost curve tends to drop off quickly.

As technology becomes more important in people's daily lives in the next century, it will become virtually invisible. In terms of consumer acceptance, the concept of "technology" is generational. Ask people over 80 about technology in their generation and you are likely to hear about the advent of radio. Ask a 60-year-old and technology is television. A 40-year-old sees technology as the computer, while a 20-year-old may not have yet witnessed anything he or she would refer to as technology.

The patients of the new millennium will have access to virtually all of the same knowledge as the providers. But will they understand what they read off the Internet, and can they trust it? Content providers such as drKoop.com and WebMD can supply valuable, peer-reviewed, and valid information. But there will always be unverified medical information on the Internet presenting treatments that may not have been subjected to the rigors of clinical trials.

■ *A NEW BREED OF HOUSE CALLS*

As healthcare entities move away from the medical center concept to one of a virtual community, consumers of healthcare will acquire the real ability to compare the quality and costs of care. Virtual healthcare will provide more alternatives for patients, and cost-competition will increase. Through Internet and two-way video connections, remote home visits by physicians and nurses will become practical.

Physicians and technicians will be able to perform routine tests and physicals in the patient's home or office via connected EKGs, EEGs, and portable telehealth units, which will include diagnosis via helmets or hats, and gloves with tactile ability. Expert systems and artificial intelligence will present caregivers with best practice options to the delivery of care.

Patients can query the health system or health plan at any time of day or night. Communication will grow increasingly digital and virtual, with multiple providers integrated to deliver care beyond anything we experience today.

▪ BEST PRODUCT PRICING

The desire to control costs and increase efficiency in the healthcare industry will motivate employers and insurers to purchase products at the best price for the best health benefits, even if those products are on the other side of the country, possibly the other side of the world.

Although it will be a controversial issue, global information technology can enable many tests and procedures to be performed "off shore" at the lowest cost site, whether out-of-state or even across national borders. The ability to source the most cost-effective health service from anywhere on the planet may be the most effective strategy in bringing the cost of U.S. healthcare under control.

Technology will enable managed care to finally coordinate treatments in the most cost-effective way. Health plans and capitated provider organizations struggle to coordinate various professionals (e.g., chiropractor, physical therapist, neurologist, orthopedist treating a patient for back pain) in a manner that is best for the patient. As commerce in the rest of the world becomes immediate, so too will patients seek providers who can coordinate and deliver services quickly and effectively. Electronic medical records will follow the patient.

▪ NEWLY FOCUSED MANAGED CARE

Clinical pathways and protocols will be automated. In the future, managing care will be real-time, electronically monitored, and evidence-based. The focus of managed care in the millennium will be high-risk people who are not acutely ill and high-cost patients who are already under care.

A major barrier to entry of competition in healthcare is risk. Employers or insurers assume risk for the costs of care under a health plan and a growing number of providers are assuming risk in some markets. Aging of the population, new technology, higher pharmaceutical use, and Medicare budget cuts are blamed for rising health costs.

Health plans that capitate providers are controlling their costs, and shifting risk. Information technology can enable healthcare providers to assess, assume, and manage global risk for the entire costs of care under a health plan. As better information and connectivity become available, providers can begin to prospectively identify the likely costs of treating their patients, and capture the savings from prevention, health promotion, and early intervention.

■ *DIFFERENTIAL PREMIUMS*

With access to deep pools of patient information in data warehouses, the concept of differential premiums may become accepted. Experience can quantify the expected cost differences in providing care to a 30-year old vs. a 60-year old, although both may work for the same company and be covered by the same health plan. This may require that commercial health plans, employers, and government pay more for some patients, but at the same time other patients may be treated for considerably less than the current rates. The treatment of patients at lower prices is one of the trade-offs when health plans and providers have access to databases of patient cost and disease experience.

Quality will continue to be the watchword for the next millennium, and technology will be the enabling force. In tomorrow's information-enabled health system, it will be possible to monitor and manage high-risk or high-cost patients as if they were receiving full-time dedicated care.

An estimated six to eight percent of younger patients and 12 to 15 percent of Medicare beneficiaries who are higher risk could be monitored more closely. Information networks can quickly and accurately make decisions about a multitude of symptoms and prescribe treatment for them as well. This futuristic scenario is possible today, for example, with new generation insulin pumps and automatic pacemaker/defibrillators.

■ *TECHNOLOGY AND THE DIGITAL HIGHWAY*

The Internet is growing from its current "garden path" state to a true information superhighway. The highway will have at least 100 lanes. Possible? No waiting for this future. A global competition is emerging between digital subscriber lines (DSL), broadband modems (through the cable company), and direct broadcast satellites. Information service providers promise a "firehose" of information and two-way communication in nanoseconds.

Healthcare IS/IT specialists are their organizations' trend-spotters when it comes to emerging technologies. Every hospital, health plan, physician office or health services provider will be connected. Entrepreneurial companies and some of the best-known healthcare organizations and health plans in America will be competing to be health information providers.

There will be an explosion of information sources and databases. Information systems specialists will be the guides to this new world of electronic technology. The fundamental question they will need to answer is how to use tomorrow's information technology to better serve their patients and the public.

33

How Will the Internet Change Our Health System?

Jeff Goldsmith

Those who make their living forecasting change in social institutions are frequently humbled by the actual flow of events. Developments that seem inevitable (such as "artificial intelligence" or the picture phone) seem to take forever to happen, while seemingly unstoppable institutions or innovations (such as physician practice management firms) suddenly collapse. Sometimes, however, innovations spring, fully blown and unheralded, seemingly from out of nowhere. The Internet is one of these.

Although health care institutions may resist the influence of network computing, eventually, the Internet is likely to accelerate the "virtualization" of health care plans and systems and help to eliminate much of the clerical burden in caregiving and insurance. The core processes in health care—interactions between physicians and patients—are likely to be rapidly and profoundly affected.

From its not-so-humble origins as an experimental, Defense Department–funded, secure data network, the Internet exploded during the late 1990s into a powerful new social institution. The adoption curve for the Internet is far steeper than that of any of the established media: Although it took radio thirty-eight years and television thirteen years to reach fifty million users, the Internet reached the same number of users in only five years. According to a 1999 Louis Harris poll, 48 percent of adult Americans—about ninety-seven million people—use the Internet to communicate with one another and to acquire information, products, and services.[1] The Internet is only incidentally a broadcast medium. Rather, it is like a flexible and powerful new nervous system for the economy and society.

One basic misperception of the Internet is that its greatest impact will be in its consumer retail applications. Consumer use is actually only the visible tip of a much larger iceberg. The underwater part of the iceberg—business-to-

Jeff Goldsmith, a health care forecaster and strategist, is president of Health Futures, Inc., in Charlottesville, Virginia. He is a member of the board of directors of the Cerner Corporation, a health care informatics company, and a director of the Essent Corporation, an investor-owned hospital management firm.

business electronic commerce—is five times larger than consumer-based e-commerce and is projected to grow at a far faster rate. According to Forrester Research, consumers spent an estimated $8 billion (out of roughly $2 trillion in overall consumer spending) online in 1998, an amount expected to increase more than tenfold to $108 billion by 2002. By contrast, businesses did more than $40 billion in Internet business with each other in 1998, an amount expected to reach $1.3 trillion by 2002.[2] In this paper I examine some of the areas of the health care system that are most likely to be affected by the spreading influence of the Internet.

■ ULTIMATE KNOWLEDGE BUSINESS

Health care services not only are the prototypical knowledge business but also are perhaps the most complex product of our economy. Just as health care organizations have struggled to assimilate earlier generations of information technology (IT), they are likely to struggle to adapt to and use the Internet.

Health care providers and systems are staggeringly inefficient at assimilating and processing information and at converting that information to knowledge. Part of the problem is that the core knowledge base of health care, biomedical science, is expanding at a geometric rate, driven by $40 billion a year in public- and private-sector research and development (R&D) spending. Also, more variability and uncertainty at the point of service exists in health care than in any other service in our economy. Although this variability does not completely defy capture, standardization, and manipulation by information systems, the technical and organizational problems associated with this process are daunting.[3]

As if this variability were not complicating enough, more complex, highly trained, and difficult people (namely, health professionals) collide at the point of service than is true in any other service in our economy. Each health profession has its unique view of the patient's needs, its own language, and an intensely territorial view of its involvement in the care process. This has created a balkanized information architecture, in which each profession has its own data system that processes and records for payment the services it provides.

The present information environment in most health care institutions is dozens of functional computing systems (such as pharmacy, clinical laboratory, billing, and accounts receivable) running different programs written in different languages on different hardware. A depressingly large fraction of these processes are mediated by paper (medical records, prescriptions, telephone message slips, and bills)—incontrovertible evidence of an early 1970s information environment.

Some health care organizations are adopting enterprisewide information systems, with a single patient identifier, a single patient record, and a common application set. As J.D. Kleinke has noted, the growth and development of enterprise systems in health care has been deeply troubled.[4] Vendors must shoulder part of the blame for promising solutions they cannot readily deliver; however, the difficulty health care organizations have had in shifting from functional to enterprise computing is, in major part, inherent in the complexity of the organizations themselves.

Indeed, it would be inaccurate to describe most health care organizations as enterprises. What they really are is collections of professions loosely and uncomfortably housed in the same physical structures. A coral reef is such a structure, much more a colony than a sentient being. As a consequence, systemic innovations are adopted very slowly. Passive resistance to change is compounded by a corrosive suspicion produced by the failure of past IT applications to materially improve productivity or processes of care.[5]

Clement McDonald and colleagues compared computer networks to a rain forest canopy, where arboreal creatures (physicians) can gather fruit (information on patients and clinical problems) effortlessly by moving across the canopy (data network) without having to climb each tree (separate data systems).[6] (The image of troupes of monkeys screaming and throwing fruit at one another is almost irresistible.)

What the Internet promises health care mangers and clinicians is a flexible, external information architecture that can reach down into the dozens, even hundreds, of health care information "silos" and extract, analyze, aggregate, and redirect data, which clinicians or managers need to make decisions. Beyond clinical uses, promising business-to-business Internet applications in health care include paperless transmission, verification, adjudication, and payment of medical claims; online marketing of health insurance to individuals and small businesses; paperless prescribing of, monitoring of, and payment for prescription drugs; medical product ordering and inventory management; and outsourcing of data processing and other management functions.

■ BARRIERS TO NETWORK COMPUTING

Sadly, many of the items listed above were achievable with technologies that have existed for years. Intranets (high-speed local-area data networks inside organizations), clinical data repositories, electronic medical claims filing, and electronic patient records all predate the Internet. Yet convincing health care managers and clinicians to use them has been difficult.

Two daunting technical challenges and a major change–management challenge stand in the way of realizing the enormous potential of network computing in health care.

Standardized coding. The first challenge is standardizing the coding and formats for clinical information. Information systems must recognize and translate different coding schemes for clinical encounters, using a medical logic engine that recognizes different clinical terminology for the same problem. Because new terminology and knowledge are being constantly created, the medical knowledge architecture must be flexible enough to permit continual updating with professional consensus. However, getting dozens of clinical disciplines and technology vendors to agree on needed standardization of clinical coding as well as on standardization of the technical specifications of information systems, so that systems from different vendors can "interoperate," is akin in complexity and politics to negotiating an international trade agreement.

Protecting privacy. The other challenge is standardizing patient identification while protecting privacy. This standardization is the essential first step in creating an enterprise health information system; it enables a hospital or group practice to consolidate a dozen or more records on the same patient into one record. Standardizing patient identification *across* health institutions is the vital step needed to create an Internet-based patient record. However, placing the medical record on the Internet exposes that record, already too accessible in paper form, to potential unauthorized access by employers, health plans, law enforcement agencies, private investigators, hackers, and others.

In the Kassenbaum-Kennedy Health Insurance Portability and Accountability Act (HIPAA) of 1996, Congress mandated that the Department of Health and Human Services (HHS) develop a unique health identifier for each individual, employer, health plan, and provider and promulgate guidelines for protecting the confidentiality of personal medical information.

When HHS issued draft guidelines recommending the adoption of a unique patient identifier in the summer of 1998, the ensuing firestorm of public criticism took the policy community by surprise. Lack of public confidence in public and private institutions' ability to prevent health information from being disclosed to employers, the courts, and law enforcement agencies, or to protect consumers from inappropriate use by health care providers themselves, was a major theme in opposition to the unique identifier.

Janlori Goldman recently reported that 27 percent of respondents to a Louis Harris poll believed that their personal medical information had been improperly disclosed. Of this group, more than 30 percent felt that they had been adversely affected by the disclosure.[7] Significant numbers of Americans pay for health care outside of insurance plans or simply avoid seeking care for sensitive problems to avoid creating a record of the problem.

The barriers to protecting medical privacy on the Internet are not technological, but rather political. Properly employed, heavy encryption and password-driven access can do the job. The real problem is a lack of public trust.

▪ PHYSICIANS: THE HARDEST SELL

The greatest barrier to realizing network computing's full potential is the same barrier that has hampered the spread of enterprise computing: persuading physicians to use these technologies. Historically, the physician has been the principal integrator of knowledge in health care. It will take a great deal of persuading to convince skeptical, time-famished clinicians that after all the broken promises of the past two decades, network computing actually can simplify and strengthen their practices. This is somewhat of a generational issue, since for most clinicians under age thirty-five, using network computing to acquire information and to communicate is as natural as breathing.

The lack of trust is even more a problem with physicians than with consumers. All too often, information technology has been imposed on physicians "from above," by alien, imperial powers (hospitals, health systems, or health plans). Vendors and information managers frequently encounter physicians' fear that information systems will be used to profile them, gather information about their practices, and discipline them or deprive them of income. It is difficult to imagine a situation less conducive to the enthusiastic uptake of a new technology than one that consumes tremendous time and energy in its adoption, while simultaneously threatening the autonomy or livelihood of the user.

However, there are persuasive reasons for physicians to adopt network computing, including the ability to increase the ease of consultation on complex cases, to reduce wasted time and effort in connecting with colleagues and patients, and to improve patient safety. Already, enterprise IT systems have demonstrated their ability to help physicians reduce adverse drug reactions.[8] Combining enterprise systems with Internet connectivity to physicians' offices, pharmacies, and pharmacy benefit management (PBM) firms could alert physicians to potential drug interactions and increase patients' compliance with drug therapy.

▪ ADMINISTRATIVE POTENTIAL

Despite the skepticism and inertia of health care managers regarding potential e-commerce applications, the Internet eventually will enable health care organizations to markedly reduce their clerical employment and improve productivity. Indeed, the maturation of enterprise computing could generate significant productivity improvements, creating the infrastructure to support network computing applications.

As administrative services are increasingly supported by computer networks, health care enterprises will increasingly outsource functions for which they can achieve economic or efficiency gains. Outsourcing in hospitals historically has been confined to hotel-type services such as housekeeping and food services. The Internet will enable outsourcing of core administrative functions such as billing and financial management, data processing, telecommunications, materials management, and human resources, as well as some clinical services such as pharmacy. There are as yet no reliable estimates on the potential productivity gains for health care enterprises from adopting network computing solutions, but my sense is that they will eventually run into the tens of billions of dollars.

■ CONSUMER APPLICATIONS

Although institutional inertia and professional skepticism seem likely to slow the adoption of network computing in health care provision, consumers have aggressively embraced this new tool for acquiring health information. According to a recent Louis Harris poll, seventy million Americans used the Internet to seek health information in 1999.[9] Seeking health information is one of the top reasons why people log onto the Internet. In doing so, consumers are bypassing both the health care delivery and health insurance systems and seeking the information they need to frame their interaction with both systems.

The traditional relationship of a physician to a patient, relative to medical knowledge, has been steeply asymmetrical. Indeed, one can think of physician income as the rent physicians extract from their command of medical knowledge. The Internet will not eliminate this disparity in knowledge, but it will enable patients to begin their dialogue with physicians at a much higher level and provide them with leverage to influence the care process.

The growing complexity of medicine and the increasing burden of micro-accountability for clinical decision making imposed by managed care have conspired to rob physicians of the time they need to remain current in their own fields. The decay rate of scientific knowledge that physicians acquire in the basic science portion of their medical education is scarily rapid. By 1998 the number of citations in the National Library of Medicine's *Medline* service was estimated at 9.2 million, growing at a rate of 31,000 new citations a month.[10]

Into this expanding knowledge vacuum charges the cyber-assisted patient. Patients have discovered that Web-based search engines and so-called health portals have given them access to the same scientific databases, clinical trials listings, new drug information, and other sources that their own physicians often do not have time to analyze carefully, along with a lot of other information of perhaps more questionable value.

The sheer volume and variability in the quality of health information on the Internet, as well as the laboriousness of acquiring it from multitudes of sources, are universally acknowledged as serious developmental problems. One wag has likened the current Internet to a "virtual Haight/Ashbury."

Many physicians with whom I have interacted resent the patients who show up with articles from the Internet. Physicians often do not have time to read all of the materials patients bring them, let alone to search the Internet themselves. The idea that physicians should rely on patients to update them on developments in their own field is a stunning reversal of the traditional information flow in medicine. Yet physicians may come to discover that some of their patients are reliable bridges to emerging medical knowledge.

Promising consumer opportunities. The Haight/Ashbury stage of the Internet is nearing an end. Free but undifferentiated content will give way to filtered, structured content. Hundreds of millions of dollars in equity capital are being invested in creating medically related Internet applications, many of which target consumers directly.

The gold standard that these firms seek is for their site/search engine/portal to become the *Yahoo!* of health care—that is, the first place consumers go to seek information or advice about health problems.[11] Aggregating "eyeballs," the odd Dali-esque e-commerce jargon for audience size, presumably creates leverage for selling advertising to firms (such as pharmaceutical and consumer products companies) that are eager to insert their commercial messages into the search process.

Another important area is giving patients access to information on quality. This information is now limited to data reported to Medicare and from consumer satisfaction surveys.[12] However, it is reasonable to expect the volume of this information to grow to include licensure and medical disciplinary files on physicians and institutions, as well as information on medical error rates. How this information is gathered, validated, and presented will be the subject of fierce controversy and contention in the coming years.

However, the most significant consumer application of the Internet is the ability to aggregate patients with common problems into "virtual communities."[13] The Internet often is the first destination of a patient newly diagnosed with a serious, chronic health problem. The patient who types "lupus" into the search box of an Internet portal is within minutes of discovering an online community of fellow lupus sufferers, which brings a framework for collective learning about how to cope with the disease independent of one's physician.

Colleagues who follow these activities closely believe that virtual communities of sufferers from various diseases eventually will pool their resources and hire clinical consultants to help them navigate the health system, as well as lobbyists to help them confront Congress, state legislatures, and health plans on coverage and payment issues.[14] This aggregation also will have significant political consequences and will complicate the already complex politics of resource allocation for research and treatment of diseases.

Patients' access to this emerging capability is predictably maldistributed by race, age, and income class. A recent U.S. Department of Commerce report found that although personal computers are in 80 percent of American homes with incomes over $75,000 a year, only 16 percent of homes with incomes less than $20,000 have them. The racial gap in Internet use is large and widening: Almost one-third of white homes are "wired," compared with less than 12 percent of black households.[15] Only 15 percent of the population over age fifty-five is online. This population's online access is particularly crucial, because the elderly not only use health services heavily but are also more likely to be isolated from one another and from caregivers.

Access through schools and libraries does mitigate some of the socioeconomic barriers to Internet access, but differences in educational level will hamper persons in lower income strata in using this powerful new tool. Strengthening access to public computing sites is the most important short-term palliative measure, but it will not be enough. Technical assistance by reference librarians, teachers, counselors, and others also will be needed. Teaching young people how to use the Internet will become a staple of health education in elementary and secondary education.

■ *BUILDING BRIDGES TO PATIENTS*

The rapid entry of new, well-capitalized actors into the traditional arena of health care has jarred both providers and insurers, which are mired, as of this writing, in serious economic difficulty. Providers see the Internet as establishing a new channel of communication with their patients, although it remains to be seen how effective that channel will be. Sadly, hospitals' efforts to leverage the Internet have been captive to their marketing departments. Many hospitals' Web sites have a depressingly "Here We Are: Aren't We Wonderful?" quality to them.

In my informal survey, few hospitals have made provision for Internet-based scheduling, insurance verification, patient history, and other functions that could ease entry into their systems, or for enabling online updates of the condition of relatives or friends in the hospital. Hospitals that approach the Internet with an eye toward redesigning their core business processes to eliminate wasted time and paperwork are probably going to be more satisfied with the results than are those that view it as a public relations device.

On the other hand, the Internet may create more options for health insurers than any other actor in the health system. As with providers, the Internet will enable insurers to eliminate many redundant clerical functions that have clogged communication with physicians and patients. The Internet can speed verification of eligibility and coverage, as well as accelerate electronic payment to providers.

However, a suite of promising consumer applications may enable health plans to alter the perception that they are adversarial to patients' interests. HealthPartners, a Minneapolis-based health plan, was one of the first to computerize its provider network information for subscribers—including location, professional qualifications, and hours of operation of provider sites—and to make it available to subscribers via touch-screen computer kiosks. When this information moved to the HealthPartners Web site (www.consumerchoice.com), the plan added consumer-satisfaction and cost information and provided (in some of its products) financial incentives for consumers to select providers in the least expensive cost tier.[16] HealthPartners executives refer to this as a "farmer's market" strategy.

While these new insurance products have not taken the market by storm, they do provide a glimpse of how electronic commerce can help insurers to regain market leverage in a wide-open-panel, consumer-choice environment.

As comparative information on quality and patient safety becomes available, health plans are the ideal purveyors of that information to their subscribers via Internet-based "maps" of the health care system. Health plans will hold providers accountable through increasingly dense and invasive comparative quality and cost information. In an open-access market, providers will gain volume not by having it directed to them by health plans through selective contracting, but by being chosen by value-conscious consumers.

Many health plans have experimented with disease management programs targeted to high-risk populations in their subscriber base (patients suffering from asthma, diabetes, congestive heart failure, and other chronic illnesses). The Internet provides a superb platform for health plans to maintain continuous, low-intensity contact with their patients via their home computers.[17] The economics may be compelling enough for plans to give patients with these diseases their own home computers and teach them how to use them.

Another significant potential Internet application is assisting patients and families in planning how to address an emerging health threat. A number of years ago John Wennberg and his colleagues at Dartmouth developed a process called "Informed Choice" for patients newly diagnosed with a threatening medical condition (such as prostate cancer) for which multiple treatment options are available. This process encourages patients and physicians to sort out the patient's objectives in treatment.

The Informed Choice process has both markedly increased patients' satisfaction with the care process and reduced the rates of invasive treatment and cost, two compelling reasons why health plans will adopt this or similar approaches.[18] Although the technology was initially based on interactive laser discs, it is ideally suited for the Internet.[19]

Health plans also may discover that giving subscribers online access to medical advice may reduce the volume of primary care physician visits and help to cut wasted motion in approving payment for services by interacting directly with patients, not physicians. They may also discover that marketing their plans directly to subscribers and businesses via the Internet could help them "disintermediate" the insurance brokers and markedly lower the cost of their product. Direct-to-consumer channels and applications promise to restructure health insurance and fundamentally alter plans' relationships with their subscribers.

■ REGULATORY ISSUES

Licensing. The traditional locus of regulation of health services and insurance—in particular, licensure of health professionals, insurance brokers, and others—has been state governments. The Internet is completely oblivious to political boundaries. The fact that consumers in one state can purchase goods or services from other states over the Internet without paying local sales taxes has already raised serious long-term fiscal policy and equity issues. These issues will eventually force a rethinking of state and local tax structure.

A similar rethinking of licensure policy may ensue. Supervision of licensure is the most powerful tool governments have in ensuring that substandard practitioners do not practice medicine. How this method of supervision remains viable in the emerging networked age is a serious policy question.

Long-distance monitoring. Internet technology allows patients in one state to be monitored, evaluated, and prescribed for in another. Major regional referral centers will develop aggressive telemedicine initiatives employing the Internet, eventually threatening the economic franchises of physicians and health systems in local communities. It is not unreasonable to expect a collision in state legislatures between protectionist local practitioners and health care organizations that intend to "practice" across regions. A similar struggle can be expected between politically powerful local insurance agents and emerging online insurance brokerages.

Pharmaceuticals. The recent emergence of e-pharmacy has raised questions about the ability of the U.S. Food and Drug Administration (FDA) and state licensure agencies to effectively control the sale and distribution of prescription drugs. The Internet spawned an almost instant black market for the drug Viagra: Physicians who never met patients face-to-face "wrote" prescriptions, which were delivered through the mail to waiting users. The combination of heavy encryption and untraceable digital cash could lead to a noticeable increase in the flow of controlled substances to illicit users, as well as a lot of potentially dangerous "self-medication." How to maintain supervision and control of prescription drugs while opening a new and valuable channel for cost reduction is a complex policy issue.[20]

Quality of information. There is much concern about the variability of quality of advice and information on the Internet. However, it is difficult to see regulation of Internet content as a policy goal worth pursuing, particularly given that filtering information and setting information quality standards is likely to be a key differentiation strategy for competing health portals and suppliers of health information. Tort liability for poor advice rendered in specific patient cases seems likely to apply to virtual medical care encounters, so the courts will provide some measure of accountability for patient-specific advice. The courts will almost certainly become involved as more invasive measures of quality and patient risk are published on the Internet, and raise questions or concerns about specific institutions.

■ COST ISSUES

Will access to medical information over the Internet increase the demand for health care and thus its cost? Certainly manufacturers of drugs, medical products, and technologies think so, as they have moved aggressively to create Web sites and to advertise in emerging e-health venues on the Internet. However, it remains to be seen if advertising on the Internet will generate sufficient measurable returns to justify large advertising expenditures for pharmaceutical and product companies. Unlike with passive media such as radio and television, consumers can simply click past Internet advertising to the content they seek.

The Internet's potential to create demand for medical services will be closely studied in the next few years. In my opinion, these studies will find that in a consumer-guided search for solutions, self-care and alternative medicine will be given equal standing with invasive, high-cost solutions to health conditions. Many consumers whose encounters with mainstream medical care yield only expensive options may find less invasive, less risky solutions to their health problems.

The Internet will also provide disease-specific consumer feedback on new treatments that may dampen demand. The Internet is a superb medium for gathering and monitoring information on adverse reactions to newly released drugs or therapies. As discussed earlier, the combination of Internet connectivity with institutional (enterprise-level) electronic monitoring of the prescribing process also has strong potential for lowering the number of adverse drug events and the associated cost.

Overall, the cost impact of the Internet may be closer to neutral than most people suspicious of technology's impact on health costs believe. Network computing may save as much money by eliminating middlemen, clerical costs, redundant processes, and medical error as it generates in increased demand for care. Interactive disease management for patients with chronic diseases may yield significant savings in the costs of avoidable care.

The Internet has a great potential to fundamentally transform both the structure and the core processes of medicine than any new technology we have seen in the past fifty years. Professional resistance to adoption of the technology and political problems associated with protecting the confidentiality of patient records pose the two biggest hurdles to fully realizing this potential. I see the Internet generating some demand for new products and services. However, that demand is likely to be counterbalanced by a more careful weighing of potential benefits, reduction in medical errors, and the elevation of less expensive substitute therapies to parity with traditional invasive medicine, as well as savings from improved disease management. As a consequence, the Internet's impact on health care costs may be surprisingly benign. The most important effect of the Internet will be to strengthen the consumer's role in relation to practitioners and health care institutions, and to create a powerful new tool to help people manage their own health risks more effectively.

Notes

1. "Americans Seek Health Information Online," *Reuters Health* (5 August 1999).
2. "The Net Imperative," *Economist* (26 June 1999): 5–11.
3. For a superb discussion of these challenges, see J.D. Kleinke, "Release 0.0: Clinical Information Technology in the Real World," *Health Affairs* (Nov/Dec 1998): 23–38.

4. Ibid.

5. For a skeptical analysis of the impact of computing on business productivity, see W. Gibbs, "Taking Computers to Task," *Scientific American* (July 1997): 82–89.

6. C.J. McDonald et al., "Canopy Computing: Using the Web in Clinical Practice," *Journal of the American Medical Association* (21 October 1998): 1325–1329. For a practical discussion of how physicians will use Internet technologies, see M. Ruffin, *Digital Doctors* (Tampa: American College of Physician Executives, 1999).

7. J. Goldman, "Protecting Privacy to Improve Health Care," *Health Affairs.* (Nov/Dec 1998): 47–57.

8. D. Bates et al., "Effect of Computerized Physician Order Entry and a Team Intervention on Prevention of Serious Medication Errors," *Journal of the American Medical Association* (21 October 1998): 1311–1316; and R. Raschke et al., "A Computer Alert System to Prevent Injury from Adverse Drug Events," *Journal of the American Medical Association* (21 October 1998): 1317–1320.

9. "Americans Seek Health Information Online."

10. P.R. Hubbs et al., "Medical Information on the Internet," *Journal of the American Medical Association* (21 October 1998): 1363.

11. For a comprehensive if breathless look at the companies developing these sites, see S. Fitzgibbons and R. Lee, "The Health.net Industry: The Convergence of Healthcare and the Internet" (San Francisco: Hambrecht and Quist, January 1999).

12. An early entrant is HealthGrades.com. See J. Morrissey, "Internet Company Rates Hospitals," *Modern Healthcare* (16 August 1999): 24. Thehealthpages.com invites consumers to rate their physicians along perceived quality dimensions. The mother lode of physician-specific information, the National Practitioner Data Bank maintained by the U.S. Department of Health and Human Services, is presently inaccessible to consumers.

13. See H. Rheingold, *The Virtual Community* (New York: Harper Collins, 1995).

14. Howard Rheingold, information technology futurist, personal communication, fall 1998.

15. U.S. Department of Commerce, *Falling through the Net III* (Washington: U.S. Department of Commerce, July 1999).

16. Aetna/U.S. Healthcare had also an early and aggressive Internet presence (www.aetnaushc.com). The firm also collaborated with the Johns Hopkins University in creating a Web health portal (www.intellihealth.com).

17. See J. Ray and J. Sydnor, "Disease Management: The Future of Managed Care" (New York: First Union Capital Markets, 12 April 1999). A pioneering, Web-based, interactive disease management effort is CHESS (Comprehensive Health Enhancement Support System), developed by David Gustafson and colleagues at the University of Wisconsin.

18. See J.F. Kasper, A.G. Mulley, and J.E. Wennberg, "Developing Shared Decisionmaking Programs to Improve the Quality of Health Care," *Quality Review Bulletin* (June 1992): 183–190. On the utilization impact, see E. Wagner et al., "The Effects of a Shared Decisionmaking Program on Rates of Surgery for Benign Prostatic Hyperplasia," *Medical Care* 33, no. 8 (1995): 765–770.

19. The company that owns the rights to the Informed Choice process, Fairview Medical Services Corporation/Health Dialog, has negotiated a half-dozen licensing agreements with health plans and is in discussion with many others.

20. See M.W. Serafini, "Drugs on the Web," *National Journal* (13 November 1999): 3310–3314.

Discussion Questions

1. In your opinion, what technological innovations used by nurses prior to World War II were particularly noteworthy? Explain.

2. Are today's nurses as inventive as their predecessors? Elaborate and cite examples.

3. What insights have you gained about the use of technology after reading the Sandelowski articles (Articles 30 and 31)?

4. Analyze the notion of surveillance as a nursing intervention and/or an intrusive venture.

5. Analyze and respond to the question: When using technology, do nurses look to care and/or care to look?

6. What are your concerns about health care technology in the new millennium?

7. What would you like health care technology to do for you?

8. In Article 33, Goldsmith asserts that the barriers to protecting medical privacy on the Internet are not technological but, rather, political. What do you think about this assertion? Elaborate.

9. What suggestions do you have for increasing the public's trust regarding the use of information on the Internet?

10. What problems do you foresee in patients' increasing use of the Internet for health-related concerns?

Further Readings

Bischoff, W.R. & Kelley, S.J. (1999). 21st century house call: The Internet and the World Wide Web. *Holistic Nursing Practice, 13*(4), 42–50.

Curtin, L. & Simpson, R. (1999). High touch strategies temper technology. *Health Management Technology, 20*(8), 34–36.

Drucker, P. (1999). Beyond the information revolution. *Atlantic Monthly, 284*(4), 47–57.

Lomax, E. (1999). Finding and evaluating medical and health information on the Internet. *Health Care on the Internet, 3*(3), 41–51.

McConnell, E.A. (1999). Health care technology: Nursing's challenge and opportunity. *Nursing Connections, 12*(4), 49–53.

Porter-O'Grady, T. (1999). From enemy to friends: Nurses and computers unite. *Nursing Management, 30*(1), 4–5.

Schloman, B. (1999). Needle in a haystack? Finding health information on the Web. *Online Journal of Issues in Nursing,* August 19: 1–7.

Schloman, B. (1999). Whom do you trust? Evaluating Internet health resources. *Online Journal of Issues in Nursing,* January 28: 1–6.

Web Site Resources for Computers, the Internet and Nursing

American Medical Informatics Association www.amia.org
American Nursing Informatics Association www.ania.org
Med Web Plus: Nursing and Medical Informatics www.medwebplus.com

General Search Engine Web Sites

Mamma www.mamma.com
Oxygen www.oxygen.com

Health Web Sites

Health A to Z www.healthAtoZ.com
HealthlineUSA www.healthlineusa.com
Healthtouch www.healthtouch.com

Professional Journal Web Sites

Computers in Nursing www.nursingcenter.com
Health Management Technology www.nelsonpub.com
Healthcare Informatics www.healthcare-informatics.com
Healthcare on the Internet www.haworthpress.com

PART THREE

ISSUES OF VULNERABILITY AND SAFETY

7

Populations at Risk

In the land of the free and the home of the brave are the tired, homeless, and worn out, all yearning for something better than what they have now. They are the vulnerable among us: people whose health and well-being are steadily eroding despite prosperous times. And they are everywhere—on busy city streets, begging; crouched in doorways; sleeping on sidewalk grates; huddled in cardboard boxes trying to keep warm. Vulnerability is the companion of young and old alike as they stand in line for food at local soup kitchens or sit in emergency departments for health care they cannot afford. And when these nameless people die in the streets, in our parks, or under freeway overpasses, vulnerability becomes their shroud.

But not all people living with misfortune look vulnerable. Their vulnerability is cloaked in respectability. They are the families crowded into hotel rooms or apartments they can barely afford. They are the elderly who must choose between food and medication. They are the single parents who move from shelter to shelter with their children in tow. They are lower- and middle-income groups fighting a losing battle trying to provide their families with basic needs. They are the people who are trying hard not to lose hope.

It is with these at-risk populations that homelessness, infectious processes, and lack of health care coverage wreak the most havoc. Yet, despite our country's improved economic climate, these issues seem to drift in and out of the public's consciousness and off the public's agenda. Instead, complacency has replaced indignation, skepticism has overshadowed need, and cutting costs has taken precedence over adequate funding. As a result, vulnerability is allowed to continue and to thrive upon the impoverished, the old, and the homeless.

Each of the readings in this chapter tells a story. For the homeless, it's the hope of finding a place to call home and the failed attempts to find one. For the uninsured, it's the fear of becoming ill and the certainty that without health coverage, there is no healthy tomorrow. For the elderly, it's the shock and disbelief that they too can become infected with HIV. For those whom tuberculosis has infected, it's knowing that this preventable disease will not respond to the drugs that in the past have contained this infection. None of these human stories has an ending. Without the collective will to find solutions to these problems, there may never be.

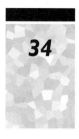

34

The Old Homeless and the New Homelessness in Historical Perspective

Peter H. Rossi

*O*ver the past decade, homelessness has received a great deal of popular attention and sympathy. The reasons for both appear to be obvious: Homelessness is clearly increasing, and its victims easily garner sympathetic concern. Our ideas about what constitutes a minimally decent existence are bound up inextricably with the concept of home. The Oxford Unabridged Dictionary devotes three pages to definitions of the word *home* and its derivatives; almost all of them stress one or more of the themes of safety, family, love, shelter, comfort, rest, sleep, warmth, affection, food, and sociability.

Homelessness has always existed in the United States, increasing in times of economic stress and declining in periods of prosperity (Monkkonen, 1984). Yet the problem has not received as much attention and sympathy in the past. Our current high level of concern reflects at least in part the fact that today's homeless are different and intrude more pointedly into everyday existence.

Before the 1980s the last great surge of homelessness occurred during the Great Depression in the 1930s. As in the present day, there were no definitive counts of the numbers of Depression-era homeless; estimates ranged from 200,000 to 1.5 million homeless persons in the worst years of the Depression.

As described in the social research of the time (Schubert, 1935), the Depression transient homeless consisted mainly of young men (and a small proportion of women) moving from place to place in search of employment. Many left their parental homes because they no longer wanted to be burdens on impoverished households and because they saw no employment opportunities in their depressed hometowns. Others were urged to leave by parents struggling to feed and house their younger siblings.

Peter H. Rossi was a professor with the Department of Sociology and acting director of the Social and Demographic Research Institute, University of Massachusetts/Amherst at the time of this article.

Reprinted with permission by the University of Chicago Press from Rossi, P., *Down and Out in America: The Origins of Homelessness.* (Chicago: University of Chicago Press) 1989.

■ *HOMELESSNESS AFTER WORLD WAR II*

The entry of the United States into World War II drastically reduced the homeless population in this country, absorbing them into the armed forces and the burgeoning war industries (Hopper & Hamburg, 1984). The permanently unemployed that so worried social commentators who wrote in the early 1930s virtually disappeared within months. When the war ended, employment rates remained relatively high. Accordingly, homelessness and skid row areas shrank to a fraction of the 1930s experience. But neither phenomenon disappeared entirely.

In the first two postwar decades, the skid rows remained as collections of cheap hotels, inexpensive restaurants and bars, casual employment agencies, and religious missions dedicated to the moral redemption of skid row residents, who were increasingly an older population. Typically, skid row was located close to the railroad freight yards and the trucking terminals that provided casual employment for its inhabitants.

In the 1950s, as urban elites turned to the renovation of the central cities, what to do about the collection of unsightly buildings, low-quality land use, and unkempt people in the skid rows sparked a revival of social science research on skid row and its denizens. Especially influential were studies of New York's Bowery by Bahr and Caplow (1974), of Philadelphia by Blumberg and associates (Blumberg, Shipley, & Shandler, 1973), and of Chicago's skid row by Donald Bogue (1963).

All the studies of the era reported similar findings, with only slight local variations. The title of Bahr and Caplow's (1974) monograph, *Old Men: Drunk and Sober,* succinctly summarizes much of what was learned—that skid row was populated largely by alcoholic old men.

By actual count, Bogue (1963) enumerated 12,000 homeless persons in Chicago in 1958, almost all of them men. In 1964, Bahr and Caplow (1974) estimated that there were about 8,000 homeless men living in New York's Bowery. In 1960, Blumberg et al. (1973) found about 2,000 homeless persons living in the skid row of Philadelphia. Clearly, despite the postwar economic expansion, homelessness persisted.

The meaning of homelessness as used by Bahr (1970), Blumberg et al. (1973), Bogue (1963), and other analysts of the era was somewhat different from current usage. In those studies, homelessness mostly meant living outside family units, whereas today's meaning of the term is more directly tied to the absolute lack of housing or to living in shelters and related temporary quarters. In fact, almost all of the homeless men studied by Bogue (1963) in 1958 had stable shelter of some sort. Four out of five rented cubicles in flophouse hotels. Renting for from $0.50 to $0.90 a night, a cubicle room would hardly qualify as a home, at least not by contemporary standards. Most of those not living in the cubicles lived in private rooms in inexpensive single-room occupancy (SRO) hotels or in the mission dormitories. Bogue reported that only a few homeless men, about 100, lived out on the streets, sleeping in doorways, under bridges, and in other "sheltered" places. Searching the streets, hotels and boarding houses of Philadelphia's skid row area in 1960, Blumberg et al. found only 64 persons sleeping in the streets.

As described by Bogue (1963), the median age of Chicago's homeless in the late 1950s was about 50 years old, and more than 90% were White. One fourth were Social Security pensioners, making their monthly $30–$50 minimum Social Security payments last through the month by renting the cheapest accommodations possible. Another fourth were chronic alcoholics. The remaining one half was composed of persons suffering from physical disability (20%), chronic mental illness (20%), and what Bogue called *social maladjustment* (10%).

Aside from those who lived on their pension checks, most skid row inhabitants earned their living through menial, low-paid employment, much of which was of an intermittent variety. The mission dormitories and municipal shelters provided food and beds for those who were out of work or who could not work.

All of the social scientists who studied the skid rows in the postwar period remarked on the social isolation of the homeless (Bahr, 1970). Bogue (1963) found that virtually all homeless men were unmarried, and a majority had never married. Although many had family, kinship ties were of the most tenuous quality, with few of the homeless maintaining ongoing contacts with their kin. Most had no one they considered to be good friends.

Much the same portrait emerged from other skid row studies throughout the country. All of the studies painted a similar picture in the same three pigments: (a) extreme poverty arising from unemployment or sporadic employment, chronically low earnings, and low benefit levels (such as were characteristic of Social Security pensions at the time); (b) disability arising from advanced age, alcoholism, and physical or mental illness; and (c) social disaffiliation, tenuous or absent ties to family and kin, with few or no friends.

Most of the social scientists studying skid rows expressed the opinion that they were declining in size and would soon disappear. Bahr and Caplow (1974) claimed that the population of the Bowery had dropped from 14,000 in 1949 to 8,000 in 1964, a trend that would end with the disappearance of skid row by the middle 1970s. Bogue (1963) cited high vacancy rates in the cubicle hotels as evidence that Chicago's skid row was also on the decline. In addition, Bogue claimed that the economic function of skid row was fast disappearing. With the mechanization of many low-skilled tasks, the casual labor market was shrinking, and with no economic function to perform, the skid row social system would also disappear.

Evidence through the early 1970s indeed suggested that the forecasted decline was correct; skid row was on the way out. Lee (1980) studied skid row areas of 41 cities and found that the skid row populations had declined by 50% between 1950 and 1970. Furthermore, in cities in which the market for unskilled labor had declined most precipitously, the loss of the skid row population was correspondingly larger.

By the end of the 1970s, striking changes had taken place in city after city. The flophouse and cubicle hotels had, for the most part, been demolished, and were replaced eventually by office buildings, luxury condominiums, and apartments. The stock of cheap SRO hotels, in which the more prosperous of the old homeless had lived, had also been seriously diminished (U.S. Senate, 1978). Skid row did not disappear altogether; in most cities, the missions still remained and smaller skid rows sprouted up in several places throughout the cities, where the remaining SRO hotels and rooming houses still stood.

■ THE NEW HOMELESSNESS OF THE 1980s

The "old" homeless of the 1950s, 1960s, and 1970s—so ably described by many social scientists—may have blighted some sections of the central cities but, from the perspective of most urbanites, they had the virtue of being concentrated in skid row, a neighborhood one could avoid and hence ignore. Most of the old homeless on skid row had some shelter, although it was inadequate by any standards; very few were literally sleeping on the streets. Indeed, in those early years, if any had tried to bed down on the steam vents or in doorways and vestibules of any downtown business area, the police would have quickly trundled them off to jail.

The demise or displacement of skid row, however, and the many other trends and developments of the 1960s and 1970s, did *not* put an end to homelessness in American cities. Quite to the contrary: By the end of the 1970s, and certainly by the early 1980s, a new type of homelessness had begun to appear.

The "new" homeless could be seen sleeping in doorways, in cardboard boxes, in abandoned cars, or resting in railroad or bus stations or in other public places, indications of a resurgent homelessness of which hardly anyone could remain oblivious. The immediate evidence of the senses was that there were persons in our society who had no shelter and who therefore lived, literally, in the streets. This change reflected partially corresponding changes in local police practices following the decriminalization of public inebriation and other court-ordered changes in the treatment of "loitering" and vagrancy. The police no longer herded the homeless into their ghettos.

Even more striking was the appearance of homeless women in significant numbers. The skid rows of the 1950s and 1960s were male enclaves; very few women appeared in any of the pertinent studies. And thus, homelessness had come to be defined (or perhaps, stereotyped) as largely a male problem. Indifference to the plight of derelicts and bums is one thing; indifference to the existence and problems of homeless women is quite another.

Soon, entire families began showing up among the homeless, and public attention grew even stronger and sharper. Women and their children began to arrive at the doors of public welfare departments asking for aid in finding shelter, arousing immediate sympathy. Stories began to appear in the newspapers about families migrating from the Rustbelt cities to cities in the Sunbelt in old cars loaded with their meager belongings, seeking employment, starkly and distressingly reminiscent of the Okies of the 1930s.

There is useful contrast between Bogue's, 1958, Chicago study (Bogue, 1963) and the situation in Chicago today. Data on the contemporary Chicago homeless was obtained in a study conducted by my colleagues and myself in 1985 and 1986 (Rossi, 1989; Rossi, Fisher, & Willis, 1986; Rossi & Wright, 1987). In 1958, there were four or five mission shelters in the city, providing 975 beds. In our studies in 1985 and 1986, there were 45 shelters providing a total of 2,000 beds, primarily for adult homeless persons.

New types of sheltering arrangements have come into being to accommodate the rising number of homeless families. Some shelters now specialize in providing quasiprivate quarters for family groups, usually in one or two rooms per family, with shared bathrooms and cooking facilities. In many cities, welfare departments have provided temporary housing for family groups by renting rooms in hotels and motels.

In some cities, the use of hotel and motel rooms rented by public welfare agencies to shelter homeless families is very widespread. For example, in 1986, New York City's welfare department put up an average of 3,500 families in so-called *welfare hotels* each month (Bach & Steinhagen, 1987; Struening, 1987).

Funds for the new homeless are now being allocated out of local, state, and federal coffers on a scale that would have been inconceivable two decades ago. Private charity has also been generous, with most of the emergency shelters and food outlets for the homeless being organized and run by private groups. Foundations have given generous grants. For example, the Robert Wood Johnson Foundation, in association with the Pew Charitable Trust, supports health care clinics for the homeless in 19 large cities, a $25 million venture. The states have provided funds through existing programs and special appropriations. And in spring 1987, Congress passed the Stewart B. McKinney Homeless Assistance Act (P.L. 100-77), appropriating $442 million for the homeless in fiscal 1987 and $616 million in 1988, to be channeled through a group of agencies.

There can be little doubt that homelessness has increased over the past decade and that the composition of the homeless has changed dramatically. There are ample signs of that increase. For example, in New York City, shelter capacity has increased from 3,000 to 6,000 over the last five years, and the number of families in the welfare hotels has increased from a few hundred to more than 3,000 in any given month (Bach & Steinhagen, 1987; Struening, 1987). Studies reviewed by the U.S. General Accounting Office ([GAO]; 1985, 1988) suggest an annual growth rate of the homeless population somewhere between 10% and 38%.

The GAO figures and other estimates, to be sure, are not much more than reasoned guesses. No one knows for sure how many homeless people there are in the United States today or even how many there are in any specific city, let alone the rate of growth in those numbers over the past decade.

The many difficulties notwithstanding, several estimates have been made of the size of the nation's homeless population. The National Coalition for the Homeless, an advocacy group, puts the figure somewhere between 1.5 and 3 million (GAO, 1988). A much maligned report by the U.S. Department of Housing and Urban Development (1984), partially based on cumulating the estimates of presumably knowledgeable local experts, and partially on a survey of emergency shelters, put the national figure at somewhere between 250,000 and 300,000. A more recent national estimate by The Urban Institute (Burt & Cohen, 1988), based on direct counts in shelters and food kitchens leads to a current estimate of about 500,000 homeless persons.

No available study suggests a national total number of homeless on any given night of less than several hundred thousand, and perhaps it is enough to know that the nation's homeless are at least numerous enough to populate a medium-sized city. Although the "numbers" issue has been quite contentious, in a very real sense, it does not matter much which estimate is closest to the truth. By any standard, all estimates point to a national disgrace.

■ *WHO ARE THE NEW HOMELESS?*

Since 1983, 40 empirical studies of the homeless have been undertaken that were conducted by competent social researchers; the results provide a detailed and remarkably consistent portrait of today's homeless population. As in the 1950s and 1960s, the driving purpose behind the funding and conduct of these studies is to provide the information necessary to design policies and programs that show promise to alleviate the pitiful condition of the homeless. The cities covered in these studies range across all regions of the country and include all the major metropolitan areas as well as more than a score of smaller cities.

The cumulative knowledge about the new homeless provided through these studies is quite impressive, and the principal findings are largely undisputed. Despite wide differences in definitions of homelessness, research methods and approaches, cities studied, professional and ideological interests of the investigators, and technical sophistication, the findings from all studies tend to converge on a common portrait. It would not be fair to say that all of the important questions have been answered, but a reasonably clear understanding is now emerging of who the new homeless are, how they contrast with the general population, and how they differ from the old homeless of the 1950s.

Some of the important differences between the new homeless and the old have already been mentioned. Few of the old homeless slept in the streets. In stark contrast, the Chicago Homeless Study (Rossi, 1989; Rossi, Fisher, & Willis, 1986; Rossi & Wright, 1987) found close to 1,400 homeless persons out on the streets in the fall of 1985 and more than 500 in that condition in the dead of winter (early 1986). Comparably large numbers of street homeless, proportionate to community size, have been found over the last five years in studies of Los Angeles (Farr, Koegel, & Burnam, 1986); New York (New York State Department of Social Services, 1984); Nashville, Tennessee (Wiegand, 1985); Austin, Texas (Baumann, Grigsby, Beauvais, & Schultz, not dated); Phoenix, Arizona (Brown, McFarlane, Parades, & Stark, 1983); Detroit, Michigan (Mowbray, Solarz, Johnson, Phillips-Smith, & Combs, 1986); Baltimore (Maryland Department of Human Resources, 1986); and Washington, DC (Robinson, 1985), among others.

One major difference between the old homeless and the new is thus that nearly all of the old homeless managed, somehow, to find nightly shelter indoors, whereas large fractions of the new homeless sleep in the streets or in public places, such as building lobbies and bus stations. In regard to shelter, the new homeless are clearly worse off. *Homelessness today is a more severe condition of housing deprivation* than in decades past. Furthermore, the new homeless, whether sheltered or living on the streets, are no longer concentrated in a single skid row area. They are, rather, scattered more widely throughout downtown areas.

A second major difference is the presence of sizable numbers of women among the new homeless. In the 1950s and 1960s women constituted less than 3% of the homeless. In contrast, we found that women constituted 25% of the 1985–1986 Chicago homeless (Rossi et al., 1986), a proportion similar to that reported in virtually all recent studies (Hope & Young, 1986; Lam, 1987; Sullivan & Damrosch, 1987). Thus, all 1980s-era studies found that women compose a much larger proportion of the homeless than did studies of the old homeless undertaken before 1970.

A third contrast between the old homeless and the new is in age composition. There are very few elderly persons among today's homeless and virtually no Social Security pensioners. In the Chicago Homeless Study (Rossi et al., 1986), the median age was 37, sharply contrasting the median age of 50 found in Bogue's (1963) earlier study of that city. Indeed, today's homeless are surprisingly young; virtually all recent studies of the homeless report median ages in the low to middle 30s. Trend data over a 15-year period (1969–1984) from the Men's Shelter in New York's Bowery suggest that the median age of the homeless has dropped by about one half-year per year for the last decade (Rossi & Wright, 1987; Wright & Weber, 1987).

A fourth contrast is provided by employment patterns and income levels. In Bogue's (1963) 1958 study, excepting the aged pensioners, over one half of the homeless were employed in any given week, either full time (28%) or on an intermittent, part-time basis (25%), and almost all were employed at least for some period during a year. In contrast, among today's Chicago homeless, only 3% reported having a steady job and only 39% worked for some period during the previous month. Correspondingly, the new homeless have less income. Bogue estimated that the median annual income of the 1958 homeless was $1,058. Our Chicago finding (Rossi et al., 1986) was a median annual income of $1,198. Correcting for the intervening inflation, the current average annual income of the Chicago homeless (Rossi et al., 1986) is equivalent to only $383 in 1958 dollars, less than one third of the actual 1958 median. Thus, *the new homeless suffer a much more profound degree of economic destitution,* often surviving on 40% or less of a poverty-level income.

A final contrast is presented by the ethnic composition of the new and old homeless. The old homeless were predominantly White—70% on the Bowery (Bahr & Caplow, 1974) and 82% on Chicago's skid row (Rossi et al., 1986). Among the new homeless, racial and ethnic minorities are heavily overrepresented. In the Chicago study, 54% were Black, and in the New York men's shelter, more than 75% were Black, a proportion that has been increasing since the early 1980s (Wright & Weber, 1987). In most cities, other ethnic minorities, principally Hispanics and American Indians, are also found disproportionately among the homeless, although the precise ethnic mix is apparently determined by the ethnic composition of the local poverty population. In short, minorities are consistently over-represented among the new homeless, compared with times past.

There are also some obvious continuities from the old homeless to the new. First, both groups share the condition of extreme poverty. Although the new homeless are poorer (in constant dollars), neither they nor the old homeless have (or had) incomes that would support a reasonable standard of living, whatever one takes *reasonable* to mean. The median income of today's Chicago homeless works out to less than $100 a month, or about $3 a day, with a large proportion (18%) with essential zero income (Rossi et al., 1986). Comparably low incomes have been reported in other studies.

At these income levels, even trivial expenditures loom as major expenses. For example, a single round trip on Chicago's bus system costs $1.80, or more than one half a day's median income. A night's lodging at even the cheapest flophouse hotel costs more than $5, which exceeds the average daily income (Hoch, 1985). And, of course, the median simply marks the income received by persons right at the midpoint of the income distribution; by definition, one half of the homeless live on less than the median and, in fact, nearly one fifth (18%) reported *no income at all.*

Given these income levels, it is certainly no mystery why the homeless are without shelter. Their incomes simply do not allow them to compete effectively in the housing market, even on the lowest end. Indeed, the only way most homeless people can survive at all is to use the shelters for a free place to sleep, the food kitchens and soup lines for free meals, the free community health clinics and emergency rooms for medical care, and the clothing distribution depots for something to put on their backs. That the homeless survive at all is a tribute to the many charitable organizations that provide these and other essential commodities and services.

The new homeless and the old also apparently share similar levels of disability. The one unmistakable change from the 1950s to the 1980s is the declining proportion of elderly, and thus a decline in the disabilities associated with advanced age. But today's homeless appear to suffer from much the same levels of mental illness, alcoholism, and physical disability as the old homeless did.

More has been written about the homeless mentally ill than about any other aspect of the problem. Estimates of the rate of mental illness among the homeless vary widely, from about 10% to more than 85%, but most studies report a figure on the order of 33⅓% (Bassuk, 1984; Snow, Baker, & Anderson, 1986). This is somewhat larger than the estimates, clustering between 15% and 25%, appearing in the literature of the 1950s and 1960s.

Physical disabilities also are widespread among the new homeless and the old. Some of the best current evidence on this score comes from the medical records of clients seen in the Johnson Foundation Health Care for the Homeless (HCH) clinics. Chronic physical disorders, such as hypertension, diabetes, heart and circulatory disease, peripheral vascular disease, and the like, are observed in 40% (compared with a rate of only 25% among urban ambulatory patients in general).

> In all, poor physical health plays some direct role in the homelessness of 21% of the HCH clients, and is a major (or single most important) factor in the homelessness of about 13%. Thus, approximately one homeless adult in eight is homeless at least in major part as a result of chronically poor physical health. (Wright & Weber, 1987, p. 113; see also Brickner, Scharar, Conanan, Elvy, & Savarese, 1985; Robertson & Cousineau, 1986).

Analysis of the deaths occurring among these clients showed that the average age at death (or in other words, the average life expectancy) of the homeless is only a bit more than 50 years.

All studies of the old homeless stress the widespread prevalence of chronic alcoholism, and here too, the new homeless are little different. Bogue (1963) found that 30% of his sample were heavy drinkers, defined as persons spending 25% or more of their income on alcohol and drinking the equivalent of six or more pints of whiskey a week.

A final point of comparability is that both the old homeless and the new are socially isolated. The new homeless report few friends and intimates, and depressed levels of contact with relatives and family. There are also signs of friction between the homeless and their relatives. Similar patterns of isolation were found among the old homeless.

■ SUMMARY AND CONCLUSIONS

The major changes in homelessness since the 1950s and 1960s involve an increase in the numbers of homeless persons, striking changes in the composition of the homeless, and a marked deterioration in their condition. The old homeless were older men living on incomes either from intermittent casual employment or from inadequate retirement pensions. However inadequate their incomes may have been, the old homeless had three times the income (in constant dollars) of the current homeless. The new homeless include an increasing proportion of women, often accompanied by their children, persons who are, on average, several decades younger. The old homeless were housed inadequately, but high proportions of the new homeless are shelterless.

Like the old homeless, the new have high levels of disabilities, including chronic mental illness (33%), acute alcoholism (33%), serious criminal records (20%), and serious physical disabilities (25%). Seventy-five percent have one or more of the disabilities mentioned.

References

Bach, V., & Steinhagen, R. (1987). *Alternatives to the welfare hotel.* New York: Community Service Society.

Bahr, H. (1970). *Disaffiliated man.* Toronto, Canada: University of Toronto Press.

Bahr, H., & Caplow, T. (1974). *Old men drunk and sober.* New York: New York University Press.

Bassuk, E. (1984, July). The homeless problem. *Scientific American, 251,* 40–45.

Baumann, D., Grigsby, C., Beauvais, C., & Schultz, D. F. (not dated). *The Austin homeless* (Final report to the Hogg Foundation for Mental Health). Austin: University of Texas.

Blumberg, L., Shipley, T., & Shandler, I. (1973). *Skid row and its alternatives.* Philadelphia, PA: Temple University Press.

Bogue, D. (1963). *Skid row in American cities.* Chicago: University of Chicago.

Brickner, P. W., Scharar, L. K., Conanan, B., Elvy, A., & Savarese, M. (Eds.). (1985). *Health care of homeless people.* New York: Springer.

Brown, C., MacFarlane, S., Parades, R., & Stark, L. (1983, June). *The homeless of Phoenix: Who are they and what should be done?* Phoenix, AZ: South Community Mental Health Center.

Burt, M. R., & Cohen, B. E. (1988). *Feeding the homeless: Does the prepared meals provision help?* Washington, DC: The Urban Institute.

Farr, R., Koegel, P., & Burnham, A. (1986). *A study of homelessness and mental illness in the skid row area of Los Angeles.* Los Angeles: Los Angeles County Department of Mental Health.

Hoch, C. (1985, December). *SROs: An endangered species.* Chicago: Community Emergency Shelter Organization and Jewish Council on Urban Affairs.

Hope, M., & Young, J. (1986). *The faces of homelessness.* Lexington, MA: Heath.

Hopper, K., & Hamburg, J. (1984). *The making of America's homeless: From skid row to new poor, 1945–1984.* New York: Community Service Society.

Lam, J. (1987). *Homeless women in America.* Unpublished doctoral dissertation, University of Massachusetts, Amherst.

Lee, B. A. (1980, September). The disappearance of skid row: Some ecological evidence. *Urban Affairs Quarterly, 16,* 81–107.

Maryland Department of Human Resources. (1986, August). *Where do you go from nowhere?* Baltimore: Health and Welfare Council of Central Maryland.

Monkkonen, E. H. (Ed.). (1984). *Walking to work: Tramps in America, 1790–1935.* Lincoln: University of Nebraska Press.

Mowbray, C., Solarz, A., Johnson, V. S., Phillips-Smith, E., & Combs, C. J. (1986). *Mental health and homelessness in Detroit: A research study* (NIMH Grant No. 5H84-MH35823-04S1). Lansing: Michigan Department of Mental Health.

New York State Department of Social Services. (1984, October). *Homelessness in New York state: A report to the governor and legislature.* New York: Author.

Robertson, M., & Cousineau, M. R. (1986, May). Health status and access to health services among the urban homeless. *American Journal of Public Health, 76,* 561–563.

Robinson, F. (1985, November). *Homeless people in the nation's capital.* Washington, DC: University of the District of Columbia.

Rossi, P. H. (1989). *Down and out in America: The origins of homelessness.* Chicago: University of Chicago Press.

Rossi, P. H., Fisher, G. A., & Willis, G. (1986). *The condition of the homeless of Chicago.* Amherst: University of Massachusetts.

Rossi, P. H., & Wright, J. D. (1987, Spring). The determinants of homelessness. *Health Affairs, 6,* 19–32.

Schubert, H. J. P. (1935). *Twenty thousand transients: A year's sample of those who apply for aid in a northern city.* Buffalo, NY: Emergency Relief Bureau.

Snow, D., Baker, S. G., & Anderson, L. (1986, June). The myth of pervasive mental illness among the homeless. *Social Problems, 33,* 407–423.

Struening, E. L. (1987). *A study of residents of the New York City shelter system.* New York: New York State Psychiatric Institute.

Sullivan, P., & Damrosch, S. (1987). Homeless women and children. In R. Bingham, R. Green, & S. White (Eds.), *The homeless in contemporary society* (pp. 82–98). Newbury Park, CA: Sage.

U.S. Department of Housing and Urban Development. (1984). *A report to the Secretary on the homeless and emergency shelters.* Washington, DC: Author.

U.S. General Accounting Office. (1985, April). *Homelessness: A complex problem and the federal response* (GAO/HRD Publication No. 85-40). Washington, DC: Author.

U.S. General Accounting Office. (1988, August). *Homeless mentally ill: Problems and options in estimating numbers and trends* (GAO/PEMD Publication No. 88-24). Washington, DC: Author.

U.S. Senate, Special Committee on Aging. (1978). *Single room occupancy: A need for national concern.* Washington, DC: U.S. Government Printing Office.

Wiegand, R. B. (1985). Counting the homeless. *American Demographics, 7,* 34–37.

Wright, J. D., & Weber, E. (1987). Homelessness and health. New York: McGraw Hill.

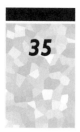

35

Helping People Off the Streets: Real Solutions to Urban Homelessness

Robert V. Hess

On a "campus" in Florida, 500 homeless men, each given just a blanket and pillow, spend an average of three months sleeping on the cement floor of an open-air pavilion in 4' × 6' "human parking spaces." In another Florida campus, participants who are willing to sleep on the floor of a large, 500-person outdoor pavilion for up to three months may be moved to the comfort of an indoor, 20-bed dormitory, where they can access needed support services.

The idea behind these campuses and others across the country is to remove as many homeless people as possible from downtown streets. Usually, these homeless campuses serve as large warehouse facilities—funded by local government, businesses, and private donations—where homeless persons can receive emergency shelter and, sometimes, support services. Often, the campuses are purposely tucked away from downtown.

Residents, business owners, and tourists, uncomfortable at the presence of the homeless, support moving them away from downtown. These feelings often apply to homeless resource centers such as soup kitchens and housing facilities. For years, organizations dedicated to assisting the less fortunate have fought a growing sense of NIMBY (not in my backyard) and anti-homelessness ordinances.

Numerous American cities—including New Orleans, La.; Orlando, Ft. Lauderdale, and Jacksonville, Fla.; San Antonio and Austin, Tex.; and Washington, D.C.—have developed campuses to address the problem of homelessness. The Center for Poverty Solutions, a nonprofit organization created in 1997 through a merger of the Maryland Food Committee and Action for the Homeless, undertook as one of its first projects a review of homeless campuses. The intent was to offer recommendations to Baltimore regarding the development of a campus for the city. What was found, however, by visiting homeless campuses in nine cities and looking at several award-winning and

Robert V. Hess is president and CEO, Center for Poverty Solutions, Baltimore, Md.

successful programs for the homeless, is that there are more effective ways to deal with this situation.

A "one-size-fits-all" campus model does not address the individual needs of the people most affected. Homeless campuses too often serve as revolving doors that warehouse poor people for a limited amount of time, then spin them back out onto the streets with no improvement in their ability to climb out of poverty. These facilities also report high incidences of vandalism and destruction of property that may be attributed in part to police depositing homeless persons at these sites against their will, as well as the dehumanizing conditions at some of these places.

Homeless campuses are just one of the latest attempts to solve or address homelessness. In some instances, agencies dedicated to assisting the homeless have created wonderful and humane ways of dealing with the people and the issues involved. Policymakers and community and business leaders, though, sometimes forget that "real" people lie at the heart of this seemingly insurmountable issue. Every person who is homeless has his or her own story and has arrived in this situation via various circumstances.

According to data from the U.S. Conference of Mayors, families constitute 38% of the nation's homeless population; 27% are children; and 14% are single women. Many have been driven to homelessness by factors such as lack of affordable housing and/or jobs that pay a living wage, domestic violence, substance abuse, mental illness, and disability.

It is not enough to simply take homeless people off the streets and hide them. The real solution is to address the reasons why they become homeless in the first place. Even if there were enough campuses to house the existing men, women, and children who are homeless, the facilities do nothing to prevent others from reaching the same plight. Housing 500, 1,000, or more homeless people in one facility not only strips them of their dignity, it disallows individualized care and tends to breed an air of intimidation and fear for personal safety, especially for families with children, seniors, and the disabled. That is not to say that emergency shelters are not needed, but, rather, that funding should be spent on planned social services to assist the homeless in receiving the help and support they need to move out of poverty.

What the homeless require are many of the same resources all people need to live. One basic misconception is that the average homeless person is lazy and does not want to work. The media reinforces the fact that unemployment levels are at an all-time low, so why are there people in this country without jobs? Survey data from the U.S. Conference of Mayors shows that this is untrue. Twenty percent of homeless Americans work full or part time, but do not earn enough to meet their most basic needs; 30% of the men and women who visit soup kitchens and food pantries are employed. Policies must be put into place to guarantee a living wage—the minimum income needed for an individual or family to meet basic needs: housing, food, health care, transportation, and clothing. For instance, economists have determined the living wage in Baltimore to be $7.70 per hour, far above the minimum wage of $5.15 per hour.

Another factor in unemployment has to do with the gap in salary and job availability for the high-tech, high-skilled workforce vs. low-skilled laborers. High demand and salaries are available for educated and experienced workers in the computer/technical industry. Employment opportunities for poorly educated or low-skilled laborers who lack technology training continue to be in the service industry, which pays significantly less and has less stability.

Furthermore, jobs that may be available may not be accessible. The urban flight so many cities have experienced in recent decades has included many businesses. Few poor or homeless families own cars, and most large cities are unable, if not unwilling, to provide transportation services to low-density suburban job centers.

Even if homeless individuals were able to find some way to get to work, who would care for their children? Safe and affordable child care is an issue for all Americans. The average family spends seven percent of its income on child care, in contrast to 25% for a low-income family. While child care expenses are part of the welfare reform initiative, just 10% of the families who qualify for Federal aid receive assistance. Every city has a waiting list of thousands of people seeking to take part in the child care assistance programs. Affordable child care must be made available so that all parents, including those who work late shifts, have access to it.

■ PROVIDING AFFORDABLE HOUSING

Why do some people choose or are forced to live on the streets? The lack of affordable housing is the major cause of homelessness. If you drive along the streets in any urban area, you will find a plethora of dilapidated buildings and unsafe housing projects. Between 1993 and 1995, the number of rental units available to very-low-income families dropped by nine percent. This translated into a loss of 900,000 units nationally. Since the Depression, most families in need of housing assistance could rely on the Federal government for help, but, in 1995, Congress ceased approving funding for additional housing vouchers. Most states now have a three-year or longer waiting period for Section 8 housing.

Over the past six years, the Federal housing budget shrank 30%, causing local housing authorities to begin targeting people with higher incomes as "preferred tenants." Making public housing more universal and less targeted toward very-low-income people makes it significantly more difficult for the homeless to move into public housing. New minimum rent requirements create yet another obstacle in finding a permanent, stable home.

Homelessness is not an insurmountable problem, but it is a challenge. The following strategies offered are meant to provide long-term support. They are based on the Center for Poverty Solutions' study of campuses and its experience with homelessness and poverty. The solution, according to the Center's report, "Helping People Off the Streets, Real Solutions to Urban Homelessness," lies in the willingness of government and community leaders to work together in promoting economic development.

Across the country, the number of emergency shelters without support services needs to be reduced while increasing the number of service-enriched transitional shelters. This entails converting the many existing emergency shelters into adequate short- and long-term transitional housing. These facilities would remain open 24 hours a day with comprehensive support services that assist people with moving into long-term or permanent housing. Support services would include job skills training, addiction recovery groups, mental health services, lavatory and shower access, telephones, and mail delivery. Long-term facilities should include job training and placement, child care, life skills training, transportation, and case management that requires clients to set clear goals and objectives. Above all, facilities must create and maintain an environment that respects the inherent worth and dignity of each individual. Cities must make the commitment to increase the number of affordable permanent housing units for families, single individuals, and people with disabilities. Successful examples can be found across the country, many of which have been funded by the Enterprise Foundation.

Some emergency shelters must be set aside to provide convalescent care beds for homeless people recently discharged from hospitals. The beds would provide a safe environment to recuperate and receive follow-up services. This would reduce the likelihood of a person experiencing complications or a relapse.

Some emergency shelters force people to leave during the day with no other place to go, only to have them return when the shelter reopens in the evening. This is especially difficult for persons who work nights and need a place to sleep in the daytime, as well as those in poor health who must face inclement weather. Baltimore has two day centers that cater exclusively to veterans or addicts. Baltimore's largest shelter for men charges residents a nightly fee and requires attendance at a religious service. It is no wonder that the homeless are forced to turn to parks, sidewalks, or libraries to seek shelter.

Cities must develop easily accessible, daytime facilities with no residential component. This would give people who are homeless a place to go during the day as well as access to programs to help restore their feelings of self-esteem, empowerment, and personal responsibility. These facilities should be relatively small (maximum capacity of about 200) and should provide housing assistance, case management, substance abuse counseling, and employment assistance. Other volunteer-based services offered by the business and social welfare community should include legal assistance, health care, dental and mental health services, and benefits enrollment. In addition, the creation of a universal system to provide every American with health care coverage would reduce the misuse of hospital emergency rooms and provide everyone with personalized health care services such as addiction counseling and treatment and disease prevention.

With Federal welfare reform legislation in place, there may be an increase in the number of homeless families as time limits are reached and families with special needs are unable to comply with work activity requirements. Emergency service providers in Baltimore are reporting a 38% increase in the number of families seeking assistance at food pantries, soup kitchens, shelters, and transitional housing facilities.

How many families will be affected in your city? Is the job market able to handle the sudden surge of low-skilled workers? In order to bridge the gap between the unskilled worker and an above-minimum wage-paying job, programs providing job training for the homeless, low-income workers, and welfare recipients must be created. These will give those most in need the training to fill living wage-paying positions. A consortium of businesses could assist in covering the costs for the programs and receive the benefit of filling vacancies with newly qualified candidates.

Lastly, a local task force should be created, bringing together community, business, religious, and government leaders to continue developing comprehensive strategies and finding creative solutions to end poverty and homelessness. Dade County, Fla., provides an excellent example of such a task force. The economic development of every city is important to creating a healthy community and improving the quality of life for all citizens. Every human being should be entitled to adequate income, affordable housing, and quality health care. If society understands this basic principle and effectively invests its resources, that inevitably will make a lasting difference.

The recommendations contained in this article have been gleaned from effective programs in communities across the country. The solutions are not particularly complicated. The problem has been and continues to be the lack of political will to help the nation's most vulnerable men, women, and children at their time of greatest need.

36

Not Gone, but Forgotten?

Romesh Ratnesar

A few minutes into his Inaugural Address, on Jan. 20, 1989, George Bush—a Republican President often derided for his inattention to domestic problems—looked out at the crowd and declared, "My friends, we have work to do." The first task: helping "the homeless, lost and roaming." Ten years later, Bill Clinton—a Democratic President often praised for his acuity on social issues—delivered his seventh State of the Union address. In the course of 77 min. and 99 proposals, Clinton didn't offer any plans to combat homelessness. He never even brought it up.

What has become of this once pressing issue? In the 1980s homelessness was widely regarded as a national emergency, one that drew heavy media coverage and gave rise to mass demonstrations (in 1986, 5 million Americans joined hands along a 4,000-mile line across the country to raise money for the homeless). That kind of public outcry led to the passage of the first and only federal law to assist homeless Americans, the McKinney Act of 1987, which authorized millions of dollars in funding for housing and hunger relief. But today that spirit is gone. In 1987 the number of articles on homelessness that appeared in the *New York Times, Washington Post, Chicago Tribune* and *Los Angeles Times* totaled 847; in 1996 those four dailies ran just 200 stories on the subject. As recently as 1991, 8% of Americans said homelessness—more than crime, the budget deficit, education or the decline of American values— was "the main problem facing the country today." Only half as many people now believe that. "Most of the emphasis today is on the feel-good," says Housing and Urban Development Secretary Andrew Cuomo, who founded a New York City homeless agency in 1986. "People don't want to focus on problems. But there's also the sense that the problem is apparently getting better."

But has it got better? Reliable estimates of the homeless population have always been hard to come by. In the early '80s Mitch Snyder, the late founder of the Center for Creative Non-Violence, an advocacy group in Washington, claimed that there were 3 million homeless in America on any given night. He later admitted that he'd made up the figure. A 1988 Urban Institute survey offered an estimate of 600,000 homeless; but after the 1990 Census, the General

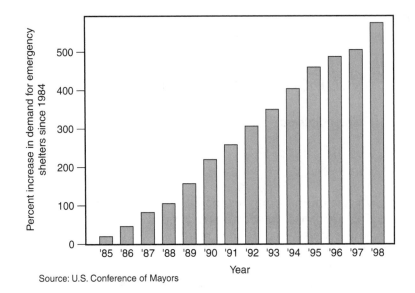

Source: U.S. Conference of Mayors

Accounting Office put the number at 300,000. A 1994 study examined computer data on shelter turnover rates from 1988 to 1992 and found that between 5 million and 7 million Americans had been homeless at one time or another during those years.

Today few reputable authorities are willing even to surmise how many people are homeless. But many researchers believe the problem is no less acute than it was in the mid-1980s. The U.S. Conference of Mayors, which publishes an annual survey on hunger and homelessness in 30 cities, says demand for emergency shelter has increased every year since the survey began in 1985, including an 11% jump in 1998. The number of people counted in Boston's annual one-night homeless census rose 40% between 1988 and 1996. Minnesota's nightly shelter population quadrupled between 1985 and 1997, and in New York City the average number of people staying in shelters climbed to 7,100 a night in 1997 after hitting a low of 6,000 in 1994. Homelessness has roiled San Francisco for much of the '90s: the Coalition for the Homeless estimates that 16,000 people are homeless there each night, twice as many as 10 years ago. Flush economic times may contribute to the problem: in many cities housing prices have soared out of reach of poor residents.

If the homeless have vanished from public consciousness in the '90s, it may be because in many cities they have vanished from sight. Cuomo attributes this to the expansion of shelters and other services; but increasingly, frustrated municipal governments are responding to the problem by cracking down on panhandling, sweeping homeless encampments out of parks and off streets and outlawing sleeping in public. At least 50 cities—from Chicago to Tucson, Ariz., to liberal Berkeley, Calif.—have antivagrancy laws on the books. Such measures only displace the homeless, however. New York's clampdown on vagrancy in Times Square, for instance, has merely pushed the encampments to the edges of the island of Manhattan.

The rise of such laws suggests that middle-class Americans have exhausted their reserves of compassion for the homeless and now see them as responsible for their own fate. "People decided that homeless people were affecting their quality of life," says Ralph Nunez, president of the New York-based Homes for the Homeless, "and they got fed up." But how fed up? In a recent survey conducted by researchers at Wayne State University, 80% of respondents said they favored increased federal spending on the homeless, and two-thirds said they would agree to a $25 tax hike to pay for homeless programs.

Ultimately, the best explanation for why Americans stopped talking about homelessness lies not in policies or public opinion but in politics. In the '80s liberal advocacy for the homeless was of a piece with Democratic outrage at Reagan Administration policies toward the poor. But the homeless issue also splintered urban liberalism, sending some working- and middle-class voters into the arms of Republicans who vowed to curtail entitlements and tighten the screws on vagrancy. To survive, Democrats revised their image as the party of the dispossessed by acceding to welfare reform, cutting aid to the homeless and courting the middle class. As liberals drifted toward the margins of the political landscape, so did the homeless.

This is not to say that government has turned its back on the problem. The Clinton Administration has spent $5 million on the homeless over the past six years—triple what was spent from 1987 to 1993. Most of the funding has gone into "continuum of care" programs that provide temporary housing and a range of services, from mental-illness treatment to job training. The approach has had some success in getting the chronically homeless on their feet, but it unsettles some advocates, who believe that the key to ending homelessness is still to boost the supply of affordable housing. In New York, 80% of homeless families who have been provided with subsidized apartments have remained intact, out of shelters and off the streets, regardless of their other problems. "No matter what is true about the homeless," says Mary Ann Gleason, executive director of the National Coalition of the Homeless, "they all have a lack of housing." That sounds like a return to the "housing, housing, housing" mantra that liberals sang in the '80s. Getting Americans to take the idea seriously again might require the return of liberalism itself.

37

Faces of the Uninsured

Siobhan Gorman

When he diagnosed Kenny Horsley with advanced skin cancer last December, neurosurgeon Joe Ordonez asked: "How long do you want to live?"

"If you'll pardon my French," answered Horsley, 48, "I want to be an old fart."

In February, when Horsley woke up from the 12½-hour operation that removed his left eye and part of his skull, Ordonez was sitting beside his bed. "I made your wish come true," Ordonez said softly. "You are going to be an old man when you die."

The nurses at Virginia Beach General Hospital call Horsley the "miracle man." But Horseley's story is not only a medical miracle, it's a financial one as well. A mover and janitor at Ewell's Furniture Store in Cape Charles, Va., Horsley can't get health insurance because his employer doesn't offer it. Nor, with a wage of $14,000 a year, can Horsley afford private insurance; he has to support Mary, his wife, and his 10-year-old daughter, Laura. Although Laura qualifies for Medicaid, Kenny and Mary don't; they make too much money.

Ordonez billed Horsley nothing for the surgery. The same goes for the surgeon who operated on Horsley's neck to examine his lymph nodes. The plastic surgeon charged $1,000 instead of $16,000. The $1,000 bill was paid with money raised by community churches and the local Lion's Club.

Kenny and Mary Horsley live frugally in this rural 1,500-person town on Virginia's Eastern Shore. "When somebody hasn't got insurance, it's terrifying. It brings you down mentally because your first thought is, 'What are you going to do?'" Horsley said. "I'm sure I'm not the only poor person in the world who is working for a living."

Of course, Horsley is right. Indeed, he is the prototypical uninsured person: a worker for a small business that does not provide insurance who makes too much money to qualify for Medicaid but not enough to afford insurance on his own. About 60 percent of the uninsured earn wages that are less than twice the poverty level, and about half work for businesses with 100 employees or fewer.

And there are a lot of Kenny Horsleys. The number of uninsured people climbed from 35.6 million in 1990 to 43.1 million in 1997, and a projection by economist William Custer of Georgia State University predicts 53 million will be uninsured by 2007 if America's economy continues to roll along, and 60 million if it doesn't.

Given these daunting numbers, targeting key groups among the uninsured may be the most manageable way for policy-makers to design solutions to the problem. "If you're going to do anything about the uninsured, you have to do it where the people are," said Paul Fronstin, a senior research associate at the Employee Benefit Research Institute, a nonpartisan research group in Washington.

Perhaps the most striking change taking place in the composition of the uninsured is the growing number of people who are uninsured because they opted not to enroll in health care plans offered by their employers. While Custer has not run projections for subgroups of the uninsured, he said several of them—including the near-elderly, Hispanic, and young adult populations—are likely to swell in the coming decade.

▪ *MAKING ENDS MEET*

Even after landing her first steady job last December as a nurse's assistant at the local health clinic in Morton, Texas, Alma Morin still couldn't get health insurance; like many, she couldn't afford the insurance premium required by her employer. Morin, 23, had recently divorced her husband after five years of a turbulent marriage and moved into a makeshift bedroom in her mother's house in Morton, a rural town in northwestern Texas.

Before she began at the clinic, though, she had found only temporary, very low paying jobs: cutting weeds in the nearby cottonfields, working the graveyard shift at Allsup's convenience store, and ringing up orders at a Kentucky Fried Chicken restaurant 30 miles from her house. She applied for Medicaid but didn't qualify because the government counted her mother's income as the "household income." Without insurance, Morin had to pay her medical bills out of her meager wages; often, she couldn't even afford to pay the $12 it cost for a visit to the doctor at the health clinic. When Morin's then-2-year-old son came down with colic in 1997, she opted to treat him herself, with manzanilla tea back rubs.

Morin remembers Dec. 7, 1998, vividly. That was the day she got the call about the full-time job. She had just completed a federally funded job-training program that paid her $5.15 an hour to take nursing classes and covered the cost of her transportation and of day care for her son. "It's an awesome job," Morin said. "I'm getting experience I probably would never get anywhere else."

Now making $960 a month, Alma can afford to pay the $12 for visits to the doctor. But the $86 monthly premium for the health insurance her employer offers remains out of the question. "We're so fixed on our budget right now, it's just too hard," she explained.

Like Kenny Horsley, Alma Morin represents a trend. In 1989, only 8 percent of the uninsured were without coverage because they chose not to take employer-offered insurance. In 1997, a quarter of the uninsured fit that description, according to a study by the Commonwealth Fund, a New York City–based foundation that supports health and social policy research. Rising employee premiums explain much of that jump, says Karen Davis, president of the Commonwealth Fund. Annual health care expenses rose from $864 in 1989 to $1,550 in 1997 for heads of households in large- and medium-size firms, the study found. For workers in small firms, the situation is worse.

Higher premiums are increasingly affecting middle-income Americans, too. About 20 percent of the uninsured live in households making $50,000 or more. Said Steven Findlay, a senior policy analyst at the National Coalition on Health Care, a Washington-based nonpartisan research group, "Earlier, even if [the premium] was 50 percent, it wasn't going to bust your budget. That's not true anymore."

▪ THE IMMIGRANT

Sitting in her immaculate but crowded efficiency apartment at a dining room table cluttered with Gerber bottles, Ana V., 26, a new mother, pauses when asked what she does when she becomes ill. Then she answers matter-of-factly in Spanish: "If I get sick, I know I can't go to the hospital, so I just go and buy something at the drugstore." Last year, when Ana was a cook at a Washington, D.C., restaurant, she slipped and fell down the stairs at work and did the only thing she could: She went to a CVS drugstore and bought pain-killing cream and Tylenol. But CVS doesn't sell medical miracles over the counter, and her back still hurts today.

Ana came to America from El Salvador in 1991 and worked as a live-in nanny for her first three years here. In 1993, she applied for and received a work permit and took a job with a cleaning service. She later got the job at the restaurant, which paid $8 an hour and offered no health insurance. Ana worked there until the restaurant burned down last December. She plans to seek work as a nanny when her 3-month-old son is a little older. Her husband has worked for the past six years as a busboy and makes on average $5 to $7 an hour with tips.

Health care became a concern for Ana in 1996, when her aunt was diagnosed with stomach cancer and died because she could not afford to treat her illness. Ana became even more concerned last September when she discovered she was pregnant. She saw her first American doctor at Mary's Center for Maternal and Child Care in Washington. Even though Mary's Center offers sharply reduced rates, Ana's bill for prenatal care had mounted to $800 by the time her son was born. She paid the debt off slowly—paying what she could each month.

Hispanics and blacks are 21 percent more likely than whites of the same economic status to be uninsured, said Allyson Hall, a program officer at the Commonwealth Fund. Although Hispanics make up 15 percent of the general working population, Hall found that they make up 22 percent of the uninsured population. And Hispanics, more than other ethnic groups, are concentrated in low-wage jobs that do not offer health insurance.

To these factors, add in the problems posed by immigrant status. "How do you reach out to the Hispanic population who worry that by signing up, they're vulnerable to being deported?" asked Ronald F. Pollack, president of Families USA, a Washington-based health care consumer advocacy group.

Ana, who is not a legal resident, does not expect the government to pay for her health care. Still, Maria Gomez, executive director of Mary's Center points out that Ana's lack of health care should concern the general public. "Those people are the same people that we depend on to cook, to clean, and to be in the kitchen when we are in restaurants. Those are the ones who are taking care of our kids when we work. Those are the teachers' aides in day care centers," she said.

■ *THE YOUNG*

Young adults such as Kevin Price, 24, are over-represented among the uninsured, and they are likely to become a larger proportion of the uninsured in the next decade.

Sitting in a Washington cafe on one of his days off, Price, an aspiring actor and professional temp, leans back and laughs when asked why he did not buy private health insurance in November 1997 after he had found it would cost him $54 a month.

"I don't know," said Price, a member of Dartmouth College's class of 1997. "I went to the medical facilities at the college once in four years, and that was after a skiing accident. I had a physical right after college [when he was still on his parents' plan], and they said I was damn healthy." He added that at the time, he figured he would find a regular job soon enough and it would offer health insurance. But that logic didn't impress his parents who continued to inquire every few months about his insurance status.

Last December, Price decided he would take a job as an administrative assistant at RegNet Environmental Services in Washington because it seemed flexible enough to accommodate his rehearsal schedule, and more important, it offered medical and dental benefits. Kevin had suspected he might have a cavity or two, but he had not gone to the dentist for fear that he was right.

While he was at RegNet, Price made about the same amount of money— $2,400 a month—he'd made as a temp *and* he had insurance. He promptly made a dental appointment. Two visits later, his teeth were clean and a cavity had been filled. His insurance covered 80 percent of the $162.50 bill. Price stuck around RegNet for another three months, before deciding to return to temping. He said he will probably sign on full time with his temp agency, Friends & Co., to qualify for some limited health care benefits. Though he has not yet asked about the details, he said, "I would guess it covers at least emergency stuff, and that's really all I care about."

Young adults are disproportionately uninsured. They make up 11 percent of the population, but 18 percent of the uninsured. In part, 18-to-24-year-olds are uninsured more often than other workers because they tend to have low-wage or short-term jobs. In part also, they are uninsured because they calculate, rationally enough, that they are unlikely to have much use for health insurance.

The numbers of young uninsured are likely to grow. The Census Bureau projects that the 18-to-24 age group, which numbers around 25 million now, will be 30 million by 2010. About one-third of those 25 million young adults are uninsured today, and if current patterns continue, that proportion will translate into 10 million in 10 years.

■ NOT OLD ENOUGH

The predicament of the near-elderly, those between the ages of 55 and 64, is that they're old enough to need regular medical care but too young for Medicare. The cost of insurance, if it's not offered in the workplace, can often be prohibitive because the near-elderly often have pre-existing medical conditions. Consider Tomasa Rodriguez, who works as a housekeeper for a family in the Georgetown area of Washington. On Dec. 8, 1998, Rodriguez, 56, woke up with piercing abdominal pain. She called a clinic, but could not get an appointment for a month. Unable to bear the persistent jabbing sensations, she called a private doctor, set up an appointment, and $190 later, was diagnosed with gallstones.

A week later, Rodriguez arrived at the hospital at 9 p.m. for her surgery and was released at 11 a.m. the next morning with a bill totaling more than $5,000. "The doctor told me, 'You have to go because if you stay, you have to pay more.'" she said. "I couldn't walk. I was in real pain. I was crying." Paying back what she can each month, Rodriguez still owes $1,500.

Increasingly, even people who had health care when they were working are losing it as soon as they retire. Since the early 1990s, employers have been cutting health care out of the retirement benefits they offer. From 1993–98, the proportion of employers who offered coverage to retirees under 65 declined from 46 percent to 36 percent, according to a study by William M. Mercer Inc., a New York City–based benefits consulting firm.

"It's a group that really can't afford not to have health insurance coverage," said Davis of the Commonwealth Fund. And as the baby boomers near retirement age, the problem is likely to get worse. "If current projections hold, you really will have a serious problem within five years with this group," Findlay said. "They're just at the breaking point now."

The Uninsured

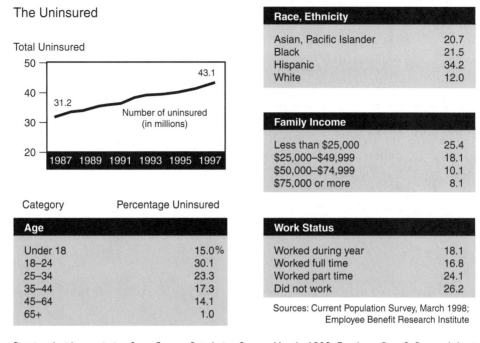

Total Uninsured

Number of uninsured (in millions)

Race, Ethnicity	
Asian, Pacific Islander	20.7
Black	21.5
Hispanic	34.2
White	12.0

Family Income	
Less than $25,000	25.4
$25,000–$49,999	18.1
$50,000–$74,999	10.1
$75,000 or more	8.1

Category   Percentage Uninsured

Age	
Under 18	15.0%
18–24	30.1
25–34	23.3
35–44	17.3
45–64	14.1
65+	1.0

Work Status	
Worked during year	18.1
Worked full time	16.8
Worked part time	24.1
Did not work	26.2

Sources: Current Population Survey, March 1998; Employee Benefit Research Institute

Reprinted with permission from Current Population Survey, March; 1998, Employee Benefit Research Institute.

■ OFF WELFARE

A smaller but expanding group of the uninsured is composed of those moving from welfare to work. In 1997, 675,000 people were uninsured as a "direct result of welfare reform," according to a recent report by Families USA. That number represents only 1.5 percent of the uninsured, but as welfare benefits continue to expire, that tally will multiply, said Pollack. "All of this is happening in a period where the economy could not be doing better." Pollack warns, so what happens in a recession?

The one positive trend among the uninsured is the increased coverage for children under Medicaid and the Children's Health Insurance Program, a federal program established in 1997 with the goal of providing health insurance for kids whose parents make too much to qualify for Medicaid. John Sheils, a vice president of the Falls Church, Va.–based Lewin Group, a health care consulting firm, estimates that of the 13 million uninsured children, 7.3 million of them are eligible for Medicaid and another 3 million are eligible for CHIP. The challenge is getting children signed up for these programs.

■ *GETTING INVOLVED*

Mary Horsley is looking for answers for those Americans, like her husband, who are uninsured and ineligible for government programs. As Kenny's ailments began to strain their marriage, Mary, 44, decided to channel her frustrations into researching the health insurance system. While cruising the Internet (she says she won't pay for cable television, but Internet access is a must), she learned about Families USA, and e-mailed the group about her family's plight. She heard right back. "It didn't help me, all those e-mails I sent to President Clinton," she said, "but Families USA responded."

Last month, the organization enlisted her to testify before Congress about her family's health insurance problems—an experience that has tapped her latent interest in politics. "I felt like I was speaking for 43 million people." Horsley said, "I'm getting really politically motivated because this is something I care about, and maybe there's really something I can do about it."

38

Myths of the Uninsured

Robert J. Samuelson

*T*he plight of the nation's 44 million uninsured demonstrates—once again—that nothing in health care is as simple as it seems. Many Americans consider the medically uninsured to be a scandal demanding attention in the 2000 presidential campaign. Bill Bradley already has a plan aiming at universal coverage for an estimated cost of $65 billion annually. But, paradoxically, some of today's uninsured already qualify for government coverage, and even providing it to everyone might not result in dramatic improvements in people's health. How can this be?

Our discussion of the uninsured is encrusted in myths. One is that health insurance is necessary to get health care. It isn't. Average health spending on the uninsured actually amounts to about 60 percent of spending on the insured, reports economist Sherry Glied of Columbia University. Some of the uninsured pay themselves; many receive free care that is subsidized by doctors and hospitals—or passed along to others in higher insurance premiums.

It's also widely believed that stingy businesses have eroded insurance by refusing to cover workers. Not really. Between 1987 and 1993, employer-based coverage did drop, from 62 percent of the population to 57 percent. But since then, it's rebounded to 62 percent. Meanwhile, the uninsured population has grown. It was 31 million (13 percent of all Americans) in 1987 and 40 million (15 percent) in 1993 before reaching last year's 44 million (16 percent).

Shrinking government coverage is one cause. The largest loss involves Medicaid: the federal-state program for the nonelderly poor. This is somewhat mysterious, because beginning in the 1980s, Congress made more children eligible for Medicaid. Sure enough, Medicaid coverage grew from 8.4 percent of the population in 1987 to 12.1 percent in 1994. But since then, it's dropped to 10 percent.

Welfare reform may partly explain the decline. Women on welfare and their children automatically qualified for Medicaid. "You went into an office, and you were told you were eligible," says Linda Blumberg of the Urban Institute. But since Congress overhauled Aid to Families With Dependent Children in 1996, welfare rolls have dropped 40 percent. More mothers work at jobs without insurance; yet, many remain eligible for Medicaid because their incomes are low. But (the theory goes) they don't sign up, either because they don't know they're eligible or because it's too much trouble.

Similar problems afflict CHIP (Children's Health Insurance Program). Passed by Congress in 1997, it gave states added funds to expand children's coverage. As a result, perhaps a third to half of the 11 million uninsured children already qualify for government coverage under CHIP or Medicaid. They simply aren't enrolled.

Declining insurance coverage also has another major cause: immigration. It is no accident that two states with very high rates of the uninsured are Texas (25 percent uninsured) and California (22.1 percent), which have huge numbers of immigrants. Many are low-skilled and poorly educated; they get jobs without coverage. Or they can't—or won't—sign up for government insurance. "The language and cultural barriers are enormous," says Leonard Schaeffer, the head of WellPoint Health Network, a large health-maintenance organization. "A lot of people don't want to be identified . . . They don't want to be in someone's computer."

But suppose—for argument's sake—that everyone gets insurance. Would people's health improve? For many uninsured, the answer is no, because they're already healthy. Two fifths of the uninsured are between 18 and 35. For most of them, insurance would protect against unexpected medical calamity. Children are an additional quarter of the uninsured. Most are fairly healthy; childhood illnesses are typically neither chronic nor critical. The real question is what happens to people with serious ailments. We don't know. No one doubts that insurance would prompt today's uninsured to visit doctors and hospitals more often. But how much this extra care would translate into better health is unclear.

On this subject, the scholarly research disagrees. A recent study from the National Bureau of Economic Research found small effects on children's health of Medicaid's expanded eligibility. A huge field trial between 1974 and 1982 by RAND concluded that more generous insurance conferred benefits only on the poorest and sickest people (about 4 percent of the population), in the form of better control of high blood pressure, for example. On the other hand, a 1993 study claimed that the uninsured face a higher risk of premature death. And a study of pregnant women in Florida found that Medicaid's expansion slightly reduced low-birth-weight infants.

In general, more insurance seems to improve Americans' health only modestly. The apparent explanation is that people's background and behavior—their genetic factors, lifestyles, diets—count for more than medicine in determining health. For the poor, this is disturbing. They are more likely than the middle class to be overweight, to smoke and to drink heavily. Among women, mothers with less than a high-school education are 10 times more likely to smoke during pregnancy than mothers with four years of college (smoking is a risk factor for low-birth-weight infants). Among adults, obesity contributes to heart disease and diabetes.

Here is the nub of the matter. Insurance coverage can be expanded, though doing so involves dilemmas. Already, a fifth of the uninsured refuse coverage from employers, mainly because it seems too expensive. The costlier private insurance becomes—because, say, government requires coverage of certain treatments—the fewer workers will buy it. Government insurance can fill the void, though this squeezes other programs. But even universal insurance is no panacea, because the real problem is not the uninsured but the poor health of the poor. The two problems aren't the same.

39

Infection With HIV
in the Elderly Population

Tracy A. Szirony

*I*nfection with HIV and subsequent development of AIDS in the population of older adults in the United States needs to be explored in greater depth. Current literature, including research-based investigations of HIV/AIDS in the elderly population is limited. McCormick and Wood (1992) relate that descriptions and details of AIDS cases in the elderly population are predominantly in the form of case reports in the medical literature.

Reports from the Centers for Disease Control and Prevention (CDC) (1996) reveal that 10% of all AIDS cases reported in the United States are in individuals older than age 50. Table 1 delineates cases of diagnosed AIDS by exposure category in people of this age group. Hinkle (1991) recognizes that

TABLE 39-1. Incidence of Infection With AIDS by Age and Exposure Category

Age	Homosexual Contact n (%)	Heterosexual Contact n (%)	Intravenous Drug Use n (%)	Hemophilia n (%)	Blood Transfusion n (%)	Total n (%)
50 to 54	14,592 (5)	2,617 (5)	5,764 (4)	162 (3)	649 (8)	27,514 (5)
55 to 59	7,985 (3)	1,754 (4)	2,541 (2)	110 (2)	649 (8)	15,512 (3)
60 to 64	4,139 (1)	1,102 (2)	1,044 (1)	103 (2)	773 (9)	8,716 (1)
≥ 65	2,527 (1)	1,235 (2)	586 (0)	126 (3)	1,741 (21)	7,682 (1)

Note: The number of AIDS cases is defined by age at diagnosis and exposure category. The numbers account for all reported cases through December 1996 in the United States. The percentages recorded indicate the percent for the identified age groups based on all age categories (CDC, 1996).

Tracy A. Szirony, M.S.N., R.N., C. is Assistant Professor of Nursing, Medical College of Ohio, School of Nursing, Toledo, Ohio.

Reprinted with permission by the *Journal of Gerontological Nursing,* October, 1999, 25(10) 25–31.

there really is no accurate way to assess the extent of HIV infection in this population because the number of infected people cannot be identified accurately. Underreporting is likely to occur, which may discount the total number of elderly people identified. In addition, it is likely that a number of older adults die without ever having been diagnosed as HIV positive.

Many articles and epidemiological data related to AIDS in elderly individuals unfortunately combine all individuals age 50 and older in one age category for identification of infection with HIV/AIDS. The current clustered age ranges for older adults with HIV/AIDS includes: 50 to 54, 55 to 59, 60 to 64, and 65 and older (CDC, 1996). Dividing the age cohort into further separate and distinct categories would help identify the epidemiology, risk factors, disease progression, and symptoms in middle age and older adults.

The purpose of this review of the literature is to increase knowledge and awareness of gerontological nurses related to older adults and HIV/AIDS. The related intent is the potential improvement of the provision of care to older adults with HIV/AIDS. Understanding the unique issues of infection with HIV in the elderly population will allow health care providers to better meet the needs of those who are ill or who may be at risk.

■ SOURCES OF INFECTION

The sources of infection with the HIV/AIDS virus need to be identified clearly and delineated for older adults so there is greater awareness among health care providers of potential risk factors and interventions so prevention and control can be implemented more easily. Adler and Nagel (1994) noted that initially older adults with HIV/AIDS most often became infected with the AIDS virus through a tainted blood transfusion. This pattern has changed since 1985 when the blood supply in the United States began to be routinely tested for antibodies to the virus. After mandatory testing began, the number of transfusion-acquired AIDS cases began to decline in all age groups.

Schuerman (1994) states that sexual contact currently is the leading cause of transmission of the AIDS virus in all age groups except for individuals older than age 65. Research completed by Gordon and Thompson (1995) found that 38% of infected older adults in their study acquired HIV/AIDS through sexual contact, 16% via intravenous drug use, and only 9% from transfusions.

■ RISK FACTORS

Although research into risk factors for the development of HIV/AIDS has been an important issue for the younger population, very little effort has been focused on identifying risk factors applicable to older adults. It is necessary to identify risk factors for individual age groups because specific interventions are essential to prevent transmission of the virus in various cohorts. A risk factor for older adults, as well as many younger adults, is that they often do not view themselves at risk for developing HIV/AIDS (Nocera, 1997). Specifically, older adults often do not use condoms as a safety measure when engaging in sexual activity because they are past their childbearing years and do not fear the potential of an unwanted of pregnancy (Luggen, 1996). The elderly population also does not consider the potential for acquiring other forms of sexually transmitted diseases routinely (Stall & Catania, 1994). In essence, the majority of older adults do not feel that they can, or will, be affected by HIV/AIDS. They do not see themselves at risk, and they may lack knowledge of the risk factors that make them vulnerable to infection. Stall and Catania (1994) present data from the National AIDS Behavior Surveys conducted between 1990 and 1991 which suggest that high-risk individuals who are older than age 50 are much less likely than individuals of the younger population to employ AIDS prevention strategies.

Wallace, Paauw, and Spach (1993), cite that homosexual or bisexual behavior is the predominant risk factor for infection with HIV in men up to age 70. In older adults who remain sexually active, it cannot be assumed that all sexual relations are heterosexual in nature. Older men who are homosexual or bisexual are much more likely than younger adults to hide their sexual preferences related to the fear of being exposed and the potential stigma associated with the disease (Lavick, 1994). This in itself may be a risk factor related to a potential lack of knowledge of the transmission of the virus during sexual contact.

It is essential to consider that it is not just older homosexual or bisexual men who may be infected with HIV. Heterosexual contact among older adults also is a risk factor that cannot be ignored. Although sexual functioning may diminish as people age, many older adults remain sexually active. Women who are past menopause are at greater risk for developing infection with HIV during intercourse because of thinning of the vaginal mucosa (Hinkle, 1991). Age-related vaginal thinning may lead to increased disruption of the mucosa during sexual activity and, thus, a greater chance of transmission of the virus through this disturbed tissue (Gordon & Thompson, 1995).

Intravenous drug use also may be a factor in the development of HIV/AIDS in the elderly population (Wallace et al., 1993). Transmission of HIV/AIDS occurs via the use of contaminated needles in all age categories (CDC, 1996), although the number of younger adults infected with HIV through contact with used needles is higher than the population of older adults who contract HIV/AIDS via intravenous drug use. The issue remains that older adults can be infected by intravenous drug use and by sharing contaminated needles (Nocera, 1997). Further research is essential to determine specific cohorts of older adults who are at risk for HIV/AIDS related to the use of intravenous drugs.

An additional risk factor specific to older adults is related to age-related decline in immune function (Scura & Whipple, 1990). Thymic involution occurs with aging, which leads to an increase in immature T-lymphocytes. Normal immune responses thus are reduced in older adults. In essence, the functional capacity of the immune system deteriorates with age, and this leads to a greater potential for various types of infections. This is a risk factor for older adults because their immune systems may not be able to combat potential infection with HIV or the resulting opportunistic infections (Hinkle, 1991).

■ *DIAGNOSIS AND PROGRESSION*

Older adults often do not obtain testing for HIV unless they are convinced by their own personal physicians that testing may be necessary (Ship, Wolff, & Selik, 1991). The questions then become:

- How many physicians are willing to suggest testing for older adults with identifiable risk factors?
- Do health care providers see the elderly population at risk for developing HIV/AIDS?

If testing is not performed, then the actual incidence of HIV/AIDS in older adults is inaccurate, and older adults who are infected with HIV/AIDS may not be identified.

Diagnosis of HIV/AIDS in the elderly population often is delayed. There is a decreased life expectancy and an increased severity of the disease process after the infection is clinically diagnosed as AIDS (Nocera, 1997). The first dilemma in diagnosis of HIV/AIDS in older adults is that members of the health care team often do not recognize signs and symptoms of HIV/AIDS in the elderly population (Hinkle, 1991). Second, older adults in this society often are not perceived to be at risk for developing AIDS. These obstacles lead to delayed diagnosis and a poorer prognosis for elderly individuals infected with HIV. El-Sadr and Gettler (1995) relate that seroprevalence studies have been targeted mainly at younger populations, and very little effort has been made to assess the extent of infection with HIV in the elderly population.

Delayed diagnosis often leads to a poorer prognosis in older adults. Current data suggest there is a shorter time between infection with HIV/AIDS and the onset of clinical symptomatology, namely opportunistic infections (McCormick & Wood, 1992). When elderly individuals are diagnosed with HIV/AIDS they most often present with advanced disease and experience a shorter length of life (Wallace et al., 1993). This shortened life span is related both to delayed diagnosis and a more rapid clinical deterioration. Skiest, Rubinstien, Carley, Gioiella, and Lyons (1996) found that because older adults were diagnosed later, the time between actual identification of AIDS and death from the disease was shorter.

One cause of the more rapid clinical deterioration is related to the decreased immune function normally found in older adults and their inability to replace T-helper cells at a rate comparable to that of the younger age groups. An increase in comorbidity also may be related to a more rapid course of the disease process and a decreased survival rate in older adults. Scura and Whipple (1990) found that among older adults who were infected with HIV, the mean time from potential exposure to the virus to testing as HIV positive was 4.2 years, with a range from 1 to 7 years. Thus, early diagnosis and treatment may be essential for improved quality of life in older adults.

■ COMMON OPPORTUNISTIC INFECTIONS

Opportunistic infections associated with AIDS often are misdiagnosed as other chronic conditions that typically affect older adults (McCormick & Wood, 1992). Signs and symptoms of opportunistic infections related to HIV/AIDS may look similar to those associated with chronic diseases commonly found in older adults. Comorbidity often masks the problem when older adults present to various health care providers with a multitude of vague symptoms, some of which may be related to an unknown infection with HIV.

Health care providers should be aware of opportunistic infections that are recognized as AIDS-defining. Wallace et al. (1993) list the five most common opportunistic infections as:

- Pneumocystis carinii pneumonia (PCP).
- Mycobacterium tuberculosis (TB).
- Mycobacterium avium complex (MAC).
- Herpes zoster.
- Cytomegalovirus (CMV).

Signs and symptoms of these infections are listed in Box 39–1. Older adults who present with symptoms suggestive of these opportunistic infections need to undergo appropriate diagnostic testing, including a differential diagnosis for chronic conditions commonly found in older adults versus those diseases which may be indicative of infection with HIV. Risk factors, possible sources of infection, and potentially unsafe behaviors should be assessed in any older adult who exhibits symptoms of any of these opportunistic infections.

■ AIDS DEMENTIA COMPLEX

AIDS has been referred to in much of the literature as the "new great imitator" (Nocera, 1997, p. 76). AIDS dementia complex (ADC) often is misdiagnosed as Alzheimer's disease when older adults develop symptoms distinctive for dementia. Neurological symptoms commonly found in individuals with Alzheimer's disease sometimes are recognized in individuals infected with HIV. Therefore, it is crucial to include testing for HIV in the differential diagnosis of dementia, as well as accurate evaluation of behavioral and functional

BOX 39–1. SIGNS AND SYMPTOMS OF COMMON OPPORTUNISTIC INFECTIONS

Pneumocystis Carinii Pneumonia (PCP)
■ Gradual onset of symptoms
■ Fever
■ Fatigue
■ Weight loss
■ Persistent dry cough
■ Shortness of breath
■ Dyspnea on exertion

Mycobacterium Tuberculosis (TB)
■ Fever
■ Cough with possible bloody sputum
■ Weight loss
■ Night sweats
■ Fatigue

Mycobacterium Avium Complex (MAC)
■ Fever
■ Night sweats
■ Weight loss
■ Nausea
■ Abdominal pain

Herpes Zoster
■ Fluid-filled blisters
■ Painful rash on the skin
■ Severe and long-lasting symptoms
■ Fever
■ Fatigue

Cytomegalovirus (CMV)
■ Symptoms vary related to site of infection:
1. Eyes (retinitis) (e.g., "floaters," decreased visual acuity, decreased peripheral vision, eventual blindness)
2. Gastrointestinal tract (colitis) (e.g., loss of appetite, dysphagia, substernal and epigastric pain, weight loss, diarrhea, fever)
3. Central nervous system (neuropathy) (e.g., tingling and pain in the hands or feet)

changes in older adults who exhibit signs and symptoms of dementia (Scarn-horst, 1992).

■ TREATMENT CHALLENGES

Late diagnosis of infection with HIV in elderly individuals leads to a variety of treatment challenges. For example, a greater number and severity of opportunistic infections may be present when the disease has progressed to an advanced stage. This, in itself, makes treatments a formidable task. Treatment is complicated further when other disease processes or comorbidity may be affecting the older individuals.

Even if the diagnosis is made early in the course of the disease, drug therapies create their own difficulties. Many older adults suffer from other conditions that require use of various medications. Drug interactions are a real concern when older adults are using drugs to treat chronic conditions and then must add other medications to treat HIV/AIDS and related opportunistic infections.

Further, drug trials of antiretroviral medications in elderly individuals currently are not available, and there are only anecdotal reports of the effects of these drugs when used by older adults. Adler and Nagel (1994) note that older adults are much less likely to tolerate the side effects of the major antiretroviral drug zidovudine (AZT). This may be because older adults metabolize many drugs differently, which may change the ability of antiretroviral agents to maintain their intended actions. Wallace et al. (1993) suggest that the use of antiretroviral agents in elderly individuals is warranted but that therapy should begin with smaller doses, and older adults should be monitored closely for any adverse effects that may occur.

■ NURSING CARE OF OLDER ADULTS INFECTED WITH HIV

Nursing care of older adults infected with HIV/AIDS can be challenging. In addition to addressing issues related to chronic conditions and problems commonly found in older adults, emphasis must be placed on the uncertainties associated with advanced infection with HIV. Older adults who are infected with HIV often experience anxiety, depression, social isolation, weakness, activity intolerance, inability to care for themselves, and issues related to loss and grieving, as well as other individualized dilemmas and obstacles.

Symptom control must be addressed as the course of the disease progresses for any individual infected with AIDS, but this is an area of specific concern for older adults who may have an ambiguous pattern of distressing symptoms. Acute symptoms must be identified and managed along with more chronic symptomatology, while continuously striving for quality of life that is acceptable to the older individuals.

Older adults with AIDS also may reach a point in the progression of the disease in which palliative care issues need to be addressed in a timely manner. As noted earlier, older adults infected with HIV/AIDS presumably will reach the end-stage of the disease process sooner than younger adults because of delayed diagnosis and treatment, as well as other health problems that complicate the clinical picture. Therefore, it is essential that all members of the health care team be experienced in the treatment of common symptoms seen in older adults with HIV/AIDS. These symptoms include:

- Anorexia.
- Weight loss.
- Fatigue.
- Decreased physical stamina.
- Diminished mental abilities.

Adequate patient education, health teaching, support, and guidance of both older and younger adults infected with HIV cannot be neglected. Concerns related to progression of the disease as well as acquired opportunistic infections should be communicated both to the individuals as well as appropriate significant others. Issues associated with sexuality and transmission of the virus also should be addressed with older adults who remain sexually active. Teaching related to current treatment measures, drug regimens, and potential side effects need to be reinforced continually. Families and significant others who are involved in the care of the individuals with AIDS should be included in the teaching process because these caregivers can reinforce what the nurses have taught.

■ PSYCHOSOCIAL ASPECTS

Psychosocial aspects of being infected with HIV/AIDS frequently are similar for both older and younger people. The stigma associated with being HIV positive, fear of telling family members, lack of support from the community and family, dwindling financial resources, and quality of life issues affect all people with AIDS. In addition, older adults often feel they may become a burden to their families and fear disclosing their sexual preferences at a late age because of rejection from family and friends. There also are a number of distinct and separate issues that are faced by older adults.

Lavick (1994) recognized the paucity of literature related to psychotherapeutic issues specifically focused on older adults. Her research identified the following psychosocial issues that may be encountered in older adults infected with HIV:

- Stage of life.
- Issues of entitlement.
- Disclosure of status to adult children.
- Historical perspective and community ties.
- Sexual issues.

Lavick (1994) also recommended the formation of a support group for older people infected with HIV. All members of her study group stated that it was beneficial to meet with other people their own age who also were infected with HIV.

The American Association of Retired Persons (1988) reported that older people with AIDS often feel isolated and lack a support network. Education, community resources, and treatment options have not been focused on the elderly population. Garvey (1994) similarly noted that older adults infected with HIV often do not use community services because they feel these services are primarily for the younger population. Reasons for lack of connection with community resources include the fear of being stigmatized and the possible lack of stamina or energy required to reveal their diagnosis at an advanced age.

■ CONCLUSION

Early diagnosis and proper treatment of HIV/AIDS in essential for the elderly population. Health care providers must assess for risk factors pertinent to the development of HIV/AIDS in all age groups of individuals they may treat. Thorough risk assessment is essential in the elderly population. Testing, education, and counseling must be offered to any individual potentially infected with the AIDS virus, regardless of age. The use of a multidisciplinary health care team approach is essential to meet goals for treatment and control of symptoms in older adults infected with HIV. Education of all staff involved in meeting the physical and emotional care needs of older adults should include a component related to older adults and HIV/AIDS.

The public health arena in the United States needs to confront the issue of HIV/AIDS in older adults. Public health measures need to be focused on educating older adults regarding their risk for infection with HIV, and community resources should be developed that will benefit this age group. Further research on issues that older adults face when infected with HIV/AIDS is critical.

References

Adler, W.H., & Nagel, J.E. (1994). Acquired immunodeficiency syndrome in the elderly. *Drugs and Aging, 4,* 410–416.

American Association of Retired Persons. (1988). Elderly and AIDS: Forgotten patients? *Modern Maturity, 17,* 6–7.

Centers for Disease Control and Prevention. (1996). *HIV/AIDS surveillance report.* Atlanta, GA: Author.

El-Sadr, W., & Gettler, J. (1995). Unrecognized human immunodeficiency virus infection in the elderly. *Archives of Internal Medicine, 155*(2), 184–186.

Garvey, C. (1994). AIDS care for the elderly: A community-based approach. *AIDS Patient Care, 8*(3), 118–120.

Gordon, S.M., & Thompson, S. (1995). The changing epidemiology of human immunodeficiency virus infection in older persons. *Journal of the American Geriatrics Society, 43,* 7–9.

Hinkle, K.L. (1991). A literature review: HIV seropositivity in the elderly. *Journal of Gerontological Nursing, 17*(10), 12–17.

Lavick, J. (1994). Psychosocial considerations of HIV infection in the older adult. *AIDS Patient Care, 8*(3), 127–129.

Luggen, A.S. (1996). AIDS in the older adult. In A.S. Luggen (Ed.), *National Gerontological Nursing Association: Core curriculum for gerontological nursing* (pp. 720–727). St. Louis: Mosby Year Book.

McCormick, W.C., & Wood, R.W. (1992). Clinical decisions in the care of elderly persons with AIDS. *Journal of the American Geriatrics Society, 40,* 917–921.

Nocera, R. (1997). AIDS and the older person. *Topics in Geriatric Rehabilitation, 12*(4), 72–85.

Scarnhorst, S. (1992). AIDS dementia complex in the elderly: Diagnosis and management. *Nurse Practitioner, 17*(8), 37–40.

Schuerman, D.A. (1994). Clinical concerns: AIDS in the elderly. *Journal of Gerontological Nursing, 20*(7), 11–17.

Scura, K.W., & Whipple, B. (1990). Older adults as an HIV-positive risk group. *Journal of Gerontological Nursing, 16*(2), 6–10.

Ship, J.A., Wolff, A., & Selik, R.M. (1991). Epidemiology of acquired immune deficiency syndrome in persons aged 50 years or older. *Journal of Acquired Immune Deficiency Syndrome, 4*(1), 84–88.

Skiest, D.J., Rubinstein, E., Carley, N., Gioiella, L., & Lyons, R. (1996). The importance of comorbidity in HIV-infected patients over 55: A retrospective case-control study. *American Journal of Medicine, 101,* 605–611.

Stall, R., & Catania, J. (1994). AIDS risk behaviors among late middle-aged and elderly Americans. *Archives of Internal Medicine, 154*(1), 57–63.

Wallace, J.I., Paauw, D.S., & Spach, D.H. (1993). HIV infection in older patients: When to suspect the unexpected. *Geriatrics, 48*(6), 61–70.

40

U.S. Faces TB Threat

August Gribbin

*T*he United States is curtailing efforts to control tuberculosis just when new lethal strains are threatening what some fear could become a public-health catastrophe. Harvard Medical School researchers have documented cases of multidrug-resistant tuberculosis, or MDR-TB, in 100 nations. Increasingly, foreign visitors and immigrants from underdeveloped countries are bringing the disease into this country.

The contagion has not yet caused dramatic spikes in health statistics or generated a stampede of concern. But TB develops slowly and not everyone who is infected develops symptoms. Then too, most Americans know little about tuberculosis, an infection that can affect various parts of the body, producing lesions and sometimes attacking the brain and spinal cord.

Typically, TB lodges in the lungs. It makes breathing difficult; induces a fierce, nagging cough; and causes exhaustion, weakness, a steady fever, nighttime sweating and bloody phlegm. Before the 1940s, "consumption," as it was called, devastated entire communities. In those days, families were split and incomes imperiled when a parent was forced into a hospital isolation ward or sanitarium to undergo harrowing treatments for months or years. Many patients had portions of their lungs collapsed or removed to save them from the disease that for decades was the nation's leading cause of death.

Then in 1945 antibiotics arrived, and the wonder drugs revolutionized treatment. Doctors eventually determined that treating patients with a combination of drugs over the course of six to nine months could cure victims 70 to 90 percent of the time. Indeed, cures were expected in most of the 18,371 active TB cases reported to the U.S. Centers for Disease Control and Prevention last year.

MDR-TB is something else, however. Drug-resistant tuberculosis have mutated and can fend off conventional medicines. Such strains are much harder to cure—often they are incurable. Physicians treat the disease by administering various combinations of expensive, infection-fighting drugs over long periods. Treating a single such patient costs $250,000—considerably more in extreme instances when a patient must be quarantined—actually isolated—for life.

Although some 8 million people around the globe contract TB each year and some 3 million die, no one knows for sure how many now have drug-resistant TB. Based on incomplete data, the World Health Organization three years ago reported 50 million cases; researchers estimate that at least 2.5 percent of these victims are infected with drug-resistant tuberculosis.

BILLIONS HARBOR TB INFECTION

Tuberculosis has caused more deaths in the world than any other infectious disease. The bacteria float on tiny, mostly invisible droplets of moisture released when a TB victim sneezes or coughs. A third of the world's population—some 2 billion people—are estimated to harbor the infection.

A small minority who inhale the bacteria quickly develop "progressive primary TB" that spreads to the lymph glands, enters the bloodstream and runs throughout the body. More often, a healthy individual's immune system fights the bacteria and captures them in what one doctor calls "caskets of calcium." People who have the inactive disease have "latent TB."

Just 10 percent of those with latent TB develop active tuberculosis, usually when another disease or infection weakens their immune systems. That happens routinely these days, for one of the infections that quickly activates TB is HIV, the human immunodeficiency virus that causes AIDS. HIV and TB go hand-in-hand. An estimated 100,000 HIV-infected people in the United States also carry the TB infection.

In the United States and other developed countries, people known to have had contact with a TB-infected individual are given a simple skin test. A clinician injects a special protein under the skin of a patient's forearm. If in 48 to 72 hours after the injection a welt forms, the patient is known to be infected.

Doctors then order chest X-rays, which determine whether the infection is active and has created cavities or lesions in the lungs. They also may take saliva samples for analysis, which can take four weeks to culture, though some labs use newer techniques that shorten the wait to two days.

Infected persons considered at risk of developing active TB generally are treated with antibiotics to ensure that they do not infect others and that their latent TB never produces the dangerous symptoms. Unless the TB bacteria infecting a person with active TB are the more recent drug-resistant strain, a properly treated victim can expect to get better within a year.

—AG

Since then, physicians studying hot spots of TB infection in places such as Argentina, China, the Dominican Republic, India and Russia have found that 7 to 22 percent carry the drug-resistant variety. That's roughly three to 10 times the expected rate. Consider that currently only 60 percent of all TB cases worldwide are ever diagnosed and fewer than 60 percent of those are cured, and the seriousness of the problem comes more clear.

"I don't want to be hysterical; I don't want to say each of us is threatened," says Barry Bloom, dean of the Harvard School of Public Health. "But there is no place from which we are distant and no one from whom we are disconnected when dealing with infectious diseases like TB."

A dire prognosis rests on several realities. Foremost is the fact that tuberculosis bacteria, including drug-resistant strains, spread with remarkable ease—by the cough or sneeze of a TB victim.

"A person with the active disease can cough in a room and leave. Someone then entering the room and breathing the air can contract the infection," explains Jim Yong Kim, who wrote the Harvard report with Paul Farmer, the principal author. TB victims riding planes, buses, trains and other public transportation carry the disease across borders, infecting fellow travelers, customs agents and others on the way. On average, each person with active TB infects 20 others.

Complicating matters further, MDR-TB cannot be determined by testing. Drug resistance is diagnosed only when the patient becomes sicker and sicker despite standard chemotherapy. As a result, MDR-TB can emerge as a significant problem even in settings with excellent TB control, as happened in Peru.

Along with many others, the Harvard researchers are calling for quick action to combat the "pandemic." The costs of fighting the new menace "are likely to be staggering," note the authors of the report, and must fall heavily on developed nations and philanthropic groups. Nevertheless, treating victims in nations where the disease already is epidemic provides the best protection for the United States—it limits the number of foreign visitors and immigrants capable of infecting Americans.

While the peril posed by the slowly building pestilence has not pierced the U.S. public's perception, none of the physicians, technicians or administrators in tuberculosis research or control questions the Harvard study's findings or conclusions. Yet there still is no visible evidence the United States is preparing to respond to the challenge, according to Kim, who believes "governments have not been appropriately concerned and generous." More important, says Bloom, "both the states and the federal government are cutting their tuberculosis programs. They're firing TB-control officers. We set up a fantastically effective anti-TB system from 1993 to the present, and now we're in the process of dismembering it."

Reichman confirms that funding for his National Tuberculosis Center has been trimmed. Other sources report cuts as well. In New York City, the TB-control budget has been slashed by 30 percent. What it comes down to, says Harvard's Bloom, is one question: "How much is our country prepared

EXPERTS SEE NEED FOR NEW DRUGS

Tuberculosis bacteria have learned to defeat the drugs commonly used to combat them; without new ones, the United States and the rest of the world is crippled in trying to quell "the emerging epidemic of drug-resistant TB," according to a recent Harvard Medical School report.

The need arises largely because patients, doctors and health officials in various parts of the world have abused the TB-treatment process. TB patients, for instance, typically must take one to four different antibiotics for six to nine months. Yet after a week or two of therapy, patients no longer can spread the disease. A week or so later, the pain eases. Then TB symptoms start disappearing.

Meanwhile, patients can experience unpleasant drug side effects, and some tend to find the regimen burdensome. They stop taking their medicine. At this point, the TB bacteria have been exposed to the antibiotics, but comparatively few have been killed. Without continued assaults from the antibiotics, the living organisms adapt. In effect, they are inoculated against the antibiotics and become immune to the drugs.

To prevent this, the World Health Organization recommended years ago that doctors and health-care workers actually watch TB patients take their medicines and assure that patients stick with the months-long program, called "DOTS," for Directly Observed Therapy Short-course. Yet the system frequently has been ignored in many countries where TB is epidemic, giving rise to numbers of cases of multidrug-resistant tuberculosis.

The four drugs commonly used to defeat TB are relatively inexpensive. But when those drugs do not work, doctors must turn to more expensive antibiotics, hoping they can chance upon combinations that will stymie the disease in given patients. Drug-resistant patients often receive as many as seven drugs daily for two years, often with mixed results. The cost of curing these patients—when they can be cured—is exorbitant.

Some researchers worry that multidrug-resistant bacteria will become immune to the substitute antibiotics, too. Thus the wish for an effective and inexpensive drug or two and for a workable vaccine—a magic bullet.

"We haven't had a new class of drugs for tuberculosis in about 25 years" and there are none in development, says Barry Bloom, dean of the Harvard School of Public Health. Along with other physicians and medical researchers, Bloom declares that drug makers are not interested in developing anti-TB formulas—the research is too expensive and there is no profit in developing a TB cure or even a vaccine, since most patients who need the medicine are poor, old or imprisoned.

Bert Spilker, senior vice president of the Pharmaceutical Research and Manufacturers of America, a trade group, disagrees with Bloom's analysis, however. "We don't conduct research specifically for a given disease," says Spilker. "We do

Continued

the research for anti-infectives in general. Most drugs found effective against TB were discovered while seeking cures for other diseases, and doctors found them active against TB."

Still, Jim Yong Kim of the Harvard Medical School asserts that something must be done. "There's talk of applying public funds to develop a vaccine" but, he says, the sums needed would be huge. "We need an altogether new way of thinking of drug development—an alternative way. It's a daunting problem. Drug companies, policymakers, public-health officials have got to get together and address this problem."

—AG

to pay to protect the future?" He asserts, "Protection means supporting treatment in poor countries to stop MDR-TB. Because when it comes here, it will be too late. There will not be much we can do at that point because the cure will be too expensive."

Discussion Questions

1. Compare and contrast the old homeless and the new homeless with respect to income, housing, age, gender, and physical and emotional disabilities.

2. What are your present attitudes about the homeless? How do they compare with the general public's attitudes?

3. When you walk past a homeless person on the street, how do you generally act?

4. Where in your community are shelters for the homeless? Are they adequate in number? If not, what community forces are at play that contribute to the shortage of shelters?

5. How many people do you know who have no health care insurance? How do they manage?

6. Under welfare reform, a great many people became employed, but then found that their health care coverage expired. What is their incentive to continue working?

7. What would be your solution to provide health care coverage to people who are uninsured?

8. Compare and contrast what Gorman and Samuelson state (Articles 37 and 38, respectively) about the realities people face in everyday life, and Samuelson's assertion that there are myths concerning the uninsured.

9. Samuelson (Article 38) contends that universal insurance is no panacea for the uninsured because the real problem is the poor health of the uninsured and the poor. Do you agree or disagree with this statement? Explain your reasoning.

10. Imagine yourself preparing for a presentation you are scheduled to give to the elderly residents in a senior facility about HIV infection. How would you begin?

11. What attitudes do you have about the elderly and the rise of HIV infection in this population?

12. What reaction would you expect from the elderly when discussing the need for protected sex? How would you plan to deal with the various reactions you may get?

13. Discuss the implications that drug-resistant tuberculosis will have on health care in this country.

14. Should people who are noncompliant about taking medication for tuberculosis be detained in an isolation ward to protect the public from the spread of this disease? Justify your answer.

Further Readings

Bernstein, N. (1999). Deep poverty and illness found among homeless. *New York Times*, 99(12), 16–19.

Cohen, C. I. (1999). Aging and homelessness. *The Gerontologist*, 39(1), 5–14.

Doran, G. (1999). I was too proud to go home. *Scholastic Scope*, 47(16), 15–17.

Lerner, B. H. (1999). Catching patients: Tuberculosis and detention in the 1990's. *Chest*, 115(2), 69–71.

Lerner, S. (1999). The uncovered. *The Village Voice*, 44(48), 27–30.

Talarico, L. D. (1998). Uncharted territory: AIDS in the older patient. *Patient Care*, 32(19), 84–96.

Wells, A. (1999). The health beliefs, values and practices of gay adolescents. *Clinical Nurse Specialist*, 13(2), 69–71.

Web Site Resources for Populations at Risk

Common Myths About the Homeless   http://www.nlchp.org
Francis J. Curry National Tuberculosis Center   www.nationaltbcenter.edu/
Homelessness: U.S. Department of Health and Human Resources
    http://aspe.os.dhhs.gov/progsys/homeless/
National Center for HIV, STD, and TB prevention   www.cdc.gov/
National Coalition for the Homeless   http://nch.ari.net

General Search Engine Web Sites

Dogpile   www.dogpile.com

Health Web Sites

AEGIS   www.aegis.com
Respect/Protect   www.respectprotect.com

Professional Journal Web Sites

Haworth Press   www. haworthpress.com
MedWebPlus   www.medwebplus.com

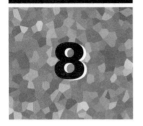

Living Longer: Are We Ready?

In past civilizations, life was short. Plagues, wars, famine, and natural catastrophes saw to that. Because people died at an early age, old age was not given much thought. Day-to-day survival was a never-ending struggle. Anything else, including the old, took too much time and effort. As one century unfolded in to the next, life expectancy increased to 40 years. Then came Otto Von Bismarck, who, in planning Germany's first pension plan during the late nineteenth century, decided that 65 was when old age began.

Today, thanks to breakthroughs in medical science, economic progress, healthier lifestyles, better nutrition, and improved public health, people are living longer and better. The average life expectancy is now 75 years, and prospects for a longer life expectancy for more and more of our population are good. Our aging population—that is, the number of people 65 and older—is growing at about six million people a year. Of that number, those 85 years and older represent the fastest growing segment of that population. Just as remarkable is the increasing number of people who have reached 100 years of age. Demographers predict that between 2010 and 2030, the number of people 65 and over will rise from 39 to 69 million. By that time, they predict there will be fewer people under 18 years of age than over 65.

The rapid growth of our aging population, however, has not brought about any significant changes in the public's attitude toward the aging. Ours is still a youth-oriented society. The marketplace is filled with goods, glamour, and glitz—all aimed at pleasing the young and well heeled. What the marketplace gives to the aging population is lip service.

In the same vein, our health care policy toward this growing segment of our population is unfocused. For the "baby boomers" who will be 65 in 2010, and for those who will be even older by that time, the lack of a clear health care policy will be especially troublesome. The impact on our health care resources will be enormous. Who will care for our aging population? What economic resources will be available for their care? What kinds of care will be needed in the next 10 to 30 years? Will Social Security still be a viable resource not only for them, but also for the younger population who will need it when they reach retirement age?

What the meaning of aging has in today's world is the first question addressed in this chapter. It is coupled with the evolution and future of Social Security as it relates to that meaning. Subsequent readings focus on the urgent need for planning the health care needs of our aging population, the implications that delay may have, and the resources needed to provide for the health care needs of the aging. Whether old age in 2010 and beyond proves that "the best is yet to be" remains to be seen.

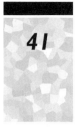

41

The Meaning of Aging and the Future of Social Security

Thomas R. Cole and David G. Stevenson

Later life in the West today is a season in search of its purposes. For the first time in human history, most people can expect to live into their seventies in reasonably good health; those over eighty-five are the fastest-growing age group in the population. Yet the words of *Ecclesiastes*—"To every thing there is a season, and a time to every purpose under heaven"—carry little conviction when applied to the second half of life.

Between the sixteenth century and the third quarter of the twentieth century, Western ideas about aging underwent a fundamental transformation, spurred by the development of modern society. Ancient and medieval understandings of aging as a mysterious part of the eternal order of things gradually gave way to the secular, scientific, and individualist tendencies of modernity. Old age was removed from its place as a way station along life's spiritual journey and redefined as a problem to be solved by science and medicine. By the mid-twentieth century, older people were moved to society's margins and defined primarily as patients or pensioners.

Because long lives have become the rule rather than the exception, and because collective meaning systems have lost their power to infuse aging with widely shared significance, we have become deeply uncertain about what it means to grow old. Ancient myths and modern stereotypes alike fail to articulate the challenges or capture the uncertainty of generations moving into the still-lengthening later years. The modernization of aging has generated a host of unanswered questions: Does aging have an intrinsic purpose? Is there anything really important to be done after children are raised, jobs left, careers completed? Is old age the culmination of life? Does it contain potential for self-completion? What are the avenues of spiritual growth in later life? What are the roles, rights, and responsibilities of older people? What are the particular strengths and virtues of old age? Is there such a thing as a good old age?

Thomas R. Cole, Ph.D., is professor and graduate program director at the Institute for the Medical Humanities, University of Texas, Galveston. David G. Stevenson is a research associate/policy analyst at the Center for Homecare Policy and Research, New York, NY.

Reprinted with permission from *Generations*, Winter, 1999–2000, 23(4) 72–76. Copyright © 2000. The American Society on Aging, San Francisco, California.

In 1979, the English writer Ronald Blythe wrote in *The View in Winter* that "the ordinariness of living to be old" was too new to appreciate. "The old have . . . been sentenced to life and turned into a matter for public concern," he wrote. "They are the first generations of full-timers and thus the first generations of old people for whom the state, experimentally, grudgingly, and uncertainly, is having to make special supportive conditions." Blythe suggested that it would soon be necessary for people to learn to grow old as they had once learned to grow up.

These perceptive remarks already have the feel of a bygone era. At the turn of the twenty-first century, the long-rising tide of modernity is turning; beneath the much heralded "age wave," uncharted postmodern cultural currents are breaking up conventional images, norms, and expectations about aging and old age. The large percentage of public economic and medical resources devoted to older people has spawned a fierce debate over intergenerational equity in shrinking welfare states. Meanwhile, writers, filmmakers, advocates, and elders are defying negative stereotypes and images of old age. Within the last decade, we have also seen renewed interest in the search for meaning in later life—variously called "conscious aging," "spiritual eldering," or "spirituality and aging." And in 1999, the United Nations' International Year of the Older Person program is making a concerted effort to emphasize that older people are active agents as well as dependent beneficiaries, sources of wisdom and guidance as well as recipients of healthcare and income transfers.

The meaning of later life is not only a matter of cultural values and personal experience; it is also linked to values and assumptions built into social policy. In our view, the current debate over the future of Social Security needs to be examined not only in the usual fiscal terms but also in moral and existential terms: What vision of a secure old age should be embedded in this cornerstone of the American welfare state? We begin with a historical review of the value tensions that have shaped Social Security since its inception and offer a brief analysis of the social meanings at stake in the current debate over the future of the program.

■ HISTORICAL ORIGINS OF SOCIAL SECURITY

Social Security has always been defined by competing values. From the program's beginnings in 1935, proponents have struck a balance between the rhetoric of offering assistance and the rhetoric of administering insurance. Although the Social Security Act included public assistance for low-income elders, Old Age Assistance (Title I) was meant to provide temporary relief until the contributory system (Title II) could take effect. In particular, President Roosevelt and his advisors thought that it was important to distinguish Social Security from welfare to ensure support for the program. Even in the midst of the Depression, "welfare" had a stigma that could have prevented the program's success.

Rather than representing a major shift in opinion about individual or governmental responsibility, income support for retirees was promoted as a logical response to the Depression. In part, the Social Security Act arose from the realization that poverty could result from factors beyond human control (Achenbaum, 1986). Individual and family misfortune did not necessarily indicate lax morals or an inadequate work ethic and, hence, was worthy of public intervention.

Yet, Social Security was also created within the context of a culture that valued independence and self-sufficiency. Economic assistance was acceptable as long as it did not compromise these principles. The underlying conflict between Social Security as insurance and Social Security as assistance reflected a deeper ambivalence between self-reliance and mutual responsibility. Americans cherished the former while recognizing the need for the latter, and Social Security had to marry both of these concepts to be successful.

In rhetoric and in practice, workers have always "earned" their right to Social Security. Benefits are based on contributions and have a direct relationship to earnings. Under this model, the government's primary role is viewed as administrative rather than redistributive. This system is equitable in the sense that individuals are treated in accordance with their individual contributions. Yet, Social Security also adheres to a broader notion of fairness by providing a minimum benefit to all who are eligible. This broader concept of public assistance is not based on individual merit but instead on membership within a larger community. The equity promoted within such a system is based on the conviction that each individual is deserving of the benefit regardless of individual circumstance. Throughout the history of Social Security, policy makers have tried to balance these two conflicting concepts of equity within the program.

■ SOCIAL MEANING OF SECURITY

How we structure our Social Security program is inextricably linked to how we define a secure old age. Security for American elders is often promoted through the ideal of choice. Choice ensures security because it supports individual control, autonomy, and independence—cherished traits in America throughout adulthood. Successful aging in this context means the combination of increased freedom in retirement with undiminished physical and cognitive functioning. It should not be surprising that many of us fail to meet this standard. Indeed, this myth of independence is perpetuated by the misguided belief that individuals should be able to fend for themselves, a belief reinforced by the popular misconception that Social Security is a contract in which the beneficiary and the contributor are perceived to be one.

Independence throughout old age and a fully funded Social Security system are in fact both myths. Most older individuals need to rely on external support at some point before they die, and Social Security is a pay-as-you-go system (current payments from younger generations go directly to older generations). Consequently, both independence in old age and the Social Security system rely on a transfer between generations. Rather than deny the existence of these transfers, we should embrace them and contemplate the relationships that are necessary to support them.

Burdenless living, independence, and self-sufficiency imply nothing about human solidarity. In fact, these ideals imply an absence of human relationships, at least in the interdependent sense. Instead of relationships, freedom is exalted as the primary good. This freedom no doubt includes the ability to conduct relationships on one's own terms—free of any necessity of exchange. Yet, as Michael Ignatieff (1984) has argued, if the welfare state serves the needs of freedom alone, it neglects the needs of solidarity and renders us "a society of strangers." As we move forward in the Social Security debate, we need to realign the values that will guide future reform and emphasize community over isolated self-reliance.

■ MEANING OF SOCIAL SECURITY

Over the years, Social Security has kept many of our nation's elderly out of poverty (poverty rates for both older men and women are about one-fifth what they would be without Social Security) and has managed to do so without high administrative cost or major scandal. However, demographic and economic projections do not bode well for the program's future solvency. Although the program is not in imminent financial crisis, policy makers point to the coming "age wave" in their push to save Social Security for future generations.

As we engage in this debate, it is important to ponder exactly what we are trying to save. What kind of program do we want Social Security to be? What ends should it serve? How will potential reforms alter the nature of the program? The inevitable cycle of dire predictions and fiscal rescue plans obscures the fact that larger questions about Social Security's meaning and purpose are often not addressed. If we want to ensure the sustainability—rather than just the affordability—of Social Security into the next millennium, we must address these more difficult questions before we proceed.

We must first decide what vision of social insurance we want to guide our Social Security program. Should we regard Social Security as a contract between and for individuals, or should it be an expression of community? Each option entails a different sense of fairness. If we envision Social Security as a contract that provides individual benefits in accordance with contributions, individual retirement accounts are perhaps a reasonable way to proceed. For many, individual accounts foster a sense of ownership and control that in turn promotes feelings of security. Regardless of the overall fiscal health of the Social Security program, each individual would have his or her own personal account. At a time when many assume that Social Security will not exist when they retire, it is easy to see the appeal of such an approach.

However, the individualized approach is deeply flawed. Individual accounts undermine the vision of social insurance as an expression of solidarity. Reliance on individual accounts subordinates the notion of mutual protection to the principle of individual choice. While this approach is consistent with the manner in which many older Americans find security, sacrificing the commitment to a basic retirement benefit for all is too high of a price to pay. If we bolster our social commitment to—and our collective confidence in—a decent minimum benefit, we would find security more easily in provisions of community than in arrangements for individual choice. Ultimately, we must reestablish the priority of sheltering individuals from risk over the ideal of personal gain.

Somewhat along these lines, some have advocated that Social Security benefits be targeted by income. Although the underlying logic of this position is appealing, the extreme of this approach—means-testing benefits—could result in the transformation of Social Security from social insurance to a welfare program. If what has happened to support for the means-tested benefit Medicaid is any indication, the widespread support that Social Security currently enjoys would dissipate considerably. A more reasonable approach is to reduce benefit payments to those with higher incomes, while maintaining a strong commitment to a decent minimum standard of living. Such an approach would be unfair from the perspective of individual equity (i.e., that individuals should receive benefits based on their own contributions), but would be beneficial for those who arguably need support the most.

Any discussion of targeting benefits naturally leads to consideration of the larger role of Social Security in retirement and, more specifically, the level of benefits Social Security should seek to provide. When Social Security began, retirement was a different entity than it is today. Average life expectancy and cultural norms about work and leisure meant that retirement was a short and unfortunate necessity. Social Security was created in part to encourage older people to retire from the workforce and to make way for younger workers. As individuals live longer and healthier lives, the possibility for an extended period of time after retirement becomes more likely. Indeed, our society has come to expect a long period of leisure when obligations of work and family life are complete.

In this context, Social Security influences retirement trends in important ways. First, the magnitude of individual Social Security benefits has a profound impact on retirement savings. The initial, modest aim of keeping older people out of the poorhouse has expanded dramatically to provide the majority of post-retirement income. Two-thirds of today's older people rely on Social Security for at least half of their total income, and even the richest quintile relies on Social Security for more than 20 percent of income. In times of scarce resources, some critics ask whether it is efficient or desirable to offer a retirement benefit that makes individual savings less necessary.

In addition, the eligibility age for Social Security benefits influences when people retire. Although the eligibility age for full benefits will increase from 65 to 67 by the year 2027, some believe that this change should be accelerated and even increased—perhaps to age 70—to reflect the improved health (and productive potential) of today's elders. Clearly, such a shift will have to grapple with cultural beliefs about when we are entitled to retire and receive pension benefits and also with such issues as job availability and age discrimination in employment.

■ *SECURITY OF SOCIAL MEANING*

Although Daniel Callahan's *Setting Limits* (1987) received less attention for its discussion of meaning and old age than for its resource allocation proposals, Callahan makes a persuasive case for the place of meaning in discussions of public policy. He argues that our modernized view of aging is hamstrung by its drive to remove the limitations of age and that it "lacks that most important of all ingredients for old age: a sense of collective meaning and purpose." Our orientation, Callahan posits, is toward an individualistic old age that gives us more of what we want (e.g., more years and less limitation) but illuminates little about the meaning and significance of those years.

The American vision of security in old age illustrates Callahan's point. As described above, we tend to feel secure when we are self-sufficient and in control. However, there are two main limitations to such an approach. First, such a standard of security is almost impossible to maintain. Second, and more important, even if we were able to maintain control until the day we die, a tenuous notion of independence does nothing to anchor our connection to a higher spiritual or ethical purpose.

If we cling to our needs and aspirations as individuals alone, we will fail to realize a deeper sense of meaning that can only be achieved through connection to the larger social and spiritual community. To achieve this kind of security—rather than just financial security—we need to develop a fundamental trust that we understand the order of the world in which we live (see Hashimoto, 1996). This cannot be done through reliance on a transitory notion of individual control. It must develop through a grounding in social relationships and spiritual beliefs.

The discussion of security almost inevitably turns to a contemplation of human need. Social Security (as well as Medicare) is premised on the idea that older Americans have a need for—and a corresponding right to—security. A narrow view of these needs can be found in the typical realm of the welfare state—food, shelter, and medical care. In this context, the provision of Social Security is important for the delivery of the monthly benefits check alone. However, as Ignatieff (1984) has argued, our needs as individuals extend beyond mere survival and include the need to achieve our potential as human beings. This realm of need includes things that the state cannot compel—love, respect, and community. It is in this gap between our claims on the collectivity and our needs *for* the collectivity where meaning can be lost.

And yet this gap between rights and needs is also where meaning is to be found. Ideals of later life are carved out of three basic dimensions of meaning: individual, social, and cosmic (Cole, 1992). We have reached the limits of what can be gained through the realm of the individual alone. It is high time that we accept the inevitable emptiness of such an approach and begin to foster our connection to the larger social and spiritual community. Our cult of independence is inevitably—and ironically—plagued by a lack of true security and, ultimately, by a lack of meaning. A truly sustainable Social Security program must be grounded in the security of shared social meanings.

Public policy has a role to play in our search for lasting security and meaning. As Social Security reform inches more and more toward a vision of individual accounts and individual equity, we must pause to consider the aspects of security that we are sacrificing in the process. Fiscal soundness matters, but it is not *all* that matters. Social Security reform and aging policy in the United States need to be socially and spiritually sound as well. Unless we look beyond the balance sheets of the future, our hopes and aspirations for growing older will be reduced to actuarial projections. We cannot afford to be so shortsighted.

References

Achenbaum, W. A. 1986. *Social Security: Visions and Revisions.* New York: Cambridge University Press.

Blythe, R. 1979. *The View in Winter: Reflection on Aging.* London: Harcourt Brace.

Callahan, D. 1987. *Setting Limits: Medical Goals in an Aging Society.* New York: Simon and Schuster.

Cole, T. R. 1992. *The Journey of Life: The Cultural History of Aging in America.* New York: Cambridge University Press.

Hashimoto, A. 1996. *The Gift of Generations: Japanese and American Perspectives on Aging and the Social Contract.* New York: Cambridge University Press.

Ignatieff, M. 1984. *The Needs of Strangers.* London: The Hogarth Press.

42

The Age Wave

Gloria Shur Bilchik

*T*ake off your rose-colored glasses, put on your bifocals, and get ready to look at health care from a more mature perspective: The Baby Boom generation is marching toward retirement age, and health care is destined to feel the crush.

Though it often comes as a personal shock to many suddenly-50 Boomers, the graying of America is no surprise to demographers. They have been tracking the upswing in America's average age and warning us about it for many years. According to the U.S. Census Bureau, when the first Boomers hit 65 in 2010, there will be 39 million Americans over the age of 65. By 2030, the 65-plus age category is expected to swell to 69 million. The most rapidly growing age group will be the 85-and-over population, which is projected to double its current size by 2025 and increase fivefold by 2050.

The effect on health care promises to be powerful. According to figures published by PricewaterhouseCoopers, older people currently use four to five times the amount of health care services used by those under 65. And while those 85 and older make up only 11 percent of today's nondisabled Medicare beneficiaries, they account for a much larger relative portion of resource usage.

The age wave has already begun. But the crest—particularly for health care—is still 10 years away. The implications are vast, and the time to start planning for them is now.

■ CHANGES IN ATTITUDE

"As the population ages, we're going to have to adopt a whole new way of looking at care," says Carol Levine, director of the Families and Health Care Project of the United Hospital Fund, New York City. "The health care system, as we know it now, is simply not prepared to handle the issues that an older population brings. And all of today's flaws will be magnified when the next wave hits."

Gloria Bilchik is a writer based in St. Louis.

A switch in orientation from acute care to chronic and long-term care will be essential, says Alan Lazaroff, M.D., of Denver's Geriatric Medical Associates. "Right now, the system is geared to rescue the elderly from the complications of chronic diseases. We need to learn to help people live, not just stop them from dying. In the future, our central principle will need to be to prevent or minimize disability."

Daniel Perry, executive director of the Alliance for Aging Research, agrees. "When we look at what robs millions of people of their ability to live on their own, we don't see big killer diseases such as cancer and heart attacks," he says. "Rather, we find unrecognized and undertreated chronic diseases of aging. These conditions will drive the cost of health care in this country for the next 50 years."

Statistics support Perry's assertion. The National Center for Health Statistics predicts a continuing rise in the cost and prevalence of chronic conditions through the mid-21st Century. In addition, a 1999 study conducted by Perry's organization found that, for older Americans who lose independence each year, the total increase in medical and long-term care expenditures is $26 billion greater than if they had maintained the ability to live on their own.

Minimizing or preventing disability means adopting an interdisciplinary approach to eldercare, says Lazaroff, because older patients' needs transcend the conventional, single-discipline approach. "In the health care model of the future, we'll work in teams, involving physicians, nurses, physical and occupational therapists, social workers, and educators," he says. "The idea that medical care is strictly a one-on-one [relationship] between a physician and a patient in a doctor's office will have to be reexamined."

This scenario also demands new interpersonal and diagnostic behaviors, says Robert Zorowitz of the DeKalb Regional Health Care Center, Decatur, Ga. As a board-certified geriatrician, Zorowitz is in the vanguard of a sparsely populated medical specialty whose influence appears destined to grow. "Doctors will have to become more sensitive to the problems specific to aging that complicate medical care—such as reduced vision and hearing loss. We'll need to look at patients, not just in terms of a collection of illnesses, but as functioning human beings. That means spending more time assessing how the patient's condition affects his or her ability to live independently and function at an optimal level."

In turn, that attitude shift calls for new emphases in medical training and research, a notion that is gaining ground. The Alliance for Aging Research recommends better medical provider training in assessing older patients' risk for disability and nursing home admission, and in finding ways to slow their transition toward lost independence. The report also calls for the health care community to close the gap between research advances and health care practice relative to the disabling conditions of the elderly.

But even medical breakthroughs will not prevent death, and the age wave will bring end-of-life issues into acute focus. "While healthy aging is going to be on the rise, we will . . . have to learn to do a better job of providing appropriate, dignified care at the end of life," says Christine Cassell, M.D., chair of geriatric and adult development at New York's Mt. Sinai School of Medicine. "It's not going to be possible to rely solely on hospices to do this work. People are going to die in hospitals. With the balance of health care shifting toward older patients, we will, at last, have to face these issues."

And if doctors, administrators, and trustees don't take the initiative, the push will undoubtedly come from another source: Baby Boomers themselves. Better informed about health care than previous generations, accustomed to a consumer's attitude and demands, comfortable with technology, and politically powerful, Boomers will exert a strong influence on the shape and style of every aspect of health care—even before they reach 65. "Baby Boomers are more focused on caring than on curing," says Larry Walker, president of the Walker Group, a governance-consulting firm in Portland, Ore. "Studies show that they value autonomy, customer satisfaction and comfort, and that they want a balance between risk and reward. As this generation ages, its focus will be on preserving quality of life. The question for hospital trustees will be, 'Which organizations will take the lead in providing the services that this generation will need and expect?'"

■ *ALTERED STATES*

For trustees, the altered state of health care promises a smorgasbord of new considerations and issues. "We'll be thinking in new frameworks, having completely new conversations, and seeking out whole new categories of information on which to base judgments," says Don Seymour, vice-president of National Health Advisors, Boston.

Many of those conversations will undoubtedly grow from the coming shifts in medical care. Boards may find themselves considering an entirely new range of expenditures, such as social programs, specialized geriatric training for nurses and other caregivers, and family caregiver support mechanisms. Trustees will also be discussing dollar allocations for physical plant alterations, such as creating larger examination rooms that can accommodate families, and reconfiguring facilities.

Over time, trustees may find themselves governing a wider-than-ever spectrum of services, business functions, and facilities. At the same time, they may be overseeing organizations that are less campus-centered, and not necessarily under the control of a single enterprise. "Both the subject matter and the shape of the health care organization are going to change," says James Roosevelt, associate commissioner of the Social Security Administration and trustee of Mount Auburn Hospital, Cambridge, Mass. "Trustees will need to assess the system's role in caring for people on a continuing basis. They'll have to keep their eyes on the mission and on their communities' needs, rather than on traditional notions of what a health system is or is not."

A critical concern in this debate will involve finding ways to knit together the right combination of services for the aging population. Analysts say that a key focus will be on allocating resources rationally. "This is a new mindset," says Seymour. "We're accustomed to a notion of stewardship that meant 'husbanding' capital resources. Now, we're moving toward a portfolio-management approach. Part of the future discussion may become, 'If there's a service needed, should we do it, and if we don't control it, with whom should we align ourselves to make sure the service is provided?'"

Debates over long-term care—facilities, services, and economics—will be front and center. It's easy to see why: The National Center for Health Statistics predicts that the number of nursing home residents will increase to 2.2 million this year, 2.6 million by 2010, and 3 million by 2020. Future watchers further predict that as many as 15 percent of the elderly population may need some form of human assistance to continue to live independently.

Finance will be high on the agenda. "Today, acute care and long-term care are funded by two separate systems. And, for the most part, we're using an acute care model to treat people with chronic conditions," says Karen Knutson, president of the American Association of Professional Geriatric Care Managers. "As more people enter the long-term care world, health systems will need to focus attention on how to achieve savings in caring for the chronically ill."

Any discussion of finance will probably come around to long-term-care insurance, too, says Mark Cohen, vice-president of LifePlans, a long-term-care insurance company based in Waltham, Mass. Cohen says that more than 500,000 new long-term care policies are written nationwide each year, and that in the next five years, the total is expected to reach 10 million.

"But just because people have long-term care policies, it may not mean that they know how to access good care," says Cohen. "So I envision some form of connection among providers and long-term care insurers, with providers managing the coordination of care for insured clients. Hospitals might even develop a system of preferred provider networks consisting of long-term care facilities."

"There is also going to be a tremendous need for geriatric care management—someone who holds the glue together," adds Knutson. Of the 1,300 corporate members of Knutson's association, 91 percent are for-profit companies. They represent more than 20,000 care managers, who offer assessment, care coordination, advocacy, placement services, caregiver support and crisis intervention. "Maybe hospitals and health systems will want to take a position in this spectrum. It's something that they'll have to talk about."

■ *ADVANCE WARNING*

The U.S. Bureau of the Census has some good news for trustees anticipating the effects of the age wave: During the next 10 years, the rate of population growth of the over-65 group is projected to be slower than at any time during the 20th century. Growth will be so slow, in fact, that the percentage of the population age 65 and over will remain near its current level for the next 10 years. It's only in 2010 that the bubble in the graph rises dramatically, with the arrival of the Baby Boomers.

Those projections mean that there is time—not to procrastinate, but to prepare. The age wave is inevitable, but current population trends do allow trustees time to deliberate about how to respond. Analysts agree that trustees should begin now to look into the major trends in their local markets—and to look further down the road to see what they may need in terms of programs, services, collaboration, and skill mixes.

With the big crunch still 10 years away, visioning is an effective way to begin preparing, says Larry Walker. "The ultimate job of trustees is to secure the future for tomorrow's consumer. To do that, you have to develop a meaningful vision—not just a series of pleasant-sounding words, and not just another conventional strategic plan."

Walker recommends developing a one-page "story" that describes the organization in 2010. "The best organizations will ask, 'Based on the demographic shifts coming to our market, what will we need to be in 2010? What unique resources will we need to serve the aging population?' Then, they'll look back to today and ask, 'Where are we now relative to that vision, with regard to leadership, collaboration, staffing, planning, and capital resources?'"

The resulting discussions may spur trustees toward restructuring or adding services, rearranging management functions, acquiring new businesses, or investigating new collaborative arrangements. Boards may even consider altering their own membership criteria, perhaps shifting the roster toward members with expertise in aging issues and long-term-care, or skill in managing change.

For forward-thinking trustees, positioning an organization for the age wave is a daunting task. But at least one observer sees a silver lining. "We talk a great deal about the burdens that older patients will bring to the health care system, and we'll never eliminate the degeneration that comes with old age," says Christine Cassell. "But let's not forget the upside: Americans over 65 have had universal access to medical care since the enactment of Medicare in 1965—making it possible for them to live longer and better than any generation before. And we've made tremendous progress in treating the illnesses that once reduced life expectancy. Let's remember: the aging of America is the greatest success story of modern medicine."

43

Ethical and Policy Considerations for Centenarians—The Oldest Old

Robert J.F. Elsner, Mary Ellen Quinn, Sandra D. Fanning, Sarah Hall Gueldner, and Leonard W. Poon

Centenarians are "expert survivors" because of their remarkable ability to overcome obstacles (Poon et al., 1992). These special people, by their very existence, are models of aging. They have lived through the Industrial Revolution, Great Depression, and world wars. They have also paid a human cost for their survival. They have experienced the death of friends and families. Many have lost children, grandchildren, and great-grandchildren, but have survived. In the United States, the average life expectancy for women is 75 years, and for men 73 years. Few people live to age 100, but the number is increasing.

In at least eight states, including Arizona, Arkansas, California, Colorado, Georgia, Nevada, Utah, and Washington, the number of 65-year-old and older residents will more than double within the next 22 years (U.S. Census Bureau, 1996). According to the U.S. Census Bureau (1998a), there were about 61,000 centenarians in the United States in 1998. This is a significant increase from the 37,000 reported in 1990, making centenarians the fastest growing segment in the United States. While the accuracy of the projection is difficult to determine, the U.S. Census Bureau's projection for 2040 is 447,000 centenarians, and 834,000 centenarians in 2050 (1998b).

This increase in the oldest-old may have important economic effects. Costs associated with care for older people are rising and are of widespread concern (Wolfe, 1993). A decade ago, Brody (1987) cautioned that the rationing of health care for the elderly should be continually examined for balance between quality of life and cost, a sentiment recently reiterated by Schnelle et al. (1999). Economics plays a critical role in staffing and other

Robert J.F. Elsner, *G.D., M.S., M.Ed., Doctoral candidate in Psychology and Research Assistant, The University of Georgia, Athens.* ***Mary Ellen Quinn,*** *R.N., Ph.D., Eta Omicron, Associate Professor of Community Nursing, The Medical College of Georgia School of Nursing, Athens.* ***Sandra D. Fanning,*** *B.S.H.E., Education Program Specialist, The University of Georgia Gerontology Center, Athens.* ***Sarah Hall Gueldner,*** *R.N., D.S.N., F.A.A.N., Beta Sigma, Director, The Pennsylvania State University School of Nursing, University Park, PA.* ***Leonard W. Poon,*** *Ph.D., Honorary, Director and Professor, The University of Georgia Gerontology Center, Athens.*

Reprinted with permission from *Image: Journal of Nursing Scholarship*, Third quarter, 1999, 31(3) 263–267.

care decisions related to insurance reimbursement and other forms of payment. "Insurance programs of past decades were developed for a medical model that emphasized rapid cures for acute disorders" (Mechanic, 1986). Belmont, Koehler, and Harris (1996) argue that we instead begin to focus healthcare economics on the long-term management of chronic illness. Battin (1987) insisted that the low quality of care for some elderly is a form of societally-sanctioned marginalization causing disproportionate deficiencies in funding and attention.

In 1988, members of the Georgia Centenarian Study (GCS) used cross-sectional and longitudinal designs to examine successful adaptation of community-dwelling and cognitively intact people in their 100s, 80s, and 60s. The investigators examined the effects of family longevity, cognition, personality, functional and mental health status, nutrition, support systems, and coping on successful adaptation. Data from 157 centenarians were included. In the 1997 phase of the study 27 surviving centenarians were examined. The accounts of three centenarians are highlighted here. To best represent the range of experiences, the stories of these three who were cognitively intact and able to communicate are presented.

"Attention is what we can give the least of "

"April" is a 106-year-old African-American woman living in southern Georgia. When we first met her at age 100, she was unloading a car full of groceries she bought with her nephew. She had lived alone in her home of many years, and was active, articulate, and happy. At the time of our second interview with her in 1995, she was still active.

When we contacted her 18 months later (1997), April had been admitted to a nursing home after breaking her hip. Because she had acceptable cognition scores for an illiterate person on the Mini-Mental Status Exam (Folstein, Folstein, & McHugh, 1975) at the previous two testings, we were disheartened to find her in bed and nearly stuporous. However, as we continued to spend time conversing with April, she became considerably more alert, and was eventually able to complete the cognitive assessment successfully.

April complained of extreme fatigue, discomfort, and inability to move her limbs. We were told by the charge nurse that the reason she was unable to move her arms or feet was that she was being chemically restrained. We asked why, and were told that she had fallen several times while trying to go to the bathroom after her hip had healed. The charge nurse stated she simply did not have the staff to assist April to the toilet each time she needed to go and that they did not want her to break her hip again. As this nurse stated, "Attention is what we can give the least of " because of staffing constraints. As a result, April voided and defecated in bed. Even though the bed was protected with pads, April was embarrassed and felt that her dignity was compromised.

April's story brings to light several important questions. It is important to note that use of chemical restraints with a resident of a long-term care facility

(LTCF) is in violation of the Omnibus Budget Reconciliation Act (1987). For example, 25mg diphenhydramine and 10mg doses of Valium were prescribed on an as-needed basis for April, yet the record revealed they were being administered at regular intervals of four times a day, an excessive dose for an 86-pound person.

Chemical usage also isolated April and made her seem demented. Indeed, the nurses had classified her as such. People with dementia are 6.4 times as likely to suffer injuries from falls compared to their nondemented cohorts (Asada et al., 1996), so if the nurses thought her to be demented, there might have been some justification for their overly cautious approach.

Institutional care is often the most appropriate care option for the demented because of difficulties in providing continuous care and safety at home (Kaplan, 1996). Kaplan's premise assumes, however, that the personnel in the facility will provide adequate attention.

We consider it a tragedy that a person who can survive for more than 100 years and recover from a hip injury at such an advanced age is put in a position she considers humiliating. Nurses' focus on the "medical-model," is a disservice to long-term residents who require care focused on sustaining functioning rather than on disease and cure. Loss of control over urinary function is a good example because of its widespread incidence. Care providers need to use interventions that promote continence for all long-term care residents (Peet et al., 1996). April's forced incontinence adversely affected her quality of life (Brocklehurst, 1993; Chiverton, Wells, Brink, & Mayer, 1996; Grimby, Milsom, Molander, Wiklund, & Ekelund, 1993; Vetter, Jones, & Victor, 1981) and caused distress (Brocklehurst, 1993; Chiverton et al., 1996) despite the availability of nursing interventions that might have helped to alleviate the problem (O'Brien, Austin, Sethi, & O'Boyle, 1991; Palmer, Czarapata, Wells, & Newman, 1997). Perhaps it would have been more helpful to April to lower her bed and place a bedside commode nearby, or to assign someone to help her to the bathroom every 2 hours (Palmer et al., 1997). These strategies of prevention and autonomy building may have increased the nurses' efficiency, while preserving April's independence. While paying attention is a constant challenge to nurses, it is not an insurmountable difficulty.

"I wanted to die in my own bed"

In northern Georgia, in a pretty little 100-year-old house, lived 108-year-old "May." May is Caucasian and had lived in her own home for more than 80 years. Legally blind for several years, she developed strategies for ensuring that she could care for herself. Her money, for example, was handled by an accountant who would give her dollar denominations in envelopes of various sizes. When shopping, she would remove bills from the various envelopes to equal the total owed. May had a good network of community support with neighbors calling on her to see if she needed help, which she rarely did.

In her home, she had systems for locating and identifying everything. She loved her home and told us on several occasions that her most sincere wish was to die in her own bed. At the first interview, we asked her if she feared falling, and being unable to get up. Her response was that she had lived and suffered long enough that she was not frightened by such a prospect.

Just before the second time we interviewed May, we learned that she had been admitted to a geriatric care facility because of her blindness. Although May protested that she was competent to live by herself, she was taken from her home. We were unable to ascertain who made this decision; May insisted it was a social worker. In any event, May told us that she thought society had sold her out by not allowing her to live her final years as she wished. Her feelings were so intense that she withdrew from further participation in the centenarian study.

Although May had enjoyed a support network in her neighborhood, she now had few visitors. Her bitterness over being institutionalized was shown in the way she treated others. Our informants indicated, during previous testing sessions, that for over 100 years she was thought of as a kindhearted, gentle person; yet in the facility she was aggressive and condescending. May told us her behavior was a reaction to her situation, saying that everyone told her she was demented and treated her accordingly, even though a formal diagnosis of dementia was not confirmed.

Collopy (1993) discussed the "intrusive beneficence" of our health care and legal systems, by which people are denied autonomy in the name of their own well-being as defined by others. Collopy (1995) raises ethical considerations for allowing independence versus imposing institutionalization, pointing out the conflict between these two views. Understanding these opposing views is essential to caring for the oldest old and others approaching the end of life (Carrick, 1999).

The inclination to classify older residents as demented is understandable, because research findings have documented that 10% of the population over age 75 exhibit some level of clinical dementia (Jorm, Korten, & Henderson, 1987; Magaziner, Bassett, & Hebel, 1987; Paykel et al., 1994; Paykel, Huppert & Brayne, 1998). Estimations of the percentage of nursing home residents with some degree of dementia are 40% to 60% (Maslow, 1991). It is not surprising, then, that premature classification of dementia might occur, forcing some older adults into unnecessary dependence.

Baltes (1996) suggests that dependency because of declines in elders is largely the result of negative attitudes in society about old age. Negative stereotyping might have kept May from dying in her own bed.

"They told me I might as well get used to never leaving here."

Despite this discouraging comment, "June" did, in fact, leave the nursing home to return to her own home. She had fallen and broken her hip while cleaning her bathroom at age 100. When she told the physicians and nurses who treated her injury how old she was, that she lived alone, and what she was doing when she fell, they thought she was confused. They found the scenario incomprehensible. It was outside their realm of expectation. June recounted her memories of the staff telling her that she would most likely never recover, never walk again, and probably never be able to leave. However, in spite of these "nay-sayers," June received excellent care. She stated that she responded to the staff because they responded positively to her, and in the end she was discharged to live with her daughter while she finished recovering.

Almost miraculously, when we next interviewed June, she was again living in her own home, cooking her own meals, and playing the piano. She once again walked in her neighborhood, thankful for physical therapy that helped her regain her strength. She holds no ill feelings toward those who told her she would never again live at home.

■ DISCUSSION

These short narratives indicate the problems and triumph of three people who lived to be 100 and those who cared for them. However, these vignettes are offered as examples based on our observations, and should not be used as generalization for all older individuals. April's quality of care was compromised to accommodate staffing constraints and limited understanding by nurses. It seems possible that May was "interred" because of prejudices about what people of specific age groups and physical conditions can do. Despite initial care provider insensitivity, June's situation represents the ideal outcome—informed, sensitive care returned her to the environment where she could survive best.

The central theme for all three was lack of individualized care and their subsequent persistent struggle to retain a voice in care decisions. These women all appear to have been stereotyped, as if all members of their age cohort are terminally ill. This attitude was recently reported by Bradley, Peiris, and Wetle (1998), who found that despite discussion and legislation, care providers are not listening to their patient as well as they need to.

Key to defining and assuring quality care is recognizing that the ultimate test of quality must come from the people who rely on our care (Kane, 1995)—in this case, people 100 years old and older in nursing homes. Faulk (1988) found that once lower-level material needs including safety and security are met, life satisfaction is increased significantly by meeting the higher level social integration needs including closeness to others, contact with family and friends, and independence. Merely meeting lower-level material needs results in incomplete care that does not enhance but detracts from quality of life.

Six goals reflecting the experiences of residents and providers in assisted living programs have been described as follows: to allow meaningful choices, to help residents stay as healthy as possible, to foster a sense of community, to structure a safe and secure environment, to provide needed care, and to offer opportunities for life-long learning (American Association of Homes and Services for the Aged, 1995). Because of their need for assistance with many tasks essential to daily life, residents of nursing homes often have limited or no control over the basic aspects of their lives. May exemplified this, having been able to care for herself at home, but then admitted to an institution because of her blindness. This situation is experienced by many people with disabilities and has been described as the "dilemma of dependency" (Ball & Whittington, 1995). Loss of control related to even necessary dependence on others translates into the loss of freedom and loss of control over personal space, possessions, information, and one's own body (Agich, 1993; Ball & Whittington, 1995). This loss may be most intense for centenarians who have lived independently.

Nurses who work in nursing homes should be aware that cognitive scores and assistance needs are fairly good predictors of subsequent falls (Asada et al., 1996). Some may also know that the most serious injuries occur in men with gait disturbance, digitalis use, and an absence of quadriceps reflex; and in women with foot deformities, and short step-length (Koski et al., 1996). What many might not realize is that activity can be associated with higher cognitive function (Christiansen et al., 1996) and that use of sensory aids for vision and hearing can increase the quality of life for older people. (Carabellese et al., 1993). These are important considerations because they can affect both the overall assessment and prognosis of a resident. In the case of May, her blindness and ill temper at being taken from her home might have made it difficult for nurses to use a standard cognitive screening test, resulting in inaccurate assessment.

All three of the determined centenarians reported a lack of meaningful, and sometimes even basic, communication with the nurses. Yet, it has been well established that effective communication with residents is an essential component of quality nursing care in the LTC setting (Steffl, 1984). There is a need to re-examine the team approach to caring for older individuals to ensure many opportunities for interaction (Charatin, Foley, & Libow, 1985; Farley, Zellman, Ouslander, & Reuben, 1999). Although nurses have many tasks to accomplish, solely focusing on tasks is inadequate. A process focus instead of a task focus might be necessary to accomplish nursing care objectives for centenarians. Interactive strategies, such as life review (Haight, 1988) can be incorporated during client bathing or grooming to help meet interpersonal needs.

All three centenarians were cognitively intact by our assessments. Certainly, all should have been treated as full partners in care decisions. It seems possible that a significant number of assessments might be done too early, too hastily, or with preconceptions about aging.

■ *IMPLICATIONS AND RECOMMENDATIONS*

Advocates for aging need to be more aggressive in enforcing laws and developing innovative policies which protect elders. Our findings, and those of other researchers (Kane & Wilson, 1993; McColl, Thomas, & Bond, 1996; Smith, Colling, Elander, & Latham, 1993) strongly suggest the need for more sensitive nurses in our long-term care system. Inadequate staffing, poor nursing leadership, and a lack of continuing education are the most likely contributors to current deficiencies.

The case histories in this study show the dilemma of trying to provide quality care with too few resources in a system that needs refocusing and adjustment to the growing older U.S. population. Wetle (1995) discusses an individual's right to proper care and informed decisions and explores the ethical concerns for nurses. These issues are also explored in recent articles by Golden and Sonneborn (1998), and Stone and Yamada (1998).

Methods for meeting the challenge of caring for our vulnerable older adults should be multidisciplinary and include policy makers, academicians, providers, family, and elders themselves. Refocusing gerontologic healthcare away from the medical model of disease and cure toward a framework of retaining and maximizing function is needed.

We propose six policy reforms to address the issues underlying the basic problems:

1. Make resident involvement in their care decisions and enhancement of perceived control integral in the caring process of elders, even the oldest and frailest.
2. Increase efforts to develop alternative models of care so that those who are not truly in need of nursing home placement have other options.
3. Increase public discussions about the issues. The balance between client-oriented goals, such as assurance of appropriate care delivery, and system-oriented goals, such as cost containment, must be met (Applebaum & Austin, 1990). Nurses must be vocal about their perspectives. Being vocal does not mean waiting for federal mandates but may mean talking to local news media personnel, being on talk shows, participating in town meetings, contacting legislators, or other such activities.
4. Explore methods of increased involvement of family and community in the care of older adults. Perhaps April's family could have become a part of her care. An option might be to develop a program of community volunteers through youth, civic, or religious groups who might regularly visit individuals such as these both before and after moves into care facilities.
5. Increase research efforts to develop and test innovative interventions that promote function and independence in both community-dwelling and institutionalized older adults.

6. Increase gerontologic education for nurses who are charged with providing care to all elders.

Friedan (1993) asserts that the principles underlying long-term care in this country deny the personhood of age. "If we are not seen as human beings but merely as 'objects' to be disposed of, warehoused until death, then restraints, drugs, are not 'abuse', but cost-efficient aids to our 'long-term care'" (p. 516).

The Georgia Centenarian Study was supported by the National Institute on Aging grant R01-MH43435. The authors thank Dr. Peter Buerhaus for his insightful comments on a previous draft.

References

Agich, G. (1993). *Autonomy and long-term care.* New York: Oxford University Press.

American Association of Homes and Services for the Aged. (1995). Residents, providers identify goals for assisted living. *Currents, 10,* 7.

Applebaum, R., & Austin, C. (1990). *Long-term care case management: Design and evaluation.* New York: Springer.

Asada, T., Kariya, T., Kinoshita, T., Asaka, A., Morikawa, S., Yoshioka, M., & Kakuma, T. (1996). Predictors of fall-related injuries among community-dwelling elderly people with dementia. *Age and Ageing, 25,* 22–28.

Ball, M.M., & Whittington, F.J. (1995). *Surviving dependence: Voices of African American elders.* Amityville, NY: Baywood.

Baltes, M.M. (1996). *The many faces of dependency in old age.* Cambridge, UK: Cambridge University Press.

Battin, M.P. (1987). Choosing the time to die: The ethics and economics of suicide in old age. In S.F. Spicker, S.R. Ingman, & I.R. Lawson (Eds.), *Ethical dimensions of geriatric care: Value conflicts for the 21st century* (161–189). Boston: D. Reidel.

Belmont, M.F., Koehler, K.N., & Harris, A. (1996). Health promotion for the elderly. In C.B. Lewis (Ed.), *Aging: The health care challenge* (261–276). Philadelphia: F.A. Davis Co.

Bradley, E.H., Peiris, V., & Wetle, T. (1998). Discussions about end-of-life care in nursing homes. *Journal of the American Geriatrics Society, 46,* 1235–1241.

Brocklehurst, J.C. (1993). Urinary incontinence in the community—analysis of a MORI poll. *British Medical Journal, 306,* 832–834.

Brody, B. (1987). Wholehearted & halfhearted care: National policies vs. individual choice. In S.F. Spicker, S.R. Ingman, & I.R. Lawson (Eds.), *Ethical dimensions of geriatric care: Value conflicts for the 21st century* (79–94). Boston: D. Reidel Publishing Company.

Carabellese, C., Appolonio, I., Rozzini, R., Bianchetti, A., Frisoni, G.B., Fattola, L., & Trabucchi, M. (1993). Sensory impairment and quality of life in a community elderly population. *Journal of the American Geriatrics Society, 41,* 401–407.

Carrick, P. (1999). Environmental ethics and medical ethics: Some implications for end-of-life care, Part II. *Cambridge Quarterly of Healthcare Ethics, 8,* 250–256.

Charatin, F.B., Foley, C.J., & Libow, L.S. (1985). The team approach to geriatric medicine. In R. Andres, E.L. Bierman, & W.R. Hazzard (Eds.), *Principles of geriatric medicine* (169–175). New York: McGraw-Hill.

Chiverton, P.A., Wells, T.J., Brink, C.A., & Mayer, R. (1996). Psychological factors associated with urinary incontinence. *Clinical Nurse Specialist, 10,* 229–233.

Christiansen, H., Korten, A., Jorm, A.F., Henderson, A.S., Scott, R., & Mackinnon, A.J. (1996). Activity levels and cognitive function in an elderly community-dwelling sample. *Age and Ageing, 25,* 72–80.

Collopy, B.J. (1993). The burden of beneficence. In R.A. Kane & A.L. Caplan (Eds.), *Ethical conflicts in management of home care: The case managers dilemma* (93–100). New York: Springer.

Collopy, B.J. (1995). Safety and independence: Rethinking some basic concepts in long-term care. In L.B. McCullough & N.L. Wilson (Eds.), *Long-term care decisions: Ethical and conceptual dimensions* (137–152). Baltimore: Johns Hopkins University Press.

Farley, D.O., Zellman, G., Ouslander, J.G., & Reuben, D.B. (1999). Use of primary care teams by HMOS for care of long-stay nursing home residents. *Journal of the American Geriatrics Society, 47,* 139–144.

Faulk, L. (1988). Quality of life factors in board and care homes for the elderly: A hierarchical model. *Adult Foster Care Journal, 2*(2), 100–115.

Folstein, M.F., Folstein, F.E., & McHugh, P.R. (1975). Mini-mental state: A practical method for grading cognitive state of patients for the clinician. *Journal of Psychiatric Research, 12,* 189–198.

Friedan, B. (1993). *The fountain of age.* New York: Simon & Shuster.

Golden, R.L., & Sonneborn, S. (1998). Ethics in clinical practice with older adults: Recognizing biases and respecting boundaries. *Generations, 22*(3), 82–86.

Grimby, A., Milsom, I., Molander, U., Wiklund, I., & Ekelund, P. (1993). The influence of urinary incontinence on the quality of life of elderly women. *Age and Ageing, 22,* 82–89.

Haight, B.K. (1988). The therapeutic role of a structured life review process in homebound elderly subjects. *Journal of Gerontology, 43,* 40.

Jorm, A.F., Korten, A.E., & Henderson, A.S. (1987). The prevalence of dementia: A quantitative integration of the literature. *Acta Psychiatric Scandinavica, 76,* 465–479.

Kane, R. (1995). *Quality, autonomy, and safety in home and community-based long-term care: Toward regulatory and quality assurance policy.* Report of a National Mini-Conference of the White House Conference on Aging. Minneapolis, Minnesota. National Long-Term Care Resource Center, University of Minnesota.

Kane, R.A., & Wilson, K.B. (1993). *Assisted living in the United States: A new paradigm for residential care for frail older persons?* Washington, DC: American Association of Retired Persons Public Policy Institute.

Kaplan, M. (1996). *Clinical practice with caregivers of dementia patients.* Washington, DC: Taylor & Francis.

Koski, K., Luukinen, H., Laippala, F., & Kivel, S.L. (1996). Physiological factors and medications as predictors of injurious falls by elderly people: A prospective population-based study. *Age and Ageing, 25,* 29–38.

Magaziner, J., Bassett, S.S., & Hebel, J.R. (1987). Predicting performance on the Mini-Mental State Examination. Use of age and education specific equations. *Journal of the American Geriatrics Society, 35,* 996–1000.

Maslow, K. (1991). Formal long-term care services and settings. In N. Mace (Ed.), *Dementia care: Patient, family, and community* (297–320). Baltimore: The Johns Hopkins University Press.

Mechanic, D. (1986). *From advocacy to allocation: The evolving American health care system.* New York: Free Press.

McColl, E., Thomas, L., & Bond, S. (1996). A study to determine patient satisfaction with nursing care. *Nursing Standard, 10*(52), 34–38.

O'Brien, J., Austin, M., Sethi, P., & O'Boyle, P. (1991). Urinary incontinence: Prevalence, need for treatment, and effectiveness of intervention by nurse. *British Medical Journal, 303,* 1308–1312.

Omnibus Budget Reconciliation Act. (1987). Public Law 100–203. Sections 4201(A), 4211(A).

Palmer, M.H., Czarapata, B.J., Wells, T.J., & Newman, D.K. (1997). Urinary outcomes in older adults: Research and clinical perspectives. *Urologic Nursing, 17,* 2–9.

Paykel, E.S., Brayne, C., Huppert, F.A., Gill, C., Barkley, C., Gehlhaar, E., Beardsall, L., Girling, D.M., Pollitt, P., & O'Connor, D. (1994). Incidence of dementia in a population older than 75 years in the United Kingdom. *Archives of General Psychiatry, 51,* 325–332.

Paykel, E.S., Huppert, F.A., & Brayne, C. (1998). Incidence of dementia and cognitive decline in over-75s in Cambridge: Overview of cohort study. *Social Psychiatry And Psychiatric Epidemiology, 33,* 387–392.

Peet, S.M., Castleden, C.M., McGrother, C.W., & Duffin, H.M. (1996). The management of urinary incontinence in residential and nursing homes for older people. *Age and Ageing, 25,* 139–143.

Poon, L.W., Clayton, G.M., Martin, P., Johnson, M.A., Courtney, B.C., Sweaney, A.L., Merriam, S.B., Pless, B.S., & Theilman, S.B. (1992). The Georgia centenarian study. *International Journal of Aging and Human Development, 34,* 1–17.

Schnelle, J.F., Ouslander, J.G., Buchanan, J., Zellman, G., Farley, D., Hirsch, S.H., & Reuben, D.B. (1999). Objective and subjective measures of the quality of managed care in nursing homes. *Medical Care, 37,* 375–383.

Smith, B.E., Colling, K., Elander, E., & Latham, C. (1993). A model for multicultural curriculum development in baccalaureate nursing education. *Journal of Nursing Education, 32*(5), 205–208.

Steffl, B.M. (1984). Communication with the elderly. In B.M. Steffl (Ed.), *Handbook of gerontological nursing* (67–72). New York: Van Nostrand Reinhold.

Stone, R.I., & Yamada, Y. (1998). Ethics for the frontline worker: A challenge for the twenty-first century. *Generations, 22*(3), 45–51.

U.S. Census Bureau. (1996). *Current population reports, special studies, P23–190, 65+ in the United States.* Washington, DC: U.S. Government Printing Office.

U.S. Census Bureau. (1998a). *Resident population of the United States: Estimates, by age and sex* [On-Line]. Available: http://www.census.gov/population/estimates/nation/intfile2-1.txt

U.S. Census Bureau. (1998b). *Resident population of the United States: Middle series projections, by age and sex* [On-Line]. Available: http://www.census.gov/population/estimates/nation/nas/npas3550.txt

Vetter, N.J., Jones, D.A., & Victor, C.R. (1981). Urinary incontinence in the elderly at home. *Lancet, ii:* 1275–1277.

Wetle, T. (1995). Ethical issues and value conflicts facing case managers of frail elderly people living at home. In L.B. McCullough & N.L. Wilson (Eds.), *Long-term care decisions: Ethical and conceptual dimensions* (63–86). Baltimore: Johns Hopkins University Press.

Wolfe, J.R. (1993). *The coming health crisis: Who will pay for the care of the aged in the twenty-first century?* Chicago: University of Chicago Press.

Discussion Questions

1. What does growing old mean to you? How do you see yourself at age 70?

2. How would you go about learning to grow old?

3. What do you think are the components of a secure old age?

4. Compare and contrast the meaning of Social Security for the elderly and for the younger population.

5. Discuss the advantages and disadvantages of individual accounts in Social Security.

6. Are Americans any more secure today than they were when Social Security began? Explain your reasoning.

7. What kind of plans would you make to prepare for the health care needs of the increasing numbers of elderly in 2010?

8. What do you think are the major stumbling blocks in preparing for the coming "age wave"?

9. If you were 70 years old, what kind of health care would you like to anticipate having?

10. What experiences have you had caring for the very old and/or centenarians? What have they taught you?

Further Readings

McCandless, N. J. & Connor, F. P. (1999). Older women and the health care system: A time for change. *Fundamentals of Feminist Gerontology, 11*(2/3), 13–27.

Mechanic, D. (1999). The changing elderly population and future health care needs. *Journal of Urban Health: Bulletin of the New York Academy of Medicine, 76*(1), 24–38.

Stipp, D. (1999). Hell no, we won't go. *Fortune, 140*(2), 102–108.

Stipp, D. (1999). Live a lot longer. *Fortune, 140*(1), 144–160.

Wagner, C. G. (1999). The centenarians are coming! *The Futurist, 33*(5), 16–23.

Weber, D. O. (1999). Age cannot wither: The golden age of the golden years. *Health Forum Journal, 42*(4), 32, 34–36.

Web Site Resources for Living Longer

American Association of Retired Persons   www.aarp.org

American Society on Aging   www.asaging.org

Coalition for Women's Health and Aging   www.womenshealth-aging.org

ElderWeb   www.elderweb.com

National Council on the Aging   www.ncoa.org

National Institute on Aging   **www.nih.gov/nia**
The Seasoned Citizen   **www.seasonedcitizen.com**
ThirdAge   **www.thirdage.com**

General Search Engine Web Sites

Go to   **www.goto.com**
LookSmart   **www.looksmart.com**

Health Web Sites

InteliHealth   **www.intelihealth.com**
Mayo Clinic Health Oasis   **www.mayohealth.org**

Professional Journal Web Sites

Geriatric Nursing   **www.mosby.com**
Journal of Gerontological Nursing   **www.slackinc.com**

CHAPTER 9

Violence: Is Anyone Safe?

Violence is everywhere. Now at levels unheard of even 10 to 15 years ago, the increase in violence has become a commonplace, ordinary event. Violence has touched everyone—young and old, rich and poor, straight and gay, white and black, Catholics, Jews, and Protestants. No one is immune, and no one is safe. These days we have come to expect "road rage," "in-your-face" confrontations, taunting, and verbal abuse. The slightest provocation can result in physical assault. Teenage gangs battle each other over violations of turf or acts of what is perceived as "dissing." People are assaulted or killed for their football jackets or their sneakers. Nothing seems to surprise us anymore.

Fear is the common coin that violence has generated. It is no longer confined to the mean streets and housing projects of our urban areas. Now, it shows up at work, down the street, next door, and even in our own homes. That violence "can't happen here" is now an illusion. It can happen here—it *does* happen here, and it's happening more than we thought possible. Is anyone safe? What are we saying about ourselves and about our country when children kill children; when an ordinary day at school includes being searched for guns and knives; and when children are escorted to and from school for fear that they will be abducted? Are these really ordinary events? Have we become *that* immune? Has the fear of violence done that to us?

In our struggle to find reasons for the causes of violence, we come up empty handed. We point to media violence, to computer games, to the lack of gun control, and to lax parenting as likely causes, but find there is no one cause. What we do sense is that somewhere in our sociocultural institutions, something has gone awry. Since our culture is expressed, maintained, and shaped through its social institutions, some core value that has guided us successfully in the past seems to have lost its meaning for us. We have relied on our legal system, schools, churches, police, and families because they are the visible reminders of our culture, reinforcing who we are, what we believe, and what we stand for. Somehow that message is not being heard as clearly as it once was.

Violence is not just a nursing issue; it's everyone's issue. We are the ones who know what violence looks like. We see it in emergency departments, in hospital rooms, and when bodies are wheeled to the morgue. But we are not just nurses, we are members of our community. It is in our communities that we must attend to the broader issues of violence that so directly affect the quality of life for all of us.

The readings in this chapter provide that opportunity. This chapter begins with an exploration of the relationship between violence and the media and how the media insinuates and exploits violence and victims of violence for its own purposes. The concluding readings focus on the victims of violence by examining the extent to which violence affects children, intimate partner relationships, and the elderly.

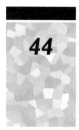

44

The Gunfire Dialogues

Thomas de Zengotita

*T*he incident at Columbine High School on April 20 arrested our attention not only because fifteen people were killed but because it consolidated our sense that school shootings say Something Important about Society. As a media event, it is related somehow to O.J. and Di and Monica, but practical preoccupation with causal "factors" distracted us, and the possibility of general synthesis was sacrificed to the need to Do Something. The essentials emerged within days of the event but flattened into cliché as the buzz of commentary echoed across our virtual polis. Still, they can be recovered.

The boy appeared in a local-folks-react piece on one of the morning shows just days after the shootings. He was white-ethnicky, pudgy and pimply, with purple streaks in his dreadlocked hair and a couple of studs in his face. He spoke with a defiant whine. He didn't condone the shootings, and he wasn't into Hitler, but he had been harassed by jocks all his life, and those kids in Colorado "at least . . . took a stand." He thought a lot of other kids like him would kind of idolize the Trench-coat Mafia.

He was right. Saturday's *New York Times* covered online discussions of the Littleton massacre. The tone was set by psychologists and Web-site executives hyping virtual communities, but quotes from the kids told the tale: "I would never personally do anything like that, but it did take guts" and "Even though I would never take someone else's life, maybe it will make people think before they open their mouths next time. . . ." The cruelty of prep and jock "culture" toward those who didn't fit in was the underlying issue for these kids. Cokie Roberts made it official that Sunday morning, and *Rolling Stone* columnist Jon Katz's Web site became a polling resource for the mainstream. The floodgates opened and commentators everywhere were publicly recalling their high school days. Cliques joined Kosovo on the national agenda.

Thomas de Zengotita teaches at The Dalton School and The Draper Program at New York University.

Sally Satel, a Yale psychiatrist, had an op-ed piece about the busloads of "grief counselors" who are as much a feature of such scenes as are SWAT teams and flower shrines. She focused on the "commodification of grief," the "unholy therapeutic alliance" between the talk-through-your-feelings-and-get-to-closure counselor and the empathic servants of the twenty-four-hour news cycle. And can anyone doubt that stricken mourners, no matter how authentic their feelings, respond at some level to implicit expectations when the cameras roll? Especially since they have seen this show on TV before; now, suddenly, they are in it.

For it is very much a show, and not only in the trivial sense that anything covered by the media becomes a show. "Senseless school shooting" is now a genre with resonance across the country because it unites universality and specificity so compellingly. There is a set: the open space of parking lots and sports fields around the one- or two-level brick-and-concrete sprawl of buildings, the school name and colors and logo—all pretty much interchangeable across the exurban landscape. There is a cast: kids made for yearbook pictures, local law-enforcement and school officials rising, or not rising, to the occasion, local volunteers in emergency services likewise, and local religious and political leaders, too. An indefinable quality of localness pervades the scene. It's the hair and mustaches, the jackets, hats and eyewear, the cars and trucks—you can feel the nearby malls and the traffic on the interstate at the edge of town. It isn't New York and it isn't L.A. It's the heartland, and everyone knows this plot: reconstructing the lives of the killers, tracking down accomplices, the community outpouring of support, the coming together, the healing process—and the rifts and recriminations as well. Likewise the spectators; we distinguish immediately between this genre and natural-disaster or horrors-of-war "shows." We know how to respond as an audience as surely as we would know how to play our roles if, God forbid, we suddenly landed a part.

"Shows" belongs in quotes because, like all things postmodern, this is a reflexive entity, and that reflexivity testifies, in its practical futility, to the power of the total phenomenon. No amount of media self-criticism makes a dent. For "*coverage* of senseless school shootings" is also a genre. The correspondents are in moved-to-the-breaking-point-but-professional mode. The anchors are in grave-demeanor-reserved-for-inexplicable-evil mode. The expert guests and other commentators are also grave, but inexplicability is not their provenance, and I-told-you-so and now-maybe-you'll-listen drives their spin toward gun control or family values or psychological-intervention programs.

The point here is not exploitation of personal pain for commercial or political gain. We are not at that familiar level of criticism. Indeed, many in the media have been moved to even more reflexive contortions because of just such concerns: correspondents asking interviewees about their grief now also ask how they feel about being interviewed about their grief. No, the point is to call attention to an emergent level of culture that transcends issue-oriented efforts to solve a social problem.

The key to the success of the show is the way everyone can identify so specifically with the set, the characters, and the plot; that is why the outpouring spreads, and innumerable other local responses are organized, or erupt, under the sign of "could it happen here?" It is like a myth played out in "real time," embracing millions of people. That is how the personal becomes the political. That is why ideologies no longer cohere and issues fragment; they can't compete with such narratives.

We come closest to addressing the situation as a whole when asking how violence in the media influences behavior. Cultural conservatives focus on permissive standards related to content, and surely that content goes way beyond anything imaginable thirty years ago. People who commit these acts always show evidence of its influence. The Littleton shooters spent a lot of time with *Natural Born Killers* and goth CDs and hate Web sites, but libertarians point out that Charlie Starkweather was inspired by comics and rock and roll, and argue that agency must be attributed to the person, not the muse. So the debate resolves itself into this question: Is the influence of today's media qualitatively different from yesterday's?

The answer is obviously yes. What is shown makes a difference. Saturation and production values matter, too. Interactivity from the killer's point of view in a graphic video game goes right to the sensorimotor brain centers. High school cliques have always been with us and jocks have always bullied geeks; the geeks now have something besides the chess club to retreat to— they have games like Doom, entire environments of testosterone-stimulating violence in which they compensate virtually for physical inequities. And compulsions of mimesis among the psychotically inclined have thresholds. This can be denied only by pointing to the fact that overall violence among teenagers, in school or out, is dramatically lower than it used to be. But that just confirms that, in an age when the organized and ritualized Fifties fistfight seems quaint, conflict-resolution programs collaborate unwittingly with computer games to nudge violence into virtuality. It also tells us that healthier kids, who never act out, cope differently with the same stimulations. What it does not tell us is that those stimulations might have powerful effects on them, perhaps just as corrosive in subtler ways.

The sheer amount of media absorbed by kids who commit such acts, the variety and intensity of its modalities, and the recurrence of specific items on their personal-favorites list tell us that something comparable in force to the oral culture Plato attacked in *The Republic* has emerged among us. Comparable in force, but very different in context and functionality. The performative Homeric narrative of pre-literate Greece provided irresistible paradigms of behavior and evaluation in an essentially tribal society. To counter the momentum of so enveloping a tradition, Plato recommended the detachments of a rational philosophy. The post-literate fusion of fact and fiction in multimedia narratives of our day are similarly enveloping, but we resist through detachments of knowingness and irony. Or most of us do. But, resistant or not, we all know what counts: being on the show.

The really decisive piece of media in the Columbine case was the tape the shooters and their friends made for a video-production course in their school. In the tape, the boys rehearsed the event they would one day—but what is the verb here? Enact? Perform? A word like that is needed. The model of plan followed by action will not apply. That model belongs to an age when events in the real world and accounts of those events in the media were essentially separate. That difference no longer exists. For the shooters knew what coverage they could expect in their second production of "school shootings." They were already and always "on"—just like the people in Hollywood and New York, pitching angles on this story to one another before the bodies were out of Columbine's library.

So we are faced with a new space for public culture somewhere between reality and simulation, between action and acting—and this holds not just for latent psychotics but for the rest of us as well. Saying, "Well, millions of kids listen to Marilyn Manson and never harm anyone" misses the point. *Those* kids are just as influenced in a *different* way by the totality that is this virtual space. They go ironic rather than psychotic. They are the "apathetic" ones, for whom politics is, at best, a field of self-expression in which certain people identify with certain issues and "promote awareness" of them—a politics in which issues have fans.

Think of it all as do followers of Nietzsche among French intellectuals. The brain and its structures, the body and its desires, meet culture directly. Inclinations and threshold are built into our neurochemistry, and stimulating content and forms of behavior are imposed by technologies of communication and the administration of daily life in routines of work and play. The more enveloping and penetrating the stimulations and routines, the more uniform and centerless the settings of our lives—and what else should we expect but occasional psychotic eruptions on a vast plain of disengagement sustained by an economy devoted to simulations?

Traditional opinion leaders don't want to see this phenomenon whole. Those in the mainstream have a piece of the action—their material interests are increasingly vested in the immaterial economy. They must see the new technologies as a force at least *potentially* for good. People on the left don't want to see it either, but, ironically, this is because the media seem to them not material enough! They cling to old bread-and-circuses, opiate-of-the-people critiques. They learned nothing from O.J. and Di and Monica. They can't believe that virtual reality is *real*. But the folks who are creating virtuality have a deeper understanding. From *The Truman Show* to *The Matrix*, a slew of recent movies is exposing the project built into these technologies. The wonder is that we don't let this surreptitious confession sink in. After all, don't these technologies have as their explicit purpose making representations more and more realistic (think computer graphics and animations) and making reality more and more representational (think Times Square and sanctioned graffiti)?

A few years ago, Benjamin Barber wrote a book that characterized posteverything culture as *Jihad v. McWorld*. He had principally in mind developments that preoccupy political thinkers—global corporate media vis-à-vis retribalization after the Cold War: Hutu killers in Nike paraphernalia and so on. Columbine showed that the phenomenon Barber described is not essentially residual, that a hybrid entity with a structuring life of its own has emerged on the planet, a life in which Serbian three-fingered salutes echo homey gangsta signs and Hitler's birthday and high school movies converge seamlessly with Trench-coat Mafia and twenty-four-hour coverage of "Terror in the Rockies." To Muslims and Christians add Hilfiger and piercing.

Half-convinced, perhaps, you ask, "What is to be done?" And the answer must be, "Don't ask *that* question so fast." For if, as a gigantic matter of historical fact, our world is becoming so intensely reflexive that distinctions between action and performance and reality and representation are eroding at every level of our lives, then that question, asked immediately, represses the realization that we are at an utter loss. And that realization might spur us to take up a challenge to our understanding, which we cannot afford to leave to prophetic digerati and deconstructing academics. Because this much can be said for certain: we are all in the show, and the show must go on.

45

The Movies Made Me Do It

Michael Atkinson

On March 5, 1995, Sarah Edmondson, the 18-year-old scion of one of Oklahoma's most prominent political clans, holed up with her 17-year-old boyfriend Ben Darras in her family's cabin with a video copy of *Natural Born Killers,* a Smith & Wesson .38, and a reported 17 tabs of acid. It's clear neither how many times they watched the film nor what the timetable had been for dropping all that dope, but, over the next two days, the teenagers road-tripped south, first shooting Hernando, Louisiana, cotton-gin manager Bill Savage, and then, the following day, convenience-store clerk Patsy Byers. Initially they had intended to go to a Grateful Dead concert in Memphis, but got the date wrong. Edmondson got 35 years; Darras got life.

Savage was DOA, and his hometown friend John Grisham raised a public stink over the Oliver Stone film, threatening to sue for product liability but never filing. Luckless, Byers was left a quadriplegic and later died of cancer, but her family's lawyer has filed a civil suit against Edmonson, Darras, Edmondson's parents, Stone, and Time Warner, maintaining that the film's creators "knew . . . or should have known" that violence would result from its being shown. In March, after bouncing around Louisiana courts, the case went to the Supreme Court and was seen as good to go.

Here comes the flood. This April, the families of three Kentucky girls left dead after the prayer-group shooting spree of 14-year-old Michael Carneal in 1997 have filed a $130 million lawsuit against no fewer than 25 parties, including the film companies involved with the film *The Basketball Diaries;* a single scene allegedly incited Carneal to action. The dream sequence, of Leonardo DiCaprio gunning down his classmates, should be immediately familiar to even those who haven't bothered seeing the film, thanks to the news coverage of the Littleton rampage. Littleton itself is destined to become the nation's mother lode of hydra-headed copycat-crime civil suits directed at the manufacturers of pop culture, just as the Klebold-Harris scenario immediately became something to mimic in high schools from coast to coast. Copycat crimes have attained front-burner notoriety, and some day soon

Reprinted with permission by *The Village Voice*, May 11, 1999, 44(18) 58–59.

Hollywood's liberty will be pitted against the perceived welfare of American children.

It's an old but neglected dynamic, and wherever you stand on the issue, itemizing the carnage attributed to the influence of movies is chilling business. After *The Birth of a Nation* hit big in 1915, the KKK enjoyed a huge resurgence and lynching stats shot up. James Cagney's psycho gangster in *White Heat* (1949) was blamed for inspiring Brit Chris Craig's 1952 shooting of a policeman. *A Clockwork Orange*'s 1971 release was followed by several rapes in England accompanied by the rapists' renditions of "Singin' in the Rain," after which Stanley Kubrick permanently removed the film from British circulation. *Magnum Force*'s murder-by-Drano was reenacted in Utah. *The Deer Hunter* precipitated a rash of fatal Russian roulette duels, a fierce love of *First Blood* sent a deranged Englishman named Michael Ryan tearing through his village commando-style, killing randomly. *Taxi Driver* spoke to John Hinckley; *RoboCop* gave ideas to two separate killers, each of whom admitted that their evisceration methods were adopted from the film. Just days after its premiere, *Money Train*, itself based in part on real incidents, inspired token-booth thieves to incinerate the clerk inside. High school footballers were maimed and killed lying down on busy highways after viewing *The Program*. *Child's Play* and its first two straight-to-tape sequels hold the record for the sheer number of dead: besides two-year-old Jamie Bulger, stoned to death by a pair of 10-year-old Chucky fans in Liverpool, and 16-year-old Suzanne Capper, burned alive in Manchester by Chucky fans who played lines of the movies' dialogues to her as she was being tortured, there is the dizzying slaughter of 35 Tasmanian vacationers by Martin Bryant, a mental patient "obsessed" with Chucky.

But for sheer inspirational force, and the highest number of captured impulse killers who have directly credited the film, *Natural Born Killers* might be the ne plus ultra of copycat-killing source material. Besides the Edmondson-Darras road trip, there have been killings in Utah, Georgia, Massachusetts, and Texas (where a 14-year-old boy decapitated a 13-year-old girl), all involving children who afterward quoted the film to friends and authorities. In Paris, a pair of young lovers, Florence Rey and Audry Maupin, led the police on a chase that killed five; supposedly, Rey said, "it's fate," à la Woody Harrelson's character Mickey, when caught. Another pair of Parisians, Veronique Herbert and her boyfriend Sebastien Paindavoine, lured a 16-year-old to his stabbing death with promises of sex, a scene right out of Stone's film. Herbert has even named the Stone film in her defense statement.

There are scores of other examples—even *Beavis and Butt-head* has its ghosts, innocent bystanders killed by child-lit fires or child-tossed bowling balls. Hunt-and-kill computer games, which provide ersatz combat training, have also been cited in the Carneal suit. Of course, in each case, the precise psychological role media played is never clear—nor can it be, until we can map a brain like a computer hard drive. In fact, some of what the press has reported about the similarities between particular murders and particular films is flat-out wrong—scores of scenes that never occurred in *Child's Play 2* were said to have been reenacted in the Bulger murder. Still, when a Georgia teen yells out "I'm a natural born killer!" to news cameras after being arrested for killing an elderly man, the tie-in is hard to ignore.

Legally, it may be impossible to prove intent on behalf of a filmmaker or a beyond-a-reasonable-doubt cause-and-effect affiliation between specific movies and specific violence. How do you account for the millions of unaffected consumers? What's equally at issue is the common cultural presupposition that the entertainment media bear no culpability for those who wreak havoc in imitation of it. Movies are movies, homicidal nuts are homicidal nuts, the crimes would occur with or without a movie's sensationalized prodding. So the wisdom goes. But is our relationship with movies so simple, or is there in fact something deeper, darker, going on? Could it be that visual media aren't merely a harmless, ephemeral diversion from reality, but a powerful factor in that reality bearing consequences we haven't foreseen?

Since most of the incidents we're aware of have children at their centers, this may prove to be true. According to University of Michigan professor L. Rowell Huesmann, an expert researcher on the relationship between violent media and violent behavior, "It's been well established that media violence makes kids behave more aggressively. Of course, there's no scientific way to evaluate how media violence may have or may have not caused real violence, but there's definitely a relationship, a 'priming' or 'cuing' of behavior for certain individuals. The reasons are well understood in psychology: even as toddlers, if we see other kids push and hit to get what they want, we imitate it, we begin to learn scripts for that behavior. In addition, there have been studies: you show images of gore to young children, they have a universally negative reaction: their heartbeat goes up, their palms sweat, and so on. You show it to them again and again, and those indications go away. They adapt, they become desensitized."

Dr. Carole Lieberman, a Beverly Hills–based "media psychiatrist," blames parental patterns of consumerism. "There's no question that parents see it happen. The *Ninja Turtles* was a significant sign: everyone could see how specific violent behaviors were derived directly from that show. But they still buy the kids the computer, the violent CD games. It's cognitive dissonance—they know, but they don't want their kids to be left out, to be unarmed."

It seems the entertainment complex knows, too: Last week, MGM announced they'd like to recall every copy of *The Basketball Diaries* from store shelves but can't thanks to a prohibitive rights agreement that lasts until June 30. Even within the Hollywood chambers, the cattle can get spooked: *Money Train* scriptwriter Doug Richardson was voted down for membership in the Academy thanks to the subway-booth torching. "Nobody would say it was because of that incident," Richardson says, "but no one would deny it. So, as a writer, am I supposed to wonder if what I'm doing is drama or pornography?

Science is going to have to get in up to its elbows in this, I think. It's a very complicated issue, and doesn't deserve sound-bite answers. Especially since there's so much suffering."

And the suffering, not of Hollywood filmmakers told they shouldn't make ultraviolent movies but of families with murdered children, may be what the debate should be about. "We could make a great step forward by simply restricting the amount of violence to which children are exposed," Huesmann says. "That's no great constitutional dilemma. I wouldn't be surprised if at this point Oliver Stone came forth and said, 'Yes, the film obviously affects some people in a certain way,' and if he did, that would be a significant first step." (Oliver Stone declined to comment.)

"Every study indicates a relationship," Huesmann concludes. "Here's a not greatly known fact: that the statistical correlation between childhood exposure to violence in media and aggressive behavior is about the same as that between smoking and lung cancer."

Research assistance: Yael Schacher

46

Media Insensitivity to Victims of Violence

Sue Carter

Watching the students who survived the Columbine High School massacre in Littleton, Colo., as they told their stories on television drove home the horror that these youngsters endured. At the same time, the saturation coverage seemed to ratchet broadcast crime coverage to a new level of intense focus on victims and their trauma. Viewers found themselves cast as unwitting voyeurs—witnessing more personal pain than they should be allowed to see.

During the first chaotic day of the incident, most broadcasts featured endlessly repeated closeups of a teenage girl choking out her account of what it was like to be under siege by her peers. Succeeding days offered a relentless succession of children recounting the terrifying details of a tragedy they barely had a chance to assimilate.

While it may be important for the media to report on violence without unduly sanitizing its impact on victims, there were times that the Colorado coverage intruded on what should have been private moments. Insensitive questions from reporters undoubtedly made these youngsters' worst days even more painful. As therapist Janna Malamud Smith wrote on *The New York Times'* Op-Ed page the Sunday after the event, "It's worrisome that these already injured students, apparently seeking comfort and attention, can be exploited for ratings."

The Columbine incident is merely the latest example of the explosion in crime coverage. Yet, it may also be a precursor of a new era of a media focus on victims that threatens to put them at even greater risk of a "second wound"—the additional trauma inflicted by insensitive and intrusive coverage.

Even as the rates of violent crime continue to decline, the percentage of news coverage devoted to it is climbing. According to George Gerbner, Bell

Sue Carter *is an associate professor in the School of Journalism, Michigan State University, East Lansing. Bonnie Bucqueroux of the Victims and the Media Program at the university assisted in the preparation of this article.*

Atlantic Professor of Telecommunications, Temple University, television networks doubled the time devoted to crime coverage between 1992 and 1993. "Moreover, *TV Guide*'s August 13, 1994, survey showed a steep increase in stories of violence, especially in local television news."

In the last three years, studies conducted by the University of Miami and the Project on Media Ownership, a research center affiliated with New York University, have underscored disproportionate crime coverage. The latter research concentrated on Baltimore TV stations and found that nearly 40% of the average 30-minute news program was devoted to crime. An examination of 17,000 local news stories broadcast during a three-month period in 1996 showed that crime is the most commonly reported category, accounting for 20% of local newscasts. Other national surveys indicate that crime occupies one-quarter of the available local news time.

The trend to more crime coverage is repeated at the national level as well. The proliferation of, and competition among, the cable news networks such as CNN, MSNBC, and Fox News, as well as the increase in primetime hours devoted to newsmagazine shows on network TV, add to the shift toward crime coverage as a top category of legitimate news. Literally hundreds of producers are scouring the country looking for victims of violence willing to talk about what happened to them. The ones who show emotion tend to receive the repeat offers, and they may be asked to appear again when a similar incident happens. Even newspapers such as *The New York Times* and *The Chicago Tribune*, which previously shied away from crime coverage, now routinely include them in their pages.

New, too, is increased reporting on the previously "hidden" crimes of domestic violence and offenses against children. "The press also is reporting in detail on sex crimes, once a taboo topic seen darkly if at all," indicates Michael Kirkhorn, who spent 14 years as an editor and columnist for five newspapers. He further notes that victim coverage is now "dramatized," perceived as a means of educating the public about the impact of violence on its victims.

While one may question some actions of the national media, remember that the bulk of news coverage is local. Troubling for victims is many local TV stations and newspapers assigning rookies to crime and breaking news, often as a trial by fire to see if they are tough enough.

The same newspaper that would never send a reporter who knew nothing of football to cover a high school game will assign an untrained reporter to interview a parent who has had a child murdered. A parent who appeared at a Victims and the Media Program presentation at Michigan State University said that an inexperienced reporter appeared at his door shortly after the father learned that his daughter had been murdered by a serial killer. The nervous young man apparently blurted out the first thing he could think of: "I know how you feel—my dog died once." While no pain compares to the loss of his daughter, the father still recoils in anguish as he tells the story.

Coverage of crime brings with it coverage of victims, frequently in dehumanizing ways and with traumatizing results. The irony is that close, intrusive coverage of the victim may be occasionally explained away as an effort to "humanize" crime. In 1994, former KCBS-TV news director John Lippman told Ted Koppel on "Nightline" that his Los Angeles station's blunt and edgy portrayal of crime and its victims was done to "put a human face on violence" in a city where homicide is commonplace.

Surveys of viewer opinion take overall media to task on the issues of trust, ethics, and, most especially, insensitivity and sensationalism. The Roper Center for Public Opinion Research conducted a survey for the Freedom Forum's Newseum in 1997 and found that 82% of those questioned expressed concern about insensitivity to victims' pain. About half of those responding found the news too biased or negative in tone. Broadcast journalists often look to tell the story through the eyes and experiences of the victim, not recognizing that he or she may be retraumatized by recounting the event and the viewer may well wish to be spared the details.

That was the case with the May 4, 1998, Los Angeles freeway suicide fed live to an audience that watched a man set his truck on fire, jump out of the vehicle with his clothes in flames, and then shoot himself with a rifle. Two stations interrupted children's programming to go live. Such a presentation is not without harm to the younger segment of the audience. A 1996 study by Joanne Cantor and Amy Nathanson in the *Journal of Communication* revealed that 37% of kindergarten and elementary school pupils in a random survey reported they had been frightened or upset by a news story on television. Moreover, the older the children got, the more scared they were. Gerbner gave a name to the phenomenon, labeling it the "mean-world syndrome." The notion is that the world, seen through the prism of TV, looks awful and harsh, and one tends to accept the view as reality—all the more so if one is young.

Far more debilitating to the victim is the personal, overstated crime reporting on local TV. The refrain that emerges from individual victims and victim groups is that invasive, in-your-face reporting revictimizes them because it underscores one of the cruelties of crime—loss of control. During a violent crime, victims lose the ability to direct their circumstances, often with devastating consequences. The local television reporter who arrives on scene, or later at the house, and thrusts forward a microphone while asking, "How do you feel?" takes away any hope of the victim's control of the interview and can even trigger post-traumatic stress disorder. PTSD is set up by a horrifying or terrible initial event. The disorder can bring with it fear, withdrawal, and sleeplessness. To limit objectionable press coverage, the National Victim Center has a list of "press no-nos" that puts off limits the coverage of funerals, videotaping and airing of body bags, and inappropriate images of victims' grief. Children are absolutely out of bounds.

A 1998 research project involving local television newsrooms in three different Michigan markets offers an interesting look at the process broadcast journalists engage in when covering crime and victims of violence. The year-long study I conducted was funded by the Poynter Institute for Media Studies in St. Petersburg, Fla. The research was based on a participant-observation look at three television stations, and several conclusions with respect to local coverage of victims of violence emerged from it.

First, there is general awareness in the newsroom by managers and reporters of public distaste for graphic and insensitive coverage, but there are no firm standards in place to guide coverage. Codes, standards, and rules that do operate tend to be applied *ad hoc*, or instituted after a story has gone awry, rather than before.

Beyond that, the temptation of the technology is substantial. Because the capability of "going live" is readily available, it is used frequently, and live shots often lead the newscasts, even if the crime reporting and victim coverage is well after the fact.

Crime and victim coverage tends to be driven by economics. Because crime is inexpensive to cover, there are more stories about crime and its victims than there are about the economy, politics, or education. The latter stories often require a greater investment of time on the part of the reporter, videographer, and producer.

In a medium governed by images of victims of crime and crime itself, coverage leans toward the shocking and can be visually grabbing. The industry practice is to "shoot tight" and capture everything on video. Then, in a display of circular logic, the prevailing view by local TV newsrooms is to use the graphic videotape "because it's there."

Competition among stations for viewers—who translate into rating points—affects the way in which victims are covered. Television stations as a group dislike being beaten by competitors to a story, and that includes all aspects of story coverage. At one station, a witness' particularly gruesome description of a victim's mutilation was aired "because the other station had it." The implication was that the other station would use it, so, not to be outdone, a reporter at the second station admitted, she had included the sound bite in her report.

■ EFFORTS TO MAKE CHANGES

In addition to guidelines set by the National Victim Center, there are other codes and standards that need to remain on local television reporters' radar scope. The Radio-Television News Directors Association has a Code of Ethics that calls upon broadcasters to reject sensationalism and to respect "the dignity, privacy, and well-being of people with whom they deal." Similar language from the Society of Professional Journalists admonishes the media "not to pander to morbid curiosity about details of vice and crime."

Occasionally, individual newsrooms will have their own guidelines on crime and victim coverage. At KEZI-TV in Eugene, Ore., it violates station policy to air tape of body bags or corpses, shove cameras into the faces of grieving survivors, or cover trials unless invited. KVUE-TV in Austin, Tex., has attempted to include some reflection in its coverage of crime and victims by establishing such threshold questions as: "Is there an immediate threat to public safety?" and "Is there a threat to children?"

These proscriptions regarding crime coverage at KVUE, though, hardly mirror what Americans are seeing in their local TV newscasts. Four-fifths of viewers have concern about reporters' lack of sensitivity. This audience represents a truly silent majority.

If viewers *are* concerned about excessive crime coverage and the effects of intrusive reporting on victims, there are ways to register displeasure, beginning with the simple and definitive step of not watching the television news program. More realistic and of greater impact is letting one's opinion be known. The old saw is that one letter represents 10 viewers. The reverbations of a pointed, well-written letter to the news director and the general manager, with copies to leading advertisers, can be substantial. While news is a service, it is not a public service. It is a commercial business and one that relies on viewer goodwill.

Savvy TV news viewing is possible. In a breaking news story that is unfolding before the audience, there is always the possibility of grim or inappropriate victim coverage. Live shots leave virtually no room for editorial control. It truly is "what you see is what you get." Live reporting puts the onus of editorship on the viewer, rather than the journalist. What if there had been a second bomb in the Murrah Building in Oklahoma City, as originally reported? What if O.J. Simpson had pulled the trigger while in the white Bronco? Could local TV news crews have dropped their signals in time and eliminated images? It is highly unlikely. In the case of children and breaking news, the responsibility is even greater for parents and teachers (remember the *Challenger* explosion?) to move quickly to cut the broadcast and address the questions children have.

The issue, though, is not to recount horror stories, but to propose solutions. The Victims and the Media Program at Michigan State University, as well as similar programs that spring up nationwide, not only attempt to educate journalism students and professionals about how to report better on victims, but to educate readers and viewers about the impact the stories have on victims—and on reporters.

The Victims and the Media Program employs the terms Act I, Act II, and Act III stories to talk about the different kinds of crime coverage. Act I stories are the breaking-news assignments that focus on gathering facts and impressions under immediate deadline, where victims can find themselves overwhelmed literally before they have had a chance to think.

Act II stories are features that occur later, typically follow-up or anniversary coverage. The reporter is not under immediate deadline, so there is more flexibility concerning opportunities for victims to set terms. Nevertheless, recounting past trauma takes a toll.

Act III stories attempt to put the incident or issue into a broader economic, sociological, historical, or cultural context. These pieces are less

TIPS FOR VIEWERS

The following list, prepared by the Victims and the Media Program at Michigan State University, is a set of situations that ought to raise red flags for viewers and readers. They identify behaviors that do not treat victims with sensitivity or fairness. Viewers and/or readers who object to such coverage can contact their local newspaper's managing editor or publisher; TV station's news director or general manager; the affiliated network; or advertisers in the newspaper or on the newscast.

An ambush or surprise interview may make sense for investigative reporting or when challenging con artists, but it has no place in victim coverage. If your local TV station shows victims slamming the door in the reporter's face too often, something is wrong with the coverage.

Too close for comfort. Telephoto lenses for video and still cameras can be used to violate victims' expected zone of privacy without their knowing how intrusive the shot will be. Let your local broadcasters or newspaper know if they go too far.

If it were your child . . . Youngsters who are victimized deserve to be heard without being patronized or exploited. The best standard is to judge the story as if it were your child being interviewed.

The blur of shock and trauma. We should wince—and protest—when it is clear that the victim being interviewed is too stunned to be an accurate reporter of events. Many victims in that condition do not even remember being interviewed.

The cliché, such as a gurney being lifted into the back of the ambulance or a casket being lowered into the ground. Challenge journalists to create fresh images to tell the story.

Victims as teasers. Many victims report feeling blindsided when TV stations use lurid footage as promos for hours prior to the newscast.

The five-second sound bite. Victims feel that they are the best experts on their own victimization. Many resent being reduced to a five-second sound bite, after which the story moves to focus on the perpetrator or interviews with "experts."

Not notifying victims. News organizations should notify victims when follow-up or anniversary stories dealing directly with them are scheduled for print or broadcast. Many victims report feeling violated and traumatized when such an article or report appears, as it often brings back painful memories. A phone call in advance helps.

common because they require a substantial commitment of journalistic resources, and they are best described as highly polished magazine-type pieces. This kind of coverage can offer victims the best opportunity to tell their stories in depth, but they also risk seeing themselves used as a prop to illustrate larger themes.

Perhaps the sole good news for victims in this changing media reality is that expanded news coverage of crime can provide victims with increased opportunities to tell their own stories. The only way, however, that this can be an empowering and therapeutic experience is when victims are assured that they can speak on their own terms. The good news for readers and viewers is that they can have an impact on coverage, registering concerns over what they see. The news for journalists is that we're watching—perhaps closer than they think.

47

The Least Among Us: Children of Substance-Abusing Parents

Joseph A. Califano Jr.

Consider the following for a measure of national self-indulgence in the midst of the longest and greatest economic boom in our history. We Americans spend more on cosmetic surgery, hairpieces and make-up *for men* than we do on child welfare services for battered and neglected children of substance-abusing parents.

A tornado of drug and alcohol abuse and addiction is tearing through the nation's child welfare and family court systems, leaving in its path the wreckage of abused and neglected children, turning social welfare agencies and courts on their heads and uprooting the traditional disposition to keep children with their natural parents.

There is no safe haven for these abused and neglected children of drug- and alcohol-abusing parents. They are the most vulnerable and endangered individuals in America. That is the grim conclusion of an exhaustive two-year analysis by The National Center on Addiction and Substance Abuse at Columbia University.

Parental alcohol and drug abuse and addiction have pushed the nation's system of child welfare to the brink of collapse. From 1986 to 1997, the number of abused and neglected children in America has soared from 1.4 million to some 3 million, a stunning 114.3 percent jump, more than eight times faster than the 13.9 percent increase in the overall children's population. The number of *reported* abused and neglected children who have been killed has climbed from 798 to 1985 to 1,185 in 1996; the U.S. Advisory Board on Child Abuse and Neglect sets the *actual* number much higher, at 2,000, a rate of more than five deaths a day.

Alcohol, crack cocaine, methamphetamine, heroin and marijuana are fueling this population explosion of battered and neglected children. Children whose parents abuse drugs and alcohol are almost three times likelier to be

Joseph A. Califano Jr. is president of The National Center on Addiction and Substance Abuse at Columbia University in New York City. He was U.S. Secretary of Health, Education and Welfare from 1977 to 1979.

Reprinted with permission by *America* magazine, April 24, 1999, 180(14) 10–12.

physically or sexually assaulted and more than four times likelier to be neglected than children of parents who are not substance abusers. The parent who abuses drugs and alcohol is often a child who was abused by alcohol- and drug-abusing parents.

Eighty percent of professionals surveyed by CASA said that substance abuse causes or exacerbates most of the cases of child abuse and neglect they face. Nine of 10 professionals cite alcohol alone or in combination with illegal or prescription drugs as the leading substance of abuse in child abuse and neglect; 45.8 percent cite crack cocaine as the leading illegal substance of abuse: 20.5 percent cite marijuana (which can hardly be considered a benign drug in this situation).

Parental substance abuse and addiction is the chief culprit in at least 70 percent—and perhaps 90 percent—of all child welfare spending—some $10 billion of the $14 billion that Federal, state and local governments spent simply to maintain child welfare systems in 1998. This $10 billion does not include the costs of health care to abused and neglected children, operating law enforcement and judicial systems consumed with this problem, treating developmental problems, providing special education or lost productivity. Nor does it include the costs attributable to child abuse and neglect that are privately incurred. These costs easily add another $10 billion to the price of child abuse and neglect.

The human costs are incalculable: broken families; children who are malnourished; babies who are neglected, beaten and sometimes killed by alcohol- and crack-addicted parents; eight-year-olds sent out to steal or buy drugs for addicted parents; sick children wallowing in unsanitary conditions; child victims of sodomy, rape and incest; children in such agony and despair that they themselves resort to drugs or alcohol for relief.

Alcohol and drugs have blown away the topsoil of family life and reshaped the landscape of child abuse and neglect in America. Parents addicted to drugs and alcohol are clever at hiding their addiction and are often more concerned about losing their access to drugs and being punished than about losing custody of their children.

■ *MOTIVATION*

For some parents, holding onto their children can provide the motivation to seek treatment. But for many the most insidious aspect of substance abuse and addiction is their power to destroy the natural parental instinct to love and care for their children. Eighty-six percent of professionals surveyed cited lack of motivation as the top barrier to getting such parents into treatment. As Alan Leshner, director of the National Institute on Drug Abuse, has observed, the addicted parent sometimes sees the child as an obstacle to getting drugs.

Parental drug and alcohol abuse and addiction have overwhelmed the child welfare system. By 1997 some caseworkers were responsible for 50 cases of child maltreatment at any one time and judges were handling as many as 50 cases a day, giving them less than 10 minutes in an uninterrupted eight-hour day to assess the testimony of parents, social workers, law enforcement officers and others in determining a child's fate.

Child welfare agencies have been forced to allocate more time to investigations, gathering evidence of neglect and abuse of children by alcohol- and drug-involved parents. This shift in focus has changed the way parents and children see caseworkers and the way these caseworkers view themselves. This shift also threatens to criminalize a process that should be driven by treatment, health care and compassion for both parent and child. The frantic response of many in Congress and the Clinton Administration is to add felonies to the Federal criminal code and throw more parents in prison—actions likely to do more harm than good for the children of these parents, who need stable and secure homes.

Few caseworkers and judges who make decisions about these children have been tutored in substance abuse and addiction. There are no national estimates of the gap between those parents who need treatment and those who receive it, but Federal Government surveys show that two-thirds of all individuals who need treatment do not get it. There is nothing to suggest that these substance-abusing parents fare any better than the general population.

As the role of substance abuse has increased, the age of the victimized children has gone down. Today most cases of abuse and neglect by substance-abusing parents involve children under five. Alcohol use and binge drinking during pregnancy are up, with at least 636,000 expectant mothers drinking and 137,000 drinking heavily. Some 500,000 babies born each year have been exposed in their mother's womb to cocaine and other illicit drugs (and usually alcohol and tobacco as well). Each year some 20,000 infants are abandoned at birth or kept at hospitals to protect them from substance-abusing parents. The proportion of children whom caseworkers place in foster care at birth jumped 44 percent from the 1983–86 period to the 1990–94 period.

Drug and alcohol abuse has thrown into doubt a fundamental tenet of child welfare workers: the commitment to keep the child with his or her natural parents. While terminating parental rights has long been viewed as a failure, alcohol, crack cocaine and other forms of drug abuse have challenged this time-honored precept.

There is an irreconcilable clash between the rapidly ticking clock of physical, intellectual, emotional and spiritual development for the abused and neglected child and the slow-motion clock of recovery for the parent addicted to alcohol or drugs. For the cognitive development of young children, weeks are windows of opportunity that can never be reopened. For the parent, recovery from drug or alcohol addiction takes time—and relapse, especially during initial periods of recovery, is common.

Bluntly put, the time that parents need to conquer their substance abuse and addiction can pose a serious threat to their children who may suffer permanent damage during this phase of rapid development. Little children cannot wait; they need safe and stable homes and nurturing adults *now* in order to set the stage for a healthy and productive life.

The cruelest dimension of this tragedy for children abused by parents using drugs and alcohol is this: Even when parental rights are terminated in a timely way for such parents who refuse to enter treatment or who fail to recover, in our self-indulgent society there is no assurance of a safe haven for the children. There are not nearly enough adoptive homes. Being in foster care, while far better than being abused, rarely offers the lasting and secure nurturing for full cognitive development—and appropriate foster care is also in short supply. More caring, responsible adults need to step forward to care for the least among us, children of substance-abusing parents.

Child welfare systems and practices need a complete overhaul. Social service providers, from agency directors to frontline child welfare workers, judges, court clerks, masters, lawyers, and health and social service staffs need intensive training in the nature and detection of substance abuse and what to do when they spot it. In all investigations of child abuse and neglect, parents should be screened and assessed for substance abuse. Caseworkers and judges should move rapidly to place children for adoption when parents refuse treatment or fail to respond to it. We need to increase greatly the incentives for foster care and adoption and the number of judges and caseworkers.

Comprehensive treatment that is timely and appropriate, especially for substance-abusing mothers, is essential to prevent further child abuse and neglect. Treatment must be part of a concentrated course that would include mental health services and physical health care; literacy, job and parenting skills training; as well as socialization, employment and drug-free housing. Since most fathers have walked out on their responsibilities, such treatment must be attentive to the fact that most of these parents are women. Where the only hope for reconstituting the natural family for the abused child rests in comprehensive treatment for the parent, it is an inexcusable and vicious Catch-22 situation not to make such treatment available.

Of course, this all costs money. Can we afford to do these things? In the most affluent nation in the history of the world, the answer is a loud and clear yes. Failure to protect these children and provide treatment for their parents who fall prey to drugs and alcohol is more likely than any other shortcoming of survival-of-the-fittest capitalism to bring the harsh judgment of God and history upon us.

In recent years, Pope John Paul II has repeatedly reminded capitalist nations to soften the sharp edges that cut up the least among them. What better way to heed that admonition than to give the needs of these parents and their children first call on the burgeoning Federal budget surplus and the money that the states are picking up from the tobacco settlement.

48

Hidden Bruises

Mubarak Dahir

Young and idealistic, Maria moved from the Southwest to San Francisco in 1990, intent on exploring her sexual identity and independence. It wasn't long before she was being wooed by a worldly woman 15 years her senior. The suitor introduced Maria to a new world filled with lesbian politics and potlucks, close-knit friendships based on feminism and sobriety, and the intriguing and exciting world of lesbian leather fetish.

Weeks after meeting, Maria and her new love moved in together. Soon after, however, what Maria had once read as attentiveness turned to obsessive jealousy. Her partner stalked her. If Maria spoke to other women, she was grabbed by the arm and dragged home, where fights punctuated by kicking, punching, slapping, hair pulling, and tackling often left Maria's body and spirit bruised. After the beatings, however, Maria's partner turned rueful, frequently buying airplane tickets so that they could visit Maria's family, something Maria longed for but couldn't manage on a $7-per-hour job.

"I was constantly afraid, hurting both physically and emotionally," Maria says now. "And yet, for a long time, I was confused, taken in by this woman's charm." Eventually, Maria become a prisoner in her own home and was even followed from room to room by trained attack dogs. One night, after discovering Maria at 3 A.M. trying to escape, Maria's partner beat her and raped her.

Activists say stories like Maria's are not uncommon. "Domestic violence is a serious health crisis in the lesbian, gay, bisexual, and transgendered communities," says Jennifer Rakowski, director of client and advocacy services at the San Francisco–based Community United Against Violence.

Statistics back Rakowski up. According to "Lesbian, Gay, Transgender, and Bisexual Domestic Violence in 1998: A Report of the National Coalition of Anti-Violence Programs," the third annual such survey, released October 5, there were 2,574 such reported cases in 1998, including two homicides. Although little research has been done on domestic violence among gays and

Mubarak Dahir is a freelance writer based in New York City.

Reprinted with permission by *The Advocate*, November, 23, 1999, Issue 799, pp. 24–29.

lesbians, most experts agree that the level equals that among heterosexuals, with anywhere from 25% to 33% of couples experiencing some form of abuse.

But despite its prevalence, gay domestic violence remains little noticed both inside and outside the gay community. While bias crime against gay men and lesbians has attracted national attention in the past year, in large part because of the murder of University of Wyoming student Matthew Shepard, domestic violence continues to remain invisible. Yet in some places the numbers for the two types of crimes are virtually the same. In New York City, fully half of the incidents of violence against gays and lesbians reported to the Gay and Lesbian Anti-Violence Project are domestic abuse cases. "That's staggering, considering we started as an organization intent on chronicling bias crimes," says Diane Dolan-Soto, domestic violence program coordinator for the project.

Moreover, experts caution that the reported figures are a mere fraction of actual abuse cases. Dolan-Soto says that although the October report gives a qualitative feel for the problem, "the numbers are starkly low. They don't give a complete picture." For starters, the report culls statistics from just ten cities.

There are host a of reasons why gay and lesbians shy away from reporting domestic violence, says Susan Holt, program manager for the Stop Partner Abuse and Domestic Violence Program of the Los Angeles Gay and Lesbian Center. As well as reasons common in abusive heterosexual relationships—such as fear of reprisal, shame, and repentance by the batterer—an additional series of hurdles and stigmas stretch before gay and lesbian victims, she and other experts say.

One of the biggest barriers to seeking help is the victim's fear of being outed. Another is the role HIV can play in the abuse. According to this year's survey, the physically disabled—including HIV-positive gay men—may be up to ten times more susceptible to domestic violence. "Some abusers threaten to withhold medications from sick partners," explains Peter Sawires, coordinator of the Family Violence Prevention Fund's National Health Resource Center on Domestic Violence, a federally funded advocacy group. "There are even cases of the batterer threatening to infect the victim."

And chances are, even if a gay or lesbian victim looks for help, there may be nowhere to turn, even in cities with large gay populations, advocates say. "There is a dismal lack of resources sensitive to gays and lesbians," says Dolan-Soto. "Most victims will be forced to go through mainstream service providers." She says that often means having to keep their sexual orientation secret or risk rejection. In New York City, she reports, only three mainstream service providers have been consistently sensitive to lesbians, and there is only one shelter for abuse victims that's willing and able to serve gay men and transgendered people. "We're nearly 30 years behind the battered women's movement," Dolan-Soto says.

Maria's case is typical. When she sought help after a year of abuse, Maria first turned to an organization for Latina victims of domestic violence, hoping the group would understand her cultural needs. "But I was told flat out they didn't have services for 'people like me,'" Maria says, still angry.

And because mainstream organizations are predicated on the heterosexual model—where 95% of batterers are men—abused gay men often have only homeless shelters for refuge and absolutely nowhere to turn for social services, notes Dolan-Soto. The assumption of heterosexuality also frequently influences how the police and courts respond to same-sex domestic violence, says Rakowski. "Because providers are so used to the female-as-the-victim, male-as-the-batterer model, there is a lot of mentality that in same-sex cases it's a fight between equals."

Maria says that while she and friends called the police on at least two occasions, her batterer was never arrested. "The police viewed it as a catfight between two lesbians, not a case of domestic violence," she observes.

With men, there is often the added social stigma about not being able to defend oneself. That was exacerbated for Ben, a Pennsylvania man, when seeking protection against his violent lover. At 6 feet 2 inches and 230 pounds, Ben confesses, "I was reluctant to go to the authorities and admit I got beat up" by a man 5 feet 10 inches and 200 pounds. "Part of it was ego," he says, "and part of it was wondering whether I'd be believed."

After nine years of intermittent violence, exacerbated by his lover's bouts of drunkenness, Ben finally sought legal protection after his lover threatened to kill him, after having thrown him to the floor and choked him. However, the police told Ben that state laws did not cover same-sex domestic violence cases. Ben's only legal alternative was to file an assault charge.

But the police advised against it. Ben says the officer told him, "The courts aren't going to be sympathetic to someone in your situation"—meaning someone gay. The officer added, "They'll throw your case out."

Ben ended up hiring a lawyer who brokered an end to the relationship only after threatening to expose the partner's history of violence to his employer—information with which the employer would be able to discern his sexual orientation. "I hated to do it that way," Ben laments, "but I felt I had no choice."

Indifference among heterosexuals is matched by continuing denial among gays and lesbians, advocates add. "Sometimes gays and lesbians are discouraged from reporting domestic violence because the community fears it will be bad public relations," says Sawires. "There's a tangible taboo against examining any kind of problem in gay and lesbian relationships, out of the real fear that someone like [evangelist] Jerry Falwell will grab on to it and distort it as another reason gay and lesbian relationships aren't healthy."

Maria says she felt "abandoned" by her lesbian friends while struggling against the violence in her relationship. "Everyone was in denial," including herself, she says, "because as lesbian feminists we wouldn't allow ourselves to admit some of us weren't treating each other any better than the heterosexist society. There was no empathy for that."

It took Maria three escape attempts, followed by months of hiding out with friends and family, before she finally broke free. "But even now," she says, "sometimes I'm still afraid to walk the streets alone."

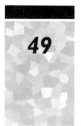

49

Elder Abuse and Neglect

Gary C. Cyphers

■ NEGLECT AND ABANDONMENT

Family members abandoned Marilyn, an 86-year-old bedridden woman, when they quickly left town after not paying the rent for three months. They left food and water, but no one knew Marilyn was still there. By the time workers came to clean the apartment, she was dead.

■ FINANCIAL EXPLOITATION

Katherine, age 80, lived alone and was somewhat confused but was able to perform activities of daily living adequately. A recent fall, though, left her physically weakened and more confused. Katherine went to live with a grandson who only sporadically was employed. Once Katherine was in his home, her grandson allowed her no contact with other family members. She lost control of her checkbook and power of attorney was given to the grandson. Katherine's valuables disappeared and most household expenses were financed by Katherine's funds. Eventually, another family member came with the police to remove Katherine from the home. Although she had wanted to get out of the situation and was upset about the misuse of her money by her grandson, she felt helpless to voice any concern or to take any action.

■ SELF-NEGLECT

Doris is legally blind and has congestive heart failure that makes activities of daily living nearly impossible. Although she is alert and at times "sharp as a tack," her judgment is increasingly poor, which threatens her health and safety.

Gary C. Cyphers is director of APHSA's Human Service Research and Information Center.

Doris' home is cluttered and filled with debris due to her hoarding, making it unsanitary and almost impossible for her to move around. An earlier apartment had been condemned because of this, which is why Adult Protective Services (APS) first became involved. Doris has no family support and is determined to remain in her current home. APS offered help from a companion aide, but Doris refused. When the APS worker visited, he determined that Doris had lost both electric and water utilities, and was becoming dehydrated and very disoriented. Medication for the congestive heart failure had not been taken in several days.

▨ PHYSICAL ABUSE

Lillian is 87 years old with multiple medical problems and an income that barely pays the bills. She has cared for her 55-year-old chronically schizophrenic daughter her whole life, but her daughter has refused to take her medication and has become increasingly agitated. A neighbor overheard the daughter physically threatening her mother and an APS worker visited the home. The worker observed a bruise but Lillian told her it was due to an accident and refused to elaborate. The worker arranged for a personal care aide, who subsequently observed a series of bruises and lacerations while bathing Lillian. When the APS worker was summoned, Lillian confided that her daughter had been hitting her and, for the first time, she feared for her life.

The plight of Marilyn, Katherine, Doris, and Lillian is in stark contrast to our optimistic view of the elderly. America's burgeoning elder population has affected every segment of the social, political, and economic landscape. Public debate of the issues surrounding the special needs of the approximately 44 million persons in this country age 60 years and over has heightened national awareness and concern. As noted in articles throughout this issue of POLICY & PRACTICE, public policies relating to such issues as affordable long-term care and quality of life are changing to meet the unique needs of the aging population.

Yet, as the public looks toward improving the lives of the elderly, abuse and neglect of elders living in their own homes have gone largely unidentified and unnoticed. The National Elder Abuse Incidence Study has shed new light on this significant problem with the finding that almost one-half million elderly persons in domestic settings were abused or neglected during 1996.

Congress directed and funded the National Elder Abuse Incidence Study as part of the 1992 Family Violence Prevention and Service Act, and it was jointly conducted by the National Center on Elder Abuse at APHSA and its research partner, Westat. The study estimates the incidence, or new occurrences, of elder abuse and neglect in domestic settings (i.e., not in institutions like hospitals or nursing homes) among persons age 60 and older in 1996. The incidence of self-neglect is also estimated.

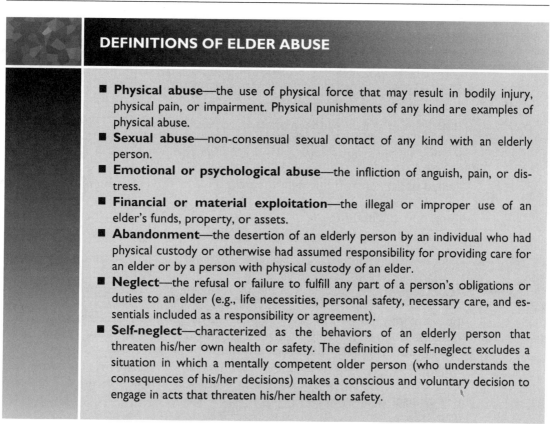

DEFINITIONS OF ELDER ABUSE

- **Physical abuse**—the use of physical force that may result in bodily injury, physical pain, or impairment. Physical punishments of any kind are examples of physical abuse.
- **Sexual abuse**—non-consensual sexual contact of any kind with an elderly person.
- **Emotional or psychological abuse**—the infliction of anguish, pain, or distress.
- **Financial or material exploitation**—the illegal or improper use of an elder's funds, property, or assets.
- **Abandonment**—the desertion of an elderly person by an individual who had physical custody or otherwise had assumed responsibility for providing care for an elder or by a person with physical custody of an elder.
- **Neglect**—the refusal or failure to fulfill any part of a person's obligations or duties to an elder (e.g., life necessities, personal safety, necessary care, and essentials included as a responsibility or agreement).
- **Self-neglect**—characterized as the behaviors of an elderly person that threaten his/her own health or safety. The definition of self-neglect excludes a situation in which a mentally competent older person (who understands the consequences of his/her decisions) makes a conscious and voluntary decision to engage in acts that threaten his/her health or safety.

▪ *STUDY METHOD*

The National Elder Abuse Incidence Study (NEAIS) used a nationally representative sample of 20 countries in 15 states and collected data from two sources in each county: reports from the local Adult Protective Services (APS) agency responsible for receiving and investigating reports in each county, and reports from approximately 1,100 "sentinels"—specially trained individuals in a variety of community agencies having frequent contract with the elderly. These 248 agencies included law enforcement (sheriffs' and municipal police departments), hospitals and public health departments, elder care providers (adult day care and senior centers, and home health care agencies), and financial institutions. The sentinel approach to collecting data is an alternative to more costly general population surveys and has been used successfully in three National Incidence Studies of Child Abuse for over 20 years. The approach is based on the belief that officially reported cases of abuse represent only a small proportion of actual episodes of abuse in the community—or the tip of the iceberg.

Historically, a major impediment to collecting uniform data on elder maltreatment nationally has been a lack of comparability of definitions of abuse and neglect among states and even among elder abuse experts. Accordingly, the first task of NEAIS was to develop standardized definitions of elder maltreatment, thus ensuring greater comparability and reliability of results.

Both APS caseworkers and sentinel agency staff were trained carefully to complete the data collection forms. Data were collected during a two-month period in each county in 1996, using staggered reporting periods to account for any seasonal variations and multiplying the results by six to annualize data. The samples of agencies and sentinels participating in the NEAIS were selected using scientific probability sampling methods to obtain a nationally representative sample. It is possible, therefore, to make valid projections from the data to calculate national estimates of the numbers of elderly who have been abused and neglected and to describe their characteristics.

▓ STUDY FINDINGS

Approximately 450,000 elderly persons, age 60 and over, were abused and neglected in domestic settings during 1996.[1] Of this number, only 71,000, or 16 percent, were reported to and substantiated by APS agencies—over five times as many new incidents of abuse and neglect (379,000) went unreported. When elderly persons who experienced only self-neglect are added, the number increases to approximately 551,000 in 1996.

Frequency of Types of Abuse

Almost half (49 percent) of the 236,500 reports of abuse, neglect, and self-neglect to APS agencies were substantiated after investigation, while 39 percent were unsubstantiated,[2] and 12 percent were still under investigation or had other outcomes. For the over 115,000 APS-substantiated reports in 1996, the largest category was self-neglect (44,168 or 38 percent). The remaining 62 percent of substantiated–APS reports (70,942) dealt with incidents in which elders were maltreated by others (called perpetrators). These nearly 71,000 elders experienced 103,000 different types of abuse and neglect[3]:

---

[1] For the most accurate estimate of the national incidence of elder abuse and neglect, researchers added reports submitted to and substantiated by APS agencies and reports made by sentinels and assumed to be substantiated.

[2] An APS agency determination of nonsubstantiation of a report of suspected abuse or neglect does not conclusively mean that abuse or neglect did not happen. Rather, an unsubstantiated report can mean that the level of proof required by that state was not sufficiently met, despite indications that abuse or neglect may have occurred.

[3] Percentages total more than 100 percent because more than one substantiated type of abuse often was reported for an incident.

- Half (49.9 percent) were neglected.
- Over one-third (35 percent) were emotionally abused.
- Almost one-third (30 percent) were financially exploited.
- One-quarter (26 percent) were physically abused.
- One out of 25 (4 percent) was abandoned.

Who Is Abused and Neglected?

Victims reported to APS have characteristics resembling those of victims identified by sentinel agencies for many categories of abuse and neglect. Women are disproportionately victims. In APS reports, women represent 60–76 percent of those subjected to all forms of abuse and neglect except abandonment, even though, overall, women represent only 58 percent of the elderly population. The greatest disparity between men and women occurred in reported rates of emotional or psychological abuse, according to APS data, with three-fourths of the victims being women. In sentinel reports, 67–92 percent of those reported as abused were women, depending on the type of abuse. According to sentinel reports, the greatest disparity between men and women was in the category of financial abuse, in which 92 percent of the victims were women.

Overall, our oldest elders (age 80 and over) were abused and neglected at rates two to three times their proportion of the elderly population (19 percent). Persons age 80 and over accounted for 52 percent of neglect victims in APS reports and 60 percent in sentinel reports. APS reports also suggest that this older group was disproportionately subjected to financial/material abuse (48 percent), physical abuse (44 percent), and emotional/psychological abuse (41 percent).

The APS and sentinel reports differ with regard to the race of abuse and neglect victims. African American elders were overrepresented in several types of abuse and neglect substantiated by APS. Despite representing 8 percent of all elders in 1996, African American elders were the victims in 17 percent of the incidents of neglect, 15 percent of financial exploitation, and 14 percent of emotional abuse substantiated by APS. Only small proportions of Hispanics and other minorities are represented in most categories of abuse reported to APS, generally less than 3 percent altogether. Sentinel data show that of those subjected to any form of abuse, fewer than 10 percent were minorities (including African Americans, Hispanics, Asian Americans, Pacific Islanders, and others).

Elders who are unable to take care of themselves were more likely to suffer from abuse. Three-quarters (77 percent) of the elderly in APS-substantiated incidents of abuse and over half (52 percent) of sentinel reports were unable or somewhat unable to take care of themselves. In comparison, a 1997 U.S. Census Bureau report estimates that only 14 percent of the elderly population as a whole have difficulties with one or more activities of daily

IF YOU SUSPECT ELDER ABUSE

If you suspect that elder abuse or neglect has occurred or is occurring to an older person whom you know, report your suspicion to the local Adult Protective Services (APS) agency. You can find the telephone number for the APS office by checking the blue government section of your phone book or by calling directory assistance and asking for the Department of Social Services or Agency on Aging. It is essential to call the office with jurisdiction over the geographical area where the elder lives.

It is also important to note that all but six or seven states have mandatory reporting requirements for a wide variety of persons, including social workers, physicians, nurses, police officers, and dentists and dental hygienists. For specific mandatory reporting requirements in your state, check with the local APS or Agency or Aging.

living. About 60 percent of elder abuse victims reported by APS have some degree of confusion, compared with the estimated 10 percent of the national elderly population suffering from some form of dementia. Finally, 44 percent of the APS-substantiated and 47 percent of sentinel-reported abused elders exhibited depression at some level, compared to the estimated 15 percent of the elders nationally who are depressed at any one time.

Elderly self-neglect also is a serious problem, with about 139,000 new unduplicated APS and sentinel reports in 1996. (Some of those described as self-neglecting were also subjected to other forms of abuse.) Women and the oldest elderly are more likely to self-neglect. Approximately two-thirds (65 percent) of self-neglecting elders reported to APS were women, who comprised only 58 percent of the elderly population. In addition, 54 percent were 80 years or older, while comprising only 19 percent of the population. An additional 20 percent were ages 75–79. The older an elderly person becomes, the more likely it is that she or he will be self-neglecting. Not surprisingly, most victims of self-neglect are unable to care for themselves (93 percent) or are confused (75 percent); many are depressed (75 percent).

Who Reports Abuse?

A wide variety of persons reported substantiated cases of domestic elder abuse and neglect to APS. Family members are the most frequent reporters (20 percent). Other categories of reporters include:

- Hospital personnel (17 percent)
- Police and sheriffs (11 percent)
- In-home service providers (10 percent)
- Friends and neighbors (9 percent)
- Victims themselves (9 percent)
- Health care providers (8 percent)
- Out-of-home service providers (5 percent)
- All others (21 percent)

In cases of self-neglect, the most frequent reporters to APS are hospitals (20 percent), friends and neighbors (19 percent), in-home service providers (12 percent), police/sheriffs (12 percent), health care providers (12 percent), out-of-home service providers, (8 percent), family members (6 percent), and all others (28 percent).

Who Perpetrates Abuse and Neglect?

Across all categories of abuse and neglect, the distribution of perpetrators by gender is almost equal, according to reports received by APS. This even distribution, however, masks gender differences by type of abuse and neglect. Women were the cause of a higher proportion of neglect (52 percent versus 48 percent by men) and neglect is the most frequent type of maltreatment caused by perpetrators (49 percent). For all other categories of abuse reported to APS, men outnumbered women as perpetrators by at least 3 to 2. Among reports by sentinels, male perpetrators outnumbered female perpetrators by 1.8 to 1. This preponderance of abuse by men is significant both in reports obtained from APS and in sentinel data.

According to both APS and sentinels, most perpetrators were younger than their victims. According to information supplied by APS, 65 percent of total perpetrators were under age 60; similar to the percentage of perpetrators under age 60 identified by sentinels. Of course, even perpetrators who are older than 60 may still be younger than the persons they abuse. Among reports to APS, the relative "youth" of perpetrators of financial abuse is particularly striking compared to other types of abuse, with 45 percent 40 years of age or younger and another 40 percent between 41–59 years old.

Relatives or spouses of the victims commit most domestic elder abuse according to APS and sentinels. Approximately 90 percent of alleged abusers were related to victims. APS data suggest that adult children is the largest category of abusers, across all forms of abuse, with proportions ranging from 43 percent for cases of neglect to nearly 80 percent for abandonment. Adult children also account for the largest category of alleged abusers in sentinel reports (31 percent). Since family members are frequently the primary caregivers for elderly relatives in domestic settings, this finding is not surprising.

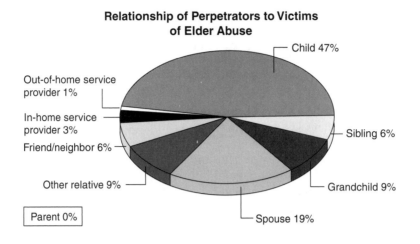

Relationship of Perpetrators to Victims of Elder Abuse

Child 47%

Out-of-home service provider 1%

In-home service provider 3%

Friend/neighbor 6%

Other relative 9%

Parent 0%

Sibling 6%

Grandchild 9%

Spouse 19%

■ IMPLICATIONS

The findings of the NEAIS raise several important issues for policy develop-ment, practice, and training in addressing elder abuse, neglect, and self-neglect. Study findings can provide a basis for designing public policies and practices, which are programmatically responsive, fiscally sound, and com-passionate. The findings can also assist practitioners, caregivers, social re-searchers, and others in identifying new approaches to reduce and prevent abuse, neglect, and self-neglect of the elderly. Because states and localities historically have had responsibility for elder abuse reporting, investigation, intervention, and services, most of the following implications are primarily for state and local governments:

- Given the large number of incidents of abuse and neglect that are unidentified and unreported, service providers, caregivers, and all citi-zens who interact with elderly people need to be made aware of and sensitized to the problem of abuse and neglect, taught to recognize the various types of abuse and neglect, and encouraged to report suspected abuse. The NEAIS has confirmed that community professionals can be trained to observe and report elder abuse and neglect.
- Physicians and health care workers are especially well placed to detect instances of abuse, neglect, and self-neglect given that even the most isolated elderly persons come in contact with the health care system at some point. The education of physicians, nurses, and other health care workers should include ways to recognize and report signs and symp-toms of elder abuse, neglect, and self-neglect and where to refer victims for other human and support services.
- An important and urgent target for policy and service planners is the abuse and neglect among the oldest elders since those age 85 and over are the most rapidly growing elderly age group.

- The western region of the nation reported the largest number of reports to APS of any of the regions. With approximately 25 percent of the U.S. population, the western region was the source of 40 percent of the reports. Additionally, almost 60 percent of the western region reports were substantiated, in contrast to an overall substantiation rate of 49 percent. More detailed study of these western states may provide information on promising policies and practices for identifying and reporting abuse that can be replicated elsewhere in the country.
- Elderly persons who are unable to care for themselves, are mentally confused, or depressed are especially vulnerable to abuse and neglect as well as self-neglect. Local community organizations and businesses need to be sensitized to recognize such warning signals among the elderly in order to mobilize the most appropriate assessment and intervention.
- Increased standardization of state definitions and general reporting procedures for elder abuse and neglect would allow a more meaningful and expedited collection and analysis of data about elder abuse, including monitoring national trends over time.
- Maintaining and enhancing a comprehensive system of services and protocols at the local level is critical in order to receive and investigate reports of elder abuse and neglect and to provide appropriate interventions and follow-up services whenever necessary.
- A national study of best practices in the elder abuse field, including effective prevention and intervention strategies and programs, could inform and guide state and local efforts.

In conclusion, NEAIS estimates almost one-half million elderly were abused and neglected in domestic settings in 1996. It further documents the

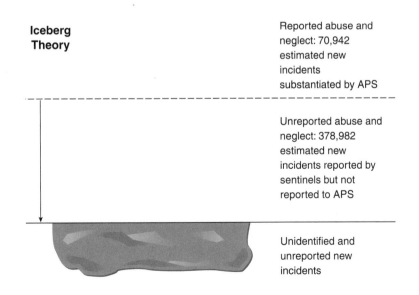

Iceberg Theory

Reported abuse and neglect: 70,942 estimated new incidents substantiated by APS

Unreported abuse and neglect: 378,982 estimated new incidents reported by sentinels but not reported to APS

Unidentified and unreported new incidents

existence of a previously unidentified and unreported stratum of elder abuse and neglect, thus confirming and advancing our understanding of the "iceberg" theory of elder abuse. The study estimates that for every abused and neglected elder reported and substantiated by APS, there are more than five additional abused and neglected elders who are not reported. NEAIS acknowledges, however, that it did not measure all previously hidden abuse and neglect, particularly among victims who do not leave their homes or who rarely interact with others in the community. Elder abuse and neglect remain the last type of family violence to be fully recognized and addressed. Our collective challenge—as policymakers, service providers, advocates, researchers, and society as a whole—is to utilize this information to improve the lives of our elder citizens.

Discussion Questions

1. Zengotita (Article 44) asserts that all of us are in the "show" when it comes to violence and that "the show must go on." Using this article as your framework, discuss the merits of this contention.

2. Analyze the merits of this statement: "The relationship between violence in the media and aggressive behavior is about the same as that between smoking and lung cancer."

3. Do parents "script" their children for violence? Support your response.

4. Where do you draw the line between children's normal growth and development and their use of pushing and hitting to get what they want?

5. What particularly offends you about media coverage of violent acts? Elaborate with examples.

6. From what you have seen on television during the past year, do you feel there is more or less appropriate coverage of acts of violence? Explain your conclusions.

7. How much media coverage is too much coverage of violent acts? Include in your response the premise of the public's right to know and the media's "feeding frenzy" in providing the public with all the details.

8. What behaviors have you noticed in children whose parents are substance abusers? Compare and contrast those behaviors with those of normal growth and development.

9. Evaluate the impact on our health care system and economy if children of substance-abusing parents are not given the care they need.

10. What aspects of same-sex violence are different from other types of domestic violence? What aspects are the same?

11. How comfortable are you in interacting with or caring for people in same-sex relationships? What contributes to your comfort or discomfort?

12. Recent accounts of elder abuse reveal that spouses and relatives commit the most elder abuse. Discuss what factors might generate elder abuse.

13. What experiences have you had in caring for elder abuse victims? What memories come to mind after your encounters with them?

Further Readings

Barnes, P. G. (1998). 'It was just a quarrel'. *ABA Journal, 84:*24–25.

Cruz, J. M., & Firestone, J. M. (1998). Exploring violence and abuse in gay male relationships. *Violence and Victims, 13*(2), 159–173.

Glass, N., & Campbell, J. C. (1998). Mandatory reporting of intimate partner violence by health care professionals: A policy review. *Nursing Outlook, 46*(6), 279–283.

Marks, A. (1999). Violence at home vs. on the street: A link? *Christian Science Monitor,* Sept. 28, 1999; 3.

Miles, A. (1999). When faith is used to justify abuse. *American Journal of Nursing, 99*(5) 32–35.

Updike, N. (1999). Hitting the wall. *Mother Jones, 24*(3) 37–38.

Vinton, L. (1999). Working with abused older women from a feminist perspective. *Fundamentals of Feminist Gerontology, 11*(2/3) 85–100.

Web Site Resources for Violence

Childhelp USA   www.childhelpusa.org
Domestic Violence and Abuse Issues   www.law.about.com
Domestic-Violence Net   www.domestic-violence.net
Elder Abuse and Aging Sites—Directory
    of Web Sites on Aging   http://www.aoa.dhhs.gov/agingsites/default.htm
Elder Abuse Prevention   www.oaktrees.org/elder/
National Center for Injury Prevention and Control   www.cdc.gov/ncipc/cmprfact.htm
Nurse Advocate: Nurses and Workplace Violence   www.nurseadvocate.org
Senate Report: Media Violence Affects Children   www.freedomforum.org

General Search Engine Web Sites

HotBot   www.hotbot.com
Metacrawler   www.metacrawler.com

Health Web Sites

CenterWatch   www.centerwatch.com
HealthGate   www3.healthgate.com
National Family Caregivers Association   www.nfcacares.org

Professional Journal Web Sites

Journal of Elder Abuse and Neglect   www.haworthpress.com
National Library of Medicine   www.nlm.nih.gov/medlineplus
Violence and Victims   www.haworthpress.com

PART FOUR

ISSUES OF HEALTH CARE REFORM

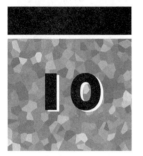

10 Delivering Health Care: At What Cost?

The idea was simple enough: The poor and elderly needed access to afford-able health care. If they allowed their health care to be managed, then they would receive improved access to the care they needed. This premise was the basis upon which Medicare and Medicaid were created, marking the beginning of health care reform.

But no one could have foreseen the tremendous cost of such an undertaking. Costs escalated more rapidly than expected. Long-term planning became increasingly more difficult because costs could not be projected, much less predicted. It was inevitable that state legislatures and Congress would have to begin a series of cost containment measures to rein in the mounting expenditures. Health maintenance organizations (HMOs) emerged as a feasible and fiscally sound venture that could continue to be affordable and still provide quality care. It was a health care bandwagon everybody wanted to be on.

Over time, however, the original concept of managed care changed. Profit making became more and more common in most HMOs, leaving many non-profit community-based hospitals scrambling for money to provide care for the poor, elderly, and underserved. For-profit hospitals merged with others and expanded their services both regionally and nationally. Managed care became a "health care industry." The corporate philosophy of HMOs shifted from services that benefited their members to services that benefited their stockholders. Patients became "customers," efficiency became a corporate mantra, and cost containment overshadowed quality care. Other changes followed. Health care fraud increased dramatically, and patients became more frustrated and more vocal about being denied the services they needed. Decisions about health care were being made by third parties—primarily insurance companies—and in some cases, HMOs dropped the elderly altogether from their health care plans. Despite these factors and the anecdotal horror stories in the media, surveys indicated that on the whole, the public seemed satisfied with their individual HMOs.

Critics of HMOs insist that other alternatives to delivering health care be explored to replace what they perceive as a health care system that is broken and beyond repair. Proponents of HMOs acknowledge deficiencies, but point to the accomplishments that managed care has made in providing affordable health care. These divergent views, coupled with the failure of HMOs to publicize their achievements, continue to fuel the debate about managed care. But however controversial managed care is, it is and will continue to be the primary source of health care in this country. *How* it can be improved is the issue before us.

This chapter begins with a discussion of the evolution of managed care and its future direction in this country. The readings that follow underscore the myths that continue to haunt managed care, the real issues that are at stake, and the underlying reasons behind the public's backlash against managed care. Given these factors, the final reading in this chapter examines where managed care is today, and what needs to be done for it to survive as a viable system of health care.

50

Managed Care Evolution—Where Did It Come From and Where Is It Going?

Aaron Liberman and Timothy Rotarius

Contrary to popular perception, managed care is not a plot developed by insurance companies or lawyers as a means of preventing Americans from securing much-needed health care. Neither is it a creation of a failed health care delivery system. Indeed, America's health services accomplishments represent a mark of excellence to which all other nations aspire. Rather, managed care represents a series of responses to certain realities within the U.S. health delivery system—some are historical, both ancient and contemporary; others are social and are based on the premises of limited availability or limited resources; and some are human—the product of corruption and greed.[1]

One thing may be certain, managed care is a product of all stakeholder groups that count themselves as representing parts of the overall system. This article shall focus on those stakeholder groups that have a significant vested interest in America's delivery system because through their work, they comprise the fabric that defines and determines the boundaries of the system.

These stakeholders include clinicians, hospitals and their management, insurance companies and other purchasers of care, pharmaceutical concerns, lawyers, and patients. The one thing each of these representative groups has in common with the others is that all have been tainted by federal regulators and the media for the excesses ascribed to the systems providing managed health services, including: (1) clinicians who have been accused of churning patients and inappropriately upcoding their procedures; (2) hospitals that have been imputed of both overbilling for provided services and supplies and routinely paying thinly veiled fees for patient referrals; (3) pharmaceutical organizations that have been accused of both setting medication prices at rates that earn them enormous profit margins and excusing away this overpricing practice as nothing more than a function of significant development costs; (4) lawyers who have been alleged to prey on the misery of elderly patients

Aaron Liberman, Ph.D., is an associate professor, and Timothy Rotarius, Ph.D., M.B.A., is an assistant professor at the Health Services Administration Program, University of Central Florida, Orlando, Florida.

and their families like vultures circling over a dead animal carcass at feeding time; (5) insurance companies that have been accused of using rating practices that capriciously increase premiums while often reflecting anything but the reality of the claims experience of their clientele; (6) medical practices that have been alleged to have violated antitrust laws through ownership of the various ancillary services and the associated physicians who have been accused of guiding every possible patient they can to that owned service in the name of quality patient care; and finally of greatest concern (7) patients who have been alleged to routinely submit or knowingly authorize the filing of fraudulent Medicare and Medicaid claims on their behalf by unscrupulous providers. In fact, two years ago, fraudulent Medicare and Medicaid claims alone were alleged to have cost taxpayers more than $15 billion dollars; the estimates of total health industry fraud that year totaled between $100 and $250 billion.[1]

Now, let the question be raised again: "Who is actually responsible for managed care?" Clearly, the answer is everyone, including those who self-righteously point fingers of blame and shame at one another while attempting to absolve themselves, their complicit responsibility for what they have begotten themselves and this society. Unfortunately, this does not represent a recent trend.

■ *HISTORICAL PERSPECTIVE*

Prior to Medicare, the emphasis of providers was twofold: improving accessibility to health care services and expanding bed capacity. Some still remember that before Medicare, when servicing those who could not afford to pay for health care services, many physicians would accept simply a home-prepared meal as barter for their professional services.

Interestingly enough, the first recorded health care program in America, which conformed to a managed care model, was started in 1798 by several East Coast shipping companies that developed pre-paid services for maritime workers in their employ. Since that time, there have been other isolated examples of programs that could be characterized as representative of managed health care models. Early programs in places as far removed as Elk City, Oklahoma, or as populous as California became the models from which more recent managed care organizations (MCOs) were developed.[2]

Following World War II, there was an acute shortage of hospital beds to treat the physical and emotional casualties of the war. The Hill-Burton Act (P.L. 79–725) was passed by Congress in 1946 during the Truman Administration to alleviate this shortage. The result was a significant expansion of hospital beds in an effort to meet the then-current health care priority of increased access to services.[3]

During the Eisenhower Administration, a National Mental Health Commission was empanelled to outline the need for an expanded bed and treatment capacity to treat the behavioral casualties of World War II and the Korean War. The work of the National Mental Health Commission was inspired by an Academy Award–winning movie entitled "The Man in the Gray Flannel Suit," which had as one of its principal themes the need for establishing community-based treatment facilities for mentally and emotionally impaired war veterans.

The Kennedy Administration saw the passage of two pieces of landmark legislation that were styled as the Community Mental Health Centers Acts of 1963. This legislation provided money for the bricks and mortar to build community-based treatment centers (P.L. 88–105) as well as for the staffing of these programs (P.L. 88–163). These laws represented the only substantive pieces of health legislation of the Kennedy White House Years.

Medicare became law in 1965, and with this legislation, health insurance for the elderly and the poor was provided through Titles 18 (Medicare) and 19 (Medicaid). Medicare and Medicaid represented the landmark legislative initiatives of Lyndon Johnson's years as President. When Medicare originally was enacted, the Social Security tax was 3.85 percent. To this was added 0.35 percent to cover Part A, the hospital care portion of Medicare. Because Medicare Part B was enacted as a voluntary program, neither Congress nor the White House Administration viewed it as requiring funding. This calculation error necessitated three adjustments in the Social Security tax rate during the next eight years. By 1973, the rate stood at 5.5 percent of the first $10,800 of income per participating employee. It was during this era that the excesses of overuse and entrepreneurialism first became painfully evident and Congress and the White House began devising strategies of cost containment—most of which were themselves expensive and doomed to failure. This was because the cost management efforts were focused primarily on limiting the amount of cost increases rather than reducing the cost of care.

The Comprehensive Health Planning Act (P.L. 89–749)[3] and the Regional Medical Programs Legislation (P.L. 89–239) were passed to encourage and foster voluntary, long-range planning. Unfortunately, rivalry and competition for funding precluded meaningful implementation of viable long-term programs. These legislative initiatives were followed by the Professional Standards Review Organizations legislation (P.L. 92–603) in 1972 and the Health Maintenance Organization Act (93–222) in 1973, which respectively introduced utilization review and precertification to the health services industry vernacular. Both of these measures had as an ultimate goal controlling the escalating cost of health services. At that time, neither legislative measure possessed an enforcement provision necessary to mandate compliance with the measures as intended by Congress and the President.

It was 1974, almost 10 years after Medicare had become a law of the land, when Congress, with White House support, enacted a substantive legislative measure with the power of enforced compliance. The law was known as the National Health Planning and Resources Development Act and it established the Certificate of Need (CON) as a requirement for the pre-approval and prior authorization of new facilities development, equipment acquisitions, and program implementation. For the first time, health care professionals were to be called to account when planning new and expanded facilities or programs. Although the Act was repealed by Congress in 1987,[3] the CON process was retained by several states as a means of controlling unnecessary facilities development.

Also in 1974, Congress enacted the Employee Retirement Income Security Act (ERISA), which was designed to protect the retirement assets of employees from overzealous and, in some instances, dishonest employers. As part of this legislation, ERISA-qualified employee health plans were granted a preemption from oversight by, and the regulatory authority of, the respective state departments of insurance.[4] This proved fortuitous for insurance carriers because the preemption disallowed punitive damages in litigation involving ERISA-qualified health insurance programs.[5] Unfortunately, this legislation also contributed to a mentality that would develop among MCOs that they were above reproach when policyholders attempted to hold them accountable for failing to act in a policyholder's best interests.

In 1983, under President Reagan, successful passage of the Tax Equity and Fiscal Responsibility Act introduced America to its first prospective payment system. Diagnosis related groups (DRGs) provided 492 separate and distinct reimbursements for designated medical and surgical inpatient conditions.[4] For the first time since Medicare's enactment, spending for health care services experienced a significant decline and the attention of legislators then turned toward free-standing, outpatient medical services as the next important cost-cutting target. In 1989, as a result of a Harvard University Study by William Hsiao and Peter Braun, resource-based relative value scales (RBRVS) were developed as a means of controlling reimbursements to physicians in medical practices that were unattached to hospitals. After a five-year test and phase-in period, RBRVS was implemented fully on January 1, 1997.[6] This left only outpatient care in a hospital setting unaffected by the cost-cutting commitments of federal authorities.

Ambulatory patient classifications, now scheduled for implementation shortly after the arrival of the new millennium, will establish a system of prospective payments for major diagnostic categories and associated ancillary services provided as part of a hospital setting.[7] Planners are now attempting to work out an articulation between hospital- and non-hospital-based outpatient services so that price shopping by providers and consumers does not overtake and compromise the benefits to be derived from the new system.

■ HISTORICAL PRECEDENT VERSUS CONTEMPORARY REALITIES

All of the legislative actions summarized thus far share one commonality: the respective initiatives were all enacted in response to America's automatic teller machine (ATM) mentality toward the ultimate federal entitlement program—Medicare. In other words, the entitlement vision created a belief that those in need of services should have unlimited access to the highest quality of care without regard to its cost. Unfortunately, the term entitlement also seems to have characterized the views of providers as much as those eligible for Medicare benefits. In short, this nation has begun to come to terms with a realization that America has reached, and perhaps even surpassed, the outer limits of its ability to subsidize a blank check approach to health services for all citizens; and unless this country is willing to accept the heavy tax requirements for such a system, difficult choices must be made.

This realization has a basis in religious precedent. The Talmud tells a story of two men of ancient times walking in the desert with one flask of water between them—one can drink and the other die; if both drink, both will die. This ancient scripture asks: "Which person should drink the water?"[11] Answer: the one holding the flask. Now, fast forward to 1996. Two men enter Southwestern Medical Center in Dallas—both are suffering liver disease, a chronic and fatal ailment without a transplant. One is a famous athlete, an icon of major league baseball; the other is a low-income person who is of minority origin. Both say: "Please help me. I'm in need of a liver." Who ultimately received the liver? The man with the flask of recognition. Despite a difference in timing of 2,000 years, very little has changed.

Managed care is unique in that it did not arise out of a specific legislative initiative but instead represents a market response, the ultimate form of which is guided by government oversight. In fact, it is the only major health services program since the advent of Medicare, which was not spawned by a formal federal government legislative initiative. As one reviews the legislation contemplated in this article, it becomes quite apparent that managed care represents an amalgamation of parts (best or worst depending on one's perspective) of several legislative acts. That is why managed care seems to have become an enduring part of the health services landscape in a relatively short period of time. It is quite likely that because of its origins, managed care in the United States will survive even its most ardent critics and their sometimes vitriolic and scathing narratives regarding its shortcomings.

Managed care today represents America's best health care hope. Perhaps it is the last opportunity for society to bring its own excesses under control. But managed care is now itself under significant scrutiny and criticism for its own hubris and its failure to serve the best interests of patients, for example, placing gag orders in the service contracts with physicians; paying bonuses to physician administrators based on the denial of needed specialist services; and the decline of acute care referrals.[8] These accusations against managed care have suggested that it is time to rethink and retool managed care to assure that its priorities are balanced between the interests of the patient in receiving timely, quality care and the commitment of the payer to achieve and maintain a healthy bottom line. Are people surprised? Are they shocked? Do they now ask how this can be? The answer quite simply is that managed care is a product of America's own citizenry and of both society's inability and unwillingness to demonstrate restraint in the use of health services. Hence, it is unsurprising that managed care itself now sits on the firing line, perceived by some as a threat to Americans' health and well-being and as a target of critical indignation.

■ WHAT MUST BE DONE

In health care, as in life, the present is both a product of the past and a precursor to the future. There are four critical adjustments that need to be made in the overall programs known as managed care: (1) patients' ability to secure acute care referrals when they are required must be assured; (2) the prerogatives of MCOs to deselect (redline) from coverage all higher risk populations must be limited; (3) the use of the profit motive to reward non-performance by service providers must be controlled; and (4) a more responsible layering of reinsurance coverage through realistic contracts both for MCOs and their associated providers must be mandated.

Simultaneously, America must prevail on providers, hospitals, physicians, and paramedical care specialists to control their penchants for excessive charging. To gore a program as well intentioned and as economically fragile as Medicare suggests an irresponsible use of the public trust. Clinicians must refrain from the plethora of unseemly practices that have been uncovered since Operation Restore Trust was implemented by the federal government.[1] In a recent article published in *The Health Care Supervisor,* the authors chronicled a host of illegitimate practices that have been uncovered since 1990. The cost to taxpayers has been significant, and by some estimates has exceeded the entire fiscal budget of most of the world's nations.[1]

If the past is a predictor of the future and the present a precursor of what is to come, is America now headed "back to the future?" The answer of course is a resounding "no." The future will present a new series of challenges along with several possibilities for correcting the new imperfections that are yet to be seen in the infrastructure of America's health delivery system.

■ CONCLUSION

Despite the pessimism sounded in pointing out past and current excesses associated with this nation's health delivery system, there is good reason for optimism laced with a good-sized dose of realism. The essential point is that each person must begin accepting greater responsibility for the consequences of his or her individual actions. For example, America has heard a warning sounded regarding the future need for long-term care. With the graying of America, it has been projected that one of the most notable challenges will be the necessity of addressing the long-term care needs of the aging population. Today, there are 2 million people in need of skilled nursing home care. By the year 2030, it has been estimated that 5 million Americans will require this form of care at an annual cost of $700 billion.[9] With an average annual cost today of $38,000 per resident,[9] the task ahead is indeed daunting. However, it is neither unreasonable nor impossible to suggest that it can be addressed effectively. To accomplish this objective, it is essential that Americans begin to accept the responsibility of protecting themselves; if one waits until age 75 to do so, it will have become too expensive and too late.[9]

In summation, citizens of America truly control the future of their health delivery system; but they must assume a more responsible posture about the realities and the limitations of that system. That means accepting also their share of the responsibility for making the system work—beyond what Medicare and individual Medi-Gap policies will pay. If Americans are to be protected through their senior years, those who can afford to do so must assure that they have established a safety net for themselves and their families. If Americans do just that much, the pressure relieved from the system will enable the U.S. government to focus on those who truly are less fortunate and who will require the social insurance support of the federal government.

A viable method of self protection today is through the purchase of long-term care insurance coverage. A person age 50 and in good health can purchase this coverage for about $50 per month or $600 per year; this includes a rider whereby the premiums paid will be refunded to the policyholder if the policy has been unused after 23 years of coverage. Some have argued that as an investment vehicle, long-term care policies are sorely lacking and a person would be better served through an equivalent investment in the stock market. If long-term care insurance represented an investment, from a Wall Street perspective, that rationale would be irrefutable. However, when one purchases an indemnity form of insurance coverage, what one is seeking is to be "made whole" in the event of a loss.[10] One is not seeking to realize a financial gain as a result of that purchase. One can neither predict nor control, with certainty, the future as it pertains to individual health and welfare. Rather, one can develop one's own safety net in the event of being confronted with health and daily living problems over which one has no control. For less than $2 per day, one can assure that one will not be faced with the necessity of depleting all of one's assets in order to secure needed skilled care as one completes the senior years.

In the future, the only people who will be able to expect additional governmental consideration are those with no visible means of support and with a lack of the mental capacity or physical ability to provide at least a portion of the necessary financing for themselves. For those poor souls, there will be inevitable gaps in the "safety net" and it is possible many may not survive the ever-present imperfections within America's health care financing structure.

Making this system of care more responsive to individual needs means adopting a responsible economic posture as well as personalized and individual ethical standards that are uncompromising. Ethics are essential to a future with both personal control over events and an opportunity to complete life independent and free of the need for public intervention. The tenets of this credo are presented for consideration as follows:

- Be honest with regard to the possibility of future health care needs in order to be truthful and forthright with others.
- Expect no more from institutions than from one's own true personal financial limits dictate.
- Ask only for that which one cannot provide for one's self and would be willing to authorize for another less fortunate person displaying similar financial circumstances.
- Work diligently to establish a health care safety net for one's self and for one's family.
- Anticipate that America's democratically developed health care practices and institutions always will exhibit inherent imperfections.
- Respect the frailties of others who must use the health care system more extensively so that one in turn can better appreciate and understand one's own limitations when they occur.
- Establish behavioral and performance expectations for others that are consistent with one's own patterns of performance and behavior.

Taking the first letter from each of the seven tenets, one spells BE AWARE. It is doubtful that one's expectations when in need of medical attention would include "a systems approach to acute treatment and ongoing care." Most, if not all, people would much prefer the treatment of a condition in a "personalized" and "caring" manner. Managed care is capable of meeting that expectation if Americans insist that it be done. The challenges today presented by managed care cannot be represented simply as systems based; they are human problems requiring Americans' involvement and insistence that they be corrected. If society does its part, it truly will have reinvented a healthier and infinitely more honest health services delivery system for the vast majority of its citizens. Now Americans have a good deal of work to do. Best wishes for our mutual success.

References

1. A. Liberman and R. Rolle, "Alleged Abuses in Health Care in the 1990s," *The Health Care Supervisor* 17, no. 1 (September 1998): 1.
2. G. Benedict, *The Development & Management of Medical Groups.* Englewood, CO: Medical Group Management Press, 1996.
3. J. Rakich et al., *Managing Health Services Organizations.* Baltimore: Heath Professions Press, 1995.
4. P. Kongstvedt, *Essentials of Managed Health Care.* Gaithersburg, MD: Aspen Publishers, Inc., 1997.
5. P. Kongstvedt, *The Managed Health Care Handbook.* Gaithersburg, MD: Aspen Publishers, Inc., 1993.

6. P. McMenamin and R. Heald (eds.), *Medicare RBRVS: The Physicians' Guide.* Chicago: American Medical Association, 1998.

7. R. Averill et al., *Development of a Prospective Payment System for Hospital Based Outpatient Care.* Wallingform, CT: 3M Health Information Systems. Published report funded by the Office of Research and Demonstrations of the Health Care Financing Administration, 1997.

8. N. Jeffrey and R. Winslow, "Aetna Told to Pay $116 Million Damages." *The Wall Street Journal,* 21 January, 1999, sec. A4.

9. H. Sultz and K. Young, *Health Care USA: Understanding Its Organization & Delivery.* Gaithersburg, MD: Aspen Publishers, Inc., 1997.

10. E. Vaughan and T. Vaughan, *Fundamentals of Risk & Insurance.* New York: John Wiley & Sons, 1999.

11. Rabbi S. Salkowitz, personal communication. Orlando, FL: February 12, 1997.

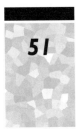

51

Managed Care: Devils, Angels, and the Truth in Between

Emily Friedman

I was on an airplane, seated next to a man who was a high-ranking executive of a major hotel chain. I was making notes for a piece I was writing about managed care. He asked what I was doing, and I told him that I was trying to analyze the backlash against managed care that had led many people to believe that all health plans were a form of the Devil Incarnate. He sniffed and said, "Well, aren't they?"

I replied by asking him how he would respond if I turned to him and snarled, "Those @!!$*&#! hotels! They're all dirty and overpriced. The room service never arrives, the fax machines don't work, and the staff are hostile and incompetent." He paled and said, "But *our* hotels aren't like that! They're very good. We have much higher standards than that!"

Touché.

That exchange is a good metaphor for what is happening in the wonderful world of managed care these days. On one side, we have a wildly pluralistic bunch of health plans that run the gamut from fast-buck profiteers to community-conscious, long-established not-for-profit entities. Many of these plans have about as much in common as I do with Sen. Jesse Helms. Yet they are all defined—and condemned—as "managed care."

These plans are also represented by very effective lobbyists and advocates. Their public relations and policy campaigns often focus on opposing any effort at regulation, no matter how mild, constantly warning that any attempt to legislate, regulate, or otherwise curb inappropriate managed care behaviors will lead to skyrocketing premiums and millions more uninsured Americans.

On the other side, we have a large and growing collection of plan members, patients, families, consumer advocates, politicians, physicians, hospital executives, other providers, policy wonks, attorneys, and journalists who paint managed care as a hideous and homogeneous monolith, an Evil Empire bent on killing patients, destroying caregivers, and wrecking the American way of life.

Emily Friedman is an independent health policy and ethics analyst based in Chicago.

Reprinted with permission from *Health Progress*, May/June 1999, 80(3) 22–26.

▥ A COLLISION OF BELIEFS

So far, the result of this collision of beliefs has been a tidal wave of negative news stories, countered by letters or editorials defending managed care; legislative initiatives in virtually every state to protect patients, providers, or both, including bills in a couple of states where there was no managed care activity at the time; a bitter debate in Congress over competing "patients' bills of rights," none of which has become law; litigation and more litigation; and growing support for federal legislation that would allow plan members or families to sue health plans for malpractice in state court, an option that most courts have ruled is barred by current federal law.

The public is confused and nervous; politicians are using managed care as a campaign issue; the plans are pleading innocent; the attorneys and consumer advocates are crying "foul"—and some 99 million people are now members, voluntarily or involuntarily, of managed care plans, according to SMG Marketing of Chicago. Among that group are about 15 percent of Medicare beneficiaries, most low-income Medicaid beneficiaries, and even hundreds of thousands of prison inmates, whose care is increasingly being turned over to investor-owned prison managed care companies. Talk about a captive population!

Meanwhile, more and more providers—especially physicians—are joining the fray, howling to anyone who will listen that health plans are ruining healthcare by forcing physicians to skimp on services, stealing doctors' income, "deselecting" physicians from plan contracts for no reason, hurting or killing patients, and profiteering like mad. One young physician of my acquaintance recently described capitation as "obscene"; another complained to me that "you can't do a decent physical on a patient in 15 minutes!"

There are more issues involved in all this than can be covered here. What I do hope to argue for is a more rational approach to the debate. There has been enough hysteria. There has been enough exploitation and opportunism. There has been more than enough lying and deception. There must be a better way to address these questions than standing around screaming at each other while trying to woo policymakers to one side or the other. We must begin to unbraid the rope of managed care that is currently being used to threaten or lynch the opposition, and try to tease out real issues from false. It might not make the debate any more pleasant, but it would certainly enhance its quality and precision.

▥ UNBRAIDING THE ROPE

I would first like to dispense with several inaccurate beliefs. One is that managed care is inherently evil and riddled with perverse incentives. Well, all payment policies are riddled with potentially perverse incentives, in and out of healthcare. Managed care is just a way of organizing health care payment and sometimes health services, and it is no more evil in concept than any other way of organizing things. Judgment must be based on how health plans behave.

The second myth is that managed care will go away if we just kick it hard enough. It won't—and if it does, it's quite certain that we will not return to fee-for-service arrangements, whose costs were even worse than managed care's, and which were almost impossible to regulate or even monitor. So if managed care doesn't work, we will likely head in the direction of a public utility or single-payer model. But that will be a long time from now; for the moment, managed care is the predominant long-term trend in healthcare.

The third myth is that angelic providers are being forced to do terrible things to patients—lie, deny, cheat, steal—by the devilish health plans. The fact is that much of this provider angst is rooted in three less innocent truths.

First, providers—physicians in particular—are seeing their net incomes decline, and they are blaming it on managed care. They are right, in part; managed care plans and entrepreneurs, seeing providers throwing money around like there was no tomorrow, realized they could move into the market and make at least one-time huge profits by extracting discounts, so they did. But the root cause of provider and physician income decline—and managed care success—is that there are far too many physicians, hospitals, and just about every other service in healthcare, and sooner or later this oversupply was going to force incomes down. All that was necessary for this to happen was for providers to lose control of the healthcare system—and they lost that to payers and employers some time ago.

Second, healthcare providers are a stodgy bunch—conservative as all get-out and change resistant to a fault (and it is a fault). Confronted with payment arrangements, incentives, rules, procedures, and policies that in many cases are wildly different from or even the opposite of what they learned in school, they rebel. We all do when faced with profound changes in how we usually do things. But that doesn't mean the changes are wrong or inappropriate; it just means they are changes.

The third underlying reason for provider—as well as patient—unhappiness is that managed care (if you can make any global characterizations about it at all) encourages more conservative healthcare practice. It also limits choice of provider, in one form or another. This leaner approach flies in the face of the "more is better" culture that pervades American society generally and medical education in particular.

This is the land of 32-ounce steaks and 17 brands of canned chili, and we like it that way. Anyone who even purports to claim that less is better and that limited choice is perfectly acceptable will face rough sledding. It doesn't matter that endless choice of provider isn't available to anyone these days except in the Medicare program, or that hundreds of thousands of patients have been seriously injured or maimed or killed by unnecessary treatments and procedures. The culture of managed care is different from the culture of the society around it, and it makes people nervous.

The final myth is that all managed care is the same. Nope. Some plans are capitated fully; some use selective capitation; most still use discounted fee for service. Most, but not all, plans are investor owned. Some are highly sensitive to their communities; others couldn't care less. Some have employed or exclusively contracted physicians; most do not. Some are regional, some national. Some spend the vast majority of their revenues on patient care; others spend far less. Some are in it for the long haul; others are here today, gone tomorrow. When you've seen one HMO, as the joke goes, you've seen one HMO.

■ THE REAL ISSUES

It seems to me that those who actually provide services to patients, as well as plan advocates, regulators, policymakers, and wonks, would be well served by jumping off their respective bandwagons of either unswerving adoration of all managed care, or mindless hatred of all managed care, and start making some distinctions. These are the issues and questions on which I think these distinctions should be based.

Plan Ownership

Two-thirds of all health plans are investor-owned, and two-thirds of all enrollment is in investor-owned plans. This sets up what is, to my mind, an irresolvable conflict between duty to investors and duty to members and patients. This is not to say—believe me!—that not-for-profit plans are all wonderful and are always honest with patients and never interfere in clinical decision making. Nor does it automatically imply that every for-profit plan is grasping every dollar it can find to send to Wall Street, regardless of the consequences. It does suggest to me that when patients and families are competing with investors for money, patients and families will lose.

The fact is, however, that most managed care is for-profit, and that is not likely to change any time soon.

There are actions providers can take in the face of this. One is to make rational decisions about which plans to contract with. If the plan has a horrible reputation, or looks and smells like a short-term "investment opportunity," don't contract with it. Furthermore, providers can share their concerns with employers, business coalitions, and other purchasers, seeking to encourage them to contract with responsible plans. It also goes without saying that ethical providers do not accept equity positions, stock, or partnerships in organizations with which they contract—that really is a perverse incentive.

Most important, if providers really think that most of the plans in their markets are more Wall Street than Main Street, they can start their own. Some provider organizations already have. The Balanced Budget Act of 1997 gave providers the chance to form provider-sponsored organizations (PSOs) that can contract directly with Medicare to provide managed care services to beneficiaries. So far, PSOs have been a non-event, with one PSO (sponsored by a Catholic organization) licensed as of the beginning of 1999. The general reason given for lack of interest in PSOs by providers is that they "don't want to take the risk." Well, fine; but then don't complain when sleazy for-profit health plans put you in compromising positions.

And by the way: What kind of health plans do providers offer their own employees? Often they contract with the very plans whose behavior they condemn in public. What kind of message does that send, especially to the employees?

Plan Structure and Risk Arrangements

As everyone knows, health plans these days come in 57 varieties—staff, group, network, IPA/broker, PPO, point of service, mixed, and on and on. They all have their advocates. My personal preference is plans that integrate the provision of health services with the *insurance* of health services, such as the old standby Kaiser Permanente. I also strongly favor the salaried practice of medicine because I think it is unfair to patient and provider alike to have a physician's income dependent on how much or how little care he or she provides to patients.

However, this model represents a tiny minority of health plans these days. The reasons are simple enough. Owning your own hospitals, clinics, and other bricks and mortar means huge overhead and great difficulty in adjusting to increases or decreases in member enrollment; you're laying people off one year and restaffing the next. Furthermore, virtually every study on the subject has found that salaried physicians' productivity is much lower than that of self-employed or other nonsalaried practitioners.

But the main problem is risk, in the insurance sense. It is much safer for a plan to contract with an employer or payer for a population of "covered lives," and then essentially sell them and their medical records to the lowest bidder while pocketing a hunk of the premium. All the risk—for cost overruns, a bad flu season, sicker-than-average patients—is shoved onto providers.

It is this issue of risk that has led to many unacceptable practices, most of them geared to making patients and providers, rather than plans, vulnerable to great financial loss. Other strategies are focused on avoiding the sick and disabled—heaven forbid that sick people should actually have coverage!

Providers should be willing and able to shoulder some, but not all, of the risk if they are contracting with an outside health plan. They should also challenge the plan about enrollment and recruitment practices, to ensure that people who are ill, or disabled, or poor, or minority are not ignored or discouraged from joining the plan. Think about it: When was the last time you saw an HMO ad on television that featured someone who was blind, diabetic, or in a wheelchair? No, it's always the "Centrum couple"—beautiful, looking like they're maybe 40, and skipping stones while on a backpacking trip. Obviously, the typical 75-year-old American.

The long-term solution, of course, is to see to it that the health status of enrollees does not result in financial penalties, by outlawing any insurance discrimination based on how sick or healthy an enrollee is. All premiums in a given area should be the same, adjusted only between regions for cost-of-living considerations. Specific plan populations should be risk-adjusted, with higher payments to plans with sicker members; Medicare is supposed to initiate this practice in 2000. And any plan found to be discriminating against people because of their health status should lose its license and eligibility to participate in Medicare and Medicaid.

Plan Priorities

What does the plan value? Where does it put most of its energy? Is it involved in subsidy of medical education, nursing education, and clinical and health services research? Does it really focus on prevention, or does it just talk the talk? Is it involved in any way in care or subsidy of the uninsured? Does it contract with "safety net" providers? Does it market its wares in all parts of the town, or only the affluent suburbs? Does it have a mission statement, and, if so, do its actions reflect that statement?

It is amazing how many managed care executives are perfectly honest (at least in private meetings) about their health plans being temporary investment opportunities. It is amazing how many are founded by people who simply pile up the requisite number of "covered lives" (often by pricing products unreasonably low), get that stock price up to the right level, and then either exercise stock options or sell out to a larger plan. There are literally billions of dollars to be made by this method. But the people could just as easily be buying and selling electronics as human beings' healthcare.

It must also be said that providers can be every bit as cynical in their motivations, with the added attraction that they are often hypocritical about it as well. At least investor types are honest about what they are doing.

Providers and patients would be well served by demanding a code of conduct—one that has teeth—for all health plans. That code should serve as the basis for granting or denying state licenses and participation in Medicare and Medicaid. There should be periodic monitoring and surprise visits. Financial records should be available for independent audit. And plans should be required to make public the priorities they claim to espouse. I think it would result in better behavior all around.

Relations With Providers

It is sadly true that many physicians and some hospitals would be perfectly willing to put up with health plan misbehavior if they could simply get a larger piece of the pie. In other words, their worries about managed care are all financial. On the other hand, physicians, nurses, and others have made legitimate complaints about health plan policies that play fast and loose with provider ethics. These include "gag clauses" (which were never in common use, but nobody knows that), alluring incentives laden with conflicts of interest, penurious capitation, simple disrespect, and ditching physicians whose practices happen to attract diabetics or schizophrenics or persons with AIDS as patients.

In judging plans and deciding which ones to do business with, providers should ask around, especially among their medical staff members, about how the plan treats them and their patients. Don't just settle for gripes about money; but take very seriously indications that plans, intentionally or not, are crippling clinicians' ability to do their jobs.

Communication With Patients

Several studies have found that the public is hopelessly confused about managed care. And small wonder; many health plan ads are deceptive, patient information materials are often a joke, and some customer service phone lines have an average time on hold of three days. In fact, I have come to the reluctant conclusion that many plans *want* to keep people in the dark. If that's the aim, they're succeeding; one recent survey by the Employee Benefit Research Institute found that 56 percent of people in health plans swear they've never been in managed care, and 6 percent of people in indemnity coverage think they're in managed care. In a recent AARP (American Association of Retired Persons) survey, 55 percent of Medicare beneficiaries reported that HMO ads were a major source of information for them about managed care.

Health plans worthy of our respect and participation tell patients the truth: that some providers are off-limits, that some procedures are not covered, that there may be a wait for appointments, that referrals to certain specialists are mandatory, and so on. This information should be in writing, at no more than an eighth grade reading level (for Medicaid patients, fifth grade level, according to a recent study). The customer service line should be staffed by people who can and will answer questions and solve problems. If emergency department use is discouraged, there must be a way for members to get information and assessments after hours. And there must be an objective process for patient appeals and grievances to be heard in a timely manner. Many of these protections are already being enacted into law; providers should be supporting, indeed demanding, such initiatives.

I would add a small pet peeve: Any plan that preaches prevention should have a policy of contacting members once a year (or whatever the recommended time interval is) to remind them that it's time for a mammogram, Pap smear, prostate or rectal exam, immunization, or other preventive service. Dentists do this; a multizillion dollar health plan ought to be able to do the same.

Resource Allocation

This is one of the best-documented measures of health plan behavior; yet few providers take advantage of it. The question is simple: How much of a plan's revenue is spent on patient care? The current range, nationally, is from 59 percent to 95 percent. I am not one who believes that money is necessarily a surrogate for quality, but it's hard to believe that the plans at the extremes of those figures provide the same access, quality, and service. Some state insurance commissioners have proposed that a minimum percentage of revenue—85 percent or so—be spent on patient care in order for a plan to operate in a state. What a great idea!

Beyond that, how does the plan allocate its money? How much of its administrative funds go to investors, executive stock options, or fancy golf outings in Fiji with legislators? Does it subsidize memberships for the uninsured poor? Does it participate in the new children's health insurance programs? Does it cover—and actually make available—hospice, rehabilitation services, long-term care, and mental health services?

Data on much of this is collected by states; in California, the state medical society makes this information available every year. Providers should be doing the same everywhere—helping the public and policymakers understand where managed care premium monies are going. But I must add an important caveat: Providers should be able and willing to answer the question of where their revenues are going as well.

Long-Term Stability

As I read the business press and note that Health Plan X is for sale, and that Health Plan Y has just gobbled up Health Plan Z, I wonder what that means for members of those plans. I know that when it happened to a plan I used to belong to, the customer service deteriorated, the number of physicians available shrank, and more restrictions appeared. For many plan members, it can mean losing a cherished physician.

Meanwhile, as the stock price zooms up and then plummets, investor-owned plans must take appropriate action to "restore Wall Street confidence." The result is a roller coaster of greater benefits, fewer benefits, better access, less access, higher provider payment, lower provider payment. In any enterprise, some volatility is inevitable; but for the investor-owned plans, the ride seems wilder than most.

For patients, families, providers, and communities, this is just unacceptable. No one can plan. No one knows which physicians or hospitals will be available. No one knows where the money is going. And as the mergers and acquisitions progress, fewer and fewer health plans are headquartered anywhere near most of their members. Try calling the Cayman Islands when you are denied a service your physician thinks you need!

The age of a plan, how long it has had its headquarters in a given place, where it operates, how many times it has merged or been acquired, and its long-term commitment to its communities are singularly important indicators of its accountability. This will become even more crucial as plans' profit margins decline, which is inevitable after artificially high one-time-only savings are achieved. Providers and patients need partners who will still be around when the big bills start coming due.

I have no illusions that these modest suggestions will bring total rationality to the war over managed care, or that acting on them will end all the problems and challenges that health plans represent. But, as former U.S. Surgeon General Joycelyn Elders, MD, once observed in another context, perhaps we can at least tone down the rhetoric. Then we can begin thinking in terms of distinctions, rather than blanket condemnations, and can clarify where we should be focusing our attention. For as managed care becomes the dominant form of healthcare reimbursement and structure, at least in our urban areas, our responsibility is to see to it that this means humane progress in healthcare. The only way to do that is to know what we are talking about.

52

What's Behind the Public's Backlash?

Gail R. Wilensky

Having spent much of the 1970s and 1980s bemoaning the rapid increases in spending on health care, the country has spent the last two years talking about various statutory provisions to "rein-in" managed care, the strategy most frequently credited with slowing down spending on health care.

While it is difficult not to feel some sense of frustration with this sequence of events, the questions raised by this issue of *JHPPL* are important to address. Is there really a backlash against managed care? Have people actually experienced problems receiving health care under their managed care plans or are they primarily concerned that they might experience problems in the future? Is this an area where the Federal government could craft legislation that would respond to the concerns of the population and if so, would it undo the advantages brought by managed care and return the country to the double digit medical inflation of an earlier period? Obviously not all of these questions can be addressed in a short commentary, but I would like to offer a few observations about the nature of the problem and some suggestions for its resolution.

■ DO PEOPLE PERCEIVE PROBLEMS WITH MANAGED CARE?

As is frequently the case in polling, the amount and degree of public dissatisfaction with managed care depends on the particular survey that is chosen. In general, however, the public indeed seems concerned about the effects that managed care is having on the quality of care delivered. According to a recent Kaiser/Harvard/Princeton Survey Research Associates (PSRA) poll, people in managed care plans are more concerned about whether their health care plan will pay the cost of an expensive treatment or do the right thing for their care than people in traditional plans. The same poll reported that substantially more people thought HMOs had decreased the quality of health care for peo-

Gail R. Wilensky, PhD., is a senior fellow at the Center for Health Affairs.

Reprinted with permission from *Journal of Health Politics, Policy and Law*, October 1999, 24(5) 1015–1019. Copyright © 1999 Duke University Press. All rights reserved.

ple who are sick than thought HMOs had increased the quality of care (Blendon et al. 1998). Nor is this survey the only instance of such reporting (Louis Harris and Associates 1997).

At the same time, the vast majority of people are satisfied with the care they receive. The percentage of people saying that they are satisfied with their care in 1998 ranged between 80 percent and 93 percent depending on the poll and type of plan they were in (*Washington Post*/ABC 1998; *Time*/CNN 1998). Even with these high percentages, there was a 10 percent gap in satisfaction between those in traditional plan versus those in managed care.

It is also interesting to note that one of the recent polls showing these high measures of satisfaction reported that almost half didn't think their satisfaction would last (Sternberg 1998). This concern about the future may in part reflect the view that "my plan" may be satisfactory but I'm not sure "your plan" is okay, which makes me worried about my plan in the future.

■ *WHAT DRIVES THE PUBLIC'S PERCEPTIONS?*

At least part of the answer to the question of why people are concerned about quality and other issues of managed care when they report such high levels of satisfaction is that large numbers are reporting problems with their health plans. Most of this type of polling data makes it difficult to assess whether the reported problems are reasonable complaints or not or whether the problems are regarded as serious or not. An analysis of some recent California polling data suggests that many of the reported problems may not have been serious or even been perceived as being major or serious (Enthoven and Singer 1998).

A more significant driver of peoples' perceptions may be the reports by other people about problems in managed care. The Harvard/Kaiser/PSRA poll reported that less than 40 percent of those who had an unfavorable view of managed care based that view on their own experience. Not surprisingly, the media has had an important role in shaping these perceptions. The same survey indicated that for 22 percent of those with unfavorable perceptions, media coverage influenced their views.

Concerns about media coverage, particularly biased media coverage as a driver of the public's perception, have been raised by the managed care industry as well as others. A recent study that attempted to assess potential bias in the media concluded there was a noticeable change in the coverage and tone of coverage over the period 1990 to 1997. While there was not a conclusion of bias in terms of all media coverage, it was noted that the tone of coverage became more critical over time. In addition, the study found that the most visible media sources had negative stories in more than half of their coverage and most often used anecdotes (Brodie, Brady, and Altman 1998). Thus the perception that the major media have been a part of the negative view of managed care is well founded.

■ *PERCEPTIONS VERSUS REALITY*

Whether or not there are significant problems with regard to the way managed care health plans function or with the quality of care delivered in managed care is a difficult question to answer. Harold Luft and his colleagues at the University of California, San Francisco have provided the best reviews of what is known in this area (Miller and Luft 1997). He reports equal numbers of significant positive and negative results for HMO performance compared to non-HMO performance but is careful to point out several caveats. There are problems caused by old data; the studies reviewed varied in scope and methods and the dimensions of performance that are reviewed are usually very limited. However, the finding of significantly worse outcomes for chronically ill elderly enrollees in HMOs reported by the carefully done Medical Outcomes Study cannot be readily dismissed (Ware et al. 1996). While this finding needs to be confirmed for larger and more representative populations of the old and chronically ill, it does suggest that research at the subpopulation level may be critical to understanding the relationship between plan types and outcomes.

■ *WHAT DOES THIS SUGGEST FOR PUBLIC POLICY?*

Even though the public is largely satisfied with their health care and there are no definitive problems with the health care that is provided by managed care plans, there is a need to respond to the public's concerns. Deciding on the response that's regarded as appropriate is likely to be more controversial.

I believe there is a need for more and better information for the public. This information should include what we know about the changes that have occurred in the health care environment, the types of plans employers and the public plans are offering, the effects of the changing delivery system, and the relationship of all of the above to quality of care. There is also a need for better information about what we know and don't know about health care outcomes, variations in health care delivery, and quality indicators.

Whether or not people will use some, all, or none of this information, at least initially, does not diminish the importance of having the information available. Over time, the chances are that more of this type of information will become increasingly used and it obviously won't be used if it's not available.

The public needs some assurances that health care plans will "play fair." Insurance commissioners presumably provide this type of assurance for plans they can regulate but some requirements for Employee Retirement Income Security Act (ERISA)–covered plans regarding information describing plans and plan benefits in clear and understandable language, and information about appeals processes and other protections also would be useful.

What may be most important, however, is to give employees a greater choice in health care plans. Many employees have only one plan offered as an employer sponsored plan. While that plan is likely to contain opt-out provisions, it will probably be far more reassuring to most employees to know they can choose to buy other plans with their pretax dollars if they don't want the plan offered by their employers. Structuring this increased choice in such a way that it doesn't push individuals into the expensive individual market or undo risk groupings will take some care. But difficult as this will be, it is far preferable to passing legislation that will substantially increase the cost of health care by forcing all plans to meet someone else's definition of the right health plan.

Unfortunately, or perhaps fortunately, since the likelihood of passing bad legislation is greater than passing good legislation, nothing much is likely to happen this year. Changing the tax laws to allow more choice would appeal to many Republicans and some Democrats, as would providing for some consumer protection but not the right to sue. For most Democrats, only consumer protection legislation that also provides the right to sue is worth passing. Otherwise having this as an election issue is likely to be preferable to having an incremental solution. Given this likely impasse, the managed care industry would be wise to use the next year or two to craft its own responses to the concerns of the public.

References

Blendon, R. J., M. Brodie, J. M. Benson, D. E. Altman, L. Levitt, T. Hoff, and L. Hugick. 1998. Understanding the Managed Care Backlash. *Health Affairs* 17(4): 80–94.

Brodie, M., L. A. Brady, and D. E. Altman. 1998. Media Coverage of Managed Care: Is There a Negative Bias? *Health Affairs* 17(1):9–25.

Enthoven, A., and S. Singer. 1998. The Managed Care Backlash and the Task Force in California. *Health Affairs* 17(4): 95–110.

Louis Harris and Associates. 1997. Poll. New York: Louis Harris and Associates, 20 August.

Miller, R., and H. Luft. 1997. Managed Care Performance: Is Quality of Care Better or Worse? *Health Affairs* 16(5):7–25.

Sternberg, Steve. 1998. Finding the Health System Unfit: Many Americans Fear the Care Won't Be There—Study: Consumers Support Legislative Fix. *USA Today,* 23 November, 1D.

Time/Cable News Network (CNN). 1998. Poll. New York: *Time,* CNN, June–July.

Ware, J. E., M. S. Bayliss, W. H. Rogers, M. Kosinski, and A. R. Tarlov. 1996. Differences in Four-Year Health Outcomes for Elderly and Poor, Chronically Ill Patients Treated in HMO and Fee-for-Service Systems: Results from the Medical Outcomes Study. *Journal of the American Medical Association* 276(13):1039–1047.

Washington Post/ABC. 1998. Poll. Washington, DC: *Washington Post,* ABC, June–July.

53

Managed Care at a Crossroads

Geoffrey E. Harris, Matthew J. Ripperger, and Howard G. S. Horn

*F*or the first time in roughly four years managed care companies appear to be reversing the negative fundamental trends that have punished earnings in recent years. Commercial pricing is in a sharp upward trend, medical loss ratios (MLRs) are improving, returns on equity (ROEs) are moving higher, and earnings estimates have been largely stable for the large market capitalization players. Unfortunately, the corresponding stock-price momentum evident in late 1998 and early 1999 suffered a dramatic reversal in late 1999, as a result of the growing intensity of societal, political, and legislative forces that threaten the managed care industry's earnings prospects and perhaps even its very existence. In fact, it would not be an exaggeration to suggest that the managed care stock universe suffered a "free fall" of virtually unprecedented proportions. In the space of several weeks the managed care universe lost roughly 20–25 percent of its value.

While the immediate impact of these forces has been on investors' perceptions and on stock prices alone, analysts are concerned that recent events could delay or even derail the fragile fundamental recovery that could improve earnings and stock-price performance. The issues confronting the industry and investors go well beyond current fundamental trends and valuation levels. What happens to managed care and financing for health care in the United States has both near-term and long-term implications for the broader health care marketplace.

■ MANAGED CARE: UNFAIRLY PUNISHED?

By most objective measures, the managed care industry has been a huge success. Health care cost trends have moderated in recent years, health care as a percentage of gross national product (GNP) has leveled off, and the overall

Geoff Harris is managing director of U.S. Equity Research at Warburg Dillon Read, a Wall Street investment firm. Matthew Ripperger is an analyst and Howard Horn is an associate at Warburg Dillon Read.

health status of the U.S. population, as reflected in growing life expectancy and reductions in infant mortality, has continued to improve. Furthermore, managed care has increased access to the health care delivery system by expanding coverage for pharmaceuticals, alternative medicine, preventive care services such as health screening, and primary care services.

Despite this track record, the industry has not only failed to capture any credit for its successes, but has consistently received bad press and has become a societal, political, and legal target. When the Health Care Financing Administration (HCFA) reduced Medicare risk rate increases as part of the Balanced Budget Act (BBA) of 1997 and some health plans responded by exiting the business, the popular press ran stories about health plans' "abandoning" seniors. No mention was made of the rate reductions as the root cause. When health plans introduced reminder cards and first-dollar coverage to increase the frequency of prenatal care, cancer screening, and basic physical examinations, the press ignored these beneficial programs. In 1996, when nearly 60 percent of plans reported that they had implemented at least one of the three most popular disease management programs (for asthma, diabetes, and congestive heart failure), the media failed to applaud them. And as health plans began to use various review programs to reduce clearly inappropriate care (such as cesarean sections and hysterectomies, driven more by income and malpractice considerations than by medical necessity), they were accused of interfering with the physician/patient relationship.

The industry's failure to earn credit for its positive contributions is the result of several factors, including (1) public-relations ineptitude; (2) fierce ideological opposition by advocates of a single-payer system; (3) clever maneuvering by the health care industry's other constituents; (4) the ongoing reluctance of our society to recognize health care as an economic resource rather than a "right"; (5) the lack of economic connection between the payer for and the user of medical services in an employer- and government-financed health care system; and (6) the large spread in industry ideology.

Public Relations Failure

While the managed care industry has been credited in the business community with reducing medical inflation, the industry systematically has failed to achieve recognition for the value it has delivered to patients. First-dollar coverage (no deductible and no copayment) has led to a dramatic expansion in coverage for and consumption of pharmaceuticals, alternative medicine services, prenatal care, immunizations, screenings, and primary care services. In fact, most of the cost savings achieved by managed care techniques have come from reductions in medically unnecessary hospital and specialist services, price concessions from providers and suppliers, and administrative efficiencies.

The fact that managed care has vastly increased access to health care has received little or no press attention. Rather, the industry has earned an image of profiteering by denying needed health care services and erecting obstacles between patient and physician. Ironically, 56 percent of U.S. health maintenance organizations (HMOs) lost money in 1998, and managed care companies have lower levels of profitability and returns on investment than many other health care industry participants have.[1]

The view that managed care companies deny services is not totally surprising, given that many managed care techniques such as utilization review, gatekeepers, and formularies clearly involve an intervention between provider and patient. Thus, the member may have the impression that cost control is more important than high-quality patient care. In addition, the industry blundered by using often poorly educated staff to carry out many of its medical management tasks. Physicians frequently complain that the utilization review person on the other end of the phone can't begin to understand his or her rationale for a given course of treatment. This frustration with the payer is then passed on to the patient with whom the physician, not the payer, has the personal history.

Managed care companies also have failed to create any relationship or brand awareness with their members. Oxford Healthplans probably came the closest to achieving a true relationship with its members through strong customer service, extensive use of nurse "hotlines," and providing coverage for innovative services such as alternative medicine. Oxford has held on to the vast majority of its membership despite severe service shortfalls and price increases in recent years.

The managed care industry also blundered by applying many of its managed care techniques equally across its membership base instead of isolating them to chronically and critically ill persons, who typically account for 70–80 percent of total medical expenditures. Thus, healthy members often were subject to the same annoying interventions as high-severity patients were but with little financial benefit to the plan and at great cost in terms of lost goodwill.

In some cases, health insurers simply stole defeat from the jaws of victory. For example, when actor Christopher Reeve sustained his horrifying injury, his health insurance company reportedly abandoned him once his lifetime benefit cap was reached, thus creating a high-profile industry enemy.[2] Suppose instead that his insurer had helped him to identify and secure additional health funds from other sources: The insurer could easily have played the role of hero and made a friend for life.

Finally, most of the cost savings achieved through the use of managed care techniques have accrued to employers instead of employees. Had employers and the industry been willing to share more of the cost savings, consumers might have taken certain inconveniences more in stride. Also, to the extent that consumers have shared in the cost savings either directly through lower premiums or indirectly through enhanced benefits, employers and health plans have not communicated these benefits to consumers very well.

The Dangerous Allure of Single-Payer Systems

In addition to suffering from its own missteps, the managed care industry, along with the entire private-sector health care financing system, has come under constant assault from advocates for universal coverage administered through a government-run single-payer system. Single-payer advocates, while largely driven by ideology, point to that fact that other nations have lower per capita health care expenditures than the United States has, without any measurably adverse consequences to health status. In fact, many European countries (the United Kingdom, Germany, and the Netherlands) have longer life expectancy and lower infant mortality than the United States despite significantly lower health expenditures as a percentage of gross domestic product (GDP).[3]

These traditional measures, however, do not adjust for the enormous demographic, socioeconomic, and value differences between the United States and other developed countries. The United States spends enormous sums of money on patients during the last months, weeks, days, and even hours of life when there is often little statistical evidence of medical benefit. In many other countries such patients would simply be made comfortable in their final hours, and the expense of a heroic procedure would be avoided. In the United States we don't let people die if there is even a remote chance of survival. While this ethic is costly, it has also resulted in major advances in medicine. Also, traditional aggregate measures of health status do not take into account quality-of-life measures. In 1997 in the United States $2.1 million was spent on reconstructive joint replacement, which might have little impact on overall life expectancy but can clearly improve quality of life.[4]

The current trend toward discrediting private-sector cost containment initiatives could serve to bolster the voice of single-payer advocates. In fact, if the Democrats win the next presidential election, we believe that a single-payer system could once again surface as a seriously considered policy solution to the new crisis in health care.

Public Relations in Other Health Care Sectors

In sharp contrast to the managed care industry, other health industry participants have done a far better job at public relations. After coming under fire from the Clinton administration in the early 1990s, the pharmaceutical industry has successfully repositioned itself in the public's and politicians' eyes as a research industry. No politician would ever suggest that we should spend less money on research, regardless of the high profit margins and returns enjoyed by pharmaceutical companies. Emphasizing the political appeal of generously funding research, the president's budget for the National Institutes of Health called for an unprecedented increased investment in medical research of $1 billion in 1999, and there is sentiment in Congress to increase spending even further.[5] Even physicians have regained some ground by positioning themselves as victims alongside their managed care patients, notwithstanding median annual earnings of $164,000 in 1997 versus $34,674 for the average working male and $24,973 for the average working female.[6] This is not to say that these constituencies do not deserve their popularity, profits, or high incomes, only that the managed care industry has missed an opportunity to achieve the same status in light of its contributions.

Unfortunately, these other sectors also have positioned themselves as adversaries to managed care. Many physicians have publicly expressed their anti–managed care sentiments, and the pharmaceutical industry has been a silent bystander while Congress debated the Patients' Bill of Rights. Their stance, however, is understandable, given that managed care companies initially created pressure on pricing, margins, and incomes in many segments of the health care system.

However, if managed care is dismantled, the likelihood of a national health insurance system administered and financed by government will increase. It is somewhat surprising and shortsighted, therefore, that the pharmaceutical industry, the American Medical Association, the Federation of American Health Systems, and others have not yet come to the defense of managed care. A single-payer, government-financed system would surely reduce profitability and returns across the entire spectrum of health care participants as it has elsewhere in the world.

In the United Kingdom, under a nationalized health care system, the pharmaceutical industry absorbed a 4.5 percent government price reduction in mid-July 1999 for drugs sold in the United Kingdom.[7] As a result, the Warburg Dillon Read Pan-European pharmaceutical team expects only low single-digit growth in Pan-European pharmaceutical sales during the next three years, versus growth in the mid to high teens in the U.S. market. U.S. pharmaceutical EBITDA (earnings before interest, taxes, depreciation, and amortization) margins average 29.24 percent, while the global average excluding the United States is 23.3 percent.[8] In addition, a national health system could have a direct negative impact on infrastructure spending and on research and development and overall capital flows into the health care sector.

An Economic Resource

Americans still have not come to terms with the fact that health care is an economic resource that must be rationed like other resources. We have put the managed care industry in the unfair position of having to make resource-allocation decisions that should be made by consumers, the government, or medical ethicists. Unfortunately, universal coverage and indemnity-style insurance are often viewed as being the same as unlimited access to health care. However, a national health insurance system would simply substitute a government rationing system for a market mechanism. A return to old-style indemnity insurance would likely result in higher medical premiums, and lack of affordability would then act as a rationing mechanism.

Disconnect Between Payers and Users

There is little direct economic linkage between consumers, providers, and financiers in our third-party payment system. As a result, consumers do not have any economic incentive to watch how the health care dollar is spent because it is not "their" money. Similarly, providers have little incentive to be sensitive to the consumer's demand curve, because they recognize that the consumer usually is not footing the bill. Attempts to better align consumers', providers', and payers' interests through vehicles such as medical savings accounts have met stiff political resistance from those who believe that such plans would benefit only the healthy rich. However, in our opinion, creating a structure in which the consumer has a financial incentive to spend wisely would act as a significant deflationary force on today's medical cost trends without compromising quality.

Large Spread in Ideology

Managed care plans do not share a common legacy, and they still operate with very different ideological and strategic approaches to the marketplace. These differences have made it difficult for the industry to join ranks to gain public and political support. Tension within the industry is illustrated by the fact that the nation's largest managed care companies do not belong to a common trade group. Although heterogeneity is not a surprising characteristic in a young and challenged industry, more unity probably would serve the health care industry well in political and public-policy circles.

■ LEGISLATION, LITIGATION, AND INVESTIGATIONS

The failure of the managed care industry to capture credit for its accomplishments has led to a significant societal backlash. Ironically, it is precisely the industry's success that has shifted the health care debate back to access and quality and away from costs. Playing on the growing public discontent with managed care, politicians and class-action lawyers have chosen their next target after tobacco: the managed care industry.

The managed care industry is under attack. Anti–managed care consumer groups are lobbying for significant regulatory and legislative changes aimed at curbing alleged managed care abuses. Politicians and legislators have responded by proposing and enacting anti–managed care legislation at both the state and federal levels. Three states—California, Georgia, and Texas—have passed laws enabling people to sue their health plans for medical malpractice with compensatory and punitive damages, and twenty-eight states have passed prompt-payment and anticapitation legislation. Many states have passed legislation mandating specific practice guidelines such as minimum lengths-of-stay for maternity care, restrictions on the application of pharmaceutical formularies, and hospital staffing ratios. Finally, sixty-eight Republicans in the House of Representatives crossed party lines to pass the Norwood-Dingell Patients' Bill of Rights that includes liability as one of its key components.

These legislative mandates are systematically removing the very tools that managed care companies and others have used to manage costs. Ironically, these techniques have yet to be proven to be detrimental to health plan members on a widespread basis. The industry has recently been hit with a number of class-action suits alleging that managed care techniques represent a breach of fiduciary duty under the Employee Retirement Income Security Act (ERISA) and fraud under the Racketeer Influenced and Corrupt Organization (RICO) Act. Fear of litigation is likely to lead managed care companies to reduce the use of medical management techniques such as utilization review and gatekeepers, which could cause the medical cost trend to rise again.

■ *THE FUTURE OF THE INDUSTRY*

Given the growing hostility toward traditional managed care techniques, the industry clearly will be forced to change. The question is whether it will have to abandon the innovations of the past decade and revert to indemnity insurance practices, or whether it will innovate again and find new ways to meet the health care needs of consumers while managing medical cost trends for employers and the government. Another key consideration is whether the industry will have the time and continued access to capital needed to innovate and to change its image, given the speed with which the legislative and legal systems are moving against current industry practices.

We believe that all constituents would be better served if health plans were to focus on the creation of efficient markets for health care services. Under such a model the health plan would no longer be viewed as an obstacle to care or as interfering in the physician/patient relationship. Rather, the health plan would be viewed as a facilitator of care, a purveyor of useful information, and a provider of helpful services. In their ultimate form health plans would no longer need to create networks or even specific insurance products. Rather, through the use of "smart cards" (credit and identification cards that are embedded with medical and financial information and have "read/write" capabilities) and the Internet, plan members would essentially create their own individualized virtual networks and products through their own choice.

The naysayers will undoubtedly say that patients are not sophisticated enough to participate this aggressively in their own medical decision making, that accurate outcomes data are too hard to collect and to interpret, that physicians will not cooperate, and that application of market forces to health care simply will not work. We acknowledge that this new paradigm would involve significant changes in attitudes among all constituents in the health care delivery system and sizable capital investments and innovation in information systems. However, we believe that it represents an option more consistent with American values of free markets, consumer empowerment, and choice than the alternative of a health care system that is heavily controlled and regulated by government.

Given the importance of innovation and capital investments to this outcome, we hope that policymakers and the public will not overreact to the shortcomings of the existing system with legislation that results in diminished access to capital. Clearly, a rush to a single-payer system would not only kill innovation in the organization and delivery of health care services but would undoubtedly have a negative impact on the future of the entire health care industry as well, including the pharmaceutical, biotechnology, and medical technology segments that offer such a bright future for the treatment and eradication of disease. If politicians and the public are able to avoid a "rush to judgment," we believe that a number of existing managed care companies can help to solve the problem.

■ ASSESSING THE MANAGED CARE COMPANIES

Large Companies

Based on our near-term view that the threat of litigation and the implementation of specific practice guidelines at the state level could lead to an acceleration in utilization and overall cost trends, we are using a selective approach to recommending stocks. It will be difficult for stocks to move higher if the fragile margin recovery that began last year is derailed by accelerating cost trends that outstrip today's rising rate increases.

We have positive investment ratings on a number of industry participants because they are large and therefore have the financial ability to invest in next-generation managed care systems. A number of these companies are already creating and implementing next-generation managed care techniques and thus are less likely to be subject to legal action or a substantive rise in costs. Companies that fall into these categories are Aetna for scale; CIGNA and WellPoint for scale and lower probability of legal action; and United-

Health Group for scale, lower probability of litigation, and next-generation managed care. We believe that companies that have used a fee-for-service model of reimbursing providers are generally less vulnerable to RICO and other suits.

Other Companies

We are concerned about the prospects for most other managed care companies in light of recent earnings results and the points articulated here. These other companies lack either the scale, the financial resources, or the vision to accomplish the changes necessary to succeed in the future. Additionally, some of these companies are experiencing near-term operational and financial problems. We believe that the only real long-term hope for these companies is to sell to one of their large peers.

We have articulated for some time now our belief that premium increases today are beginning to outstrip medical cost increases for the majority of the publicly traded managed care organizations. The result has been a downtrend in MLRs for the universe of publicly traded companies. Historically, relative stock-price performance has had an inverse correlation with MLR trends. That is, stocks have outperformed the market when MLRs were declining and underperformed the market when MLRs were increasing. Given ongoing capacity withdrawals and an attempt by the industry to improve profitability, we expect premium trends to continue a sharp upward acceleration over the next several years. In addition to improving MLR trends, earnings estimates have been stable to rising for the larger players, returns of equity appear to have bottomed out, and the ratio of operating cash flow to net income appears to be improving, which suggests a rebuilding of reserves.

Unfortunately, we believe that recent legislative and legal events could delay or derail the fragile industry recovery by creating an upturn in medical utilization. The capital investment that companies will need to transform themselves into next-generation managed care entities will be substantial.

Only the large managed care players will thrive, because they have the ability to invest in systems and adapt to the changing operational paradigm. In our opinion, small companies will have less opportunity as the industry changes, because of their lack of scale and size, unless they are able to leapfrog the competition through tremendous innovation. This could contribute to another round of consolidation as companies try to preserve franchise value and membership.

Notes

1. "Over Half of HMOs Lose Money for Second Consecutive Year," *Medical Benefits*, 15 September, 1999, 3.

2. Reeve's difficulties with insurance are documented in a variety of places, including "Dana and Chris Reeve," *Ladies' Home Journal,* November 1999, 240.

3. W.B. Schwartz, *Life Without Disease* (Berkeley, Calif.: University of California Press, 1998).

4. "Orthopedic Implants: 'Off and Running,'" *Med-Pro Month* (October 1999): 286.

5. "A Dramatic, Unprecedented Increase: President Unveils 1999 Budget for NIH," *NIH Record,* 24 February 1998 (http://www.nih.gov/news/NIH-Record/02_24_98/story04.htm).

6. American Medical Association, *Socioeconomic Characteristics of Medical Practice,* 1997–1998, (Chicago: AMA, 1998); and U.S. Bureau of the Census, "Money Income in the United States: 1998," *Current Population Reports,* Series P-60 (Washington: U.S. Government Printing Office, 1998).

7. K.H. Koch et al., *European Pharmaceuticals Handbook* (New York: Warburg Dillon Read LLC, 1999), 5.

8. Ibid., 7.

Discussion Questions

1. Medicare has been termed "America's automated teller machine." Is this an accurate description of Medicare? Discuss.

2. Managed care has been described as "America's best health care hope." To what extent do you agree or disagree with this statement?

3. How realistic are Americans about the responsibilities and the limitations of managed care?

4. There are many myths surrounding managed care. With which of those myths do you agree or disagree? State your reasons.

5. What are the pitfalls of a managed care health plan that is investor owned?

6. How can you ascertain whether your managed care program focuses more on its investors than on its patients?

7. What is your assessment of the media's role in the public's perception of managed care?

8. Why has managed care failed to capitalize on its successes?

9. What would happen to our health care system if managed care were dismantled? What alternatives are available?

10. What do you predict will be the future of managed care in this country?

Further Readings

Bonyman, C. G., Jr. (1999). Muddled care managed care. *Health Affairs, 18*(5), 264–266.

Peak, T. & Barusch, A. (1999). Managed care: A critical review. *Journal of Health and Social Policy. 11*(1), 21–36.

Rodwin, M. A. (1999). Backlash as prelude to managing managed care. *Journal of Health Politics, Policy and Law, 24*(5), 1115–1127.

Terry, K. (2000). Where's managed care headed? *Medical Economics, 77*(7), 244–256.

Thorpe, K. E. (1999). Managed care as victim or villain? *Journal of Health Politics, Policy and Law, 24*(5), 1061–1071.

Vladeck, B. C. (1999). Managed care's 15 minutes of fame. *Journal of Health Politics and Law, 24*(5), 1207–1211.

Web Site Resources for Delivering Health Care

Managed Care Central   www.familiesusa.org/managedcare
Managed Care Information Center   www.themcic.com
Medicare Health Plan   www.medicare.gov
Medicare HMO   www.medicarehmo.com/mcmnu.htm

General Search Engine Web Sites

Metacrawler   www.metacrawler.com
Microsoft Network   www.msn.com

Health Web Sites

Combined Health Information Database   www.chid.nih.gov
Medicare Rights Center   www.medicarerights.org
PharmInfoNet   www.pharminfo.com
U.S. Department of Health and Human Services   www.healthfinder.com

Professional Journal Web Sites

Managed Care Magazine   www.managedcaremag.com
MedWebPlus   www.medwebplus.com

Economics: Dollars and "No Sense"?

The English writer Izaak Walton once said, "Look to your health; and if you have it, it is . . . a blessing that money cannot buy." These days, money can't buy even that. Health, nowadays, comes at a price many people cannot afford.

This is a time of economic contradiction. We have new drugs that have improved our lives enormously, yet many people do without because they cannot afford them. We live in a time when, despite the convenient proximity of local drugstores, people travel to Canada or Mexico to buy their drugs for less money. We live in a time of unparalleled prosperity, and yet people living below the poverty level spend 50% of their income on medications. We have unlimited food choices, yet choices for many people are limited; they either eat or buy medications. We live in a time of low inflation, yet drug costs have risen four times the rate of inflation this past year alone.

Undoubtedly, drug coverage for Medicare and Medicaid recipients is a "hot-button" issue in this country. The escalation of drug costs and grossly inadequate drug coverage are hard to ignore. The problem has been evident for a number of years, and it's not only growing, it's getting worse. The future will be a gloomy one for millions of people if a solution is not found quickly.

Why is something so obviously in need of a solution taking so long to accomplish? Two words come to mind: *money* and *politics*. The pharmaceutical industry is much admired in the corporate world for its ability to reap large profits for the drugs they produce and market. Because their drug patents give them a monopoly, pharmaceutical companies can charge whatever they want—and they do. However they may justify drug costs, their bottom line is profit making and plenty of it. Their lobbying efforts in Congress, for example, cost them a small fortune, but if these efforts delay or defeat any legislative measure that would adversely affect their profits, the cost is well worth it.

The political arena is no less contentious. Partisan debate, growing controversy, and a flurry of proposals of one sort or another swirl in and around the halls of Congress. The general theme in Congress is not *if* there will be a drug coverage benefit, but *how* it will be fashioned. Congress must overcome several key obstacles to arrive at a solution, including eligibility, cost containment, affordability, and financing. Whether an election year will bring about these needed changes is anyone's guess. Delaying the solution will only worsen the problem. And then what?

The economic ramifications of Medicare reform and its political resolution are the focus of this chapter. The emphasis of the readings in this chapter include an overview of Medicare's evolution and role in our country's health care, problems of cost containment, financial limits of health care, and several proposals for Medicare reform. When equitable and affordable solutions are found, then Medicare reform will be the blessing of health that money can buy for all its recipients.

54

Healing Medicare

Laura D'Andrea Tyson

Before enactment of Medicare in 1965, few elderly persons had reliable health insurance. When insurance was available, it was expensive and limited, and its renewal was uncertain. As a consequence, nearly 50 percent of the elderly had no health insurance at all, and faced bankruptcy from the costs of serious illness. Medicare provided all elderly Americans 65 or older with health coverage if they or their spouse had worked in a job subject to payroll taxation. As a reliable source of basic health insurance for the elderly, the Medicare program has been a tremendous success. Today, however, Medicare faces formidable challenges: an inadequate benefits package, an inefficient system of delivery, and a long-term budget gap.

In principle, getting rid of the inefficiencies would help expand coverage and reduce the budget shortfall. But how to achieve these goals is the subject of political and technical dispute.

Incomplete Coverage. Medicare was designed according to the medical and insurance practices of the mid-1960s. It excludes prescription drug coverage, "catastrophic" coverage (for conditions requiring long-term care), and coverage for many preventive services—all features of most private insurance plans. Medicare's deductibles and co-payments for inpatient hospital services are higher than most private plans. Compared to private health insurance in the United States, not to mention universal coverage abroad, Medicare's benefit package is parsimonious.

As a result of gaps in its benefits, Medicare covers only about 50 percent of total health care spending by the elderly. Less affluent households must devote more of their income to health spending than richer ones—or go without care. This regressivity is offset to some extent by Medicaid programs, which help low-income Americans cover their Medicare premiums, co-payments, and deductibles and buy prescription drugs. However, these programs are limited to the poorest Medicare beneficiaries, and coverage is incomplete.

Laura D'Andrea Tyson is Dean, Haas School of Business, University of California at Berkeley.

Wasted Resources. Medicare's current structure, which relies on price controls to limit costs, fosters inefficiencies. Providers maximize income by encouraging utilization of services to compensate for their controlled prices; beneficiaries have weak financial incentives to use Medicare services in a cost-sensitive manner. Neither the Health Care Financing Administration (HCFA), the agency responsible for running Medicare, nor Congress can readily adjust the prices of tens of thousands of medical services to reflect rapidly changing market and technological conditions. So Medicare prices can diverge from market prices for long periods of time. Price controls also produce a strong inducement for fraud among Medicare suppliers. The free choice of provider, so popular with Medicare beneficiaries, is also an obstacle to the efficient management of care. Current law prevents HCFA from using such efficiency-enhancing measures as competitive bidding, selective contracting with preferred providers, and disease and case management techniques common to the private health care system. Legislative efforts to allow HCFA to use such techniques have been effectively blocked by supplier groups.

Medicare's inefficiencies are reflected in large and persistent regional differences in Medicare costs per beneficiary, differences that cannot be explained by living costs or demographics. At least one-quarter of the four-to-one regional differences in Medicare spending per capita is the result of differences in patterns of medical practice and utilization of medical services, with no observable effects on regional health outcomes. So reducing inefficiencies in the current Medicare system can slow spending growth without reducing the quality of care. The question is how—and how much?

A Budget Gap. Even with its meager benefits package and even after significant spending cuts mandated by the Balanced Budget Act of 1997, Medicare faces a long-term budget crunch. Medicare's financing difficulties reflect both the aging of the population and the growth of overall health care spending. By 2030, Medicare enrollment will double from 40 million to 80 million Americans. On average, medical outlays for persons aged 65 and older are nearly four times as large as outlays for persons aged 19 to 54. But changing demographics are not the main source of Medicare's projected growth. Rather, increases in per capita Medicare spending are driven by technological breakthroughs in medicine and their increasing utilization. Barring unforeseen—and highly unlikely—changes in medical technologies that significantly slow the growth of overall health care costs, the Medicare system will require additional revenues.

▦ THE POLITICS OF REFORM

The 1997 budget agreement mandated deep cuts in projected Medicare spending over 10 years mainly through the usual price-control mechanisms. The agreement also enhanced the ability of Medicare beneficiaries to choose among traditional fee-for-service Medicare, health maintenance organizations, and preferred-provider organizations, and broadened the number of experiments testing the applicability of such private-sector techniques as competitive bidding and case management to Medicare. In addition, the budget deal established a bipartisan commission to recommend financial and programmatic reforms to address Medicare's long-term challenges.

The commission split along partisan and philosophical lines. For a variety of reasons—most notably the absence of an immediate Medicare crisis—a supermajority of the commission's 17 members was unable to agree on recommendations, and the commission ended in the spring of 1999 without issuing a final report. Nonetheless, the commission's deliberations and the Clinton administration's July 1999 proposal in response are instructive for what they reveal about the likely direction of Medicare reform in the future. The major issues dividing the commission were drug benefits, the role of competition in a reformed Medicare program, and long-term strategies for reducing the budget gap.

■ DRUG BENEFITS

Four out of five senior citizens are prescribed at least one daily drug treatment, and one in five takes five prescribed drugs per day. Per capita spending on drugs by the elderly is more than three times that of other adults and nearly 10 times that of children. On average, an elderly American spends more than $600 per year on drugs, with one in 10 spending more than $2,000 per year. Despite the obvious need for prescription drugs, about 35 percent of the elderly have no drug insurance. The remaining 65 percent obtain some drug coverage, much of it incomplete, through three channels: Medicaid (which affects only the 20 percent of the elderly living below the poverty line), supplemental insurance policies provided by former employers, and private insurance plans. The resulting patchwork system is riddled with inequities, inefficiencies, and excess administrative costs. Only about 30 percent of employers currently offer retiree health benefits, and that number is steadily declining. Annual premiums already exceed $1,000 for supplemental policies with limited nondrug benefits and an annual cap of $1,250 on drug spending. The majority of elderly Americans, whose annual incomes are less than $25,000, cannot afford such bare-bones Medigap policies.

According to a recent analysis by the National Academy of Social Insurance, a Medicare drug benefit will cost between $10 billion and $24 billion annually, depending on its terms. Adding prescription drug coverage to Medicare as a purely voluntary option won't work because of the "adverse selection" problem: The relatively healthy, whose premiums are needed to subsidize the sick, will tend not to buy drug coverage absent a generous government subsidy. Those most likely to choose the drug coverage option are those most likely to incur significant drug costs. But without an insurance pool that includes both the well and the sick, the sick would face astronomical and unaffordable premium costs.

According to the federal government actuary, a subsidy of about 50 percent of the premium price would be necessary to convince the majority of beneficiaries to enroll voluntarily in a Medicare drug coverage program, thereby solving the adverse selection problem. Without an adequate subsidy, this problem could be solved if all Medicare beneficiaries were required to participate in such a program. But mandatory participation is not viewed as a viable political option, in light of the resounding defeat of efforts to add a mandatory catastrophic-care option to Medicare in the late 1980s.

A related problem is that generously subsidizing Medicare drug coverage with federal dollars will drive out billions of private dollars already spent through employer-provided plans and private policies, increasing federal spending without a commensurate increase in prescription drug coverage. To many skeptics, this "substitution" of federal dollars for private dollars is simply wasteful. But there is no way around it if the adverse selection problem is to be resolved.

If Medicare did cover prescription drugs, how would they be priced? The federal government uses price controls for other services covered by Medicare. Would the price control mechanism be extended to drugs? If so, how would the government set the prices it would pay for drugs over time, and how would it deal with the rapid introduction of new drugs? Concerns over government price controls are the major reason the drug industry remains strenuously opposed to adding drug coverage to Medicare, and the industry stands ready to exercise its substantial political clout to stop it. Indeed, the industry even opposes a compromise solution, which would allow the same private beneficiary providers that act as drug purchasers for HMOs to act as drug purchasers for Medicare.

The chairmen of the National Bipartisan Commission on the Future of Medicare, Senator John Breaux and Congressman Bill Thomas, proposed a new subsidy to the poorest elderly (those with annual incomes of less than $11,000) for the purchase of limited drug coverage through private plans. The Democratic members of the commission rejected this recommendation on grounds of efficiency and equity. First, given the meager proposed subsidy, the unresolved adverse-selection problem would price drug coverage out of range for many low-income beneficiaries. And second, limiting a new Medicare drug subsidy to the poorest beneficiaries would violate Medicare's basic structure as a social insurance program available to all elderly Americans regardless of income.

Both criticisms helped shape the proposal for Medicare drug coverage offered by the Clinton administration in July 1999 and the proposals currently championed by Vice President Al Gore and Bill Bradley in their presidential campaigns. All three introduce a new voluntary Medicare prescription drug benefit, with a generous federal subsidy. The Clinton administration and Vice

President Gore offer a voluntary program in which the government would pay half of the costs of prescription drugs for each beneficiary, up to a total of $5,000 with no deductible. Additional subsidies would be available for elderly with incomes below 150 percent of poverty, fully covering the premiums and cost sharing for those with incomes below 135 percent of poverty. To strengthen the incentives to participate, these plans would ensure that, even after the $5,000 cap is hit, beneficiaries would continue to receive price discounts on drug purchases. To counter concerns that Medicare drug coverage would drive out private coverage, the Clinton-Gore plans also provide financial incentives for employers to retain prescription drug benefits for retirees.

Bradley's plan does not cap overall drug benefits, but it does have a deductible and more stringent co-payment requirements. Although the latter features provide stronger incentives to discourage unnecessary drug expenditures than do the no-deductible Clinton-Gore plans, such features are unlikely to win favor with the Medicare beneficiaries who prefer first-dollar coverage. Even with these incentives, the absence of an overall cap means that Bradley's drug plan is about twice as expensive as Vice President Gore's.

Despite these and other technical differences between the Clinton-Gore and Bradley drug coverage proposals, all three of them share an important feature. They eschew price controls, relying instead on the negotiations between private benefits managers and drug companies to determine the prices to be charged to Medicare beneficiaries. Medicare would operate much like HMOs that rely on such managers to negotiate drug prices for their covered patients. Because of its sheer size, however, Medicare would have significant clout in such negotiations—which is why the drug industry remains opposed.

Similar opposition to Medicare's bargaining strength has also blocked numerous proposals to allow Medicare to engage in competitive bidding to determine the prices of other covered services rather than to pay a set of controlled prices to "any willing provider" of such services. If Medicare is to move away from its antiquated and increasingly ineffective system of price controls, it will have to be granted the ability to pick and choose among providers and to exercise purchasing power against drug companies just as private plans do.

This conclusion motivated the Clinton administration to recommend that Medicare be allowed to adopt techniques already proven effective in the private sector at controlling costs without impairing the quality of care. These techniques include preferred-provider options in which beneficiaries are charged lower prices if they choose service from designated high-quality providers, competitive bidding and selective contacting in purchases of goods and services, and capitated disease- and case-management techniques in contracts for the treatment of high-cost chronic diseases like diabetes and coronary heart disease.

▨ COMPETITION AND MARKET REFORM

Most members of the National Bipartisan Commission on the Future of Medicare were convinced of the necessity of enhancing Medicare's ability to negotiate with private providers, except in the area of drugs. But a majority of commission members wanted to go even further by allowing private plans to compete directly with one another and with HCFA in the provision of all Medicare benefits. The purpose of such competition would be to encourage more efficient, cost-sensitive decision making by both producers and consumers in the Medicare program. Producers would be encouraged to become more efficient because they would be allowed to compete with one another for Medicare dollars. Consumers would be encouraged to become more cost conscious because they would be allowed to choose among competing plans for their Medicare services and to pay lower Medicare premiums if they chose lower-cost plans. Both economic logic and the experiences of the Federal Employees Health Benefits Program and other employer-sponsored programs allowing beneficiaries a choice among comparable insurance plans on the basis of price indicate that a similar system for Medicare could generate cost savings over time. There is, however, considerable uncertainty about the magnitude of this potential effect.

The competition approach espoused by the majority of commission members had two defining features. First, all plans granted permission by the government to compete for Medicare beneficiaries would be required to offer the same specified set of benefits as those in the standard fee-for-service Medicare plan. This condition was necessary to guarantee that competition among plans would be based on price and quality, not on coverage. Second, the government would make a contribution toward the payment of the premium of the plan chosen by each beneficiary, with the remainder paid by the beneficiary. The government's contribution would be set as a percentage of the weighted average of the costs of all plans, including the standard HCFA fee-for-service plan, competing to provide Medicare benefits. Setting and adjusting this percentage over time would be key political decisions, determining how Medicare costs were shared among beneficiaries and taxpayers. At least initially, commission members proposed setting this percentage at about 88 percent, the federal government's current share in Medicare spending per beneficiary.

The commission's competition approach preserved Medicare's entitlement to a specified set of benefits, allowed beneficiaries to pay lower premiums for plans covering such benefits at lower prices, and imposed a specified share of the risk of rising Medicare costs to its beneficiaries. Such an approach, which has come to be called a "premium support" approach in the health care field, should not be confused with a voucher approach. In a voucher system, such as the one proposed by the Republican Congress in 1995, the government would pay a fixed dollar amount to each beneficiary toward the purchase of a private plan without specifying the benefits to be covered. A voucher model would replace the Medicare entitlement to a package of specified health benefits with an entitlement to a government subsidy to purchase private health coverage. And if the value of this subsidy were set in nominal dollar terms, as the 1995 Republican plan proposed, all of the burden of rising health care costs would be borne by the beneficiaries.

Although the premium-support approach has several desirable features, it also has some serious downside risks. First, like any system based on choice in insurance markets, this approach would enhance the ability of providers to isolate the sickest population into small high-cost pools. This risk could be mitigated with a mandate that each participating health plan accept all Medicare beneficiaries who apply for coverage, and charge them the same premium regardless of difference in their age, sex, disability status, and other health risk indicators. The government's premium contribution to different plans would then be "risk adjusted" to vary depending on the risk characteristics of their enrollees, but the premium contributions of all enrollees choosing a particular plan would remain the same.

Second, given significant regional differences in health costs, there could also be significant regional differences in the premiums of private plans competing to provide such services in a premium-support system. This risk could be mitigated with an adjustment of the government's premium contributions so that Medicare beneficiaries would not be required to pay more for the same package of services because they lived in high-cost regions or because there were few competing plans in their regions.

Third, if the government's premium contribution were set as a percentage of the weighted average costs of participating plans, including traditional fee-for-service Medicare, and if its costs grew more rapidly than the costs of alternative plans, then those choosing the fee-for-service option could face significant increases in their premiums. As a result, although the Medicare entitlement to a specified set of services would be protected under the premium-support approach, the Medicare entitlement to receive these services with unlimited choice among providers in a fee-for-service setting would not be. Given the strong preference of the elderly, particularly those who are older and sicker, for choice among providers, and given mounting public skepticism about managed care, the risk of eroding Medicare's entitlement to an affordable fee-for-service option is the major reason for virulent opposition to the premium-support approach. Such an approach is based precisely on the idea that beneficiaries choosing more expensive plans would pay more while those choosing cheaper ones would pay less. This would mean that Medicare beneficiaries with limited incomes would be encouraged to choose low-cost plans and could be priced out of high-cost plans, including the fee-for-service plan to which they are currently entitled in the Medicare program.

The July 1999 Clinton plan proposed a compromise, allowing greater competition and choice in Medicare services while guaranteeing that beneficiaries selecting Medicare's traditional fee-for-service program continue to pay only the premium required by current law. The president's plan introduced a new "competitive defined benefit program," which, like the premium-support model, would allow private plans to compete with one another and with HCFA to offer a specified set of Medicare benefits. In contrast to the current Medicare+Choice system, in which the government pays managed-care providers a flat payment based on the costs of Medicare's fee-for-service plan, in the competitive defined-benefit model, the government would pay private plans on the basis of their actual price bids. Payment to competing plans on the basis of such bids has been used successfully by private employers and the Federal Employees Health Benefits Program to enhance efficiency and contain program costs. In the Clinton plan, beneficiaries could choose among plans offering Medicare benefits at prices lower than the cost of HCFA's traditional fee-for-service program, and they would be allowed to keep 75 percent of the resulting premium savings, with the remainder going to the Medicare program. Those who chose a more expensive plan than the traditional one would pay the full additional cost of their selection. And the government would continue to rely on price controls and whatever private-sector management techniques it was authorized to use over time to control the costs of the traditional fee-for-service program.

In contrast to the premium-support model, the president's competitive defined-benefits model would preserve Medicare's entitlement both to a specified set of benefits and to fee-for-service medicine with unlimited choice among providers. The preservation of the latter entitlement would come at the price of considerably smaller savings in projected Medicare expenditures. Indeed, the administration estimated that the savings resulting from its competitive defined-benefits plan would only amount to about $8 billion over its first 10 years. In contrast, the commission estimated that premium support would save $66 billion over its first decade. And over the long run, the commission optimistically assumed that the efficiencies fostered by premium support would slow Medicare spending about a percentage point per year. Even the most ardent proponents of such an approach among academic economists warn that its aggregate savings are likely to be far smaller and insufficient to resolve Medicare's long-run financing gap.

■ MEDICARE'S FINANCIAL HEALTH

As an additional measure to slow the long-run growth of Medicare spending, the chairmen of the commission recommended a gradual increase in the age of eligibility for Medicare from 65 to 67, to conform to Social Security's gradual increase in the age of eligibility to 67, by 2022. According to commission estimates, the proposed increase in the eligibility age for Medicare would eliminate about one-quarter of the projected gap between Medicare Part A expenditures and revenues by 2030. But this financial improvement would come at the cost of an increased number of uninsured Americans. According to recent estimates, between 10 percent and 20 percent of Americans aged 65–66 would lose health insurance if Medicare's age of eligibility were increased to 67, which would in turn aggravate one of the glaring failings of the American health care system: the large and growing number of the uninsured.

In contrast to the commission's proposal, the Clinton plan left Medicare's eligibility age at 65 and allowed Americans between ages 55 and 65 to purchase Medicare coverage at an actuarially fair market price. The new buy-in option was designed to pay for itself while addressing the problem of uninsured older Americans. In recent years, the number of uninsured has been growing most rapidly among Americans aged 55–65, who are twice as likely to have health problems as the 45–55 age cohort.

Neither the commission's recommendations nor the president's plan proposed introducing income testing into Medicare premium payments. Income testing might be justified on the grounds that Medicare has become a distinctively regressive system over time, with poorer elderly both paying a larger fraction of their disposable income for health and utilizing Medicare services less extensively than richer elderly. But in order for there to be significant Medicare savings from income testing, either the high-income threshold for paying a higher premium would have to be set quite low or the income-related premiums would have to be set quite high. The former approach would require politically sensitive increases in premium payments for a large fraction of the Medicare population. The latter would encourage the more affluent elderly to choose private coverage over Medicare, undermining its social insurance function and relegating it to a program primarily for the poorer, sicker population.

Medicare requires major reforms. Incremental measures that rely on tightening arbitrary price controls will only increase dissatisfaction with the Medicare program from providers, beneficiaries, and taxpayers. Given the dramatic changes that have occurred in the health care system since 1965 when Medicare was first introduced, at least four types of changes in Medicare are warranted.

First, a meaningful prescription drug benefit must be added to Medicare on a voluntary basis, with the government relying on private benefits managers as intermediaries to negotiate drug prices. Second, Medicare must be granted authority to use modern management techniques to pick and choose among providers and plans based on their cost and quality of service. Third, to encourage greater efficiency in the Medicare program, private plans must be allowed to compete with HCFA and with one another to provide a specified benefits package on the basis of price and quality, and beneficiaries must be allowed to share in the savings resulting from choosing low-cost plans. This condition implies that Medicare must be reinterpreted as an entitlement to a government subsidy and choice among competing health care plans for coverage of specified benefits, not as an entitlement to unlimited selection among providers in a fee-for-service setting. Finally, if Medicare's unintended regressivity is to be reduced, its premium should vary with income, and the higher premiums paid by high-income beneficiaries should be used to finance an expansion of benefits for low-income beneficiaries.

Even with structural reforms that encourage more competition in the Medicare program, its costs per beneficiary should be expected to continue to rise at about the same pace as per capita private health care spending. And without unforeseen changes in medical technology, both kinds of spending will continue to grow faster than the overall economy. Reform proposals that assume or require that per capita Medicare costs grow more slowly than private health care costs are neither credible nor justifiable. The reason for reforming Medicare is to reduce its inadequacies, inequities, inefficiencies, and projected financing gap, not, as some alarmists would have it, to save the American economy from toppling under the weight of Medicare spending.

A modified and phased-in premium-support approach such as the one proposed by President Clinton, along with the addition of a prescription drug benefit and a limited degree of income testing, is a sensible yet cautious way to begin modernizing Medicare to meet its real challenges. Even these structural reforms will not solve Medicare's longterm financing gap. But the economy is strong enough to provide decent health care for America's elderly, and we can find the additional revenues to do so.

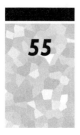

55

What Price Coverage Reform?

Aimee L. Stern

*I*n the year 2005, an eight-year-old boy falls off his skateboard and requires knee-replacement surgery. An 80-year-old man also wants a new knee so he can ski at Aspen this winter. Who gets the surgery? A cardiac patient who 10 years ago would have spent seven days in the hospital is discharged in three and a half. Where does he go, and who monitors his care? Medicare creates a voucher program and funnels the elderly into private HMOs. But this results in a dramatically lower reimbursement rate for hospitals. How will they make up for the lost income?

These three questions illustrate the coverage issues that will increasingly be major points of contention. The U.S. is now facing the worst health care crisis in its history, and Baby Boomers will surely be hit the hardest. The first wave of aging Boomers will reach retirement age by the year 2010, at the same time Medicare is predicted to face a trillion-dollar deficit. Health care costs are growing at 2.5 times the rate of inflation. And at their current rate of savings, few Baby Boomers will have enough retirement income to finance their own health care, according to Richard Lamm, former governor of Colorado, and professor of public policy at the University of Colorado in Denver.

Coverage reform, which began in earnest in the mid-1990s, is expected to continue at a rapid pace well into this century. Yet no matter what reforms are made, hospitals are going to be under enormous pressure to cut costs and services while providing high-quality medical care to aging communities. In this brave new world, trustees will be taking on greater oversight responsibilities than ever before.

"Trustees have tremendous opportunities to be influential as public spokespeople and to influence policy at a grassroots level," says James Roosevelt, associate commissioner of the Social Security Administration, and trustee of Mount Auburn Hospital in Cambridge, Mass. "We already see that

---

Aimee Stern is a business writer based in Washington, DC.

Reprinted from *Trustee*, January 2000, 53(1) 24, 26–27 by permission. Copyright © 2000 by Health Forum, Inc.

the most effective trustees are deeply involved in their communities and in touch with their needs and concerns."

In this century, health care organizations will focus largely on three critical issues: quality of life, quality of care, and the quality of the health care business. Here are some suggestions for how trustees can start to prepare.

▪ QUALITY OF LIFE

As society ages and people live longer, each generation will face a unique set of problems. As many elderly people begin to live well into their nineties, their Baby Boomer children will find themselves pulled in different directions: struggling to care for aging parents, struggling to send their children to college, and struggling to retire comfortably. Younger generations will most likely be asked to pay much higher taxes to support programs such as Medicare and Social Security.

When an aging society has fewer and fewer systems to support it, huge inequities can arise. Major ethical questions must be addressed over the issue of whether one generation should pay for the well-being of another, and, if so, to what extent. Society will have to examine systems that cut back on some health services. Lamm says that society will have to confront the significant question of whether age should even be a consideration in the delivery of health care.

Most Americans can now obtain health care services that are deemed necessary by their doctors, no matter how old or how sick they are. But at some point "who gets what?" will have to be addressed. Policymakers will begin asking questions such as, "Why should 44 million people go without health insurance when the wealthy get Medicare for free?"

There are no easy answers to these questions, and trustees will find themselves right in the middle of the debates. To prepare, Paul Hofmann, Ph.D., advises trustees to open up a dialogue with the communities they serve. A two-pronged approach may be the best way to go, says Hofmann, senior vice president of the health care industry practice at Aon Consulting, San Francisco, and a former hospital CEO. First, trustees need to learn more about the needs of local consumers; secondly, they need to educate them about the tough issues that their hospitals face.

One place to look for solutions is in Oregon, which took a proactive approach to reducing its number of uninsured. The state began by informing the public that it would have a limited number of dollars to spend on health care, and that it wanted to spend them wisely. Then it sponsored a series of town meetings with various hospital representatives and the people they served to engage them in a debate about what types of services should be state financed. The result was a plan that both constituents and politicians supported.

"Oregon's approach is not a panacea, but examining what the state did can help trustees get started," says Hofmann. "The state scrutinized how to deliver the appropriate services to different age groups and created a model for how to do it."

Trustees also need to let the general public know just how hard a job hospitals have today and explain some of the issues they will face in the future. Most people know very little about what goes on inside a hospital. Lamm says hospitals should invite the public, the media, and their local government representatives for a series of seminars explaining how hospitals handle emergencies, what kinds of care are available, and what investments they've made to improve quality of care. He believes the public often takes medical care for granted, so it's important to demonstrate that a hospital is a complex organization that struggles to provide quality care on a limited budget.

■ QUALITY OF CARE

For many hospitals in the last decade, cutting costs was a matter of survival. Hospitals began seriously cutting back in the mid-1980s when Medicare introduced DRGs (diagnosis-related groups), which set specific amounts of time patients should stay in the hospital per DRG. When a Medicare patient is discharged before the time limit expires, a hospital makes money. When the patient stays longer than the pre-set length of stay, the hospital often must eat the cost. In addition, the Balanced Budget Act of 1997 placed further restrictions on what hospitals could charge Medicare for various services.

As a result, many hospitals have been pushing hard to reduce the number of days patients spend in their facilities. When a public outcry was raised over women who were discharged the day after childbirth, some states mandated minimum-stay requirements. Pregnancy and childbirth are political hot potatoes, and legislators can score points by addressing them. But as costs skyrocket, hospitals are expected to push for abbreviated inpatient care for a broad range of conditions, no matter how much ill will the decisions may garner.

The fact is, shorter hospital stays are perfectly reasonable for many patients and procedures. But problems arise when hospitals do not address where patients will go after discharge, or monitor their level of follow-up care. Often, once patients are transferred to skilled nursing facilities, the hospital takes an "out-of-sight, out-of-mind" approach. Wanda Jones, president of the New Century Health Care Institute, San Francisco, points out that skilled nursing facilities are not always equipped to handle post-operative patients. Staff in these facilities are often trained in rehabilitation rather than the acute care management needed by post-operative patients. As a result, patients don't always get the care that they need, which can leave the hospital vulnerable to potential litigation if something goes wrong.

Jones recalls a presentation she saw given by the chief financial officer of an Arizona hospital. The CFO bragged that, while the recommended length of stay for cardiac patients was seven days, she managed to push them out of the hospital in just three-and-a-half days, making cardiac care a very profitable DRG. But the CFO could not explain what kind of care patients received in the skilled nursing facility where they were transferred after leaving the hospital.

Jones suggests that trustees address shortened stays by asking management, "What happens to those patients once they leave us?" Every hospital has written patient care guidelines and medical protocols that must be followed. Trustees should examine these protocols and have a medical professional explain them. Otherwise they will not know how the staff is cutting corners.

In addition, hospitals must recognize that they cannot offer as comprehensive a range of services as they once did, says Ken Kaufman, head of his Northfield, Ill., consulting firm. He recommends that trustees help management determine what services the community needs and figure out which of these it can afford to deliver. "The crunch is very serious now and will only get more so in the future," he says. "Hospitals must be highly directed in the things they do. They should decide what they do well and get out of the other services if they can."

■ QUALITY OF BUSINESS

Expect that in this century Medicare will push for privatizing a wide array of services. It will shift much of the responsibility for the elderly to HMOs and other entities and issue vouchers that will allow senior citizens to pay providers directly. Seniors may welcome this move because it will simplify their paperwork and allow them access to a wider range of services. However, hospitals, which are used to getting Medicare payments directly from the government, may see a dramatic drop in the amount of reimbursement they receive for services delivered, according to Uwe Reinhardt, the James E. Madison Professor of political economy at Princeton University.

Remember, Medicare is a not-for-profit program, points out Reinhardt. He says that only 2 percent of Medicare funds go for administrative costs, while 98 percent go directly to hospitals. Managed care organizations, on the other hand, use 15 to 20 percent of their premiums on marketing, administration, and returns to investors. Reinhardt expects that managed care organizations will pass along these costs to hospitals by lowering their reimbursement rates.

Trustees can take a number of approaches to ensure that their hospitals are prepared for the cutbacks. First they can study markets where privatization has already begun. Since California was one of the first states to embrace managed care, it is way ahead of many others in its evolution. Reinhardt suggests that trustees invite the CFOs of organizations such as Sacramento-based Sutter Health Systems or San Francisco–based Catholic Healthcare West to speak to the board and discuss how they are coping with privatization. These voices of experience may provide potential solutions that the board has not yet considered.

In addition, Kaufman says, hospitals may want to look to the corporate world for ideas. Most corporations have five- and 10-year "battle" plans that create likely scenarios and provide guidance on potential responses if those scenarios play out. Hospitals should draw up battle plans, too, and be prepared to change strategy as the market changes.

He suggests that trustees:

- Develop a better understanding of the hospital's strategic direction and work to shape that direction so it is flexible enough to respond to changing market dynamics
- Create a financial plan that measures and monitors the types of changes that have an impact on hospitals, such as Medicare payment adjustments
- Ensure that analytical tools, such as modeling and forecasting software, are available for conducting long- and short-range planning

The next few decades will be both a trying and exciting time for hospitals and their boards. Trustees will be in the forefront of creating health care systems that can survive and thrive well into the next century. "Trustees are in a wonderful position to help Americans frame the questions that will shape health care policy in the new millennium," says Lamm. "Charlie Brown says there is no problem so big you can't run away from it. Well, it's the hospital trustee's job to make sure we start facing up to the health care crisis today."

56

Problems With the Medicare Drug Benefit Plan ... And What Can Be Done

John C. Goodman and Merrill Mathews, Jr.

President Clinton has outlined a new prescription drug entitlement for people on Medicare, the federal health insurance program covering 39 million seniors and the disabled. The plan would:

- Pay half of all prescription drug costs, with no deductible, up to a maximum of $2,000 in expenses (i.e., the government would pay as much as $1,000) beginning in 2002, growing to a maximum of $5,000 in expenses (or $2,500 for the government) by 2008.
- Charge participating seniors $24 per month, increasing incrementally to $44 per month by 2008.
- Allow any Medicare beneficiary to join, with the expectation that 31 million eventually would enroll.

According to the White House, beneficiaries would pay a total of $110 billion in premiums over 10 years, while the federal government would kick in $118 billion (or $168 billion, according to the Congressional Budget Office).

Although Congress considered including a prescription drug benefit in 1965 when it created Medicare, concerns over additional costs and the paucity of advanced drugs undermined support for the benefit. So why do it now? Before Congress passes legislation extending such benefits, tough questions need to be answered.

Is It Needed? Today, seniors have access to a wide range of beneficial prescription drugs for both acute and chronic conditions. Many of the drugs are affordable for all but the poorest seniors, but some are very expensive. However, about 65% of Medicare beneficiaries have a prescription drug benefit to help them with those costs. Nevertheless, the White House expects the large majority of seniors—about 80%—to shift to the government plan because it will seem so cheap. Of course, the only reason it will seem cheap is that taxpayers will be subsidizing it.

John C. Goodman is President of the National Center for Policy Analysis and Merrill Mathews, Jr., is Vice President of Domestic Policy at the Dallas-based public policy think tank.

Reprinted with permission from *Consumers Research Magazine*, September 1999, 82(9) 16–19.

Who Will It Help? Ironically, the plan gives little help to seniors with low or high drug costs. But it's ideal for someone in the middle. Since seniors initially will pay $24 per month, or $288 per year, in premiums to get the benefit, they won't gain unless they have more than $576 in drug costs. (At exactly $576, the benefit—$576 ÷ 2 = $288—exactly equals the premiums.) And the total benefit is only $712 ($1,000 benefit minus $288 in premiums).

On the other hand, since the government will initially pay only $1,000 toward each senior's prescription drug costs, those with catastrophic costs—say, $12,000 a year or more—will get little help.

The president's plan also calls for paying the premiums and co-payments for those below the poverty level. But is that necessary? Low-income seniors already qualify for Medicaid as well as Medicare—and Medicaid provides drug coverage for 88% of them. While the president talks about helping the poor, he really is creating a middle-class entitlement.

Is It Fair? The plan redistributes wealth from the "have-nots" to the "haves." Young, low-income families will be taxed to pay the $118 billion subsidy paid by the federal government. However, people age 65 and older have more assets and more after-tax income per capita than those under age 65.

Will the Program Worsen Medicare's Financial Crisis? Medicare is already facing a long-run funding crisis twice the size of Social Security's. Although recent changes in the program and a strong economy have postponed collapse of the Part A Medicare trust fund until 2015, the tax burden is expected to soar in future years. By the time today's college students reach retirement age, Medicare taxes will have grown from the current level of about 5.35% of payroll (the 2.9% payroll tax which funds Part A plus the general revenue subsidy to Part B) to almost 14%. In order for these students to collect their own benefits, future workers—most of whom are not yet born—will have to pay one out of every seven dollars they earn (almost as much as they will pay to support Social Security) just to cover medical bills for the elderly.

Adding an expensive benefit to Medicare will only increase the burden on future generations.

What Will It Do to Drug Spending? Whether, on balance, seniors spend more under the president's proposal is still an open question, at least in the short term. If seniors who already have comprehensive prescription drug coverage drop their plans for the president's less comprehensive but less costly program, they may spend less. And those with no coverage who join the president's plan may spend more. But since coverage under the president's plan is scheduled to grow over time, the long-term effect will almost surely be increased spending.

One reason is utilization. When people are insulated from the cost of something, they tend to spend more. For example, according to a recent article in the health policy journal *Health Affairs:*

- Medicare beneficiaries without prescription drug coverage, on average, spend about $432 per year on drugs, all of it out-of-pocket.

■ Seniors with coverage spend about $691 per year on prescription drugs, with $232 coming out of their own pockets.

Can Managed Care Hold Down Costs? President Clinton has proposed turning to large pharmacy benefit management firms (PBMs) as a way of achieving economies of scale to hold down costs. PBMs in each geographic region would bid on providing the service to all Medicare enrollees, and the federal government would grant monopoly status to the successful firm. PBMs would purchase the drugs in large quantities at discounted prices and supposedly pass the savings on to seniors.

Currently, about 170 million Americans are in some form of managed care and many of them acquire prescription drugs through PBMs. However, concerns are growing that some PBMs sacrifice quality for quantity. PBMs are under contract to the drug companies, which tie payments to sales volumes of particular drugs. According to the American Medical Association's drug policy director Joseph Cranston: "The motivation is to sell that product, possibly at the expense of the right clinical decision." Thus the problem with PBMs appears similar to that with HMOs: the goal of controlling costs is sometimes achieved by sacrificing quality.

Are Price Controls Next? If the president has underestimated the program's cost or utilization or overestimated the budget surplus, Congress will be forced to raise premiums, raise taxes or impose price controls on drugs. The last option would be the most politically appealing—and the most devastating to research on and availability of new drugs.

Is the President Making the Problem Worse? Clinton administration policies have been reducing the number of seniors with a drug benefit by cutting reimbursement rates to Medicare HMOs. Some managed care plans got only a 2% increase in 1999, even though health care costs have been rising about 7%. As a result, many of the largest HMOs dropped out of some Medicare markets, leaving some 450,000 seniors, many of whom had drug coverage, scrambling to find new Medicare HMOs. Another 325,000 seniors may be dropped this year.

For the seniors who cannot afford the prescription drugs they need—and some cannot—it makes sense to consider a targeted solution rather than a broad-based new entitlement imposed on a financially strapped program.

To paraphrase P. J. O'Rourke from several years ago: You think drugs are expensive now, wait until the federal government decides to make them affordable.

■ . . . AND WHAT CAN BE DONE

In what follows, we propose four simple solutions that require no new taxes and no new government spending.

Solution #1: Free Medigap. The design of Medicare violates almost all the principles of sound insurance. The program pays too many small bills the elderly could easily afford on their own, while leaving them exposed to thousands of dollars of potential out-of-pocket expenses. For example, about 360,000 Medicare beneficiaries spend more than $5,000 out of pocket every year on Medicare-covered services. In addition, Medicare's failure to cover prescription drugs encourages the elderly to turn to more expensive (hospital and doctor) therapies.

In order to limit their financial exposure, about 75% of seniors acquire, either through a former employer or private purchase, supplemental (medigap) insurance, which pays many or all of the expenses Medicare does not.

However, federal law imposes Medicare's insurance philosophy on medigap insurers. Like Medicare, medigap policies must cover small-dollar items such as the Part A and Part B deductibles, but they need not cover the largest bills. Coverage for drugs is an option.

Were insurers given more freedom, they could create plans responsive to the needs of the market. Specifically, if insurers were free to forego coverage of many routine expenses, they could offer more generous drug coverage—with no increase in premiums (see example that follows).

Solution #2: Free Medicare. The combination of medigap insurance and Medicare is very wasteful. In fact, health economists estimate that seniors with both types of coverage spend about 30% more on health care than those with Medicare alone. Private plans could create an alternative that provides more coverage for less cost.

For example, some 16% of seniors have shifted out of traditional Medicare and into private-sector HMOs. These HMOs are required to cover everything that Medicare covers, but most cover much more. A recent survey found that 95% of Medicare HMOs provide their enrollees with a prescription drug benefit.

However, the Clinton administration and a Medicare bureaucracy hostile to any challenge to its power and authority have combined to halt and even reverse the trend. As mentioned before, after the administration cut reimbursement rates to Medicare HMOs this year, many HMOs dropped out of the program, leaving some 450,000 seniors, many of whom had drug coverage, scrambling to find another HMO or return to Medicare. Another 99 HMOs intend to leave next year, affecting 325,000 more seniors.

The Clinton administration also has blocked other options for seniors. The Medicare+Choice program is supposed to give the elderly the full range of non-HMO options available to the nonelderly, including fee-for-service insurance and Medical Savings Accounts. Yet none of these options currently exist.

What could the private sector do for the elderly if given a chance? A Milliman & Robertson analysis concludes that with the average amount Medicare currently spends on each senior, a private plan could in principle establish a $1,585 across-the-board deductible and cover hospital, physician, and drug costs above that deductible. Although a deductible of that size seems like a lot of money, many seniors are already spending $1,500 to $2,000 a year for medigap coverage. While medigap insurance could eliminate the deductible, a better option for seniors would be to take the money they currently spend on medigap premiums and put it in the bank. (See the next solution.)

FACTORS BEHIND PRESCRIPTION SPENDING

Over the past five years, prescription drug expenditures have grown significantly, both in total and as a share of all health expenditures. Prescription drug spending grew, on average, from 1992 to 1997 by 11% a year compared with a 5% average growth rate for health expenditures overall. Drug spending during that same period also consumed a larger share of total health care spending—rising from 5.6% to 7.2%.

While total drug expenditures depend both on the prices paid and the volume used, the recent spending increases appear to have more to do with stepped up volume than price. A precise determination of how much is due to volume versus price increases is not possible since only data on the retail pharmaceutical prices are widely available. The actual prices paid are often lower than retail levels, as insurers, PBMs, and other purchasers negotiate significant discounts from manufacturers and other suppliers. Market changes in recent years have likely altered the size of those discounts.

Several factors have contributed to increased prescription drug use and the resulting spending increases: namely, more individuals have third-party drug coverage, new drug therapies have been introduced into the market, and manufacturers have marketed drugs more aggressively through advertising directly to consumers.

The increase in private insurance coverage for prescription drugs is a likely factor accounting for the rise in utilization. In the decade between 1987 and 1997, the share of prescription drug expenditures paid by private health insurers rose from almost a third to more than half.

The development of new, more expensive drug therapies—including new drugs that replace old drugs and new drugs that treat disease more effectively—also contributed to the drug spending growth. The average number of new drugs entering the market each year has grown from 24 at the beginning of the 1990s to 33 now. Similarly, biotechnology advances and a growing knowledge of the human immune system are significantly shaping the discovery, design, and production of drugs. Advertising pitched to the lay consumer has also likely upped consumers' use of prescription drugs. Between March 1998 and March 1999, industry spending on advertising grew 16%, to $1.5 billion.

—*U.S. General Accounting Office*

Solution #3: Free Roth IRAs. Roth IRAs permit people to set aside up to $2,000 a year after taxes in retirement accounts that grow tax free. After age 59½ the funds can be withdrawn without penalty for any purpose, including medical expenses. Since the elderly by definition satisfy the age test, Roth IRAs could potentially serve as "backended" Medical Savings Accounts for the elderly.

However, there are two small problems.

First, the law prohibits taxpayers from depositing more in a Roth IRA than they receive in earned income in any year. Since only about 18% of those age 65 and over work (and therefore have earned income), this restriction excludes the vast majority of seniors.

Second, unless deposits are held for at least five years, the interest earned is not tax free. Clearly this restriction discourages the type of annual deposits and withdrawals that are needed for health care.

The solution is to allow seniors to deposit the maximum in their accounts (regardless of the amount they earn) and let them use the funds at any time without tax consequences—provided that the Roth IRA backs up a Medicare or (even better) a Medicare+Choice private health plan.

Solution #4: Free the States. More than half the states have high-risk pools that permit uninsured people who have been denied health insurance to obtain coverage for a reasonable premium. This concept can also be used to solve some of the problems of seniors. For example, 13 states already provide low-income seniors with prescription drug assistance and many more states are considering similar legislation.

By their nature, high-risk pools require subsidies. So where would the new money come from? A potential source is unused antipoverty money—currently restricted to food stamps, Medicaid and other welfare programs. Congress should free the states to use these funds to provide prescription drug high-risk pool insurance for the elderly poor.

These proposals would impose no new taxes (or "premiums") and would cost the government nothing. At a time when Medicare is in financial trouble, it makes much more sense to look at smaller, less expensive, targeted solutions for seniors who need help.

57

Free Health Care Does Not Exist

Thomas Sowell

Since virtually everything is called a "crisis" these days, perhaps we should not be surprised to hear about a health-care "crisis." Still, those of us old-fashioned enough to believe that words should have meaning may wonder just what this crisis consists of.

Are we getting worse health care than in the past? Worse than the rest of the world? Worse than we would like?

The answer to the first two questions is clearly "no." Doctors today can cure or prevent diseases that were virtually a death sentence in the past. People from other countries—even rulers of some other countries—come here for medical treatment, while few Americans go overseas to get medical care.

■ WHAT THE "HEALTH-CARE CRISIS" BOILS DOWN TO

If our standard is whether we are getting worse than we would like, that applies to virtually everything, not just health care. I could be driving a newer, more powerful and more luxurious car. I would like to have a body like Arnold Schwarzenegger's, a brain like Einstein's and a voice like Pavarotti's.

While some things, like brains and voices, are gifts of nature, even these can usually be improved if we sacrifice the time to work on them. Other sacrifices, whether of money or time, can improve other things. The real problem is that we are not willing to make some of these trade-offs.

Fine. But don't turn it into a "crisis" because what you want has a cost. Everything has always had a cost.

Virtually every aspect of the so-called health-care crisis boils down to the fact that everybody wants somebody else to pay for health care.

Thomas Sowell, PhD, a senior fellow and economist at the Hoover Institution, is a national syndicated columnist and author of Race and Culture.

Reprinted with permission from *Human Events,* January 1, 1999, 55(1) 14.

Health Maintenance Organizations (HMOs) have been criticized for getting mothers out of hospitals too soon after childbirth. But HMOs cannot force any mother to leave a hospital. They can only stop paying and let others decide whether it's worth the cost to continue staying. Alternatively, the HMOs can charge higher fees and cover longer stays.

The basic underlying fact that is not going to change is that medical care is costly, whether those costs are paid by HMOs, the government, the patients or anybody else. We can try to pretend that these costs don't exist or hope to force somebody else to pay them, but none of that changes the costs of the fact that they have to be paid.

With our country's record prosperity, surely it is not too much to expect adults to face up to trade-offs. We are not talking about going hungry so that a child can have an appendix removed. We are talking about not eating out as often, or not buying so expensive a watch, so that a mother can spend another day or two in the hospital.

■ *GREAT GAME FOR POLITICIANS*

Politicians see all this very differently. They leave trade-offs to economists, who don't have to get elected. Politicians win votes by passing laws creating "rights" for patients to get this or that, without either providing any money to cover the costs or expecting the patients to cover the costs.

It is a great game for those in the business of getting reelected. But the costs don't disappear, no matter how much they are shuffled around.

When the government tried to shift the costs of medical care for the elderly onto HMOs, the HMOs started getting rid of elderly patients. Whether HMOs, are good, bad or indifferent, they are just one way of delivering medical care. If there are better ways, people are free to find them. What is not free are more medical "rights."

How did we ever get into the present mess in the first place? There was a time when a patient simply went to a doctor and paid for treatment. The costs and the trade-offs these would entail were very plain to everyone. If it was worth it to get a broken arm fixed, but not worth it to go in every time you had the sniffles, then you made such choices accordingly.

Employer-paid "fringe benefits" began during World War II, as a way to get around government-imposed wage and price controls, when employers needed to hire more people but were prevented from attracting them with higher pay. Politicians found it expedient to exempt these benefits from the heavy taxes they put on money income. From this has followed the grand illusion of something for nothing, which has created needless problems in health care, as it has in so many other aspects of life.

Discussion Questions

1. What factors contribute to Medicare's inefficiencies? How would you resolve them?

2. Explain the regional differences in Medicare funding. What inequities stand out?

3. What do you think is the fairest way to provide drug coverage to Medicare participants? How politically popular would your solution be?

4. How would you refute the arguments against drug coverage?

5. What factors would contribute to Medicare's financial health? Which one would most likely be approved by Congress?

6. Should wealthy people continue to receive Medicare for free? Should they be made to subsidize people who are not insured? State your reasons.

7. What does "quality of life" mean to you? How do you plan to ensure that you have quality of life?

8. What can or should be done to provide drug coverage and maintain the stability of Medicare? Elaborate with examples.

9. Evaluate the fairness of the various proposed drug coverage plans.

10. Compare and contrast the various solutions proposed by Goodman and Mathews (Article 56) with respect to economic feasibility and fairness.

11. What is the major premise behind the contention that free health care does not exist?

12. What tradeoffs would you make in order to have affordable health care coverage?

Further Readings

Feder, J. & Moon, M. (1999). Can Medicare survive its saviors? *The American Prospect,* May/June, 44:56–60.

Holmer, A. F. (1999). Drug expenditures: Take off the green eyeshades. *The National Journal, 31* (46), 3329.

Moskowitz, D. B. (1999). The double edge of a Medicare drug benefit. *Business and Health, 17*(99), 18.

Rother, J. (1999). A drug benefit: The necessary prescription for Medicare. *Health Affairs, 18*(4), 20–22.

Sullivan, K. (1999). Bad prescription. *The National Journal, 31*(3), 27–32.

Worth, R. (1999). America's real drug problem. *The Washington Monthly, 31*(12), 21–24.

Web Site Resources for Economics

Alliance for Health Reform   www.allhealth.org
Guide to Health Economics   www.healtheconomics.com
Health Care Financing Administration and Medicare   www.hcfama.org
Medicare Watch   www.medicarewatch.org

General Search Engine Web Sites

Northern Light   www.northernlight.com
Yahoo   www.yahoo.com

Health Web Sites

Family Doctor www.familydoctor.org
Health Insurance Association of America   www.hiaa.org
We Media   www.wemedia.com

Professional Journal Web Sites

Medical Economics   www.medec.com
Nursing Economics   www.ajj.com

12 Politics: Do We Make a Difference?

Politics is not a neutral word. The mere mention of politics these days conjures up images of unsavory, unscrupulous people trying to outwit and take advantage of others. Today's political climate does little to change that perception. Dubious fund-raising practices, soft money, and a Congress mired and immobilized in partisan bickering have left the public feeling battered and betrayed by the very process that is supposed to work for them. The outcome of this feeling is obvious: Politics has become a joke and has "turned off" a large segment of the public. As a result, many people have become cynical about politics in general and politicians in particular. That cynicism has spread into the polling booth. Each year, fewer and fewer people bother to vote. They drop out of the political process feeling that nothing they say or do will make the slightest difference. Without their participation, the status quo of politics continues, the disenchantment grows, and "politics as usual" remains the only game in town.

Despite it all, politics is an essential process. We engage in it because, as Aristotle once said, "Man is by nature a political animal." In the arena of everyday life, not one day goes by that doesn't involve us in some sort of political interaction. At home, at work, in our churches, and schools, we persuade, cajole, influence, and negotiate one thing or another. Our government does the same thing, but on a much larger scale. Who gets what, how they get it, and when they get it are all a part of the political process. The arena is bigger, but so are the issues.

The political process within our government is not an easy road to tread. It's convoluted, slow, cumbersome, and maddening. But it's ours and it works. It is through this process that we learn what the specific concerns of an issue are, whom it will benefit, who might be left out, and what costs are involved. Health care is one of the major issues being examined and debated in Congress. Given the increasing number of people reaching their 65th year soon, the health care debate must focus on how to provide care for our burgeoning aging population. Congress knows that it must do something soon, because of the growing number of aging individuals. The elderly have gained a great deal of political clout over the years, primarily because there are so many of them and because they vote. The aging are, by far, the largest block of voters in our country, and are the most vocal and adamant in making clear what their needs are. The baby boomers, who were protesting for various causes in the 1960s, will add their voices to this already vocal and politically active group. And Congress is beginning to listen. The cynic may say that Congress started listening only because 2000 was an election year. The pragmatist may respond by saying, "So what? It's the outcome that counts." And so it does.

The focus of this chapter is the political process as it relates to health care issues. Nursing's evolution as a political force is detailed in the opening reading of this chapter. In the readings that follow a general overview of the political process is provided, together with its problematic applications to health care and some of the solutions needed to influence the outcome of these issues.

58

Nursing's Past, Present, and Future Political Experiences

Bethany A. Hall-Long

Contemporary public policy shifts and political opportunities make it important for the nursing profession to revisit the efforts of its political pioneers. Such historical inquiry can reveal "old truths about nursing's past and shed light on its emergence, helping to determine whether as a profession it has grown up or just grown older" (Church, 1985, p. 188) in the public policy arena. In addition to reviewing some of nursing's political roots, an examination of nursing's policy research and political activities can offer insight to the profession for improved political transformations.

Since the nursing profession is 97 percent female, much of the battle that nurses have had to fight to gain recognition in the policy process has been for women's rights. Among the many women's groups and female dominated professions, nursing has been one of the premiere political forces. "Nurses organized the first major professional association for women, edited and published the first professional magazine by women, and were the first major professional group to integrate black and white members" (Bullough & Bullough, 1984, pp. 41–42). Despite the profession's earlier organizational capabilities, the female profession of nursing "represents 67 percent of the health care providers in the United States, and very few are in positions where they can influence health policy making" (Sohier, 1992, p. 63).

The small cadre of contemporary nurse leaders in politics (De Back, 1990; Milio, 1989) continue to face extensions of public health and nursing practice policy issues that their earlier predecessors also encountered. Although not exhaustive of all politically astute nurse leaders, critical players in nursing's political establishment and American Women's History can be traced to such leaders as Nightingale, Barton, Dock, Wald, and Sanger.

At the time of this article, Bethany A. Hall-Long, Ph.D., R.N.C., was an assistant professor at the Center for Health Policy, College of Nursing and Health Science, George Mason University, Fairfax, VA.

Reprinted with permission from *Nursing & Healthcare: Perspectives on Community*, Jan/Feb 1995, 16(1) 24–28. National League for Nursing, Publishers.

Florence Nightingale is known as the wealthy young British woman who founded the nursing profession during the Crimean War era. Her efforts have earned her the title, "consummate political nurse" (Goldwater & Zusy, 1990, p. 6). She was influential in the reformation of hospitals and in crafting and implementing public health policies for the British Sanitary System (Kalisch & Kalisch, 1982). Florence Nightingale was the first nurse to exert political pressure on government and remains among a small cadre of politically renowned nurses.

During the American Civil War, the school teacher who volunteered as a nurse, Clara Barton, was responsible for organizing the nursing services. She is not only known for her role in improving battlefield health care, but also for establishing the American Red Cross. Barton's persuasion of Congress in 1882 to ratify the Treaty of Geneva so that the Red Cross could perform humanitarian efforts in times of peace has had lasting impressions on national and international policies (Kelly, 1991).

By the turn of the 19th century, America was influenced by such politically skilled nurses as Margaret Sanger, Lillian Wald, and Lavinia Dock. Margaret Higgins Sanger, a public health nurse in the Lower East Side of New York, was instrumental in addressing health issues of factory workers, especially women. Her experience with a large number of unwanted pregnancies among the working poor facilitated her role in promoting public birth control education and accessibility. Despite the legal and social ramifications, she opened the first birth control clinic in America in Brooklyn. Her political activism has had a lasting impact on women's health care policies (Kelly, 1991).

Like Nightingale, Wald was a wealthy young woman who took a different path from most women in her social class. The path she chose led to the improvement of the welfare and health of women and children in the United States. She cofounded the Henry Street Settlement House in New York, which was devoted to providing health care, social services, and education to the sick poor. One of Wald's greatest contributions came with her political ingenuity and pressure to see the creation of the United States Children's Bureau. The Bureau was established by Congress in 1912 to oversee fair child labor laws that facilitated the well being of the country's children (Kelly, 1991).

Wald's friend, Lavinia Dock, was a prolific writer and political activist who was among the early feminists. She was a devoted suffragette who eagerly participated in protests and demonstrations until the 1920 passage of the Nineteenth Amendment to the U.S. Constitution which allowed women to vote. In addition, she waged a campaign for legislation to allow nurses versus physicians to control the profession. In 1893, with the assistance of Isabel Hampton Robb and Mary Adelaide Nutting, she founded the very politically active organization, the American Society of Superintendents of Training Schools for Nurses of the United States and Canada, a precursor to the current National League for Nursing (NLN) (Goldwater & Zusy, 1990; Kelly, 1991).

■ NURSING ORGANIZATIONS MANIFEST THE CYCLICAL NATURE OF INTEREST GROUPS

The value of organized efforts among nurses was recognized during the late 19th century. The National Associated Alumnae of the U.S. and Canada and American Society of Superintendents of Training Schools of the U.S. and Canada were formed in the 1890s. These groups were the precursors of the current American Nurses Association and National League for Nursing respectively. Nursing alumnae groups were formulated mostly in response to state licensure requirements, standards of education, and welfare issues of nurses (Kelly, 1991). The leaders of the groups, typical of other female occupations of that time, were mostly older and unmarried. These dedicated women actively tried to gain influence in the male-dominated hospitals and colleges.

Over the years, the number of nursing organizations have dramatically increased. Expository works reflect how nursing associations or interest groups have played a positive role in influencing and promoting nursing practice and public health policies (American Academy of Nursing, 1987; Bullough & Bullough, 1984; Kelly, 1991). Political effectiveness of organizations is influenced by organizational skills, resources, and incentives. Divisiveness and turf battles have been known inhibitors of the nursing interest groups' political capabilities for years (American Academy of Nursing, 1987; Raymond Rich Associates, 1946). However, nursing associations have become increasingly aware of the need for intraprofessional interaction and consensus on public policy positions.

"Nursing organizations have not remained static. They have arisen in many forms; they have competed for members, powers . . . they have differentiated and diversified; they have merged; some have declined and died. . . . Changes happened in response to a multitude of variables within and external to the profession" (American Academy of Nursing, 1987, p. 1). Thus, nursing shares with other disciplines and professions the cyclical nature and central role of interest groups. Some are national and international organizations, while others are regional, state, local, or specialty-focused. Despite their differences, all organizations are in a dynamic relationship with their legal, economic, social, technological, and political environments.

An example of this progressive involvement in the political arena was displayed by the organizational steps leading to the ANA's Political Action Committee (ANA-PAC). In 1971, a small group of nurses in New York State formed the Nurses For Political Action (NPA), a nonpartisan, nonprofit association of registered and practical nurses. The NPA was set up to influence state and national policy makers, to educate other health care professionals and the public about nurses and health policy, and to recognize nurses' role in the health care delivery (*American Journal of Nursing*, 1972). The NPA was appointed as an ad hoc committee of the ANA's Board of Directors in 1973 to investigate the establishment of a policy arm for the ANA. In conjunction with state political action groups and the NPA, an independent arm of ANA, the National Coalition for Action in Politics (N-CAP) was formed. The N-CAP's focus was on educating, assisting, and stimulating political education and participation of nurses as well as nonpartisan fund raising (*American Nurse*, 1974; *American Journal of Nursing*, 1971). In 1986, the N-CAP became part of the ANA and was renamed the ANA-PAC.

Effective alliances among nursing associations have been formed and include such entities as the Tri-Council for Nursing, the National Federation of Specialty Nursing Organizations (NFSNO), and the Nursing Organization Liaison Forum (NOLF).

The Tri-Council for Nursing originated in 1981 and was composed of the American Nurses Association (ANA), the National League for Nursing (NLN), and the American Association of Colleges of Nursing (AACN). In 1985, the American Organization of Nurse Executives (AONE) joined the alliance without any change in title. The collective efforts of these groups such as the Tri-Council for Nursing have played an important role in advancing the profession and the nations' health in the policy arena (Carty & Cherry, 1989). According to the American Academy of Nursing (1987), the Tri-Council for Nursing "grew out of a succession of efforts to respond to the multiple interdependencies and the need for a more unified approach by the nursing profession to its publics" (p. 22). A major intent of the alliance is to facilitate coordination and communication on key professional issues and activities as well as to assist with promoting concordance on federal legislation of mutual concern.

Similarly, NFSNO is a loosely structured alliance of nursing specialty organizations. Its members range from large national organizations (e.g., the American Association of Critical-Care Nurses) to very small groups (e.g., National Intravenous Therapy Association). Since its origins in 1981, NFSNO's focus has been on coordinating efforts of practice, education, and other areas of mutual concern among nursing organizations. In 1985, NFSNO decided to include only clinical specialty organizations as members and to exclude large multipurpose nursing organizations such as the ANA or NLN.

NOLF is another coalition of nursing organizations that attempts to give a unified approach to national policy issues and nursing interests. ANA, in collaboration with representatives from a number of other nursing organizations, established NOLF in the early 1980s. NOLF, a diverse forum within the ANA, meets at least annually to promote concerted actions by national nursing organizations. Its members can include organizations that are also part of the NFSNO alliance such as the American Critical Care Nurses Association.

■ RESEARCH ON NURSING'S POLITICAL SOCIALIZATION STILL IN ITS INFANCY

The nursing profession, like other female professions, is using a number of political efforts to influence policy development while attempting to eliminate sexist images. Women in society are becoming more and more actively involved in local, state, and national politics and the 1990s have been deemed the decade of women in politics.

Despite such progress, women's deliverance from apolitical images and behavior has been slow. Whicker, Jewell, and Lovelace (1989) describe how women have made some inroads in obtaining elected political office at the state (13.9 percent of positions) and local (17.1 percent of positions) levels. The authors discuss women's political paradox of constituting 53 percent of the population, yet possessing only a small fraction of elected offices at all levels of government. With the 1992 elections, U.S. Congressional records were broken in regard to the number of women winning elections. Women comprised 11 percent of the 435 members of the U.S. House of Representatives and seven percent of the 100 members of the U.S. Senate. Most significantly, 1992 saw the election of the first African-American woman to the U.S. Senate (Carol Moseley Braun, D-Illinois), and the first nurse to the U.S. House of Representatives (Eddie Bernice Johnson, D-Texas).

An increased number of anecdotal articles on public policy education, socialization, participation, and research (Batra, 1992; Buerhaus, 1992; Sharp, Biggs, & Wakefield, 1991) have appeared in the nursing literature. However, actual policy studies in nursing have minimally increased since Milio's (1984) comprehensive literature review which found sparse nursing policy research in nursing and no nursing policy analysis research by nurses. Research on nursing's political socialization, education, and participation levels is in its infancy. In developing nursing administration curriculum, Scalzi and Wilson (1990) surveyed 184 top-level, U.S. nurse executives in home health, acute care, long-term care, and occupational health settings. They found that law and health care policy were ranked as the most time consuming and most important by nurse executives regardless of the practice setting. The role of education and socialization in health policy and politics was deemed essential for future nurse administrators.

Barry's (1989) descriptive research study of the political socialization processes of 33 nurses in specialized policy-making roles in the state and federal governments found that nurses involved in policy making were not "typical" of employed nurses. They, like other political pioneers in nursing, tended to be older, not married, childless, and had higher levels of formal education. In addition, Barry found that formal nursing education had not been a major factor in socializing these nurses for their political roles. The majority of the nurses had acquired an interest in the public policy process after they had completed basic nursing education as a result of interactions with non-nurses immersed in the public policy process.

Hanley (1983) underscored the need for political education in all generic and continuing education nursing programs to enhance the influence of education and political behaviors. Her exploratory study found that nurses with baccalaureate-level education were as active as teachers and engineers in such political behaviors as voting, campaigning, communal activity, and protest. Building on Hanley's work, Gesse (1989) examined education as a predictor of the political participation of nurse-midwives who belonged to the American College of Nurse-Midwives. She found that the members' political behaviors, particularly voting, increased after involvement with the political activities of the American College of Nurse-Midwives. However, contrary to Hanley's study, education was not identified as a predictor of political participation.

Hayes and Fritsch (1988) found a significant relationship between nurses' political attitudes and the amount of their political activity. Their descriptive correlational study of 250 registered nurses in Massachusetts revealed that the early political socialization and education of nurses boosted nurses' political attitudes and eventual political participation. In addition, higher levels of education and professional organizational membership were associated with greater participation.

In 1988, Daffin examined the political expectations and participation of registered nurses (n = 447) in Alabama who were employed in clinical practice, academia, and administration. Of her sample, 91 percent expected politically active nurses to participate in the nine political roles of voter, monitor, negotiator, networker, leader, spokesperson, campaigner, lobbyist, and player. However, only 26 percent of the sample indicated that they actually participated in these roles. Nurse administrators had the highest political expectations and participation, and were trailed by the nurse educators who were followed by the nurse clinicians. Daffin concluded that although nurses have high political expectations, they primarily are limited to their political role of voting.

Archer (1983) explored the political participation activities of over 500 nurse administrators in home health, hospitals, and schools of nursing. The three political activities observed most frequently among her subjects were voting, writing letters to legislators, and belonging to and/or serving on community or nursing organizations or boards. Ninety-four percent of Archer's participants felt that nurses were not as active politically as they should be. In turn, they listed potential reasons for their low political participation which included inadequate political socialization and education, apathy, divisiveness among nursing's associations, and the lack of knowledge of and skills in the political process.

To fill the void of political frameworks in nursing, Hall-Long (1993) devised a public policy process model. The Tri-Council for Nursing's political efforts with the 1991–1992 Nurse Education Act's reauthorization was used as the exemplary case to test the model. Analysis of the data gathered from interviews and questionnaires collected from 15 participants, representing the Federal Government and the Tri-Council for Nursing, supported the utility of the model in analyzing the political process at the national level. Ancillary findings of this case study furthermore revealed that organized nursing often perceived its effectiveness and frequency of select political strategies in a more favorable rating than did govermental respondents.

■ A UNITED VOICE IS MORE POLITICALLY POWERFUL THAN FRAGMENTED ECHOS AND DIVERSE APPEALS

A number of political implications can be extracted from nursing's political pioneers, organized efforts, and policy studies. Nurses at the bedside, in academia, and administration are affected on a daily basis by public policy. Thus, the inclusion in such debates demands that all nurses be proactive in the earliest stages of policy development. Individual nurses can influence policy decisions at all intergovernmental levels, and organized nursing's unified efforts such as with *Nursing's Agenda for Health Care Reform* (Tri-Council for Nursing, 1991) will be critical to exerting nursing's influence early on in the political process. In addition to these policy development efforts, nurses need to strive to promote better political strategies. As previously discussed, these strategies entail improved public policy education, socialization, and general participation.

Specific strategies can include: integration of public policy courses and/or content into nursing curriculum; active socialization and recognition of nurse educators, administrators, and clinicians for public policy participation; taking part in organizational or professional legislative networks and/or grassroots initiatives; establishing educational or work experiences in diverse public policy-making settings at the local, state, and federal levels; conducting public policy research; giving testimony at public hearings; assisting with campaign efforts, and running for public office. Nurses have direct experience and a thorough knowledge of the health care needs of individuals, families, and communities. The profession represents experts in addressing the diverse health care needs of the country's underserved and most vulnerable groups. Nurses need to now collaborate with the public and media in engineering policy positions that promote the nation's health as well as the public policy-making role of the nursing profession.

In turn, organized nursing needs to unite on the public policy front. A united, central voice is much more politically powerful than fragmented

echoes and diverse appeals. Coalitions among nursing organizations and professional and consumer groups can provide many opportunities to advance
nursing's policy agenda and "victories."

Obviously, the implications for positive political change are enumerable.
Following the lead of our political pioneers risk-taking behavior, contemporary nurses need to face the political challenges of the 21st century to guarantee representation around the public policy–making tables. Once around
these tables, political voices and power will be welded to the nursing profession and to the consumers they represent.

References

American Academy of Nursing (AAN). (1987). *The evolution of nursing professional organizations: Alternative models for the future.* Washington, DC: American Academy
of Nursing.

American Journal of Nursing. (1972). Nurses political action group formed. *American
Journal of Nursing, 71*(10), 1784.

American Nurse. (1974). N-CAP: Nursing's political action arm. *American Nurse, 6*(6),
1, 12.

Archer, S. (1983). A study of nurse administrator's political participation. *Western
Journal of Nursing Research, 5*(1), 65–75.

Barry, C. (1989). *A descriptive study of the political socialization processes of nurses in
specialized roles in federal and state governments.* Dissertation Abstracts International (University Microfilms No. 89-19002).

Batra, C. (1992). Empowering for professional, political, and health policy involvement. *Nursing Outlook, 40*(4), 170–176.

Buerhaus, P. (1992). Teaching health care public policy. *Nursing & Health Care, 13*(6),
304–309.

Bullough, V., & Bullough, B. (1984). *History, trends, and politics of nursing.* Norwalk,
CT: Appleton-Century-Crofts.

Carty, R., & Cherry, B. (1989). National Center for Nursing Research. In C.E. Lambert
& V.A. Lambert (eds.), *Perspectives in nursing: The impacts on the nurse, consumer, and society* (pp. 254–277). Norwalk, CT: Appleton & Lange.

Church, O. (1985). New knowledge from old truths: Problems and promises of historical inquiry of nursing. In J. McCloskey & H. Grace (eds.), *Current issues in nursing* (2nd ed., pp. 182–189). Boston, MA: Blackwell.

Daffin, P. (1988). *Similarities and differences in political expectations and participation
among nurses in clinical practice, education, and administration.* Dissertation Abstracts International (University Microfilms No. 89-09780).

De Back, V. (1990). Nursing needs health policy leaders. *Journal of Professional Nursing, 6*(2), 69.

Gesse, T. (1989). *Education as a determinant of political participation of nurse-midwives.* Dissertation Abstracts International (University Microfilms No. 89-09780).

Goldwater, M., & Zusy, M. (1990). *Prescription for nurses effective political action.*
Philadelphia, PA: Mosby.

Hall-Long, B. (1993). *A policy process model: Analysis of the Nurse Education Act of
1991–1992* (doctoral dissertation). George Mason University, Fairfax, VA.

Hanley, B. (1983). *Nurse political participation: An in-depth view and comparison with women teachers and engineers* (doctoral dissertation). The University of Michigan, Ann Arbor.

Hayes, E., & Fritsch, R. (1988). An untapped resource: The political potential of nurses. *Nursing Administration Quarterly, 13*(1), 33–39.

Kalisch, P. & Kalisch, B. (1982). *Politics of Nursing.* Philadelphia, PA: Lippincott.

Kelly, L. (1991). *Dimensions of professional nursing* (6th ed., pp. 423–426). New York, NY: Pergamon Press.

Kessler, T. (1989). Research and policy formation: Is there a fit? *Journal of Professional Nursing, 5*(5), 246.

Milio, N. (1984). Nursing research and the study of health policy. In *Annals of Nursing Research.* New York, NY: Springer.

Milio, N. (1989). Developing nursing leadership in health policy. *Journal of Professional Nursing, 5,* 315–321.

Raymond Rich Associates. (1946). Report on the structure of organized nursing. *American Journal of Nursing, 46*(10), 648–661.

Scalzi, C., & Wilson, D. (1990). Empirically based recommendations for content of graduate nursing administration programs. *Nursing & Health Care, 11*(10), 522–525.

Sharp, N., Biggs, S., & Wakefield, M. (1991). Public policy: New opportunities for nurses. *Nursing & Health Care, 12*(1), 16–22.

Sohier, R. (1992). Feminism and nursing knowledge: The power of the weak. *Nursing Outlook, 40*(2), 62–93.

Tri-Council for Nursing. (1991). *Nursing's agenda for health care reform.* Washington, DC: American Nurses Association.

Whicker, M., Jewell, M., & Lovelace, L. (1989). *Women in Congress.* Unpublished study, Virginia Commonwealth University, Richmond, VA.

59

Washington: Will Congress Stop Playing Politics With Health Care?

Michael Pretzer

Before Impeachment Saturday, the Democrats were acting as if they had won the November election. But all they really did was exceed everyone's low expectations, then stand around while the GOP's commander in chief, Newt Gingrich, shot himself one last time.

The Republicans were acting as if they had lost. But mostly they failed to meet their own—and history's—high expectations. They still have majorities in the House and Senate, and they might prove more effective without the mercurial and mouthy Gingrich at the helm.

The truth is that neither party won or lost. Americans didn't give Democrats or Republicans a mandate. No full speed ahead. No take a hike.

Instead, Americans sent a straightforward, if somewhat scolding, message: Cut the crap. Drop the curtain on the slimy soap opera. Get on with real business.

But that raises the question: What do Americans want Congress to do about health care? What do they think is serious business? The voters didn't offer a lot of clues.

Just before Election Day, President Clinton got all huffy about health-care reform. Turn your vote into a referendum for the Patients' Bill of Rights, he told the electorate.

But Americans didn't heed his call. According to exit and post-election polls, they based their voting more on the economy, education, Social Security, and taxes.

For some strange reason, Americans have become skeptical of elected officials' attempts to reform health care. In a recent poll conducted for the American Association of Health Plans, 68 percent of respondents said that candidates who push for managed-care regulations do so for political gain—not for the benefit of patients. That attitude may have surfaced in the election. According to *The Wall Street Journal*, the majority of candidates who advocated a tighter rein on managed care lost.

Also troubling: On issues such as Medicare, Americans seem unrealistic and ill-informed. Fewer than 25 percent think Medicare is headed for a crisis,

Reprinted with permission from *Medical Economics*, January 11, 1999, 76(1) 83–91.

while nearly 30 percent think the program has only minor problems or none at all. Only 20 percent have heard about the Medicare+Choice program. Roughly two-thirds are eager to expand Medicare—to cover prescription drugs and long-term home care and to serve 62- to 64-year-old seniors.

For better or worse, Congress will have to lead rather than follow when it deals with health care this year.

◼ UNFINISHED BUSINESS, PART ONE

To say that Congress did nothing about health care in 1998 is only a slight exaggeration. To be precise:

- It appropriated more than $168 billion for the Health Care Financing Administration to use (wisely, we presume) this year. That's a 7.4 percent increase from 1998.
- It gave the National Institutes of Health $15.6 billion. That's a 14.6 percent increase, and $819 million more than the administration had requested.
- It passed a law requiring health plans that cover mastectomies to also cover breast-reconstruction surgery. (The driving force behind the mandate was New York Republican Alfonse D'Amato, who lost his bid for re-election to the Senate.)
- It reformed Medicare's troubled home-health payment system.

But on the big issues, those bundled as patients' rights, Congress went round and round without getting anywhere. The public had it pegged: Proposing a patient-protection act was nothing but a campaign strategy in 1998.

Could it be different in 1999? Maybe. The next national election is 22 months away.

Last year, the patient rights that were debated included:

- Access to easily understood information about a health plan and its benefits.
- Access to information about financial arrangements between a plan and its physicians.
- A prudent-layperson standard for coverage of emergency services.
- Access to appropriate specialty care.
- Quality-assurance programs for health plans.
- A ban on provider gag clauses.
- A grievance-and-appeal procedure for treatment decisions.
- Confidentiality of medical records.
- Health-plan liability in instances of malpractice.
- A reasonable appeals process for terminated providers.

The Democrats, convinced that they hold the high ground on health-care issues, are eager to revive the patients' rights debate. Senate Minority Leader Tom Daschle, D-SD, says a patient-protection act is the party's highest priority this year. Expect Rep. John D. Dingell, D-MI, and Sen. Edward M. Kennedy, D-MA, who sponsored the Democratic version of the act last year, to do so again. This time, though, they and their colleagues may be more willing to compromise on some issues to get a bill passed.

Republicans, who haven't been overly enthusiastic about patients' rights, may finally be warming to the subject. This time a year ago, another Republican, Rep. Charlie Norwood, a dentist from Georgia, was talking tough. He wanted to give patients the right to sue managed-care plans that are protected by ERISA, but the idea didn't sit well with his GOP colleagues. Last summer, Norwood caved in to party pressure and endorsed the House Republicans' watered-down patient-protection act. Now Norwood's back on his soapbox, pushing for a law that would hold managed-care plans liable for medical decisions.

Norwood and sympathetic Republicans may be able to join with Democrats to get the House—where Republicans lost five seats—to pass a patient-protection act that includes managed-care liability. But the Senate, which refused to even consider a protection act in 1998, certainly won't endorse the contentious provision. If Congress is to enact a patients' rights bill at all, it'll have to stick to the more agreeable issues: access to information, grievance procedures, and the prudent-layperson standard for ER coverage.

■ THE UNINTENDED CONSEQUENCES OF MEDICARE+CHOICE

In 1997, Congress created Medicare+Choice, a program that was to give seniors several alternatives to standard fee-for-service and HMO Medicare. All sorts of managed-care arrangements were envisioned, arrangements that would simultaneously make seniors happy and keep medical costs in check.

Medicare+Choice, which went into effect this month, hasn't worked out as planned. In fact, it could more aptly be called Medicare minus choice. At the end of 1998, 40-some managed-care plans pulled out of Medicare—two or three a year is typical—and about 50 others reduced their services. Nearly 50 new managed-care plans have applied to enter the Medicare market, according to HCFA, and about 25 plans that already serve Medicare say they'll expand. But the pluses won't nearly offset the minuses. More than 400,000 seniors will be affected by managed care's pullout, and as many as 50,000 beneficiaries could be left with no HMO option at all.

The managed-care industry blames the government for this predicament. "There are serious structural problems—payments, compliance, and transition issues—that need to be addressed with the new Medicare+Choice program," says Karen Ignagni, president and CEO of the American Association of Health Plans. "Decisive steps can and should be taken now to prevent this situation from having an even greater impact on Medicare beneficiaries."

Others blame the clock. HCFA has been preoccupied with getting its computer systems and claims carriers ready for 2000 and hasn't had the time or the manpower to fully develop the regulations for Medicare+Choice. Moreover, HCFA has to put tight deadlines on managed care because Congress put tight deadlines on HCFA.

In Washington, there's plenty of finger-pointing and sniping. Congress may become concerned enough to revisit the issue—to hold hearings or even amend the Medicare+Choice laws. A debate over new legislation could trigger another battle among providers for shares of the Medicare pie.

Meanwhile, seniors may be asking themselves, Who cares? A study released a few months ago by the Office of Inspector General (OIG), Department of Health and Human Services, found that seniors are losing interest in managed care. Although awareness of HMOs among seniors increased from 70 percent to 79 percent from 1995 to 1997, those who said they might join one declined from 35 percent to 23 percent. Forty percent said they'd be willing to hear more about the managed-care options—down from 64 percent in 1994.

One survey doesn't prove that enthusiasm for HMOs is waning, of course. But it wouldn't be the first time that the public is thinking one thing while Congress is thinking another.

▇ UNFINISHED BUSINESS, PARTS TWO AND THREE

Last year Sen. Don Nickles, R-OK, the majority whip, sent shivers up the spine of organized medicine. He pushed hard for a bill called the Lethal Drug Abuse Prevention Act. The legislation failed, but Nickles has promised to revive it in this session of Congress.

The bill has two purposes. It would prohibit physicians from using controlled substances, such as morphine, to assist in acts of suicide. And it would protect doctors who prescribe these drugs for the relief of pain. Hard to argue with such noble causes, right?

The way organized medicine sees it, danger lurks just beneath the high-mindedness. How will government enforcement agencies determine whether a physician is trying to relieve the pain of a terminally ill patient, or terminate the patient's painful life? It's a slippery slope that could make doctors even more reluctant to prescribe narcotics. "We fear this bill could have the unintended consequence of increasing the already too-large numbers of patients dying in severe, constant pain," says Robert B. Copeland, chair of the board of regents at the American College of Physicians–American Society of Internal Medicine.

Bills such as Nickles' could also result in Drug Enforcement Administration sleuths poring through your files—which brings to mind another issue that Congress will almost surely take up this year: the protection of medical records. If Congress takes a pass, the responsibility of regulating electronic medical records will fall on the shoulders of HHS. Hard to imagine the Republicans letting the Democrat-controlled executive branch loose on this one.

In the past, a number of congressmen introduced bills relating to the confidentiality of medical files. Right now, Sen. Bob Bennett, R-UT, has cornered the market with his Medical Information Protection Act, which applies to both paper and electronic records. The bill gives patients guaranteed access to their own files, and makes it illegal except in certain circumstances for the files to be disseminated without the patient's permission. Organized medicine has given the bill, as written, mixed reviews. Supporters praise it for allowing records to be used for legitimate research; opponents, including the AMA, criticize its ambiguous language.

■ *LOOKING AHEAD TO MEDICARE 2008*

The big event of the year probably will not involve the passage of legislation. It'll be the issuance of a report. By March 1, the National Bipartisan Commission on the Future of Medicare is to make its recommendations for putting Medicare on firm financial footing. Under the current structure, Medicare's Part A trust fund is projected to go bankrupt in 2008.

The commission has 17 members, including nine members of Congress and one congressional staffer. Talk to any 10 people in Washington, and five will tell you that the commission may get something done because a majority of its members are politicians. They understand how Congress works and will make recommendations accordingly, goes the argument.

The other five people will tell you that the commission won't get anything done because it contains so many politicians. How, they ask, will someone like Rep. Jim McDermott, D-WA, a psychiatrist who has been a champion of a national single-payer health system, and someone like Rep. Bill Thomas, R-CA, who thinks medical savings accounts are a gift from heaven, ever agree on anything?

We'll see.

Last year, the commission had it easy. It listened—at hearings in Washington and at town meetings across the country. It heard the AMA say that Medicare's tax-based funding system ought to be replaced by one based on private savings. It heard Physicians for a National Health Program say that a single-payer system would solve many of Medicare's financial problems by putting all Americans under one system. It heard the National Coalition on Health Care say the answer to Medicare's problems is a voucher system (each beneficiary gets money to buy his own private health insurance). It heard the Society of Thoracic Surgeons say that "focused clinical systems" would deliver better care to seniors than large health plans. It heard the American Association of Health Plans say that HMOs could serve seniors better if they weren't so heavily regulated.

In December, the commissioners stopped listening and started talking—among themselves. By March, we'll all know what they had to say.

Then it'll be Congress' turn. "Medicare reform will be one of the most pressing health-care issues addressed in the next Congress," predicts Sen. Bill Frist, R-TN, a thoracic surgeon and a member of the commission. "After we've had time to appropriately evaluate this information, I believe we'll be able to enact fair, affordable, and effective reforms."

But Frist is probably a bit too optimistic. "There'll be a lot of debate on the issue," says Rep. John Cooksey, R-LA, an ophthalmologist. "Structural change, however, probably won't occur until sometime after the 2000 election."

■ THE UNINSURED: A PROBLEM THAT WON'T GO AWAY

If Congress does indeed take matters seriously this year, it'll have to face the biggest health-care problem in America.

The ranks of the uninsured are growing. In 1997, more than 43 million people—18.3 percent of the non-elderly population—had no health insurance. The year before, the figure was around 41 million.

If Congress attacks the problem, it probably will take only a few small steps: make health insurance 100 percent tax-deductible for the self-employed, for instance, or set up a system that lets private organizations (like religious groups and labor unions) negotiate health insurance deals for its members as employers do now.

Congress isn't likely to take a big leap, but Cooksey plans to give the legislators a shove. He's writing a bill that would offer tax deductions to those who buy health insurance and provide tax credits or vouchers to people who can't afford insurance. "The current employer-based health-care system, is flawed," says Cooksey, who will introduce his bill later this year.

■ NEW REGULATIONS AND REVIEWS

Last summer, HCFA postponed the implementation of its new guidelines for documentation of evaluation and management services. But the guidelines, which elicited a torrent of objections from physicians, haven't gone away. HCFA is still working on them, with limited help from the AMA. According to the latest projection, they'll be finalized this year or early next.

This spring, OIG will release its third annual audit of Medicare payments. The previous reports established a certain pattern. First, Congress expresses outrage at the amount of improper billings and reimbursements. Second, medicine attacks OIG's auditing methodology and frets that Congress and the public will blame doctors for gaming the system. Third, HCFA announces new initiatives to fight improper billing—as well as outright fraud and abuse. Fourth, physicians become more anxious. Fifth, business goes on as usual. Then the next year's report, new congressional outrage, etc. Maybe OIG will report a brighter billing-and-payment picture this time, and the pattern will be broken. But probably not.

In 1999, OIG will review several aspects of physicians' Medicare billing practices. HCFA will tinker with the practice-expense component of physician Medicare fees; phase two of the resource-basing of practice expenses goes into effect January 2000. The agency will work toward "administration simplification," a set of regulations that affect the transmission and security of electronic medical data.

Everyone's going to be busy—and a little worried. A storm cloud hangs over the federal government, and nowhere is it darker than over HCFA. The government must ready its computer systems for 2000. The General Accounting Office, which is monitoring the federal agencies' progress, hasn't given HCFA's Y2K work good marks. If HCFA doesn't get its act together quickly, physicians could be looking at lengthy delays in Medicare reimbursements a year from now.

▓ *GETTING REAL ABOUT HEALTH CARE*

According to syndicated columnist David S. Broder, health-care issues remain unsolved because "the problems are real but the solutions are not." A realistic discussion of health care must include three things: cost, coverage, and quality.

"All three are inextricably linked," Broder writes. "But Washington has chosen to deal with them one at a time—and by doing so, it has almost guaranteed that realistic solutions will not be found."

In a few short years, we've gone from Clinton-care, which was mostly about coverage, to patient protection, which is mostly about quality. Will 1999 be the year Congress seriously considers cost, coverage, *and* quality?

No. Neither Congress nor the public is ready yet. Last November, Americans told legislators to get real. But they didn't mean *that* real.

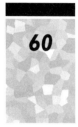

60

They're Here, They're Gray

Aimee Howd

Americaʼs 77 million baby boomers are aging. The first of them turned 50 on Jan. 1, 1996. Fifteen years into the third millennium they will become the largest generation of retirees in American history. For more than a decade gerontologists, economists and demographers have been warning public-policy makers that when this mammoth generation hits retirement the United States will have a crisis on its hands.

Public-policy makers, in turn, have quaked in their tasseled loafers at the thought of tangling with age 50-plus voters. Seventy-seven percent of those 65 and older—more than any other age group—turned out at the polls in 1996. Although they are divided roughly 60/40 Democrat and Republican, nothing galvanizes them like a threat to their own interests. The American Association of Retired Persons, or AARP, claims more than 30 million members, nearly 2,000 staffers, an annual budget of half a billion dollars and is regarded as the most successful lobby in the capital.

The numbers of those over 65 will increase by 47 percent during the next decade alone. And scientific and medical advances promise boomers the longest average life span of any generation in history, as a new politics of aging affects every aspect of domestic and foreign policy.

Sen. Charles Grassley, the Iowa Republican who chairs the Senate Special Committee on Aging, called a hearing in November—published as "The Babyboomers Are Coming: Aging in a New Millennium"—to look at the impending age wave. "It's already the most politically sensitive issue Congress deals with," Grassley tells **Insight.**

First among the hot buttons of aging politics, of course, are Social Security and Medicare. At the Aging Committee hearing, ranking member Sen. John Breaux, a Louisiana Democrat, remarked: "While strengthening these programs is essential, the retirement and health-care programs are only two pieces of a much bigger puzzle. The size and distinct character of the boomers will not only create a sense of urgency to current issues but create a whole new set of aging issues."

Half of baby-boomer households have a total net worth of just $10,000, so it already is clear that most haven't saved enough to sustain the high standard of living to which they're accustomed—especially if Social Security benefits are cut. It also is clear that those benefits will be sustainable only by major tax increases for their working children and grandchildren, further reducing savings by succeeding generations.

In the 20th century the number of Americans older than age 65 increased from 3 million at its beginning (when life expectancy was just 47 years) to 33 million at its close (when life expectancy reached 80 years). The U.S. Census Bureau predicts that by 2035 the aged will number 70 million. And increased life expectancies have been matched by decreased birthrates, down from 3.8 during the baby boom after World War II to 2.1 today. Thus, the ratio of workers to retirees has fallen drastically even as elder benefits have risen to 33 percent of the federal budget—a per-capita expenditure for the elderly 11 times that for children.

Baby boomers are busy caring for their own children as well as their aging parents, confronting their own mortality and recognizing that their retirement years are approaching. The more thoughtful among them are seeing the tensions between their own likely reliance on government benefits and their concern for their children.

Baby boomer Terri Kelly turns 50 this month and qualifies for the seniors discount at the Kentucky Fried Chicken fast-food chain. A homemaker and a bus driver for the Head Start program in the small town of Kirksville, Mo., she is no political hobbyist but, as her parents aged, she began to follow federal aging policy. Kelly says that unlike millions of Americans who mark the milestone of turning 50 by handing over their dues to join an advocacy group for the aged (most often the AARP), she doesn't see any reason to fund advocates for status-quo retirement entitlements.

"The entitlement system is going to get top-heavy when we [baby boomers] get there. The younger people are going to have to pay more and more out of their checks, because there will be more retirees compared to workers," says Kelly, whose two sons entered the workforce this year at ages 20 and 21. "It's going to put too much of a burden on the next generation. They'll resent it. It's just not right."

Add to Social Security costs the taxation for Medicare, the lack of trained elder-care providers and other long-term care concerns and, as a political issue, these problems begin to look like a fiery pit.

Seniors who are thinking of the costs of policies they advocate now in terms of future generations have formed some alternative lobbying groups, including 60 Plus Association and the American Seniors Coalition. And a September 1999 Zogby poll not only showed wide support across party lines and racial groups for allowing people to invest their Social Security taxes in privately owned individual retirement accounts, but found they were more likely to vote for candidates who support such privatization in this year's elections.

Yet Social Security reform frightens politicians and the status quo is still on a collision course with the actuarial future. Doomsayers prophesy an all-out intergenerational war, pitting baby boomers against generation Xers to scrap over zero-sum resources. Less febrile analysts simply are asking how a democratic society can balance the benefits everyone wants to provide to the elderly with the costs of those benefits to their children and grandchildren.

In 1994, investment banker Peter Peterson, a former Commerce secretary, adviser to presidents and chairman of the Council on Foreign Relations, served on Clinton's bipartisan Kerrey-Danforth Commission on Entitlement and Tax Reform. The commission issued a report, endorsed unanimously by its 20 Democratic and Republican congressional members, which published the blistering conclusion that without reform the costs of just five programs—Social Security, Medicare, Medicaid and federal civilian and military pensions—would exceed total federal revenues by 2030. This, of course, means that not a dime would be available for any other program, from national defense to education. In an interview with **Insight,** Peterson notes that "for the first time [Democrats and Republicans had] agreed on the scope of the crisis."

But because the issue was so politically volatile the commission expired without making concrete proposals for change. To this day, Peterson reports, almost everyone involved in public life remains too afraid of the political cross fire to risk advocacy of the public-policy adjustments needed to disarm the time bomb.

In his important new book, *The Grey Dawn,* Peterson says there is a "growing disjuncture between what leaders know must be done and what policy changes they are willing to take to the voters." He tells **Insight,** "One of the profound philosophic questions is can a democracy like ours deal with a silent, slow-motion crisis that isn't going to have an impact in the current election cycle. Will we undergo pain to solve a problem for someone else's gain five years in the future?"

Peterson points out that the obvious elements of America's aging crisis are only a drop in the ocean of a global aging crisis that will change international relationships of the entire developed world. According to government figures, its full force will begin breaking during the next five or 10 years throughout Japan and Western Europe, where (barring sizable immigration) the population will shrink to half its present size in the next 50 years. The ratio of working taxpayers to nonworking pensioners is 1-to-3 in developed nations; by 2030, it will fall to 1.5-to-1 or lower, barring reforms.

As the capital of older developed nations is poured into pensions and the countries grow desperate for workers, will younger developing nations find that the balance of power has shifted into their hands? Within developed nations will culture wars erupt under the pressures of immigration and labor shortages? What does a power shift mean for the international security commitments of a weakened developed world?

"I keep wondering if some young political leader isn't going to see this problem coming and instead of formulating it as 'greedy geezers vs. the young' create a new political coalition, based on general interest in behalf of the future in which the young and the old join forces around a common future," says Peterson. "It sounds idealistic, I know. And it's certainly not present now."

But in the midst of cost and crisis questions surrounding the new old population, unprecedented opportunities also emerge. Ken Dychtwald, psychologist, gerontologist and author of the newly released book, *Age Power: How the 21st Century Will Be Ruled by the New Old,* sees the pros and cons in the aging of his own generation. "Sixty-five years as a marker of old age has become obsolete. Let people choose to retire when they are ready and when they can afford to, instead of using a cutoff age [of 65] set in Germany when average life expectancy was 45," he argues.

With 50 soon to be the average age of the nation's population, people will have new choices about how to invest their longer and healthier lives. Dychtwald points out that 40 million retirees spend an average of 43 hours a week watching TV. "I think that we think of the elderly the wrong way," says Dychtwald. "We think of them as lost souls, as decrepit men and women who need our charity above all. I think of them as fascinating wise men and women who have an abundance of resources that could be helping to nourish America."

Discussion Questions

1. If any one of our past nursing leaders were here today, how do you think she would judge our present-day efforts in politics?

2. Discuss the factors that contribute to the lack of participation by nurses in politics.

3. In what ways are you politically active in school or in your community?

4. If nurses fail to be of one voice about their profession and health policy, who will speak for them?

5. What do you think it would take for Congress to stop playing politics with health care? Elaborate.

6. In your opinion, why are elderly people so ill-informed about Medicare and Medicare+Choice?

7. Which aspect of Medicare do you feel is in most need of reform? State your reasons.

8. Does our democracy have the will to deal with health care problems during an election year? What will it take?

Further Readings

Bellandi, D. & Hallam, K. (1999). Lobbies work hard during congressional recess. *Modern Healthcare, 29*(35), 2–3, 14, 16.

Birmbaum, J. H. (1999). Follow the money. Hard money. Soft money. Lobbying money. Which buy Washington? *Fortune, 140*(11), 206–208.

Frank, B. (2000). Taps for caps: Budget myth and realities. *The American Prospect,* February 14; 21–23.

McClymont, M. (1999). Hearing old voices. *Elder Care, 11*(6), 8–12.

Meier, E. (1999). Political activities for rainy days. *Nursing Economics, 17*(3), 181–184.

Stone, P. H. (1999). Kinder, gentler arm-twisting. *The National Journal, 31*(29), 2080–2081.

Web Site Resources for Politics

E.politics   www.epolitics.com
National Political Index   www.politicalindex.com
Politics 1   www.politics1.com
PoliticsOnline   www.politicsonline.com
Votenet   www.votenet.com

General Search Engine Web Sites

Excite   www.excite.com
Lycos   www.lycos.com

Health Web Sites

Caresoft   www.caresoft.com
USA Healthcare   www.usahealthcare.org/index.shtml

Professional Journal Web Sites

MedWebplus   www.medwebplus.com
Revolution Magazine   www.revolutionmag.com

PART FIVE

ENVISIONING THE FUTURE

13

Back to the Future

Most of us are fascinated by the future. We like to think of ourselves as forward looking, leaving the past as an entertainment for incurable nostalgics. In a society where nothing lasts for long and built-in obsolescence is a way of life, history is considered by many as just another "throw away." Not so. The health care problems we face are not new or obsolete. Our history tells us that; the future tells us nothing. To make our future a reality, we must learn from the lessons of the past. Being able to envision the future comes from using the building blocks of the past to create a foundation of lessons that can be used to shape our future.

Nursing's history is a treasure trove of experiences rich in courage, risk taking, and purpose. Throughout this book readings from our history illustrate those experiences and the evolution of thought and progress within nursing. In their totality, they illuminate the past and, with the lessons they provide, nourish our future. And what lessons might they hold for us? That depends on what we're looking for. Do they illuminate our way and guide us to the future? Is nursing's history merely a weary rehearsal of mistakes that we are destined to repeat? How has nursing changed over the years? Are the sequences of events in nursing's history such that we can foresee what our future might be? What does our history tell us about our profession and ourselves?

Opening the door to our history allows us to discover and reflect upon the early days of nursing and what it was like back then. What were the concerns of nurses in those times? The first reading in this chapter is an account of what nursing was like and what nurses did in those early days. Some similarities are present, but the differences illustrating the evolution of nursing practice since those early days are remarkable. Other questions come to mind. What was nursing like 40 years ago? What were nursing's issues back then? What were nurses' hopes for the future? Were those hopes realistic? How were they met? Were they met at all? Are the concerns of nursing still the same? What hasn't changed in nursing? Those are some of the questions that come to mind as the remaining readings are explored. Starting with the year 1950, and continuing over a span of several decades, nurses and other health care professionals share their hopes for the future. What they have to say connects us to what was, what came to be, and, ultimately, to what may be. Their voices speak of common concerns and problems, many of which are with us still. Above all, they speak with voices of hope and promise. The themes that emerge are the threads that bind us to nursing's history and from which we weave its future.

61

A Backward Glimpse

Anne A. Williamson

I well remember when the ambitious little *Journal* appeared on the horizon, for at that time—1900—I was well started on private nursing in New York City, having graduated in 1896 from what was then the New York Hospital School of Nursing, now affiliated with Cornell University.

I remember how hard nurses worked at that time. People thought we were superior beings who could go on indefinitely, sometimes twenty-four hours out of the twenty-four. In those early years we cared for maternity patients in private homes and apartments. Once, when I pointed out to a patient that her apartment was rather small for the birth of a baby, and suggested that she go to the private patient's department at Sloan, she felt insulted and said she would not disgrace her baby by having it born in a hospital!

Many operations were done in the home in those days. The first case I had after I graduated was for a very well-known surgeon. He gave me his printed instructions and the address of the patient, and that was all I had to help me, except what I had read about operations in "Clara Weeks." I went to the house the day before the operation and started in. Carpets had to be taken up—they were nailed down in those days—the floor scrubbed, pictures removed, the walls wiped down, curtains removed, and the windows washed. When I finished the "spring cleaning," I hunted all over the house for basins and pitchers enough for a major operation; these I left to soak in bichloride in the bath tub. The next day we moved the kitchen table in and went to work. For the anesthetic, we made a cone of newspaper, put in a wad of cotton or gauze, and poured the ether or chloroform on it. You may wonder how we ever had satisfactory results with such primitive methods, but the patient made a wonderful recovery.

Anne Williamson, R.N. (New York Hospital School of Nursing, now associated with Cornell University) was associated with the California Hospital, Los Angeles in the capacity of director of social service. Many of the changes in nursing which she refers to here she has described in her book, Fifty Years in Starch.

Often we would go to houses where there was no plumbing, no gas, and of course no electric light. We used kerosene lamps or candles and quite often I had to hold the lamp over the incision in order that the surgeon could see distinctly. Can you imagine what the fire department would think of such a procedure today? But we never had an accident.

Some of the hospital operating room procedures would also seem unusual now. I remember especially the sponges we used. They were real sponges—we called them "elephant ears"—and my hands were almost parboiled from wringing them out of hot water. We never could be sure they were surgically clean. Once during an operation I squeezed some sand out of one. I managed to drop it on the floor and go on as if nothing had happened, although the supervisor gave me a look that hinted dire consequences. The "dressing-down" she gave me when the operation was over made me so angry that I never did tell her why I dropped the sponge.

We treated maternity patients differently in those days, too. When I think of all the clothes the babies wore—the tight band around the abdomen, the long petticoat that was folded about the feet so the baby could not kick and get a bit of exercise, and then the long dress. And those long binders we put on the mother—one hundred and fifty safety pins in each!

Nurses uniforms also are more sensible now. We no longer wear long skirts that pick up all the dirt on the floor, or high starched collars, or the stiff cuffs that we were not allowed to take off unless we were giving a tub bath. If we should appear in those outfits today we would look like the pictures in the old nursing books. In fact, one day I put on my old student nurse uniform to have a picture taken, and as I was walking down the corridor of the hospital I heard a visitor say, "My, look at that nurse. Doesn't this hospital ever progress?"

When we graduated, $25 a week for a private duty nurse was considered the height of affluence, and for the most part it was for an all-night-and-day job. It took the greater part of fifty years to increase it to $11 for an eight-hour day. Now nurses can live a normal life like other professional women; most large hospitals have adopted the forty-hour week, salaries have certainly improved, and nurses no longer think it is unethical to consider the financial aspects of their professional work.

In addition to everything else, the status of the student nurse has changed a great deal in the past fifty years. I can well remember the long hours of duty, the classes and lectures in the evening after a hard day on the wards, and the pernicious habit—in some hospitals—of sub-letting (so to speak) the students as special nurses for private patients. Sometimes they were assigned to twenty-four-hour duty with very sick patients; a cot was put in the room but there was no chance to use it. Most students nowadays, however, are assured a real professional education. More attention is given to the social life of the nurse and the absurd rule that student nurses and interns must not meet socially—a rule that was impossible to enforce because everyone broke it—has been relegated to the dark ages.

Doctors now treat nurses in a far more professional manner than they did fifty years ago. The time has passed when a nurse was told to give the white pill at six o'clock, the powder at bedtime, and the pink capsule when the patient asked for it. I used to feel like a small child when I received an order like that.

Another conquest that has been made during the past fifty years is the attitude of the United States Government towards the professional nurse. I served in the war with Spain in 1898 and I remember how nurses who volunteered for the service were turned down at first. Finally public opinion and the activity of the newspaper reporters were responsible for nurses being accepted, under the auspices of the Red Cross, for the camp hospitals where typhoid was raging. The nurse furnished her own uniforms, her equipment, and many other things needed by her patients.

In World War I, nurses were not only accepted but encouraged to volunteer, but they lacked true officer status and were still dominated by the petty officers, especially by the top sergeant who felt that he was in charge. By World War II, however, not only were nurses enrolled with the beginning rank of second lieutenant, but before the war was over they had received full commissioned status.

More than fifty years have now come and gone since I first practiced nursing. I can forget the hard knocks of those early days when I realize that it was those hard knocks that helped to raise our profession to where it stands today. We are going on to bigger and better things. It has been a privilege to have worked alongside of many famous nurses who have blazed the trail and who are with us no more. If they were with us now, I know that they would share my satisfaction in knowing, not that we have arrived, but that we are "on the way."

62

Looking Ahead With the Nursing Profession

Leonard A. Scheele

*F*orecasting the future of any social institution is bound to be a compound of interpretation of historical developments, observation of current trends, and of wishful thinking. A forecast is also a view from a single point in time, and the factors contributing to the prediction may at the very moment be undergoing marked alterations. Especially is this true in a period of rapid and violent change, such as the era in which the whole world is living. Rather than forecast the future of nursing, therefore, I should like to set forth some of the current trends and their possible results.

In considering these trends, I am struck by the similarity of the problems affecting nursing, medicine, dentistry, pharmacy—in fact, all of the health professions. Possibly each group has some problems which appear to affect it uniquely; but if we study these problems minutely we are likely to conclude that they are similar to those in the related professions. I like to think of nursing, not as a separate element in health services, but as an integral part of the whole; to think of nurses, not merely as specialists, but as integral members of the health team. The possibilities in nursing, as I see them, are therefore similar to those in other health professions.

■ THE FORCES SHAPING OUR HEALTH SERVICES

The course of events in nursing, as in other types of health service, is being shaped by powerful social forces which arise outside the professions. Among the forces that are directly affecting the health professions, the following are of major importance:

Dr. Scheele's position as surgeon general of the Public Health Service, Federal Security Agency, enabled him to keep in close touch with the nursing profession; viewing health problems from an overall standpoint, he was well qualified to discuss the possible developments of nursing.

1. The growth of the nation in population, education, and wealth, which increases the effective demand for health services of all kinds.
2. The desire of the consumers to have a responsible share in the planning, organization, and administration of their health services.
3. The aging of the population which increases the volume of long-term illness and thus increases the need for services.
4. Advances in medical science and technology which increase the complexity and costs of facilities and of many types of service. (Conversely, advances also reduce the amount of service required in some situations and make possible new, large-scale services at lower unit costs. For example, the introduction of antibiotics has greatly reduced the amount of work involved in the treatment of infectious diseases.)

The nursing profession itself—along with other professions—also helps to shape our health services. As stated in the recent report of the Expert Committee on Nursing of the World Health Organization, nurses—the "final agents" in health service—determine in large measure the quality of the care which reaches people. It is interesting to note that the nations with the finest health records possess both medical and nursing personnel of high quality. Increasingly, nurses also contribute to planning with individuals and groups. A recent British report[1] states that "the nurse with her disciplined training and many-sided humanity has a contribution to make to policy-making on questions of health and welfare and in the wider field of public affairs." And so I say that the nursing profession itself is a force which molds our health services.

■ MORE EFFECTIVE USE OF PERSONNEL

In a recent study of a New England hospital, it was found that head nurses were spending from 20 to 25 per cent of their time on such duties as the floor clerk of a hotel usually performs. The same situation has been revealed in studies conducted in other parts of the country. In other hospitals, it has been found that more than 50 per cent of the nursing care is provided by unclassified auxiliary personnel.

These findings strikingly indicate that more effective use of personnel is essential. It is not likely that a great increase in the amount of service per patient will be possible. The major improvements in quality of service must then derive from improved administration.

The nurse is also part of the larger team dedicated to care of the sick and to promotion of human health. Up to the present time the nurse has been given too few educational and work opportunities to participate in a many disciplined team, in which her judgment as well as her technical skill is sought. Several developments indicate that the nurse will be used increasingly as a member of a medical or public health team representing a variety of special knowledges and skills. The home care program for chronically ill patients at Montefiore Hospital, for example, places the hospital nurse in a teamwork relationship not only with the physician, but also with social workers, physiotherapists, and visiting nurses. In public health programs, nurses are being brought into team relationships with social workers, health educators, nutritionists, school teachers, sanitarians, and other personnel. Clinical research requires not only highly skilled nursing, but teamwork of a high order among clinicians, laboratory scientists and technicians, nurses, and all others engaged in the project. The recent expansion of clinical research in chronic diseases is likely to continue; as a result, more nurses will be needed on research teams.

The development of community nursing services also is a growing trend. The co-ordination of public health nursing, visiting nursing, and home care programs has been under way in some of our larger communities for a number of years. As programs for care of the chronically ill expand, the opportunities for group nursing, health supervision of elderly people, case finding in the families of patients, and education of patients for convalescence and rehabilitation will increase.

■ THE NURSE AND THE COMMUNITY

Nursing, like all other health services, is a social institution and its future cannot be considered apart from the society in which it functions. The type, scope, and organization of services depend upon the decisions of the community in which the services are provided.

In the United States, the local community is the social unit immediately responsible for determining and supporting its health services; but the local community itself is a part of larger communities, the state, and the nation. On these the local community calls for leadership and assistance.

This interplay of national, state, and local influences is what gives American community life its remarkable characteristic of unity in infinite variety. Up to the present time, this American trait has been reflected in a tough resistance to the imposition of rigid patterns, whether on the part of national official agencies or national voluntary and professional organizations. In many cases, state organizations also are resisted or disregarded by local communities even when proposed changes seem to be urgently needed. The greatest challenge to leaders in every walk of life, in national, state, or local organizations, is to preserve the stability and individuality of the local community, without encouraging static and negative attitudes.

Nursing has never relinquished its basic preoccupation with the patient; but the struggle for standards, qualifications, decent conditions of employment, and professional recognition has grown more intense and has been fraught with greater difficulties in recent years. Inevitably, the problems of nursing have produced a certain amount of separatism, as have similar problems in medicine, dentistry, pharmacy, and other professions involved in the provision of health services.

The professions on the whole have not yet learned that social problems cannot be solved effectively by any one group, and that society has a primary responsibility in solving these problems. Moreover, the professions have not fully recognized that community leaders can contribute sound thinking, fresh viewpoints, and practical aid to the solution of professional problems. The presence of leaders in public affairs on several advisory councils of the Public Health Service has demonstrated this truth to our organization.

In the past three years, there has been a striking increase in citizens' groups concerned with planning and action for better community health services. It is probable that this trend will continue with gathering impetus, as the demands for health services increase. Moreover, the scope of problems which come under the purview of community organizations for health is likely to increase. Whereas action in recent years has been focused largely on community hospital facilities and local health units, care of the chronically ill and aged will gain major importance.

The public also is aware of the shortages of health personnel; but for the most part, the awareness is not buttressed by understanding of the specific problems of recruitment, education, employment, and distribution of personnel. Once the citizens realize that the facilities and services they are planning cannot materialize without personnel, they will undoubtedly give these problems a high priority on their agenda, and they will recognize that the community, too, has a responsibility in financing the education of health personnel. They will look to the health professions for information, advice, and cooperation—not for direction or for ready-made plans conceived without reference to the community's needs, aspirations, and resources.

If the professions meet the public forthrightly in attempts to solve common problems, benefits will flow back and forth across the conference table. It should be said, however, that the mere participation of all groups concerned does not insure effective solutions. Only when the participants lose some of their identity and learn to think and act as a group, focusing upon the problem, will their proposals be pertinent, widely accepted, and put into operation. Too often, professional leaders in the health field assume the attitude of teacher, assigning the role of pupil to leaders in other fields and in public affairs. Too often, civic leaders are recruited to some professional cause as a "front" to assure community acceptance and prestige. Sooner or later, the professions will come to realize that neither of these attitudes will achieve the desired results. Only when the professions sit down as real partners with other leaders to solve problems in relation to the consumers' needs and resources, will the public and the professions work out the most effective and satisfying plans for health services.

The nurse is an invaluable member of a health planning group. She becomes a leader of real stature when she brings to the group her rich experience in service to human beings and in association with her nursing colleagues, leaving at the door of the conference room a little of her professional pride, and a few of her preconceived ideas of standards and functions.

The trends toward greater public participation in health affairs and toward greater professional participation in community affairs are here to stay. From my point of view, they are the most encouraging trends in sight. With increased support from the community, increased recognition by other professions, and greater demands for service from every quarter of the globe, the future of nurses and the nursing profession looks very bright.

63

Nursing in the Decade Ahead

Maryann Bitzer, Nancy Milio, and Hildegard Peplau

Computers have entered our lives . . .

Maryann Bitzer

Since 1951 when the first commercial model began operating in the U.S. Census Bureau, computers have made a remarkable impact upon many areas in our society. Their use in specialized areas has contributed to man's journey to and exploration of the moon, while their widespread use in business has added what might be called a "dunning letter syndrome" to man's list of frustrations.

Nursing as a profession, though not one of the first areas to be affected by computers, will by no means be the least affected. The computer's capacity for record keeping, information retrieval, and decision making will be in evidence throughout hospitals from medical record libraries and laboratories to nurses' desks in the coming decade. At their desks nurses will have on-line access to computers to assist them in planning patient care.

Maryann Bitzer was an instructor in nursing fundamentals, medical-surgical nursing, and social science. In 1963, she began work in computer-assisted instruction and in 1966 began directing a project in computer-based education for nurses at Mercy Hospital School of Nursing, Urbana, Ill. She earned a B.S. and an M.S. in educational psychology at the University of Illinois, Urbana.

Nancy Milio is best known for her work in Detroit's ghetto with the Mom's and Tot's clinic, which she described in the Journal in March 1968 and in 9226 Kercheval, a book published in 1970 by the University of Michigan Press, Ann Arbor. Ms. Milio, a graduate of the College of Nursing, Wayne State University, also earned an M.A. in sociology at Wayne and a Ph.D. in sociology at Yale University, New Haven, CT.

Practitioner, master teacher, lecturer, and writer, Hildegard Peplau, was president of the American Nurses Association and professor of psychiatric nursing at Rutgers University, New Brunswick, NJ. She is probably best known as a teacher of many generations of psychiatric nurses and for her book, Interpersonal Relations in Nursing. She earned a diploma at the Pottstown, PA Hospital School of Nursing, a B.A. at Bennington College, VT., and M.A. and Ed.D. degrees at Teachers College, Columbia University. During 1969–1970, she was interim director of the ANA.

Computers, already in use in medical research and diagnosis, are beginning to be of real value in the care of critically ill patients. Monitoring of cardiac intensive care patients, preprocessing electrocardiograms and X-rays, processing anesthesia and surgical data, obtaining obstetrical intensive care information are but a few current uses being reported. Large, time-shared systems, while providing patient monitoring, can provide numerous other functions simultaneously.

Computer-based education (CBE), is one important aspect of computer use which will make major changes in society and in man himself. Data gathered in studies of CBE over a 10-year period indicate it is likely that nurses of the future will receive at least some portion of their basic education via computer-based education systems. With computer terminals located in classrooms, libraries, dormitories, or homes, nurses will be able to interact with a large, remote computer system. Computers will provide them with information in written, pictorial, or verbal form and produce computerized simulations of patients and problem situations. Using the keyset of computer-connected terminals, nurses will control their own progress through lesson material and type comments, questions, and responses to questions. Using their own approaches to problems, they will be able to perform experiments, gather data, and evaluate their own work.

Computers will process responses, judge them in a variety of ways, and indicate the results immediately. Although a single computer system will serve thousands of students simultaneously, it will still provide each student with material suited to his learning ability and interest. The computer also will be capable of concurrently teaching a variety of courses while providing diverse services to other medical areas.

A nurse may find that orientation to her job will, in part, be provided by way of a computer terminal located at her place of employment. At the same time, other nurses, participating in inservice education programs will keep abreast of new developments in the health field through new study units programmed each week. In another section of the hospital, a diabetic patient will be able to sit at a terminal and practice menu planning with an instructional program prepared by a nutrition therapist. Meanwhile, a new patient at a terminal in the admitting office will provide his personal and medical history through a computer interview.

Assistance to the medical staff with the monitoring of critically ill patients, the pathology department with their research, and the teaching staff with the education of students, employees, and patients are only a few of the many uses of the computer in a medical center.

Though much of this work is still in beginning stages, all indications are that computers are likely to play an integral part in assisting members of the health professions to provide comprehensive health care to people. Not only will computers provide efficient services to each member of the health team but, with terminals in homes, a large part of the population in any given area can be instructed in health practices, thus giving preventive medicine an additional impetus.

Nursing has a choice of perspectives . . .

Nancy Milio

Nursing in this decade can choose to move in one of two major directions. It can continue its rightfully termed "navel-gazing" activities, its concern with itself as a profession, making it increasingly ingrown and isolated. Or, it can lift its sights to a broader perspective of major concern for health care in the United States, and thereby accept its share of responsibility for the record set by health professionals in this country, a deplorable record when compared with more than a score of other nations in the world, most of whom are far less technologically advanced than we.

The ingrowness fostered by profession*alism*—an overconcern with the accoutrements of a profession—has characterized nursing for longer than some of us can remember. It has led to overspecialization, and the financial, prestigeful, and organizational rewards that go with it for the few and the opposite for the many, all labelled "nursing personnel." It has been based on the assumption that more nurses, more and higher college degrees in nursing, or even better paid nurses make for better health care. That assumption has never been proved, and, indeed, some studies suggest that it is false. We know that more funds *per se* have not improved health care, witness Medicare and Medicaid.

Our fetish for professionalism has led to an emphasis on institutions rather than the community, an emphasis which is reflected in the recent report of the National Commission for the Study of Nursing and Nursing Education. This report is disappointing because among other things, it assumes that health care means "sickness care" and, therefore, clinical training and specialization is the focus in preparation for nursing.

A more timely perspective for nursing would result if we focused on health rather than on sickness. Basic nursing education must include an understanding of and practice with intergroup and interorganizational relations. It must give nurses an opportunity to comprehend the sociocultural and political-economic influences which produce sickness and affect the health care settings in which they practice. The understanding of interpersonal concepts now taught is simply not sufficient for a broader perspective.

Then graduate work, as one option, could prepare nurse-clinicians. But another important option ought to be programs to prepare a kind of nurse-organizer-planner-manager who could focus on the group and organizational aspects of health care, from local ghettos to the national political economy.

If nurses so prepared were available, nursing would not have to fret over not being called upon by health planning groups. If nursing had developed concern and definitive principles about health care reorganization, it would not *wait* to be called upon. A nursing profession which looked outward would long since have been among the leaders of planning national health insurance legislation. It would be working on means to implement a fundamental reorganization of health care services, including the involvement of all social and economic groups. It would be opening the profession to the disadvantaged and to older persons by developing educational programs which recognize beginning practice in the health field, work as a community aide, for example, and credit this work toward professional education. It would be publicly criticizing the use of financial and organizational resources for ultraspecialized medical technology which benefit the few, while millions want for the minimum of preventive health care.

With such a perspective nursing might attract the growing able group of women now concerned with the women's liberation movement, the more socially aware men and women from economically disadvantaged groups, as well as activist youth from affluent families.

Few will doubt the direction nursing is likely to take unless the scattered members of the profession who hold non–status quo views can mobilize themselves and lead nursing in a more socially relevant direction.

Nurses as a collectivity must take a stand . . .

Hildegard Peplau

When it is difficult to distinguish between trend-based projections and wishes for the future of nursing, both ought to considered. One thing is certain: changes now occurring in this society coupled with the efforts of nurses will reshape nurses' work.

Nursing has come a long way since 1900; it is now on the verge of being a profession, fully recognized as such by other disciplines and by the public; it has been moving slowly but steadily toward becoming an independent health service, one that complements and interdigitates with the services of many other disciplines—medicine, social work, psychological services, and the like. Coincidentally, the "pyramid" view of the patient care disciplines is yielding slowly to the "pie" concept. Colleagueship is evolving; the expertise of each health professional, from his "wedge of the pie," shared and interrelated, all together comprise the "patient care" or "health maintenance services" society needs. In the decades ahead, this shift in concept will be more clearly recognized and implemented. For nurses to participate fully, the reshaping of basic nursing curriculums will need to include theory and practice related to nursing care of the ill and nursing practice directed toward health maintenance.

Improved patterns of health care will surely emerge both from the widespread present concerns and concerted efforts by all the health disciplines to bring about more useful systems of delivery of health services. The economics of health care and the relationship between costs and full utilization of those professionals in short supply will dictate both shared responsibility and revised systems. In this regard, reconsideration of Lydia Hall's concept put into practice at Loeb Center, New York, N.Y. would be useful—a view very much ahead of its time. This concept holds that what is needed for the critically ill is a well-organized, equipped, and thus expensive, medical science center in which medicine is the primary, authoritative profession. Thereafter, often in a matter of a few days, patients require a less costly nursing science center, in which professional nursing is the primary discipline. The effectiveness and economy of this two-step delivery system has been demonstrated.

Several new phrases are being introduced into everyday language and being acted upon, coined to spur recognition that intelligence, competence, and social responsibility are, indeed, not sex linked: "women's liberation," "be all that you can be," "rescue the female brain," and the like. As these cliches catch on, nursing which now is a predominantly woman's profession will certainly benefit.

In the decade ahead we can expect more nurses to seek graduate education and, thus, more clinical specialists in the various components of nursing and more researchers will become available to enlarge the development now barely begun of the scientific practice aspects of nursing.

As the anti-intellectualism that plagues nursing gives way and wider social respect for the female intelligence emerges, new forms of independent striving can be expected. Greater public demand for new types of health services, efforts toward population limitation, and the concept of career-and-marriage for women, will contribute toward greater independence of nurses. Private practice of nursing in all clinical areas will increase. Partnership group practices of physicians *and* nurses will develop, the nurse retaining her own professional identification and collecting her own fees for services. These services will be both of remedial and health maintenance kinds.

Nurses have demonstrated a singularly significant individual commitment to direct nursing care of sick people. Witness the outstanding record of registered nurses everywhere to the poor, the needy, the sick and the injured, under conditions of peace, war, and civilian emergencies. However, in order to achieve their social aims of improving the health of this society, nurses will need to recognize and participate in a second and equally important aspect of the commitment which society expects of a professional. The young, particularly, recognize that pollution of the water and air, slum housing, ineffective educational systems, hunger, war, and other such hazards to healthy living must also be the concern of the health professional. While the individual nurse can certainly take some local action with regard to these problems, changes in the direction of improved conditions for healthy living are more likely to occur when the collectivity takes a stand. The American Nurses Association is the mechanism through which individual nurses—contributing their dues, expert opinions, and efforts—can address themselves to the larger social issues that impinge upon health. The nursing profession, as an organized collectivity of individual nurses, is remiss when it does not speak—at the state and federal levels—on matters that pertain to health. And it cannot speak effectively unless all registered nurses commit themselves to support this effort.

In the decades ahead, nurses in greater numbers will slowly but surely recognize their need for ANA—their need to pool their money and power in order to effect social changes that are essential to strengthening nursing practice and making nursing a viable force in health affairs at the policy making level in this society.

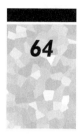

64

The Future of the Nursing Profession

Luther Christman

The commonly accepted belief that the past is prologue holds for forecasting the future of health care as well as for other phenomena. For example, a child born in 1982 could expect to live 74 years, an increase of 24 years over a child born in 1900.[1] This substantial increase in life span will show another large increment by the end of this century.

The lengthening of the average life span occurred in three different stages that grew out of the steady accumulation of scientific knowledge. The first stage ran from roughly the turn of the last century to the late 1930s and can be classified as an era of sanitation. Development of immunological techniques took place during this period, and the ravages of the highly contagious diseases and their concomitant secondary effects were markedly curtailed. The second state, which lasted well into the 1960s, was the era of antibiotics. The combined advances of the two eras eliminated all the quick killers and left to be solved the slow disease processes such as cancer and cardiovascular, renal, and endocrine diseases. The third stage of technological innovation will enable the effective management of these relatively slow-killing forms of disease, a condition that appears to have given rise to attacks against the technological imperative by science writers, economists, and bureaucrats.

A brief review of the effect of each of the three stages may place them all in a perspective that permits more rational discussion and prediction. Development of immunological techniques and antibiotics had a major impact in curtailing the forces that produce ill health until the capability of each particular form of endeavor reached its limits. Each was cost-effective. The same can be said of technology except that its full capability has not yet been demonstrated. Refinement of present technology, the development of new and simpler equipment, and occasional major breakthroughs are occurring.

At the time of this article, Luther Christman, R.N., Ph.D., F.A.A.N., was Vice President for Nursing Affairs and Dean of the College of Nursing at Rush-Presbyterian-St. Luke's Medical Center, Rush University, Chicago, Illinois.

Reprinted with permission from *Nursing Administration Quarterly*, 1987, 11(2) 1–8. Copyright © 1987, Aspen Publishers, Inc.

Over time, the costs of technology decline, and its use creates additional healthy years of life as the primary disease process is further controlled. Although the loss of brain cells, nephrons, and other important cells takes place unremittingly with age and death is inevitable, various ways will be found by means of vitamins and other chemicals to retard the aging of cells. In essence, society may soon be approaching the analogue of the parson's one-horse shay.

■ *NURSING IN TODAY'S ENVIRONMENT*

When considering the possible dimensions of the future role of the nursing profession, one must first examine current social phenomena and trends. No professional role exists in a vacuum or grows in isolation. Instead, roles develop to meet the expectations of others. It might be said that professional roles are invented by society to supply the services that can be rendered only by those with specialized knowledge. Society gives certain rights and privileges to these roles but, in turn, it exacts certain obligations. The professions that most effectively fulfill those obligations are most apt to obtain the rewards given for maintaining an adequate supply of services.

Effective Nursing Requires Advanced Training

Almost everyone is keenly aware of the rapid expansion of knowledge and the growth of technology. Both developments greatly affect all professionals. Daily confrontation with a constantly expanding stream of new and complicated information is creating uneasiness in all types of practitioners. So rapid is the creation of new knowledge that many patients probably are being treated by obsolete methods every day. What are the implications for nurses of this set of conditions? One imperative is that all nurses must form positive attitudes toward continued and advanced study. Scientists who have studied the rate at which knowledge is expanding predict that the lifetime of all knowledge will shrink so dramatically that most persons will not have current information. Thus, the knowledge that most persons possess will become outmoded almost faster than they are able to acquire new knowledge, so that many of people's actions will be based on obsolescent information.

Because of the tremendous rate at which scientific knowledge is accumulating, it is not risky to predict that the clinical doctorate will become the entry level requirement for the practice of nursing. If nurses wish to have parity on the health team, they must have equally rigorous clinical preparation.

Expert knowledge is a prime means by which power, influence, and economic rewards are secured. The laws governing the practice of nursing in all of the states will be modified greatly when this level of preparation is the common denominator. Imagine how different the milieu of care will be when every nurse, every patient, every hospital administrator, and every physician addresses all nurses as "Doctor."

The debate over requirements for entry-level practice of nursing has moved beyond the tediousness of stereotypic argumentation among nurses to one of more serious import. If one correctly reads the signs of the future of health care, the issue of entry level has assumed a higher level of abstraction—can nursing survive and grow as a profession without university education as a mandate for the basic level of preparation? For too long a time, nurses have drawn invidious comparisons between themselves and other nurses at different entry levels. In the process, they almost seem to have been oblivious to what is happening to educational preparation in the entire health field. Nurses are the only health care practitioners who have a weak academic background at the entry level. They are the proverbial low ones on the totem pole when compared with all other health professionals. What is more, the gap in knowledge between other health professionals and nurses is increasing. The entry-level preparation of physicians and dentists aside, clinical psychologists acknowledge nothing less than the doctorate; dietitians insist on a baccalaureate degree, and growing numbers are enrolling in graduate study. Similar levels of preparation are required for beginning physical therapists, occupational therapists, medical record librarians, and medical technologists. Social workers and hospital administrators recognize master's preparation and above as the nominal education, while pharmacists are required to obtain a professional doctorate as the basic preparation. Thus, the social mandate for health care practice is preparation not at the baccalaureate level but at higher levels. Are such levels of preparation necessary for the provision of health care?

One does not need a crystal ball to foresee that unless nurses have levels of education comparable to those of other prominent health care providers, nurses will become the babysitters for the other professions. If the continuing disparity in scientific and theoretical background between nurses and other health care professionals is not corrected, nurses may find themselves in the position of making the other professions look good instead of directly serving patients and improving the practice of nursing. One cannot have a poor educational background and maintain much influence over the form and direction of the health care delivery system. A worrisome prediction under these conditions is that the nursing profession may fail to attract its share of bright young minds and thus may be doomed to mediocrity. Nurses may protest that they are being ignored because they are primarily women, but that assertion is self-deluding. Men in the nursing profession have the same general attitudes and behaviors. Most of the health care professions mentioned above include large percentages of women who have found the time and means to obtain the appropriate education.

Effective Nursing Means Training in High Tech Skills

That opportunity knocks but once is a long-surviving adage. The specifics of many new and unusual developments in the health care system are relatively unpredictable. All that can be predicted is that those who may now appear over-prepared but who are ready to manage change in the best and most efficient fashion will succeed. Time and events will not wait for nurses. Nurses either will be ready or will be passed over by those more qualified. Furthermore, much of what will become interesting and exciting in the care of patients will transfer almost unnoticed until such new practices become regular features of the health care delivery system. The only certainty is that each new spin-off from science and technology will require sophisticated knowledge. The possessors of the required expert knowledge will become the prime participants in the provision of care; those without such knowledge will have secondary status. The growth of knowledge in the basic sciences is exponential. It is on university campuses that strong links with scientific research and channels for the dissemination of new knowledge provide the possibility of developing the scholarly and professional approaches to learning so necessary to accommodating new knowledge readily.

Nurses with less than a university education are far removed from links with new knowledge and probably are being taught obsolete knowledge throughout their entire basic preparation. Thus, they begin their careers with a significantly weak, questionable base of scientific knowledge. Because most nurses involved in the direct care of patients do not have a university education, they lack the fundamental knowledge that can facilitate the discovery of new and imaginative patterns of nursing care delivery systems.

The false ideologies of technical and professional nursing have demonstrated the fallacy of thinking that nurses can be alert users of science for the welfare of patients if they do not share a common base of scientific knowledge and understanding. Nurses will not be able to overcome the lag time in using sciences effectively until a large number are prepared at the doctoral level. A ratio of 1:5 at the master's level and 1:20 at the doctoral level is probably a basic necessity now to deal effectively with new scientific developments until the profession becomes fully prepared by means of doctoral education to pull its weight in the health care delivery system.

In all likelihood, the economic well-being of nurses has been severely hampered by the presence of so many small, local, nonbaccalaureate programs. Because employers can staff their hospitals with a minimum number of registered nurses supplemented by additional, less qualified nursing personnel, they do not find it necessary to compete on the open market for nurses in the same way they do for all other types of professional staff. The climate for this kind of economic exploitation is furthered by the adamant stance of faculty members who wish to perpetuate categories of training below the baccalaureate level. If all nurses were educated in universities, the economic law of supply and demand would operate as it does for all other types of educated persons that communities need.

Launching a professional career is far different for persons who have a doctoral degree than for those who do not. The ease of moving to more advanced levels is apparent. The sheer satisfaction of having levels of knowledge similar to those of colleagues on the health team, the adequacy of that base for absorbing new knowledge, and the capability of using sophisticated methods of science are all intrinsic satisfactions that stimulate interest in the job at hand. In addition, a base is formed for pursuing employment that permits the two career family to flourish with less strain than otherwise.

This state of affairs is both stimulating and alarming. The challenge is exciting. Nurses, if properly prepared, will have the potential for treating patients in a sophisticated manner not thought possible even a few years ago. On the other hand, nurses will also have to commit a sizable portion of time to organized study. The license a nurse holds will become more a license to study than a license to practice. Adopting this style of life may be difficult for some nurses. A certain aura of antiintellectualism has always been apparent within the profession. Nurses with advanced and specialized knowledge frequently have been suspect. Such an attitude is not as ingrained or widespread in the other major health professions, where the reverse is usually the case.

Nursing students graduating today have more than 40 years of practice ahead of them because the mandatory retirement age will be eliminated. During this period, changes in the delivery of health care will be more extensive than in all of history. Just the introduction of one product of technology—the computer—will change the whole methodology of giving care. Hospitals will go on-line so as to be able to use massive computers. Central computerized laboratories will replace existing individual hospital laboratories. Many patient-monitoring devices will likewise be centralized. Consultation with expert nurses from other areas of the country will be routine. By merely putting in a request, physicians, nurses, and others will receive almost instant print-outs of current information about the management of any clinical problem. Hospitals will have an entirely different staffing pattern. Only expertly trained personnel will be necessary. The intense pressure for numbers of personnel will be replaced by a search for quality and competence.

The bulk of the care will be programmed through the computer in a highly individualized and scientifically precise way based on all of the known data on the patient, including all data undergoing change through automatic monitoring, accumulated information in the national (international) data-bank about the patient's disease entity, and the clinical insights of the care providers. The massive numbers of people required to staff the infrastructure of support services will be markedly reduced or replaced, to a considerable degree, by robots and computer operation. Nurses' stations will not be needed. Release from such requirements will make possible a more imaginative type of architecture. Construction will be designed more appropriately around what is best for patients.

The voluminous medical charts for patients that now exist will be unnecessary. All the clerical work that encroaches on the time of nurses and physicians will be substantially reduced through computer programming. Management strategies will change considerably. Furthermore, computer-assisted managerial techniques will reduce the number of managers necessary to operate health care facilities. In addition, each manager and each health care provider of whatever profession will be monitored continuously for every error of commission and omission. A state of perfect accountability will be in place. All acts of excellence will likewise be recorded. Thus, quality assessment will be automated. This methodology may replace peer reviews. Renewal of licensure could be based on these data. National norms of performance could be established for licensure renewal based on meeting or exceeding these norms rather than on more flimsy continuing education credits.[2] It is only a matter of time until computerized means are available for measuring professional performance with a high degree of accuracy. All professional persons will be living in the proverbial fishbowl. Fortunately, all new information will be stored in knowledge banks that will be easily accessible so that all types of providers will learn how to be their own teachers.

▥ FUTURE WORK OF NURSES

More Time for Holistic Patient Care

It is certain that the work time of nurses will undergo great revision. What will nurses be doing? For one thing, freed from ritual and routine, from the problems of coordination, and from endless paperwork, they will have much more time to devote to patients. Nurses will attend professionally to all the psychosocial problems that persons usually have when they are ill, effectively draining off the anxiety of a patient with such life-threatening illnesses as myocardial infarction, attending to the depression and other mixed emotions of a patient with terminal carcinoma, and assisting a dying patient's family through their grief. In essence, nurses will be expected to acquire the skills needed to deal very sensitively with the wide range of emotional reactions to illness that are expressed in patients' behaviors.

Nurses will spend considerably more time as health teachers. Since the entire population of the country is becoming much better educated, most patients will be able to act as intelligent collaborators in their health care instead of as passive recipients of attention. A test of the capability of nurses to facilitate this constructive movement will be how well nurses can establish the rapport necessary to ensure success in this endeavor. As leisure time increases, families, if adequately assisted, are likely to become more involved in caring for ill family members. Because of better education and mass communication, patients and their families will be capable of making fairly accurate estimates of the quality of care they are receiving.

Need for Clinical Investigative Ability

In the future all nurses will be expected to have clinical investigative ability. Relatively few nurses will be full-time researchers, but application of the scientific method to problems of practice will be common place. Because nursing care is an applied science, all nurses will have to obtain some research training. Consequently, the means of transforming scientific knowledge into improved nursing care will be a major concern for nurse practitioners.

The clinical management of each and every patient will take the form of a mini-research design. What is now labeled the nursing process will be replaced by the more rigorous practice of using the methods of science for each clinical act. The more generalized concepts of nursing care plans and of conditioned and restricted behavior as prescribed by procedure books will fade into oblivion. Scientific rigor will be developed to a very high order. Thinking and behavior will be integrated into complex levels of sophistication in each practitioner.

New Dimensions in Nurse–Physician Relationship

The relationship between physicians and nurses will take on new dimensions. As nurses become better educated, the knowledge gap between nurses and physicians will decrease as the knowledge overlap increases. As a result, nurses will be capable of working as close collaborators with physicians on the clinical designs of patient care. From such interaction, many novel and useful formats of care are certain to evolve. Furthermore, through collaborative research, the entire system of delivering care to patients will undergo extensive reorganization. The studies being done by behavioral scientists, industrial engineers, and economists are furnishing enough knowledge to change radically many of the organizational inefficiencies in the health care system.

New Forms of Health Care

Health care will assume new forms. Most physicians and nurses focus on the management of episodic illness or crisis. In the future, this preoccupation will be less emphasized. Nurses and physicians will collaborate in programs to prevent illness and maintain health rather than seek patients only when they are ill. The economic rewards of practice probably will be tied more closely to keeping the population healthy than to attending to the cure process. Furthermore, advanced technology will enable patients to receive much of their care in their homes. Telemetry, sensoring devices, and the richer preparation of providers will make this feasible. This development, too, will require that nurses be prepared at much higher levels because they will be working as solo practitioners in the patient's home.

None of the foregoing is highly imaginary. All of the trends commented on here have already been initiated in some form or other. New and more startling innovations certainly exist in the minds of some researchers. As studies follow on studies, the cumulative effect is dramatic. The push of science, sparked by the work of inquisitive scientists, shows no signs of abatement.

■ TOMORROW'S TRENDS AND TODAY'S NURSES

What does all this mean for today's young students and for nurses already in the field? To compete successfully in this technological age, many deficits in knowledge will have to be overcome. Computer-assisted nursing practice will require that nurses possess a richer base of knowledge, including more training in mathematics and statistics and in biophysical and behavioral sciences. Nurses will have to learn techniques for using computers effectively and acquire the understanding needed to translate research findings into improved care. Since nurses will have much more time to work closely and intimately with patients, they will have the opportunity to refine their practice, in all its dimensions, to a notable extent.

The direction of future progress will be controlled not by health care providers but by worldwide developments in science and technology. Providers will adapt to these changes by retraining, by constant pursuit of new knowledge, by preparation that is wider and deeper than has been the case historically, and by a greater interdependence of effort. If the concept of the past as prologue has any validity, it only exists as a highly speeded up version of events as the spectacular growth of science acts as a catalyst to heighten the momentum of the rapidity of change.

As John Naisbitt and others have documented, we are moving into a postindustrial world of knowledge.[3] The cybernetic culture will be the dominant ethos. The sophistication of the hardware and software of the computer era has barely begun. Computer technology will be a major tool enabling radical reconstruction of the health care system. As Stanley Lesse has so imaginatively described in his recent book, *The Future of the Health Sciences*, the use of this technology will reorder the system.[4] He envisions a system in which citizens will monitor their own care in precise ways. Technology, in essence, will be the primary care modality. Vast storage banks of scientific data will be available to make this new form of primary care and the lifelong monitoring of each person's health a certainty.

It is conceivable that there will be a sharp reduction in demand for health care professionals. There may be intense competition for employment both within and among professional groups. Probably only the most competent will enjoy full career patterns. Those who are complacent and do not read the signs well will pay the costs of their disregard. Others who are caught up in the excitement of change and keep pace with developments in knowledge will experience an exhilaration of accomplishment that cannot be imagined.

Regardless of the individual reaction of each nurse to the awesome developments in science, the inevitability of remarkable change confronts the profession. All of us must be aware of that reality. The best outcomes for patients and for nurses will be achieved if we are active in enriching knowledge as the basis of practice in proportion to the expansion of knowledge. Adjustments of less quality will be maladaptive and make the future of the profession problematic.

References

1. National Association for Home Care. "Attempted Dismantling of the Medicare Home Health Benefit." Report to Congress, Washington, DC, July 21, 1986.
2. Christman, L. "The Future of Nursing is Predicted by the State of Science and Technology." In *The Nursing Profession, A Time to Speak,* edited by N.L. Chaska. New York: McGraw-Hill, 1982, pp. 802–06.
3. Naisbitt, J. *Megatrends.* New York: Warner Books, 1982.
4. Lesse, S. *The Future of the Health Sciences.* New York: Irvington, 1981.

Discussion Questions

1. What common themes are expressed in the nursing readings from the 1950s through the 1990s? What areas differ?

2. What themes and/or goals for nursing's future have not yet been realized? What reasons may account for this?

3. Will nursing, as it is known now, become extinct in this technological age? Elaborate.

4. What predictions do you have for nursing's future?

5. Given today's realities in health care, how do you see nurses functioning in the future?

6. How would you *like* to see nurses function in the future?

7. What do you see as the major issue between how nurses function today and how you would like to see them function in the future?

Further Readings

Barnum, B. J. (1987). Nursing: Now, then and maybe again. *Nursing Outlook, 35*(5), 219–221.

Dickerson-Hazard, N. (1998). Nursing in the next millennium: Where are we as a profession? *Vital Speeches of the Day, 64*(16), 493–497.

Donley, R. (1996). Nursing at the crossroads. *Nursing Economics, 14*(6), 325–332.

Keeling, A. W. & Ramos, M. C. (1995). The role of nursing history in preparing nursing for the future. *Nursing and Health Care Perspectives on Community, 16*(1), 30–34.

O'Neil, E. (1999). The opportunity that is nursing. *Nursing and Health Care Perspectives, 20*(1), 10–14.

Styles, M. (1987). The tarnished opportunity. *Nursing Outlook, 35*(5), 229.

Web Site Resources for Back to the Future

American Nurses Association   www.ana.org
Brownson's Nursing Notes   http://members.tripod.com/~diannebrownson/
National League for Nursing   www.nln.org
World Future Society   www.wfs.org

General Search Engine Web Sites

The Big Hub   www.thebighub.com
Go   www.go.com
Netcenter   www.netcenter.com

Health Web Sites

Medicine Net   www.medicinenet.com
Thrive Online   www.thriveonline.com
WebMD   www.webmd.com

Professional Journal Web Sites

The Futurist   www.wfs.org
MedWebplus   www.medwebplus.com
Online Journal of Issues in Nursing   www.ana.org

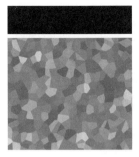

INDEX